Handbook of Pharmacy Healthcare

Diseases and patient advice

SECOND EDITION

Edited by

Robin J Harman

BPharm, PhD, MRPharmS
Independent Pharmaceutical and Regulatory Consultant
Farnham, Surrey, UK

Pamela Mason

BSc, MSc, PhD, MRPharmS
Independent Pharmaceutical Consultant
London, UK

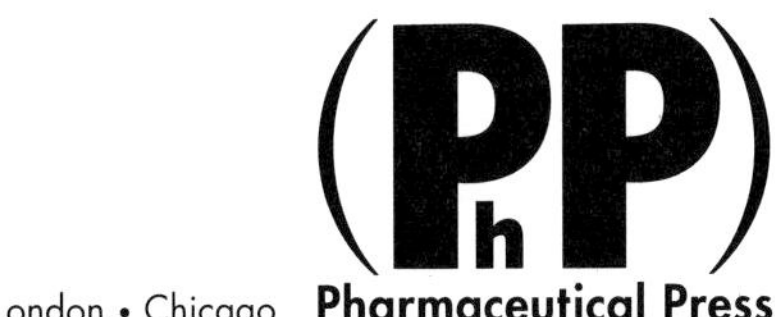

London • Chicago Pharmaceutical Press

Published by the Pharmaceutical Press
Publications division of the Royal Pharmaceutical Society of Great Britain

1 Lambeth High Street, London SE1 7JN, UK
100 South Atkinson Road, Suite 206, Grayslake, IL 60030-7820, USA

First edition published 1990
Second edition published 2002

Text design by Barker/Hilsdon, Lyme Regis, Dorset
Typeset by Type Study, Scarborough, North Yorkshire
Printed in Great Britain by The Bath Press, Bath

ISBN 0 85369 507 5

A catalogue record for this book is available from the British Library

Contents

Preface

THIS IS THE SECOND EDITION of the *Handbook of Pharmacy Healthcare*. Edited by Robin Harman, the first edition was published in 1990 as one of a new series of books to replace *The Pharmaceutical Handbook* and *The Pharmaceutical Codex*.

The aim of this second edition remains unchanged, i.e. it is designed to provide a comprehensive but concise account of a wide range of diseases for which medicines are prescribed or for which non-prescription medicines are bought over the counter and to help pharmacists to apply that knowledge to the benefit and care of patients.

Pharmacists have expertise in medicines that patients are receiving, but to communicate effectively with patients and provide good pharmaceutical care, they also need knowledge of the diseases for which those medicines are used. By using **Part A** of the *Handbook* pharmacists can obtain a concise summary of the causes, symptoms and treatment of different diseases, from which they can provide information to patients. The range of diseases covered remains essentially the same as that in the first edition, although the detail has been changed to reflect current knowledge, and the range is intended to be comprehensive. Although many of the diseases included are unlikely to be encountered by pharmacists on a regular basis, their inclusion is justified on the grounds of completeness and because incidents can occur in which a particular disease or condition may achieve prominence.

The structure of the book has remained unchanged partly for the benefit of those familiar with the first edition to continue to find information easily, although each chapter has received attention and been updated appropriately. Moreover, several new chapters have been included in this edition. In **Part B**, which covers the management of specific patient groups, there is a new chapter on pregnancy. Pharmacists can make a significant contribution to this group of patients who are usually particularly receptive to advice about their health at this stage of life. There is a new chapter on diagnostic tests in recognition of the fact that pharmacists are often asked questions by patients who may be concerned and confused about what a certain type of test involves, why it is used and what the results may mean.

Whatever stage of your pharmacy career you are at – student, pre-registration trainee or qualified pharmacist – it is hoped that this book will help with the understanding of disease, and more importantly, that it will help pharmacists communicate that information to patients. Today, even more than when this book was first published, pharmacists are recognised by the public and other health professionals as a reliable source of advice on a range of healthcare matters.

Robin J Harman
Pamela M Mason

May 2002

Acknowledgements

The editors wish to thank the contributors who wrote certain of the chapters for the first edition of this book and updated them for this edition:

Clive Edwards, BPharm, PhD, MRPharmS
Responding to symptoms

Michael H Jepson, BPharm, MSc, PhD, FRPharmS, MCPP, MinstPkg, DHMSA, FIPharmM, MBIRA(hon)
Communication, counselling and concordance

All diagrams are reproduced from the *Sourcebook of Medical Illustration,* Parthenon Publishing, 1989. Photographs were supplied by Science Photo Library, London, Mike Wyndham Medical Picture Collection and the *Pharmaceutical Journal*.

About the editors

Robin J Harman, PhD, MRPharmS, has been an independent pharmaceutical and regulatory consultant since 1998, and has published extensively within the pharmaceutical and medical sectors. He is editor of the second edition of the *Handbook of Pharmacy Health Education* (Pharmaceutical Press, London, 2001). From 1990 to 1998, he was Editor-in-Chief of *The Regulatory Affairs Journal* and *The Regulatory Affairs Journal (Devices)*, which provide information to the pharmaceutical and medical devices industries respectively. Previously, he was an Editor in the Department of Pharmaceutical Sciences at the Royal Pharmaceutical Society of Great Britain. He was author of the first edition of *Patient Care in Community Practice: A Handbook of Non-medicinal Health-care* (Pharmaceutical Press, London 1989) and edited its second edition (Pharmaceutical Press, London, 2002). He was also editor of the first edition of the *Handbook of Pharmacy Health-care: Diseases and Patient Advice* (Pharmaceutical Press, London, 1990).

Pamela Mason, BSc, PhD, MRPharmS, has been an independent pharmaceutical and nutrition consultant since 1994. She writes regularly for the *Pharmaceutical Journal* and for other pharmaceutical organisations. She is the author of *Dietary Supplements* (Pharmaceutical Press, London, 2001), *Locum Pharmacy* (Pharmaceutical Press, London, 1998) and *Nutrition and Dietary Advice in the Pharmacy* (Blackwell Science, Oxford, 2000). She is editor of *Tomorrow's Pharmacist*, the *Pharmaceutical Journal*'s annual publication for students and preregistration trainees. Between 1989 and 1994, she worked as an editorial assistant on the *British National Formulary* and as a writer of training material at the National Pharmaceutical Association. She has nearly 20 years' experience as a practising community pharmacist in Manchester, North Wales and London.

Part A

Fundamentals of disease

Introduction

Pharmacists have traditionally been involved almost exclusively with the therapeutic use of medicines, and their expertise in this field is well recognised. However, this role cannot be considered in isolation from an awareness of the diseases for which medicines are administered. To provide this essential foundation for the use of medicines, **Part A** of the *Handbook of Pharmacy Healthcare* details the fundamentals of disease.

A knowledge of the causes and symptoms of disease is an essential prerequisite for an understanding of the rationale for, and mechanisms of, drug treatment, and this fact is used as the basis for therapeutics teaching in many undergraduate pharmacy courses. As part of the learning process it is also useful to be aware of the classification of disease, and recognition of this fact has been adopted as the starting point for the presentation of the disease monographs in **Chapters 1 to 13** inclusive. Diseases have been classified according to their occurrence in the body, using the same classification of body systems as that contained within the *British National Formulary* (BNF). The reasons for linking this book so closely with the BNF are twofold. First, its frequent use means that many pharmacists are familiar with this classification. By following the same classification, it is hoped that readers will quickly gain familiarity with the *Handbook*, and its effective use may be expedited. Secondly, a conscious decision was made at the outset of compilation of the *Handbook*, to omit references to specific examples of medicines used to treat a particular disease. Instead, the reader is referred to the relevant class of drugs in the BNF (usually in an analogous chapter) where detailed information can be found. Duplication of information is therefore minimised and the clear distinction in emphasis of the two books between diseases and medicines is maintained.

The chapters containing disease monographs (Part A) have been subdivided into further classification. These have been derived from detailed consideration of *The Merck Manual*, 17th edition (M H Beers and R Berkow (eds), Merck Research Laboratories, New Jersey, 1999), and the *World Health Organization International Statistical Classification of Diseases and Related Health Problems (ICD) Volumes 1, 2 and 3,* 10th revision (WHO, Geneva, 1992). Where more than one classification is possible for a particular disease (based on its local manifestation or its occurrence as a complication, or on a generalised underlying disease process), the classification determined by the WHO as the underlying disease process has been selected for this book.

The disease monographs have been written concisely and provide a brief but detailed summary of the major aspects of each disease. Each monograph has been divided into three sections: definition and aetiology, symptoms, and treatment.

The **aetiology** of diseases can be influenced by a wide variety of factors. Infections can be contracted by personal contact with others; environmental causes are becoming increasingly recognised; and genetic predisposition (i.e. autosomal and recessive traits) can be a determining factor (e.g. cystic fibrosis and inborn errors of metabolism).

In recording the **symptoms** of each disease, no attempt has been made to define their relative occurrence, other than to specify whether one or more symptoms is predominant (e.g. diarrhoea in cholera; petechiae in thrombocytopenia). Equally, although non-specific symptoms (e.g. malaise, fatigue and nausea) are mentioned, by definition their occurrence cannot be definitely correlated with that disease. What is more important is the sequence of development and the range of symptoms which, when considered together, provide a composite picture that is characteristic of a particular disease. Certain disease states benefit from illustration with black-and-white photographs.

To enable pharmacists to recognise the diverse range of diseases of which many common symptoms can be a component, and to assist them in assessing the possible causes of an individual symptom, symptoms recorded in the disease monographs have been collated into **Part C, Symptoms and disease identification**. A discussion of the criteria for selection of symptoms in this list can be found in the Introduction to Part C.

To emphasize the patient and disease aspects of the book, as opposed to therapeutic aspects, general classes rather than specific examples of medicines are detailed in the **treatment** section of disease monographs. The only exceptions to this general rule are instances where a specific medicine is used. For further information, readers are referred to the appropriate section within the BNF in which detailed data about medicines and their use may be found. **All cross-references specified within the treatment sections are to the BNF.**

Pharmacists are often asked for advice about organisations that patients suffering from a particular condition can join, or from whom information may be sought. The tremendous importance and reassurance that patients can derive from contact with others in a similar predicament should not be underestimated. To help pharmacists readily identify those organisations which have an interest in a particular condition, many disease monographs are supplemented by the names of one or more relevant self-help organisations. Full details (including UK address, telephone number, email and website and a brief summary of aims and services) of the main organisations are given in Chapter 20.

Each chapter in Part A (except Chapters 5 and 8) includes an illustrated description of relevant anatomy and physiology. Most pharmacists will have studied biology (including human biology) before entering undergraduate pharmacy, but it was deemed useful to include in each chapter a brief resumé of those anatomical and physiological systems referred to within the disease monographs. It must be stressed, however, that these sections are not intended to provide a comprehensive discussion of anatomy and physiology, for which there are innumerable excellent specialised textbooks (*see* Selected bibliography and reference sources).

Introduction to anatomy and physiology

Many of the terms used within the disease monographs refer to anatomical positions in relation to another organ or tissue within the body. Medically, these relationships may be given directional terms, some of which are described below. Organs within the body may also be described in terms of planes or sections, illustrating the direction in which an organ lies or in which vessels pass. All of these terms are based on a person in a standing position looking forward (frontal position), and are commonly grouped in pairs of opposites.

Directional terms

Superior	above or higher, situated nearer to the top of the head
Inferior	below or to the base of the body
Anterior/ventral	closer to or on the rear surface of the body
Posterior/dorsal	closer to or on the rear surface of the body
Midline	an imaginary vertical line down the centre of the body
Medial	closer to the midline or the middle portion
Lateral	further away from the midline to towards the side
Ipsilateral	on the same side (of the body)
Contralateral	on the opposing side (of the body)
Proximal	nearer to the point of attachment (e.g. of a limb to the trunk)
Distal	further away from the point of attachment (e.g. the distal convoluted tubule in the kidney is further away from the glomerulus than the proximal convoluted tubule)
Superficial	on or toward the surface of the body or of an organ
Deep	further away from the surface of the body or of an organ

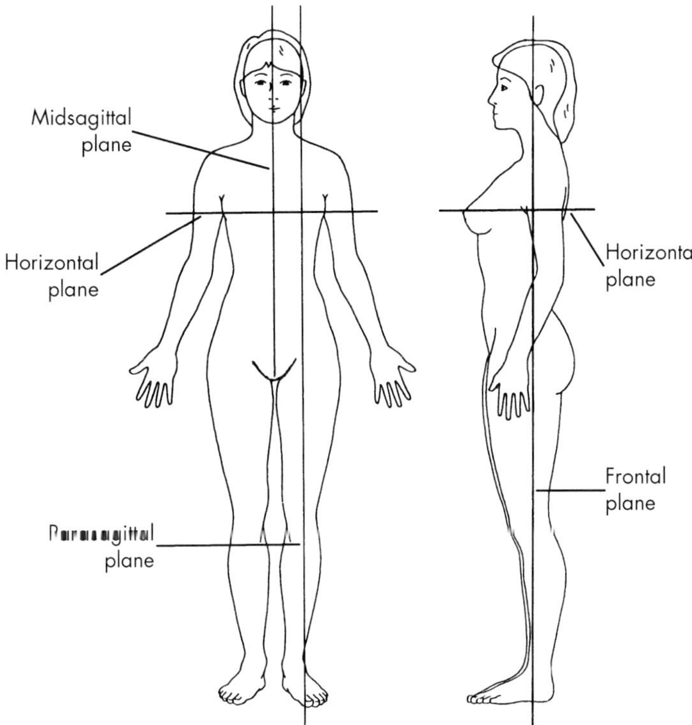

Figure 1 Planes of the body.

Planes

Medically, nomenclature also exists for the different planes of the body. These imaginary flat surfaces may be considered to dissect the body into regions and may be used to describe the predominant direction in which an organ lies (Figure 1).

Vertical planes are described as sagittal, and may be midsagittal or parasagittal. A midsagittal plane passes through the midline and divides the body into two equal halves. A parasagittal plane is parallel to the sagittal plane but the division produces two unequal portions. A further vertical division may be considered with the body turned at a right angle to the frontal position. A vertical division down the side of the body produces the frontal plane which divides the body into anterior (front) and posterior (rear) portions.

A horizontal (transverse) plane is situated at right angles to the sagittal plane and divides the body into superior (upper) and inferior (lower) portions.

Common names and anatomical terms

Pharmacists act at the interface between the medical world and the general public. They have to be capable of communication with medical practitioners, nurses and other medical personnel who may be familiar with a comprehensive medical vocabulary. They also have to be able to impart information to members of the public for whom an aura of mystique, and sometimes confusion, may exist around medical terminology. Pharmacists must therefore be able to readily interconvert medical and lay terminology, and the list in Table 1 is intended to provide a guide to the most commonly used terms.

Table 1 Commonly used medical terms

Common name	Anatomical term	Common name	Anatomical term
Head		**Limbs – upper**	
Head	cephalic	Arm pit	axillary
Neck	cervical	Arm	brachial
Skull	cranial	Front of elbow	antecubital
Face	facial	Back of elbow	olecranal
Eye	orbital or ocular	Forearm	antebrachial
Ear	otic	Wrist	carpal
Cheek	buccal	Palm	metacarpal
Nose	nasal	Thumb	pollex
Mouth	oral	Fingers	digital or phalangeal
Chin	mental	Anterior surface of hand	palmar or volar
Trunk – front		Posterior surface of hand	dorsal
Chest	thoracic	**Limbs – lower**	
Breast	mammary	Thigh	femoral
Navel	umbilical	Front of knee	patellar
Hip	coxal	Hollow behind knee	popliteal
Groin	inguinal	Leg	crural
Pubis	pubic	Calf	sural
Trunk – rear		Ankle	tarsal
Shoulder	acromial	Toes	digital or phalangeal
Back	dorsal	Great toe	hallux
Loin	lumbar	Sole of foot	plantar
Buttock	gluteal	Heel of foot	calcaneal

1

Gastrointestinal and related disorders

1.1 General disorders

Appendicitis

Definition and aetiology

Appendicitis is acute inflammation of the vermiform appendix, commonly caused by obstruction of the mouth of the lumen of the appendix. It occurs most frequently in children over five years of age and in adults of 20–40 years of age. Apart from hernia, it is the most common reason for a severe acute abdominal pain. There is an approximately 0.1% fatality rate.

Symptoms

Appendicitis usually starts with referred, colicky, central abdominal pain, which may be only moderately severe; anorexia, nausea and vomiting, and mild fever may develop within 1–2 hours of the onset of the pain. Classically, the central pain shifts to the right iliac fossa within 6 hours (Figure 1.1), becoming persistent and steady. The pain is accentuated on movement, deep breathing and coughing. There is referred pain in the right lower quadrant.

Other symptoms include constipation, dysuria and abdominal tenderness; diarrhoea is relatively uncommon. Complications include perforation, which may lead to peritonitis, formation of an appendix mass palpable in the right iliac fossa and abscess formation.

Treatment

Treatment is by appendicectomy, which can be carried out by laparoscopy, permitting a quicker recovery.

Constipation

Definition and aetiology

Constipation is defined as increased difficulty and reduced frequency of evacuation of hard stool, and may be chronic or acute. It may be accompanied by a feeling of incomplete evacuation. Any definition of constipation must take into account the widespread social and societal variation in what constitutes normal frequency of defecation. It can vary from three times a day to once every three days. Failure to appreciate this normal variation has led to widespread and unnecessary laxative use.

Simple (chronic) constipation is usually due to lack of dietary fibre or poor bowel training. Acute constipation implies a definite, sudden change in bowel habit. It may be due to organic causes (e.g. mechanical obstruction by impacted faeces, paralytic ileus or a sudden decrease in exercise levels). If the acute change in bowel habit persists for some weeks, colorectal cancer or other causes of partial bowel obstruction may be responsible.

Constipation can also be caused by systemic conditions (e.g. debilitating infections, hypothyroidism, parkinsonism, hypercalcaemia, spinal

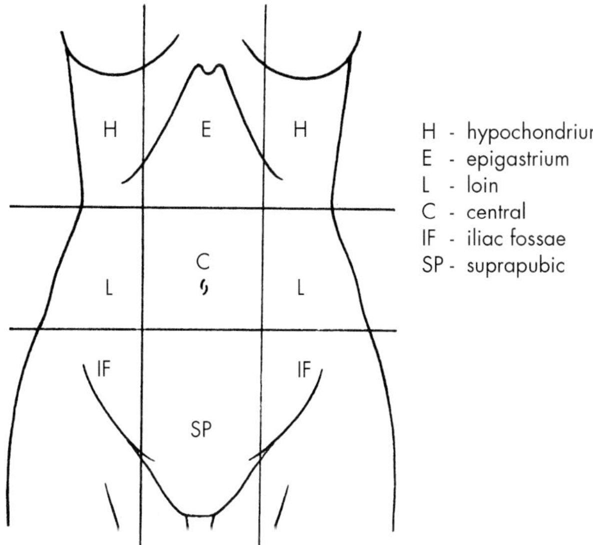

Figure 1.1 Diagram of the abdominal region.

lesions and depressive disorders) or local nervous action disturbances (e.g. anal fissures, haemorrhoids, proctitis, irritable bowel syndrome, diverticular disease, megacolon and diminished muscle tone, particularly in the elderly). Pregnancy and the presence of other pelvic masses may also be contributory factors. Constipation may be a side-effect of drug administration and laxative abuse.

Treatment

Most cases of constipation can be successfully treated by dietary adjustments alone. Long-term constipation should be treated by increasing the bulk of intestinal contents with the use of a high-fibre diet (e.g. bran) and increased fluid intake. Artificial means using bulk-forming laxatives (BNF 1.6.1) may also be effective. If these measures are unsuccessful, stimulant laxatives (BNF 1.6.2), faecal softeners (BNF 1.6.3) or osmotic laxatives (BNF 1.6.4) may be used. Bowel cleansing solutions are not treatments for constipation.

Diarrhoea

Definition and aetiology

Diarrhoea is characterised by an increased frequency, an increased fluidity of defecation or an increased volume of faecal output, or a combination of the three. The colon reabsorbs between 1.5 and 2.0 litres of water each day from the bowel contents as they pass along the large intestine; only 150–200 mL is excreted in the stool mass. Any event that reduces the amount reabsorbed has a significant impact on stool consistency.

Diarrhoea may be caused by a disorder of the stomach, biliary system, small or large bowel, a systemic illness (e.g. hyperthyroidism or diabetes mellitus) or the ingestion of drugs, toxins or poisons. Psychological disturbances can also produce diarrhoea.

In its acute form it may be caused by food poisoning, dietary indiscretion, by bowel infection (viral, bacterial or parasitic) or ingestion of bacterial toxins. Traveller's diarrhoea is normally caused by bacterial toxins, in particular by pathogenic *Escherichia coli*, *Campylobacter* or *Shigella* species.

Chronic diarrhoea may be due to malabsorption, Crohn's disease, diverticular disease, ulcerative colitis, malignant disease, protozoal or occasionally helminthic infections, disturbances of intestinal motility (e.g. irritable bowel syndrome) or to the effects of drugs. Pseudomembranous colitis may develop after antibacterial therapy and cause acute or chronic diarrhoea.

Faecal impaction occurs mainly in the elderly and may give rise to spurious diarrhoea, which alternates with constipation.

Treatment
Treatment is directed if possible to the underlying cause. Prophylaxis is not usually recommended. For symptomatic treatment in adults a fluid-only diet may be sufficient, although antidiarrhoeal adsorbent powders or mixtures (BNF 1.4.1) may be useful in mild diarrhoea. Antimotility drugs (BNF 1.4.2) may be given in more severe cases. Bulk-forming drugs (BNF 1.6.1) remove excess fluid and control faecal consistency in patients with an ileostomy or colostomy. The risk of dehydration in severe diarrhoea is especially high in the very young, the old and choleraic patients, and rehydration should be carried out by means of oral rehydration therapy (BNF 9.2.1) or, if necessary, by parenteral preparations (BNF 9.2.2) for fluid and electrolyte imbalance. Spurious diarrhoea may be overcome through evacuation of the rectum by the administration of laxatives (BNF 1.6) or by manual removal.

Diverticular disease

Definition and aetiology
A diverticulum is a small saccular mucosal pouch, which distends outwards from the external muscle wall of the gastrointestinal tract. Diverticula occur most commonly in the sigmoid colon, but may also develop in other regions of the gut (e.g. oesophagus, duodenum and small intestine). Their incidence appears to be associated with diets low in fibre and with prolonged raised pressure within the colon. The disease occurs much less frequently in vegetarians. Inflammatory complications of diverticular disease are rare but potentially dangerous.

Diverticula occur only rarely in people under 30 years of age. Their occurrence increases with age, and more than 50% of those over 70 years of age may have diverticula present, albeit usually asymptomatically.

Symptoms
The occurrence of diverticula is frequently asymptomatic, and they are only detected on unrelated pelvic investigation. It has been estimated that only 10% of diverticula produce symptoms, and only 1% require surgery. Symptomatic diverticular disease is characterised by abdominal pain and altered bowel function (e.g. diarrhoea, constipation or both). Pain, located usually in the left iliac fossa, may be relieved by defecation.

Inflammation may be associated with abdominal tenderness, fever and constipation; an inflammatory mass may be present. Symptoms may also arise from complications which include abscesses, fistulas (e.g. to the bladder or vagina), peritonitis, rectal bleeding and intestinal obstruction.

Treatment
Symptomatic diverticular disease may be treated with a high-fibre diet, bran supplements, bulk-forming laxatives (BNF 1.6.1) and antispasmodics and other drugs altering gut motility (BNF 1.2).

In the event of inflammation or associated complications, bed rest, fasting, intravenous nutrition (BNF 9.3) and intravenous antibacterial drugs (BNF 5.1) are indicated. Opioid analgesics (BNF 4.7.2) may be required for severe abdominal pain. Surgery may be necessary for complications, failure to respond to treatment or recurrent attacks.

Gastritis

Definition
Gastritis is defined as inflammation of the gastric mucosa, which may be acute or chronic.

Acute gastritis

Definition and aetiology
Acute gastritis may result from irritation due to drugs (e.g. salicylates and non-steroidal anti-inflammatory drugs), alcohol, corrosive agents, irradiation, bacterial toxins (e.g. staphylococcal) or can be associated with bacterial infection (e.g. salmonellal infections). Stressful events (e.g. trauma and surgery) may also precipitate symptoms.

Symptoms
Acute gastritis is usually asymptomatic, but anorexia, epigastric pain, and nausea and

vomiting may occur. Gastritis is an important cause of upper gastrointestinal haemorrhage, which is characterised by haematemesis or melaena. Acute gastritis due to the ingestion of corrosive materials is characterised by severe chest and epigastric pain; haemorrhage, vomiting, hypotension, shock and perforation may occur.

Treatment
Conservative measures include removal of the causative agent (e.g. cessation of alcohol intake and avoidance of non-steroidal anti-inflammatory drugs). Antacids (BNF 1.1) may be required in symptomatic patients. Severe bleeding associated with acute gastritis is treated with intravenous administration of fluids (BNF 9.2.2), antacids (BNF 1.1), gastric aspiration and lavage. Blood transfusion may be necessary. Surgery is associated with high morbidity and mortality, and is avoided if possible.

Chronic gastritis

Definition and aetiology
The causes of chronic gastritis are not clear but are thought to include autoimmune diseases (e.g. thyroid disease, Addison's disease and diabetes mellitus) and prolonged gastric irritation. *Helicobacter pylori* has been implicated as a cause of non-autoimmune disease. Chronic gastritis occurs commonly in association with peptic ulceration, cancer of the stomach, and following gastric surgery. The condition has also been reported in megaloblastic anaemia and iron-deficiency anaemia.

Symptoms
Chronic gastritis varies in severity. It may affect only superficial tissue or cause a variable degree of glandular atrophy. Metaplasia frequently occurs in atrophic gastritis. Uncomplicated forms are usually asymptomatic although anorexia, epigastric pain, nausea and vomiting, and hypochlorhydria or achlorhydria may occur.

Treatment
Treatment is not usually necessary for uncomplicated chronic gastritis. Dyspepsia may be relieved by antacids (BNF 1.1) even if hypochlorhydria is present. Iron-deficiency anaemia (BNF 9.1.1) or megaloblastic anaemia (BNF 9.1.2) should be treated with replacement therapy.

Gastroenteritis

Definition and aetiology
Gastroenteritis is a group of clinical syndromes characterised by acute inflammation of the stomach, intestine or both. It may be due to food poisoning, and bacterial, viral or protozoal infections.

In food poisoning, gastroenteritis is due to ingestion of food contaminated by bacterial enterotoxins and bacteria which invade the gut mucosa. Non-bacterial causes include ingestion of poisonous or chemically contaminated food (e.g. mushroom poisoning from *Amanita* toadstools and solanine poisoning from green potatoes).

Bacterial gut infections are varied in aetiology. Epidemics of infantile gastroenteritis may be caused by enteropathogenic strains of *Escherichia coli*. Viral infections are a common cause of gastroenteritis and are usually due to rotaviruses in young children.

The ability to withstand the symptoms of gastroenteritis depends upon age and whether there are any other debilitating illnesses present at the same time.

Symptoms
Nausea, vomiting and diarrhoea are classical symptoms. Abdominal pain and fever may also be present. In severe cases, dehydration, prostration and shock may develop. Incubation periods and clinical features vary according to the causative toxin or bacteria. The incubation period for *E. coli* in infantile gastroenteritis is 8–48 hours, and diarrhoea and vomiting may lead to dehydration and severe illness. Alternatively the illness may be mild, and vomiting and malaise absent. The incubation period for rotaviruses is 24–72 hours, and gastrointestinal symptoms are frequently preceded or accompanied by upper respiratory symptoms (including otitis media). Diarrhoea, vomiting or both often occur and the illness is usually self-limiting, lasting between three and eight days.

Treatment
Gastroenteritis is treated by the oral administration of fluids (BNF 9.2.1) to prevent or redress dehydration, and by avoidance of solids until symptoms have subsided. In severe cases, intravenous administration of fluids (BNF 9.2.2) may be required. Antidiarrhoeal drugs (BNF 1.4) may be given as an adjunct to fluid and electrolyte replacement, but in general should not be used in infants or children. Antibacterials are generally unnecessary in simple gastroenteritis and may prolong symptoms.

Ileus

Definition and aetiology
Ileus is a condition in which the transit of intestinal contents by peristalsis is arrested or severely impaired. Paralytic (adynamic) ileus is due to functional failure of normal intestinal peristalsis. It commonly occurs post-operatively following abdominal surgery. It may also occur in patients with acute pancreatitis, ischaemic gastrointestinal disease, choledocholithiasis, peritonitis and external trauma, or may be induced by ganglion-blocking antihypertensive drugs.

Mechanical ileus is mechanical or organic obstruction of the small intestine or colon and may be complete or partial (subacute obstruction). It is commonly caused by fibrous bands and adhesions, hernias, malignant disease, impacted faeces or inflammatory bowel disease.

Symptoms
The symptoms vary according to the site and extent of the obstruction. They include abdominal distension, colicky pain, anorexia, constipation, and nausea and vomiting; dehydration and shock may develop. Different parts of the gastrointestinal tract are affected by paralytic ileus post-operatively to varying extents. The ileum regains motility within several hours, but the stomach may not resume normal emptying for 24 hours. The colon may remain stagnant for 48–72 hours.

Complications of ileus include strangulation or infarction, leading to gangrene, perforation and peritonitis. Complete mechanical obstruction is fatal if untreated.

Treatment
Paralytic ileus is usually self-limiting and is initially treated conservatively. Recovery may be expedited with intravenous fluid replacement (BNF 9.2.2) and gastric aspiration. Mechanical ileus is treated similarly but surgery should be carried out as soon as the patient's condition allows.

Immediate surgery is required for strangulation or infarction. Parasympathomimetics (BNF 1.6.2) are used rarely for paralytic ileus, and should be avoided if organic obstruction is present. Opioid analgesics (BNF 4.7.2) may be required, and antibacterial drugs (BNF 5.1) should be given if peritonitis is present.

Infantile colic

Definition and aetiology
Infantile colic consists of spasms of severe griping pain, which increase in intensity to a peak, remit for a short period, and then recur. The condition may arise in the stomach, intestines and kidneys. For that arising in the ureters, *see* Renal calculi and colic, or in the biliary tract, *see* Cholecystitis.

Intestinal colic may be due to relatively trivial causes (e.g. swallowing air), emotional upset and over- or under-feeding. It may, however, also be associated with more serious complaints (e.g. food poisoning and intestinal obstruction).

Symptoms
Infants in the first months of life are commonly affected by intestinal colic. It is characterised by paroxysms of crying associated with pulling up of the knees and irritability in an otherwise thriving infant. Attacks commonly occur in the evening, but unlike crying caused by loneliness or a soiled napkin, are not usually relieved by picking up the child. The excessive crying may itself cause swallowing of air, creating a recurring cycle of cause and effect.

Treatment
Non-drug remedies include lying the infant on his abdomen or changing feeding equipment or technique. Persistent colic may be treated with antimuscarinic antispasmodics (BNF 1.2). Dicycloverine (dicyclomine) is contraindicated

in infants under six months of age, by which age colic should only rarely still be a problem.

Irritable bowel syndrome

Definition and aetiology

The irritable bowel syndrome (IBS) is a chronic motility disorder that can involve the entire gastrointestinal tract but with no demonstrable organic cause.

Symptoms

It is characterised by recurrent episodes of abdominal discomfort, pain and altered bowel habit. The pain may be colicky or a continuous dull ache and is commonly related to food intake. It may be relieved by defecation or on the passage of flatus. There may be a history of diarrhoea or constipation, or alternating diarrhoea and constipation; the faeces may be described as 'marbles', 'pellets' or 'rabbit droppings' (scybala) and mucus may be present. In some cases, the predominant symptom is constipation; in others, it is diarrhoea. Rectal bleeding does not occur unless haemorrhoids or other lesions are also present.

Other symptoms include abdominal distension and flatulence which may be related to the intake of food. Non-intestinal symptoms (e.g. fatigue and headache) are thought to be psychosomatic. Symptoms may be aggravated by emotional stress, anxiety or depressive disorders. Diagnosis is made by suspecting IBS to be the cause of the patient's symptoms and excluding other causes.

Treatment

Many patients are reassured when the benign nature of the condition is explained. Treatment may consist of a high-fibre diet (e.g. bran). Drug therapy should be avoided if possible, but bulk-forming drugs (BNF 1.6.1) may be required for constipation, and antidiarrhoeal drugs (BNF 1.4.2) may occasionally be necessary. Antispasmodic drugs and other drugs altering gut motility (BNF 1.2) may be required for abdominal colic. Underlying anxiety or depression should be treated.

Ischaemic gastrointestinal disorders

Definition and aetiology

Ischaemic gastrointestinal disorders may be acute or chronic. They vary from mild ischaemia with superficial necrosis that causes no permanent damage, to massive ischaemia and infarction. Ischaemia may result from arterial occlusion due to atherosclerosis with or without thrombosis, embolism or less commmonly aortic aneurysm or polyarteritis nodosa. Other causes include thrombosis of the mesenteric vein (e.g. as a complication of abdominal surgery or cirrhosis of the liver), and hypotension occurring as a complication of shock.

Acute intestinal ischaemia

Definition and aetiology

Acute intestinal ischaemia occurs primarily in older patients with degenerative cardiovascular disease.

Symptoms

The onset is usually abrupt, but may be insidious. It is characterised by colicky abdominal pain in the right iliac fossa, which later becomes constant, severe and diffuse. Other early symptoms include diarrhoea which may be bloody, nausea and vomiting, anxiety, dyspnoea, pallor and sweating. Later symptoms include anuria, cyanosis and hypotension followed by necrosis, leading to infarction, gangrene, peritonitis, shock and death.

Treatment

Treatment consists of intravenous administration of fluids (BNF 9.2.2) to correct fluid and electrolyte imbalance and intravenous antibacterial drugs (BNF 5.1). Blood is also given if necessary. Surgery should be carried out as soon as possible; resection of the intestine is usually necessary, but embolectomy or thrombectomy may reduce the length of intestine that has to be resected (e.g. in patients who are already compromised by cardiovascular disease). The mortality rate is high.

Chronic intestinal ischaemia

Definition and aetiology
Chronic intestinal ischaemia is usually associated with extensive atherosclerosis involving at least two of the visceral arteries. It may progress to acute intestinal ischaemia.

Symptoms
It is characterised by chronic postprandial abdominal pain (usually occurring 20–60 minutes after eating), which is unrelieved by antacids. As the condition progresses, the patient becomes afraid to eat and marked weight loss occurs.

Treatment
Treatment consists of surgical reconstruction of the arteries.

Focal ischaemia of the small intestine

Definition and aetiology
In focal ischaemia of the small intestine, only a segment of the small intestine is affected (the 'focus'), causing local ulceration which, on healing, leads to stenosis. It may be caused by vascular disorders (*see above*) or may be due to a strangulated hernia, blunt trauma to the abdomen or irradiation. Drug-induced ulceration (e.g. from ingestion of potassium salts) is another important cause. A rare cause is localised vasculitis secondary to infections or collagen disorders.

Symptoms
Focal ischaemia is characterised by colicky abdominal pain occurring 2–3 hours after eating, associated with nausea, abdominal distension and occasional vomiting.

Treatment
Treatment consists of surgical resection of the obstructed segment.

Ischaemic colitis

Definition and aetiology
Ischaemia of the colon may be widespread or segmented. It may be caused by vascular disorders (*see above*), by venous occlusion, or may be associated with colorectal cancer, colonic prolapse or volvulus.

Symptoms
It is characterised by abdominal pain in the left iliac fossa and nausea and vomiting, followed by the passage of loose faeces darkly stained with blood.

Treatment
Treatment consists of intravenous administration of fluids (BNF 9.2.2) and intravenous antibacterial drugs (BNF 5.1). Surgical resection may be required if a stricture develops or if there is evidence of peritonitis, persistent bleeding or an underlying colonic disorder (e.g. malignant disease). However, more than 90% of cases resolve spontaneously.

Megacolon

Definition
Megacolon is a condition in which there is acute or chronic dilatation of the colon.

Congenital megacolon

Definition and aetiology
In congenital megacolon (Hirschprung's disease), the absence of neurons in a distal portion of the colon results in a narrowed segment that is not able to undergo normal peristaltic movement. This 'bottleneck' effect produces dilatation of the normally innervated colon proximal to the affected segment.

Symptoms
The condition usually presents in the first few days of life and is characterised by severe constipation, abdominal distension, vomiting and poor feeding. Presentation in the later weeks of life is associated with mild constipation, which dates back to the neonatal period; anorexia and failure to thrive may also be present. If only a very short section of bowel is involved, the presentation may be delayed into adult life.

Treatment
Congenital megacolon should be treated by resection of the affected portion of bowel,

although temporary colostomy may be necessary to relieve acute obstructions.

Acquired megacolon

Definition and aetiology
Acquired megacolon is dilatation that occurs as a result of chronic constipation. It usually occurs in mentally retarded or psychotic children and in infirm or elderly subjects.

Symptoms
Symptoms are similar to those of congenital megacolon, although faecal incontinence due to impacted faeces is also common.

Treatment
Acquired megacolon is treated with rectally administered laxatives (BNF 1.6), followed by retraining of bowel habits.

Peptic ulceration

Definition and aetiology
Peptic ulcers develop through loss of tissue of the mucosa, submucosa and muscularis mucosae in regions of the gastrointestinal tract exposed to gastric secretions that contain acid and pepsin. They may occur in the lower oesophagus, the stomach (gastric ulceration), and the initial few centimetres of the duodenum (duodenal ulceration). It was once thought that ulceration results from an imbalance between the damaging actions of acid and pepsin, and the mucosal defence mechanisms. However, two major causes of the disruption to the mucosal normal defence mechanisms are now commonly accepted: the presence of certain drugs (e.g. aspirin and other anti-inflammatory drugs); and the chemicals produced by *Helicobacter pylori*, which infects the duodenal mucosa.

Gastric ulceration

Definition and aetiology
Gastric ulcers may be benign or malignant. Benign gastric ulcers are usually single, circular or semicircular discrete breaks in the gastric mucosa, which frequently penetrate deeply into the muscularis mucosae. The most common cause of gastric ulceration is infection with *H. pylori*. Acute or chronic ingestion of aspirin or other anti-inflammatory drugs may also cause the condition.

Symptoms
Gastric ulcers are characterised by localised epigastric pain, which may become worse after eating; unlike duodenal ulcers the pain is worse during the day, although differentiation on clinical grounds is unreliable. Other symptoms include anorexia, nausea and vomiting, excess salivation and weight loss. Acute or occult haemorrhage or perforation are the commonest complications and are sometimes the presenting features. Relapses after healing occur less frequently than in duodenal ulceration.

Treatment
Treatment is as described below under duodenal ulceration. Surgery may also be required for persistent, bleeding, malignant ulcers or ulcers which fail to heal.

Duodenal ulceration

Definition and aetiology
Duodenal ulcers usually occur as benign, single, circular breaks in the mucosa of the duodenal bulb. The strongest factor in the development of duodenal ulcer is the presence of *H. pylori*. Increased acid secretion also occurs, which predisposes towards duodenal ulceration. Smoking, being of blood group O and genetic considerations may be other aetiological factors. Duodenal ulceration is very common, affecting 10–15% of the population at some time during their lives.

Symptoms
Duodenal ulceration is typically characterised by epigastric pain, which is often localised. The pain may be described as gnawing, burning, boring, aching, or as a sensation of pressure, heaviness or hunger, and may be mild or severe. The pain may be relieved by food, but commonly recurs 2–3 hours after eating and is worse at night. Nausea and vomiting are relatively uncommon unless there is severe pain or pyloric

stenosis. Haemorrhage may occur, causing haematemesis, melaena and iron-deficiency anaemia. Perforation will produce severe acute pain, collapse and peritonitis. Haemorrhage, perforation or both may occur in patients without previous symptoms. Duodenal ulceration is frequently associated with spontaneous remissions and relapses.

Treatment

The treatment of duodenal and gastric ulceration has been evolving since the discovery of *H. pylori* as a causative agent. Therapy has focused on eradication of the bacteria by the macrolides antibiotic clarithromycin, in combination with a broad-spectrum antibiotic (e.g. amoxicillin or metronidazole) and a proton pump inhibitor (BNF 1.3).

Conservative treatment to be undertaken simultaneously comprises rest, avoidance of gastrointestinal or mucosal irritants (e.g. smoking and alcohol), small and frequent meals, going to bed with an empty stomach. Symptomatic treatment with antacids (BNF 1.1) may be helpful. Surgery is a less frequently used option compared with previously due to greater success with drug treatment. It still has a role in the treatment of acute complications (e.g. haemorrhage and perforation) and for unsuccessful medical treatment.

Acute erosive ulceration

Definition and aetiology

Multiple superficial ulcers may develop in the oesophagus, stomach or duodenum of acutely stressed patients, particularly after major trauma, extensive burns or during shock or hypoxia. These 'stress ulcers' can also develop in patients whose upper gastrointestinal mucosa is damaged by alcohol or non-steroidal anti-inflammatory drugs.

Treatment

Antacids (BNF 1.1) and ulcer-healing drugs (BNF 1.3) may be used for the prophylaxis and treatment of stress ulceration. There is no place for the antibiotic therapy used in treatment of gastric and duodenal ulceration.

Polyps

Definition and aetiology

A polyp is a growth that protrudes from a mucous membrane. Polyps found in the large intestine are usually adenomas with malignant potential. Their origin is uncertain, but their incidence has been linked to dietary factors that alter the flora of the colon and cause the production of carcinogens through bacterial action. Genetic factors may also be important (e.g. in familial adenomatous polyposis).

Symptoms

Polyps frequently occur asymptomatically and tend to be diagnosed on associated investigation. They vary considerably in size, and occur singly or in groups. The greatest incidence is in the rectum and sigmoid colon. The most common symptom is rectal bleeding which, if persistent, may cause mild anaemia. In familial adenomatous polyposis, there is a widespread covering of polyps over the lining of the colon and rectum.

Treatment

A polyp should be removed for assessment of the tissue type. Follow-up is necessary to monitor for the development of adenocarcinoma. The very poor prognosis of familial adenomatous polyposis may be improved by continuous monitoring. Total proctocolectomy with ileostomy formation or ileo-anal anastomosis may be necessary in severe cases that may progress to carcinoma.

Pyloric stenosis

Definition and aetiology

Congenital hypertrophic pyloric stenosis is the obstruction of the pyloric outlet (pylorus) of the stomach due to thickening of the pyloric muscle. It occurs most commonly in neonates. It is not usually present at birth but develops over the initial four to six weeks of life. It is thought to occur genetically through a complex multifactorial inheritance, affecting siblings and children of childhood sufferers. It affects about 2 per 1000 live births, with occurrence in three or four times as many males as females.

Acquired pyloric stenosis may occur in adults through inflammation or fibrosis of the pylorus as a late complication of chronic peptic ulceration or malignant disease.

Symptoms

Congenital hypertrophic pyloric stenosis, which most commonly arises in first-born males, usually produces symptoms within the first weeks of life. It is characterised by vomit (without bile) projected up to a metre, constipation, dehydration, weight loss and hunger. Rarer and less severe forms may not be detected until early adult life. Acquired pyloric stenosis occurs in adults and produces vomiting (several hours after eating) and weight loss, both of which may be associated with a long history of ulceration and its symptoms.

Treatment

Treatment consists of intravenous nutrition and fluid and electrolytes (BNF 9.2), followed by corrective surgery. Hypertrophied muscle may be divided surgically in the congenital condition or the obstruction bypassed in the acquired form.

1.2 Oesophageal disorders

Achalasia

Definition and aetiology

Achalasia (cardiospasm) is a rare idiopathic condition in which there is a failure of peristalsis in the oesophagus combined with a failure of relaxation of the cardiac sphincter. It may be caused by local nerve cell degeneration.

It begins usually between 20 and 40 years of age, but can progress slowly and insidiously for months or years.

Symptoms

Achalasia is characterised by dysphagia; chest pain may also occur. Nocturnal regurgitation of undigested food, which occurs in about 30% of patients, may produce pulmonary aspiration leading to lung abscess, bronchiectasis or pneumonia. Distal oesophageal cancer is a late complication in 5–10% of cases regardless of treatment.

Treatment

Achalasia may be treated by dilatation of the cardiac sphincter, but surgery (cardiomyotomy) may be necessary.

Dyspepsia

Definition and aetiology

Dyspepsia (indigestion) is a collection of symptoms which may occur shortly after eating or drinking. Acute episodes may be due to overindulgence in food or alcohol. Chronic dyspepsia may occur in peptic ulceration, hiatus hernia, reflux oesophagitis, chronic gastritis, cholecystitis or ischaemic heart disease; it may also occur independently of any pathological change (non-ulcer dyspepsia). Dyspepsia is aggravated by heavy smoking, stress and anxiety and may be psychosomatic.

Symptoms

The major symptoms are epigastric discomfort, chest pain or both. It may be accompanied by a feeling of fullness after eating, heartburn, abdominal distension, flatulence, eructation, anorexia, and nausea and vomiting; a change in bowel habit may also be reported. Eructation may occur in anxious patients due to aerophagia.

Treatment

Dyspepsia may be treated with antacids (BNF 1.1); antispasmodics and other drugs altering gut motility (BNF 1.2) may also be useful in non-ulcer dyspepsia. The use of more complex drugs (e.g. H_2-receptor antagonists and proton pump inhibitors or agents to eradicate *Helicobacter pylori* (*see* Peptic ulceration) is not recommended. Lifestyle changes (e.g. stopping smoking, moderating alcohol intake and eating regularly, avoiding foods which aggravate the problem) are commonly beneficial.

Dysphagia

Definition and aetiology

Dysphagia is an awareness of difficulty in swallowing, due to solids or liquids not passing smoothly from the oesophagus to the stomach. It should be differentiated from neurotic dysphagia (globus hystericus) in which there is a feeling of a lump in the throat that is not associated with swallowing, but often with severe emotional stress (e.g. anxiety or grief).

Dysphagia may be due to lesions of the mouth or tongue. Neuromuscular disorders of the pharynx (e.g. myasthenia gravis and bulbar palsy) or of the oesophagus (e.g. achalasia, systemic sclerosis and diabetes mellitus) may be aetiological factors. Other causes include extrinsic pressure (e.g. mediastinal glands and thyroid enlargement) or intrinsic lesions (e.g. foreign body, benign or malignant strictures and pharyngeal pouch).

Treatment

Treatment may involve dilatation or surgery.

Gastro-oesophageal reflux disease

Definition and aetiology

Gastro-oesophageal reflux disease (reflux oesophagitis) is a condition in which reflux of gastric and duodenal contents into the oesophagus, caused by incompetence of the lower oesophageal sphincter, produces inflammation. It is commonly associated with hiatus hernia, but may occur independently of any anatomical abnormality, particularly in the obese and during pregnancy.

Symptoms

It is characterised by heartburn or chest pain (which may be confused with cardiac pain) and is aggravated by stooping or lying down. Pain may occur whilst eating or drinking. Other symptoms include regurgitation of gastric contents into the mouth and dysphagia of solids. Hoarseness and nocturnal cough or wheeze are signs of pulmonary aspiration. Complications of reflux oesophagitis are few, but may include oesophageal erosions and shallow ulcers. Resultant blood loss may produce iron-deficiency anaemia; rarely, deep oesophageal ulcers may develop, producing severe pain radiating to the back or neck. Oesophageal strictures are a further complication.

Treatment

Treatment consists of elevation of the head of the bed, avoidance of stooping and tight clothing and administration of antacids (BNF 1.1). Ulcer-healing drugs (BNF 1.3) and metoclopramide (BNF 1.2) may also be used. Patients should be advised to lose weight and avoid alcohol, caffeine, smoking and any foods (e.g. chocolate, fatty foods and onions) which aggravate symptoms. Food and drink should also be avoided late at night, before retiring. Dilatation may be required if strictures are present and surgery indicated for resistant cases.

Hiatus hernia

Definition and aetiology

Hiatus hernia is the upward protrusion of the gastro-oesophageal junction of the stomach into the thorax. The most common form (constituting 90% of cases of hiatus hernia) is the 'sliding' form; in the less common 'rolling' form, a part of the stomach only is carried upward into the thoracic cavity alongside the oesophagus.

Hiatus hernia is common in obese subjects and during pregnancy; rolling hernias occur more frequently in women than in men and the incidence increases with age.

Symptoms

Most patients with hiatus hernia are asymptomatic. If symptoms are present, they are usually related to reflux oesophagitis and include heartburn, chest pain and regurgitation; chest pain without reflux oesophagitis may also occur and cause confusion with cardiac pain. Haemorrhage may occur with both types of hiatus hernia, leading to iron-deficiency anaemia. Rolling hernias may produce vague chest discomfort and occasionally become incarcerated or strangulated.

Treatment

Patients with hiatus hernia presenting with symptoms of reflux oesophagitis are treated for this latter condition. Surgery may be required if symptoms persist and for rolling hernias to avoid the risk of incarceration or strangulation.

Oesophageal varices

Definition and aetiology
Oesophageal varices often arise as a consequence of portal hypertension (e.g. in cirrhosis of the liver).

Symptoms
Bleeding may occur, resulting in haematemesis or melaena. However, massive haemorrhage may occur, leading to shock. Symptoms of the underlying liver disease (e.g. ascites, hepatic encephalopathy, hepatomegaly and jaundice) may be present.

Bleeding varices may also occur in the veins of the stomach.

Treatment
Treatment is by transfusion, and administration of vitamin K (BNF 9.6.6) and certain posterior pituitary hormones (BNF 6.5.2). Sclerotherapy may be used; if bleeding persists, emergency surgery may be necessary. Treatment of the underlying liver disease may be required.

1.3 Non-specific inflammatory bowel disorders

Crohn's disease

Definition and aetiology
Crohn's disease is a chronic granulomatous and inflammatory disease of unknown cause affecting any part of the gastrointestinal tract, particularly the terminal ileum. The disease most commonly begins in young adults, and remissions and relapses occur during its course. It affects about 7 per 100 000 of the population. Some cases may not be distinguishable from ulcerative colitis.

Symptoms
It is characterised by abdominal pain, chronic diarrhoea, mild fever and weight loss. In some cases, the symptoms may mimic those of appendicitis. Rectal bleeding occasionally occurs in colonic forms of the disease. Fistulas and abscesses commonly occur and may penetrate the intestine in the abdomen or perianal region. Non-intestinal complications include anaemia, aphthous stomatitis, arthritis, erythema nodosum, growth retardation in children and nutritional deficiencies. Eye, hepatic and renal complications may also occur. In children, and more rarely in adults, non-intestinal symptoms may predominate in the absence of abdominal pain and diarrhoea.

Treatment
No specific treatment is available for Crohn's disease. Diarrhoea and anaemia may be treated symptomatically. Rest and treatment with corticosteroids (BNF 6.3.2) may be of value. Antibacterial drugs (BNF 5.1) may be required in the presence of overwhelming infection or abscess. Sulfasalazine may be helpful in suppressing colonic disease and azathioprine has been used for maintenance (BNF 1.5). Intravenous nutrition (BNF 9.3) or elemental diets may produce remission or be required during acute relapses. Surgery may be required, but is often complicated by fistula and abscess formation. Relapses often occur.

Self-help organisation
National Association for Colitis and Crohn's Disease

Toxic megacolon

Definition and aetiology
Toxic megacolon is an acute dilatation of the colon (principally affecting the transverse and ascending colon), which may occur as a complication of ulcerative colitis or, more rarely, of Crohn's disease.

Symptoms
It is characterised by abdominal distension and tenderness, dehydration, diarrhoea, fever, malaise and tachycardia, and may lead to perforation, peritonitis and septicaemia.

Treatment
It is treated by intravenous administration of fluids (BNF 9.2.2), 'nil by mouth', discontinuation

of antidiarrhoeal drugs, gastric aspiration, intravenous antibacterial drugs (BNF 5.1), and intravenous corticosteroids (BNF 6.3.2). Surgery (colectomy) should be carried out if there is no response to medical treatment within 24–48 hours and can considerably reduce the overall mortality.

Ulcerative colitis

Definition and aetiology

Ulcerative colitis is a chronic condition of unknown cause in which there are changes in the structure of the mucosa and submucosa of the wall of the colon, with widespread inflammation and superficial ulceration. It always affects the rectum, where the inflammatory process appears to begin (or rectosigmoid area) and from which it usually spreads proximally to a variable extent. The disease most commonly begins between 20 and 40 years of age, although it may occur at any age. It affects between 10 and 12 per 100 000 of the population.

There is an overlap between ulcerative colitis and Crohn's disease, and 10% of cases cannot be differentiated. Ulcerative colitis is twice as common as Crohn's disease.

Symptoms

Symptoms vary from diarrhoea in mild disease to septicaemia, dehydration and malnutrition in severe forms. Diarrhoea, with blood and mucus in the faeces, is a common sign, although if the disease is confined to the rectum there may, paradoxically, be constipation. Tenesmus and pain frequently precede defecation; abdominal cramp may be due to colonic spasm. Other common symptoms are anaemia, anorexia, fatigue, fever and weight loss. Remissions and relapses occur in most patients, although a small number have chronic disease. Gastrointestinal complications include toxic megacolon, perforation, severe haemorrhage, pseudopolyposis, fibrous strictures and cancer. Rectal complications may occur (e.g. abscesses and fistulas), though they are less common than in Crohn's disease. Non-intestinal complications include erythema nodosum, pyoderma gangrenosum, rashes, arthritis, aphthous stomatitis and eye disorders. Ankylosing spondylitis, liver and biliary diseases, and growth retardation in children have also been associated with ulcerative colitis.

Treatment

Symptomatic treatment may be required, with intravenous administration if necessary, to correct deficiency of electrolytes (BNF 9.2), vitamins (BNF 9.6), minerals (BNF 9.5) and other nutrients. Blood transfusion may be necessary for anaemic patients and antibacterial drugs (BNF 5.1) may be required for treatment of infections. Corticosteroids, sulfasalazine and azathioprine are used in the treatment of ulcerative colitis (BNF 1.5). Symptoms of mild ulcerative colitis may be relieved with antidiarrhoeal drugs (BNF 1.4), but these should be used with caution in moderate or severe disease because of the risk of precipitating ileus or toxic megacolon. Regular follow-up examinations (sigmoidoscopy and colonoscopy) should be made to detect the possible development of colorectal cancer, which has a much greater incidence in patients with a long (more than 10 years) history of extensive ulcerative colitis. Surgery is required for cases unresponsive to medical therapy.

1.4 Malabsorption syndromes

Coeliac disease

Definition and aetiology

Coeliac disease (gluten-sensitive enteropathy, idiopathic steatorrhoea or non-tropical sprue) is a chronic disorder of the small intestine in which there is an unusual sensitivity to gluten, sometimes associated with secondary lactose intolerance. It is a common disorder, having an incidence in the UK of approximately 1 in 1500. Coeliac disease may occur in children or adults and is sometimes familial, with 10–15% of siblings being affected. Dermatitis herpetiformis is a related condition.

Symptoms

It is characterised by abnormalities of the jejunal mucosa, which cause malabsorption and steatorrhoea. The malabsorption leads to weight loss and deficiency of minerals and vitamins. Other non-specific symptoms include fatigue, malaise, abdominal distension, anaemia, aphthous stomatitis, bone pain and oedema.

Treatment

In most cases, avoidance of foods containing gluten (e.g. those prepared from wheat, rye, barley and oats) results in normal intestinal function, but the disease returns if gluten is again ingested. A range of gluten-free foods is available (BNF 9.4.1 and Appendix 7). Some medicines (e.g. tablets) may be prepared with gluten-containing ingredients and should be avoided. Administration of nutritional supplements (BNF 9.1, 9.5 and 9.6) may be necessary if deficiencies occur.

Self-help organisation

Coeliac Society of the United Kingdom

Short-bowel syndrome

Definition and aetiology

The short-bowel syndrome is a term used to describe the effects which may occur after extensive surgical resection of the small intestine. Up to 60% of the small intestine may be resected without causing the syndrome.

Symptoms

Symptoms depend upon the length of residual small intestine, the site of resection, and the presence or absence of residual disease. It is characterised by malabsorption with associated nutritional deficiencies. Resection of the ileum allows the passage of bile salts and fatty acids into the colon. The resultant interference with water and electrolyte absorption may lead to diarrhoea, steatorrhoea and gallstone formation. Megaloblastic anaemia may follow ileal resection. There may be an increased risk of renal calculi, due to increased oxalate absorption. Jejunal resection may cause gastric hypersecretion, which may lead to peptic ulceration.

Treatment

Treatment consists of intravenous administration of fluids in the early post-operative period (BNF 9.2.2), intravenous nutrition (BNF 9.3) if severe diarrhoea is prolonged post-operatively, and antidiarrhoeal drugs which reduce motility (BNF 1.4.2). Oral feeding should be introduced gradually and elemental diets (BNF 9.4.2) may be useful. Patients should be encouraged to take frequent small meals, and a relatively high calorie intake may be necessary to avoid the effects of malabsorption. Minerals (BNF 9.5) and vitamins (BNF 9.6) may be required for deficiencies and pancreatin supplements (BNF 1.9.4) for pancreatic insufficiency.

Tropical sprue

Definition and aetiology

Tropical sprue is a chronic malabsorption syndrome which occurs in patients who live in or have visited the tropical areas (e.g. the Caribbean, southern India and South-east Asia). Its aetiology is unknown.

Symptoms

It is characterised by diarrhoea or steatorrhoea, abdominal discomfort and distension, anorexia, malabsorption and weight loss. Glossitis and stomatitis are common, and pigmentation of the skin and oedema may occur. The condition may have an acute onset with severe diarrhoea, fever, and blood and mucus in the faeces; remission may occur on leaving the tropics. Malabsorption may lead to vitamin deficiencies and megaloblastic anaemia.

Treatment

Treatment consists of administration of a tetracycline (BNF 5.1.3), folic acid and hydroxocobalamin (BNF 9.1.2). Treatment should be continued for at least six months and relapses may occur. Antidiarrhoeal drugs (BNF 1.4.2) may be necessary and intravenous administration of fluids (BNF 9.2.2) may be required in acute illness. Mineral (BNF 9.5) or vitamin (BNF 9.6) supplements may be required for other nutritional deficiencies.

Whipple's disease

Definition and aetiology

Whipple's disease is a rare malabsorption syndrome, which usually occurs in men between 30 and 60 years of age. It is caused by a bacterium, *Tropheryma whippelii*, which infiltrates the mucosa of the small intestine.

Symptoms
It is characterised by arthritis, steatorrhoea and weight loss. Other common symptoms include abdominal pain, clubbing of the fingers, fever, lymphadenopathy, nutritional deficiencies, skin pigmentation and weakness. Anaemia may develop.

Treatment
Treatment consists of prolonged administration of antibacterial drugs (BNF 5.1) and correction of nutritional deficiencies (BNF 9.3 and 9.4).

1.5 Liver disorders

Cirrhosis of the liver

Definition and aetiology
Cirrhosis of the liver (Figure 1.2) is a group of chronic diseases of multiple aetiology. It is characterised by destruction of parenchymal cells, loss of their normal lobular structure with widespread fibrosis, and regeneration of the remaining cells to form nodules. Chronic alcohol abuse and viral infection with hepatitis B and hepatitis C are common causes of cirrhosis in the western world. Congenital causes include hereditary haemorrhagic telangiectasia and inborn errors of metabolism (e.g. hepatolenticular degeneration and haemochromatosis, which are both inherited and treatable causes of cirrhosis). Some cases are of unknown origin (cryptogenic cirrhosis). Prolonged cholestasis may lead to biliary cirrhosis. Cirrhosis can also result from adverse reactions to drugs (e.g. isoniazid, methotrexate and methyldopa).

It is the third most common cause of death in the western world in people between 45 and 65 years of age after cardiovascular disease and cancer.

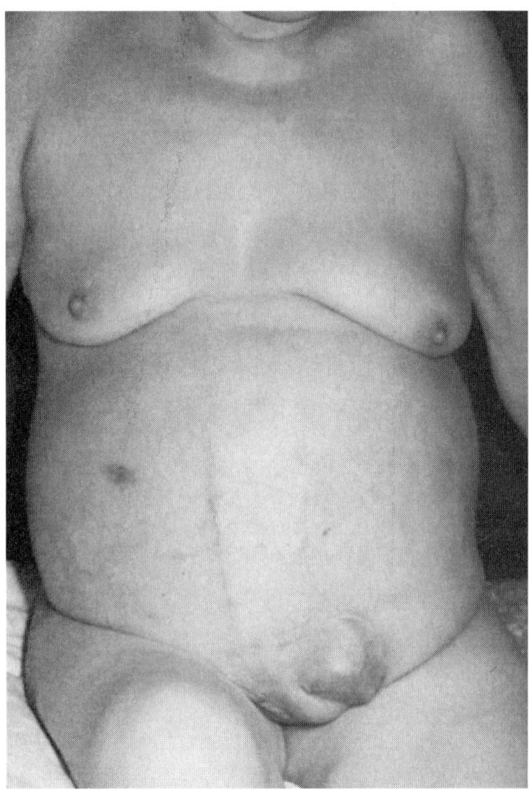

Figure 1.2 Cirrhosis of the liver. (Reproduced with permission of Science Photo Library.)

Symptoms
The disease may have a long latent period and be far advanced before symptoms appear. The disturbance of liver architecture may produce a blockage of venous flow causing portal hypertension. This gives rise to ascites, with abdominal distension and pain, oesophageal varices resulting in haematemesis and splenomegaly. The disturbed liver structure may also lead to biliary obstruction, with associated jaundice and pruritus.

The loss of liver cells and an inefficient blood supply to the regenerated cells results in liver-cell failure, primarily affecting the metabolism of ingested substances. Toxic products of protein metabolism may cause hepatic encephalopathy leading to coma, and the toxic effects of drugs are increased and prolonged.

Other metabolic consequences of liver-cell failure include oedema, impaired synthesis of albumin and various clotting factors, and delayed breakdown of hormones (e.g. hydrocortisone and oestrogens). Excess quantities of these hormones can lead to the formation of spider telangiectasia, erythema of palms and soles and, in the male, gynaecomastia and atrophy of the testes. Other clinical features include whitened nails (having a pink area at the tip), finger clubbing, glossitis, paraesthesia, parotid-gland enlargement, pyrexia, muscle wasting and weight loss. In some patients, the regenerative activity in the hepatic

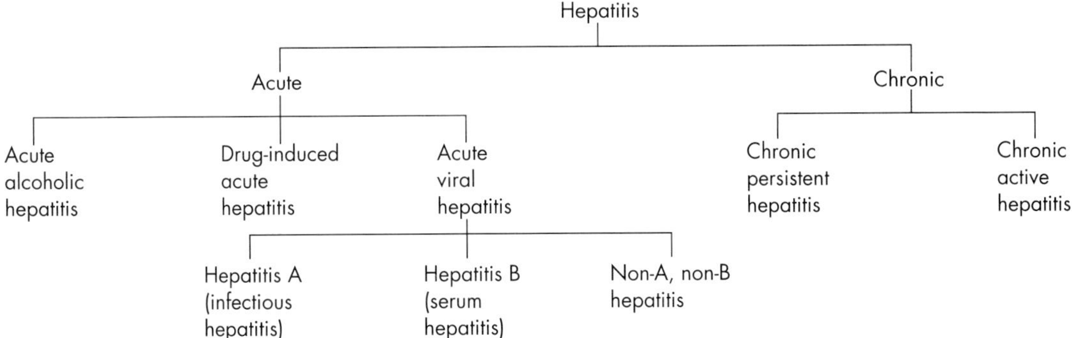

Figure 1.3 Classification of hepatitis.

nodule becomes neoplastic, resulting in hepatoma.

Treatment

Since the disease process cannot be reversed, treatment is designed to prevent further fibrosis and limit the development of fluid retention and encephalopathy. A diet rich in energy and protein should be given unless encephalopathy is present, when protein intake should be limited. In general, alcohol should be avoided.

Hepatic coma due to encephalopathy is prevented or treated by reducing the absorption of toxic nitrogenous substances from the intestine. This is achieved by reducing protein intake and reducing the bacterial population of the gut by administration of antibacterials (e.g. neomycin, BNF 5.1.4). Salt intake should be restricted when ascites or oedema are present, and potassium-sparing diuretics (BNF 2.2.3) administered if required. In severe ascites, abdominal paracentesis may be required.

Surgery may be required when cirrhosis is due to obstruction of the bile ducts. Pruritus, which is most commonly associated with cirrhosis caused by biliary obstruction, may be relieved by the use of antihistamines (BNF 3.4.1) and colestyramine (BNF 1.9.2). Corticosteroids (BNF 6.3.2) may relieve symptoms and prolong life when used in the active phases of the disease, particularly if there is evidence of progressive active hepatitis.

Self-help organisations

British Liver Trust
Children's Liver Disease Foundation

Hepatitis

Definition and aetiology

Hepatitis is an inflammatory condition of the liver characterised by diffuse or patchy hepatocellular necrosis. It may be acute or chronic (Figure 1.3). Acute forms may be due to viral infections, alcohol, drugs or toxins; if they persist, chronic episodes can develop.

Acute viral hepatitis

Definition and aetiology

Acute viral hepatitis may be caused by at least four specific viruses: hepatitis A virus (HAV), hepatitis B virus (HBV), hepatitis D virus (HDV) and hepatitis C virus (HCV) (formerly called non-A, non-B hepatitis virus). More rarely, yellow fever and infectious mononucleosis together with cytomegalovirus, herpes simplex virus or rubella virus infections may lead to an acute hepatitis syndrome.

HAV is usually spread by faecal–oral contamination (e.g. of food), although transmission by blood transfusion is also theoretically possible. Outbreaks occur sporadically, but small epidemics may develop in institutions. More significant outbreaks can accompany large movements of population (e.g. in war). There also appears to be an increased incidence among promiscuous homosexuals. The incubation period is from two to six weeks. There is no carrier state.

HBV is usually transmitted in transfused blood or plasma, by the use of non-sterile needles and syringes, by sexual intercourse, oro-genital contact or by contact with infected secretions. High-risk groups include haemophiliacs, homosexuals, drug addicts, haemodialysis patients, and healthcare and laboratory personnel. The incubation period is from one to six months. Some patients may become asymptomatic carriers. Exposure at birth transmitted from a mother to the child results in persistent infection in the child.

HDV can only reproduce in the presence of HBV. It is seen primarily in intravenous drug abusers and haemophiliacs.

HCV is the major cause of post-transfusion hepatitis and is common in drug addicts and other needle-users. The incubation period is 2–23 weeks. Many patients become carriers.

Symptoms

The first (prodromal) phase of HAV is usually rapid in onset and characterised by mild fever, malaise, anorexia, nausea and vomiting, abdominal distension, rashes and arthralgia. Classically, the patient may describe a loss of taste for coffee or tobacco. After 3–10 days jaundice may rapidly develop, the fever subsides, and the patient feels better. The stools are pale, the urine is dark, and hepatomegaly occurs, accompanied by mild splenomegaly, in about 20% of cases. In elderly patients there may be disorientation and confusion. Jaundice usually subsides after two to four weeks. However, in many patients, especially children, jaundice does not develop and the illness is perceived as a non-specific influenza. The prognosis is usually good, but complications (e.g. acute hepatic necrosis, hepatic cirrhosis and aplastic anaemia) may occur.

Clinically, HBV follows a similar pattern to HAV, but tends to be more prolonged and to have a greater mortality. Up to 90% of patients with HBV recover completely. About 1% may develop acute hepatic failure (fulminant hepatitis), characterised by progressive mental changes, deepening jaundice and the development of encephalopathy. Some patients will become chronic carriers of the infection, or develop chronic persistent hepatitis or chronic active hepatitis. HBV has also been associated with the development of primary hepatocellular carcinoma.

The presence of HDV is suspected if exceptionally severe symptoms occur in HBV infection.

Most cases of HCV infection are asymptomatic and only become apparent when they have reached the chronic phase and a patient is tested routinely for anti-HCV antigens. Cirrhosis develops in 20% of HCV patients, which can proceed to hepatocellular carcinoma.

Treatment

In most cases of acute viral hepatitis irrespective of the causative agent, no special treatment is required. Patients should be advised to rest; bed rest may be required for severe lethargy but does not accelerate recovery. A diet low in fat but high in protein and carbohydrate should be instituted. Corticosteroids should not be given unless there is prolonged jaundice. Alcohol should be avoided throughout the course of the acute illness. The condition is infectious during the prodromal phase, and strict personal hygiene is important in preventing the spread of infection. Contacts may be given normal immunoglobulin (BNF 14.5) for prophylaxis, following which protection lasts for about three to six months, depending on dosage.

Hepatitis A vaccine (BNF 14.4) is available as an alternative for the protection of close family. Other groups who may benefit from immunisation include laboratory staff who work directly with the virus and travellers to high-risk areas. Hepatitis B vaccine (BNF 14.4) is used for prophylaxis in individuals at high risk of contracting the infection. A combined hepatitis A and hepatitis B vaccine is also available (BNF 14.4).

Accidental contamination with hepatitis B virus-infected blood may be treated by passive immunisation with specific hepatitis B immunoglobulin (HBIG) (BNF 14.5).

Acute alcoholic hepatitis

Definition and aetiology

Acute alcoholic hepatitis is characterised by diffuse hepatic inflammation (fatty and hyaline) and necrosis, and is a precursor of cirrhosis.

Symptoms

Patients may present with symptoms similar to those of acute viral hepatitis, although unlike acute viral hepatitis, cholestasis may be a dominant early feature.

Treatment
There is no specific treatment, but patients should be advised to abstain from alcohol and adopt a well-balanced diet. About 10% of cases will proceed to cirrhosis in spite of abstention from alcohol.

Self-help organisation
Alcoholics Anonymous

Drug-induced acute hepatitis

Definition and aetiology
Certain drugs and chemicals can cause an idiosyncratic acute hepatitis, which may mimic the broad clinical spectrum associated with acute viral hepatitis. Examples of offending agents include halothane, isoniazid, methyldopa, gold, rifampicin, paracetamol and sulphonamides.

Treatment
Most patients will make a complete recovery provided the responsible agent is identified and withdrawn.

Jaundice

Definition
Jaundice (icterus) is a yellow discoloration of the skin, sclera and mucous membranes caused by the accumulation of bilirubin. Depending on the cause of the jaundice, bilirubin may be conjugated (in the liver cell), water-soluble and excreted in the urine (conjugated hyperbilirubinaemia); this occurs in cholestatic jaundice. In other forms of jaundice (e.g. haemolytic), the bilirubin is unconjugated, water-insoluble and not excreted in the urine (unconjugated hyperbilirubinaemia). In all types, tissues and fluids throughout the body (except mucous secretions) accumulate bilirubin.

Cholestatic jaundice

Definition and aetiology
Cholestatic (obstructive) jaundice is caused by obstruction in the bile ducts (extrahepatic) or between the liver cells and bile ducts (intrahepatic), and results in conjugated hyperbilirubinaemia. Numerous drugs and chemicals may cause intrahepatic cholestatic jaundice (e.g. phenothiazines, anabolic steroids and, more rarely, oral contraceptives). Intrahepatic jaundice may also occur in primary biliary cirrhosis, in pregnancy and in rare inherited disorders. Extrahepatic cholestatic jaundice may be due to gallstones, strictures, pancreatitis or malignant disease.

Symptoms
The condition is usually insidious in onset, of variable intensity, and characterised by pruritus and anorexia. The faeces are pale or clay-coloured and contain excessive amounts of fat, and the urine is dark.

Treatment
Treatment is related to the cause, and in extrahepatic obstruction, surgery may be necessary.

Haemolytic jaundice

Definition and aetiology
In haemolytic (acholuric) jaundice, excessive destruction of erythrocytes results in the release of more bilirubin than the liver can metabolise. It may be due to excessive fragility of the erythrocytes, as in certain congenital diseases (e.g. sickle-cell anaemia and beta thalassaemia) or it may be caused by toxin-producing microorganisms, haemolytic poisons, megaloblastic anaemia or circulating erythrocyte antibodies. Jaundice is likely to be particularly severe in neonates with haemolytic anaemia, and if the plasma bilirubin concentration is not controlled, kernicterus may develop. Haemolytic jaundice may develop as a result of the administration of drugs (e.g. methyldopa). Mild unconjugated hyperbilirubinaemia may also occur in the absence of liver disease or overt haemolysis (Gilbert's syndrome, a hereditary disorder affecting approximately 2% of the population).

Symptoms
The faeces may be darker than normal and there may be splenomegaly.

Treatment
Treatment depends on the cause of the disease, but surgery and the administration of corticosteroids may be required.

Hepatocellular jaundice

Definition and aetiology
Damage to the parenchymal cells of the liver may occur due to acute viral hepatitis, acute alcoholic hepatitis or drug-induced hepatitis. As a result, the cells fail to take up bilirubin, conjugate it, and pass the complex to the bile ducts. Congenital abnormalities and deficient enzyme systems are also causative factors.

Symptoms
Intrahepatic cholestasis may develop. The onset of jaundice is usually rapid and the disease varies from mild to severe.

Treatment
Treatment depends on the underlying cause, but generally surgery is of no value and should be avoided.

Physiological jaundice

Definition and aetiology
Physiological (neonatal) jaundice due to hepatic immaturity is a common condition, particularly in premature neonates. It usually appears after the first 24 hours in full-term neonates and after 48 hours in premature neonates.

Treatment
It may be treated by phototherapy.

Kernicterus

Definition and aetiology
Kernicterus is degeneration of brain tissue in neonates. It is caused by bilirubin crossing the blood–brain barrier as a result of high plasma concentrations of unconjugated bilirubin (unconjugated hyperbilirubinaemia), and is usually associated with haemolytic disease of the newborn. This is now rare due to careful monitoring during pregnancy and the use of anti-D (Rh_0) immunoglobulin in rhesus-negative women who have previously carried a rhesus-positive baby.

Symptoms
The development of kernicterus in full-term jaundiced neonates may be characterised by drowsiness, anorexia, vomiting and convulsions. In premature neonates there are usually no clinical symptoms other than jaundice. It may be fatal or result in permanent brain damage.

Treatment
Plasma bilirubin concentrations should be monitored in jaundiced neonates. Phototherapy may be effective in alleviating hyperbilirubinaemia and is used in the prevention of kernicterus, but exchange blood transfusion may also be required.

1.6 Biliary-tract disorders

Cholangitis

Definition and aetiology
Cholangitis is inflammation of the bile ducts (Figure 1.4), usually due to bacterial infection. It is commonly associated with gallstones partially obstructing the common bile duct or biliary strictures. It may be mild and intermittent or severe (suppurative cholangitis).

Symptoms
Cholangitis is characterised by malaise, fever and chills, followed by pain (which may be colicky and severe) in the right upper quadrant of the abdomen. Vomiting, cholestatic jaundice and pruritus may also ensue; the urine becomes dark and the faeces are pale. Recurrent attacks may result in the formation of an hepatic abscess. Suppurative cholangitis may lead to septicaemia and shock.

Treatment
Treatment consists of parenteral antibacterial drugs (BNF 5.1) and intravenous administration of fluids (BNF 9.2.2) to correct fluid and electrolyte imbalance. Surgery may be required to remove bile-duct stones (choledochotomy) and the gall bladder (cholecystectomy) or for surgical repair of a biliary stricture.

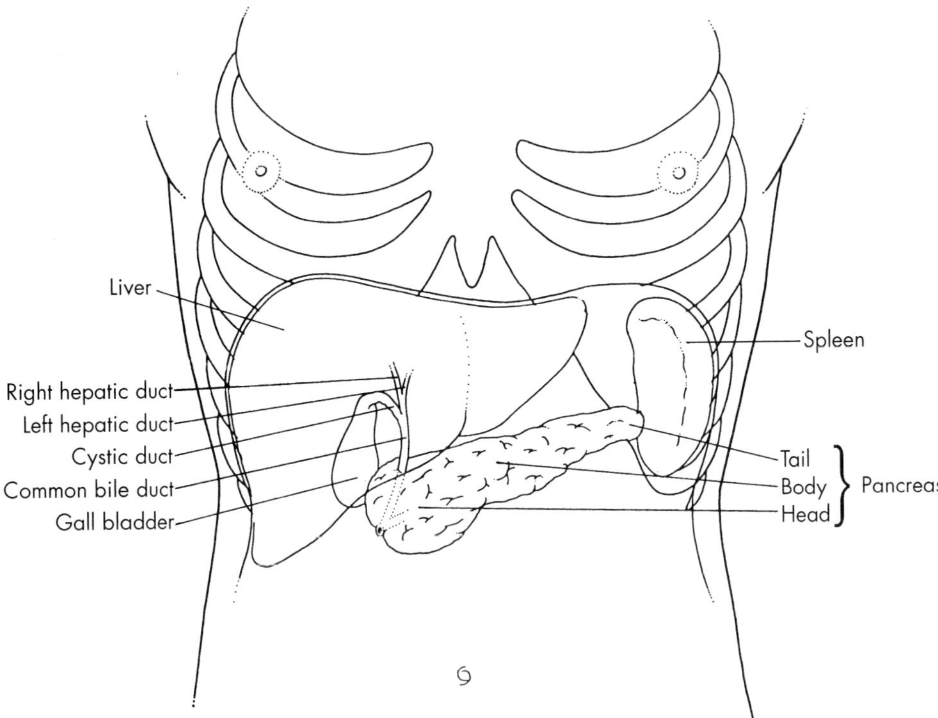

Figure 1.4 Accessory digestive organs.

Cholecystitis

Definition

Cholecystitis is an inflammatory condition of the gall bladder, which may be acute or chronic.

Acute cholecystitis

Definition and aetiology

Acute cholecystitis occurs at the same time as gallstones in nearly all patients. It results from the toxic effects of retained bile on the gall bladder wall, following the obstruction of the outlet (cystic duct) of the gall bladder by a gallstone. Secondary bacterial infection frequently occurs.

Symptoms

Acute cholecystitis is characterised by severe pain of relatively sudden onset localised in the right hypochondrium or in the epigastrium. The pain is continuous and often radiates to the back. In uncomplicated cases it gradually subsides over a period of 12–18 hours. Flatulence and nausea are common and mild fever may occur. Persistent vomiting and jaundice may be present, but are more likely in obstruction of the common bile duct. Complications include empyema of the gall bladder, cholangitis, gangrene and perforation, which may lead to abscess formation, fistulas or peritonitis.

Treatment

Treatment consists of parenteral opioid analgesics (BNF 4.7.2), intravenous administration of fluids (BNF 9.2.2), and for all except mild cases, treatment with antibacterial drugs (BNF 5.1). Surgery may be required urgently if complications develop; otherwise cholecystectomy is performed after the acute symptoms have resolved, either within two to three days or after an interval of two to three months.

Chronic cholecystitis

Definition and aetiology
Chronic cholecystitis is the most common form of gall bladder disease resulting from gallstones. It usually develops insidiously, but may follow an attack of acute cholecystitis.

Symptoms
It may be characterised by recurrent attacks of biliary colic or by recurrent episodes of constant right hypochondrial or epigastric pain. The pain may radiate to the right shoulder or the back and lasts for periods ranging from about 15 minutes to several hours. It commonly occurs after a meal or wakes the patient at night, and symptoms are frequently related to the ingestion of fatty foods. However, in a significant number of patients the symptoms are vague and ill-defined and include abdominal discomfort and distension, nausea, flatulence and intolerance of fatty foods. Complications include acute cholecystitis, passage of stones into the common bile duct (choledocholithiasis), pancreatitis, formation of fistulas, gallstone ileus, and rarely cancer of the gall bladder. Occasionally the accumulation of mucus and gallstones produces hydrops, which is characterised by constant right hypochondrial discomfort and a tender mass, without the occurrence of acute cholecystitis.

Treatment
Treatment consists of surgical removal of the gall bladder (cholecystectomy) for established cases of chronic cholecystitis. If the diagnosis is in doubt (e.g. vague symptoms associated with a well-functioning gall bladder containing stones), conservative treatment may be tried (e.g. weight reduction and a low-fat diet). Drugs acting on the gall bladder may also be used (BNF 1.9.1).

Gallstones

Definition and aetiology
Gallstones (cholelithiasis) are stones formed in the gall bladder. Gallstone disease is common and the incidence increases progressively with age. The stones may be classified as cholesterol stones, bile-pigment stones or mixed stones.

Cholesterol stones are usually solitary, large and faceted. They are thought to be associated with raised biliary cholesterol secretion and diminished bile acid synthesis. Racial differences, diet, drugs (e.g. oral contraceptives) and gastrointestinal disease (e.g. Crohn's disease) also influence the development of cholesterol stones. Bile pigment stones are either composed purely of bile pigment or of bile pigment and calcium. Pure pigment stones are black, hard and brittle; they are commonly found in patients with haemolytic anaemia, cirrhosis of the liver, chronic bile-duct obstruction and malaria. Stones formed of bile pigment and calcium are brown, soft and pliable and have been associated with infections of the biliary tract. Mixed stones, composed of cholesterol, bile pigment and calcium are usually multiple and faceted.

Gallstones occur more commonly in women and obese subjects. It has been estimated that about one in five of all people of under 65 years of age have gallstones.

Symptoms
The majority of gallstones remain in the gall bladder and may be asymptomatic (silent gallstones). If the neck of the gall bladder becomes obstructed by a gallstone, biliary colic will occur and acute or chronic cholecystitis may develop. Multiple small stones may cause intermittent episodes of biliary colic when a small stone passes into the common bile duct (*see below*). If the bile duct becomes obstructed, cholestatic jaundice may develop. Other complications of gallstones include cholangitis, biliary cirrhosis, and development of an internal biliary fistula. Acute pancreatitis and cancer of the gall bladder have been associated with gallstone disease. Patients with uncomplicated gallstones may complain of abdominal discomfort and distension, flatulence and intolerance to fatty foods, but it is uncertain whether these symptoms are directly related to the gallstones.

Treatment
Gallstones may be treated surgically by removal of the gall bladder (cholecystectomy). Certain patients with cholesterol stones may be treated with chenodeoxycholic or ursodeoxycholic acid (BNF 1.9.1).

Choledocholithiasis

Definition
Choledocholithiasis is the occurrence of gallstones in the common bile duct.

Symptoms
Classically, it is characterised by biliary colic, cholestatic jaundice and fever. It is commonly associated with cholangitis, in which case fever and chills are present. Nausea and vomiting occur frequently and pruritus may be severe. Choledocholithiasis may, however, be asymptomatic or present with only one of the classical symptoms. Prolonged choledocholithiasis may eventually lead to obstructive biliary cirrhosis.

Treatment
Treatment consists of surgical removal of the gallstones (choledochotomy) and cholecystectomy if the gall bladder is present. In some cases, the stone may be removed from the bile duct using an endoscope. Parenteral antibacterial drugs (BNF 5.1) may be required if cholangitis is present, and intravenous fluids (BNF 9.2.2) may be required for fluid and electrolyte imbalance.

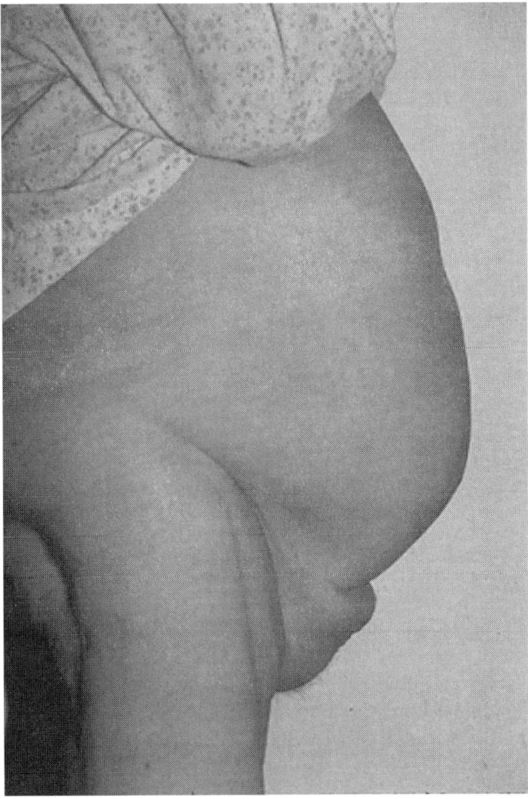

Figure 1.5 Ascites. (Reproduced with permission of Dr P Marazzi/Science Photo Library.)

1.7 Peritoneal disorders

Ascites

Definition and aetiology
Ascites is the accumulation of fluid within the peritoneal cavity. It is most commonly caused by cirrhosis of the liver, malignant disease, advanced congestive heart failure or tuberculosis. Other causes include obstruction of the hepatic vein, hypothyroidism, hypoalbuminaemia (e.g. as a result of nephrotic syndrome), ovarian disease, pancreatitis and inflammatory diseases of the peritoneum.

Symptoms
Symptoms may include abdominal pain and distension (Figure 1.5), dehydration, dyspnoea and muscle wasting. Minor occurrences of ascites may be asymptomatic.

Treatment
Treatment consists of bed rest, adoption of a low-sodium diet, and restricting fluid intake if required. If the condition does not improve, potassium-sparing diuretics (BNF 2.2.3 and 2.2.4) may be given. Drainage of fluid may relieve severe discomfort and shorten the period of hospitalisation.

Peritonitis

Definition and aetiology
Peritonitis is the acute inflammation of the peritoneum. It is usually caused by bacterial infection secondary to gastrointestinal perforation, and may be localised or diffuse. Common causes of localised peritonitis are appendicitis, Crohn's disease, diverticular disease, peptic ulceration,

salpingitis and chemical irritation (e.g. in severe acute pancreatitis). A common causative organism is *Escherichia coli*.

Diffuse (generalised) peritonitis may result from a ruptured appendix, perforated peptic ulcer or perforation of the colon (e.g. due to infarction, obstruction or ulcerative colitis).

Tuberculous peritonitis may accompany pulmonary tuberculosis, while rarer causes are fungal or parasitic infections.

Granulomatous peritonitis may develop postoperatively from the presence of starch and magnesium oxide used to reduce the stickiness of surgical rubber gloves.

Symptoms

Bacterial peritonitis is usually characterised by acute abdominal pain and tenderness, dehydration, fever, hypotension, ileus, nausea and vomiting and tachycardia. These symptoms are not always present, however, particularly in elderly patients and in patients undergoing corticosteroid therapy. Complications include abscess formation, oliguria (occasionally leading to acute renal failure) and shock. In tuberculous peritonitis, the development of symptoms is often insidious, but may include anorexia, fever, malaise and weight loss. Abdominal distension and ascites are present in about 70% of cases. Fungal peritonitis usually occurs only in immunosuppressed patients.

Treatment

Peritonitis should be treated with antibacterial drugs (BNF 5.1), intravenous administration of fluids (BNF 9.2.2), gastric aspiration and opioid analgesics (BNF 4.7.2). Blood transfusion may be required. Surgery should be carried out as soon as possible to correct the underlying cause.

1.8 Anorectal disorders

Anal fissure

Definition and aetiology

An anal fissure is an acute lengthways tear or a chronic circular ulcer in the epithelial lining of the anal canal. Acute tears are usually caused by large hard faeces or are idiopathic. They may also arise through childbirth and diarrhoea (e.g. in Crohn's disease). Young children may also develop acute tears. Chronic fissures comprise circular or elliptic ulcers, which are secondary to fibrosis due to chronic infection.

Symptoms

Patients with a chronic anal fissure may report an external skin tag (sentinel pile). Painful symptoms are produced by all fissures, particularly during defecation. Marked spasm of the anal sphincter and slight bleeding may also occur.

Treatment

Adoption of a high-fibre diet (e.g. bran), administration of faecal softeners (BNF 1.6.3) and application of topical soothing agents (BNF 1.7.1) are all beneficial and are used in conjunction with rectal dilators. Bathing in warm salt water may also provide relief. Surgery may be necessary for chronic fissures.

Anorectal fistula

Definition and aetiology

An anorectal fistula (fistula in ano) is a hollow fibrous tract, usually connecting the anal canal or rectum to an opening in the perianal skin. It may result from the rupture or surgical drainage of an anorectal abscess, or be due to Crohn's disease, diverticular disease, tuberculosis, sexually transmitted disease, malignant disease or anal fissure. In neonates, fistulas are congenital and are more common in boys. Rectovaginal fistulas may also occur, arising congenitally or following radiotherapy, pelvic surgery, childbirth or malignant disease.

Symptoms

Continual discharge of pus, blood, mucus and occasionally faeces through the perianal opening results in discomfort, irritation and pruritus ani. Pain from an underlying abscess may also be present.

Treatment

Soothing preparations (BNF 1.7.1) may be applied topically, but surgery (fistulotomy) is the only effective treatment.

Haemorrhoids

Definition and aetiology

Haemorrhoids (piles) are varicosities of the network of veins which line the anus and rectum (haemorrhoidal plexus). They are commonly caused by straining as a result of constipation, low-fibre diets and pregnancy.

Haemorrhoids may be internal or external. Internal haemorrhoids, which do not prolapse, are termed primary (or first-degree); those which prolapse on defecation but withdraw again are termed secondary (second-degree); and permanently prolapsed haemorrhoids are referred to as tertiary (third-degree) haemorrhoids. External haemorrhoids (a subcutaneous haematoma at the anal verge) often leave a permanent protruding fold or skin-tag.

Symptoms

The principal symptom is the discharge of bright red blood from the rectum, which at first occurs only on defecation but later may occur independently of bowel action. Persistent blood loss may lead to a secondary anaemia. Soreness, pruritus ani, discharge of mucus and pain on defecation may occur. Haemorrhoids which have prolapsed and thrombosed are painful and may become infected or gangrenous.

Treatment

Treatment consists of the adoption of a high-fibre diet, the use of faecal softeners (BNF 1.6.3), and the application of soothing preparations (BNF 1.7.1). Warm salt baths may give symptomatic relief. Patients should be instructed in hygienic measures and to replace protruding piles after defecation. Uncomplicated internal haemorrhoids which bleed may be treated by injection of a rectal sclerosant (BNF 1.7.3). Rubber-band ligation and cryosurgery are also used. In the presence of complications (e.g. prolapse), haemorrhoids require surgical treatment (haemorrhoidectomy).

Proctitis

Definition and aetiology

Proctitis is an inflammation of the rectal mucosa. Infectious proctitis may be caused by *Shigella* spp. or sexually transmitted diseases (especially in male homosexuals). Non-infectious causes include radiation injury, trauma, ischaemia or chronic inflammatory disease (e.g. Crohn's disease). Ulcerative proctitis (haemorrhagic proctitis) is a form of ulcerative colitis in which inflammation is limited to the rectum.

Symptoms

It is characterised by rectal bleeding, discharge of mucus, tenesmus and anal or perianal soreness. The frequency of defecation may be increased, but the faeces are often normal or hard and dry. Anaemia may occur, but other systemic symptoms are rare. Remissions and relapses are common.

Treatment

Treatment of proctitis depends on the underlying cause. In infectious proctitis the infecting microorganism should be identified and treatment directed accordingly. Ulcerative proctitis may be treated with corticosteroid suppositories or enemas or with sulfasalazine (BNF 1.5). Treatment may be supplemented by adopting a high-fibre diet to avoid hard faeces and applying soothing preparations (BNF 1.7.1).

1.9 Pancreatic exocrine disorders

Cystic fibrosis

Definition and aetiology

Cystic fibrosis is an inherited disease affecting infants, children and young adults. It is characterised by the widespread secretion of abnormally viscid mucus and by sweat containing high electrolyte concentrations. It is transmitted by an autosomal recessive gene. Approximately 1 in 20 people carry the gene and 1 in 1600 Caucasian births are affected. The precise genetic abnormality has been identified, located on 250 000 base pairs of genomic DNA on chromosome 7q. There has been a steady improvement in the survival rates of those diagnosed with cystic fibrosis due to better clinical management, and the number of adults with cystic fibrosis doubled between 1971 and 1991.

Symptoms

Respiratory-tract disorders and pancreatic insufficiency are the most important manifestations, but symptoms vary in severity. Bronchial obstruction, recurring respiratory-tract infection, bronchiectasis, emphysema, and pulmonary insufficiency leading to cor pulmonale are respiratory complications. Pancreatic insufficiency may be asymptomatic, although the pancreatic ducts become blocked. Diabetes mellitus and hepatic changes may also occur. Meconium ileus may be the presenting symptom in the newborn, indicating intestinal obstruction. Vitamin deficiency is likely due to malabsorption. Other common symptoms include diarrhoea, steatorrhoea, failure to thrive despite hyperphagia and rectal prolapse. The prognosis beyond early adulthood is poor due to progressive pulmonary and pancreatic degeneration, although the outlook has steadily improved over recent years.

Treatment

Drug treatment comprises the administration of pancreatin supplements (BNF 1.9.4), parenteral fat-soluble vitamins (BNF 9.6), and appropriate high-dose antibacterial drugs (BNF 5.1). Bronchodilators (BNF 3.1) may also be necessary. Mucolytics (BNF 3.7) have been used, and drug treatment for diabetes mellitus may be required. Bronchodilators, mucolytics and antibacterial drugs delivered via a nebuliser in the home are gaining in popularity. Foods for special diets (BNF 9.4.1 and Appendix 7) are available, and surgery may be needed for intestinal obstruction. Physiotherapy with postural drainage is beneficial for pulmonary symptoms and needs to be a daily routine.

Self-help organisation

Cystic Fibrosis Trust

Pancreatitis

Definition

Pancreatitis is inflammation of the pancreas. It may be acute or chronic.

Acute pancreatitis

Definition and aetiology

Acute pancreatitis is an inflammatory and sometimes haemorrhagic process in the pancreas. Ischaemia and activation of proteolytic enzymes result in damage to the pancreas and surrounding tissues. More than 80% of hospital admission cases are caused by biliary-tract disease and alcoholism; the remainder are due to drugs (e.g. thiazide diuretics, azathioprine, and overdosage with paracetamol). Abdominal surgery, viral infection and a crush injury (e.g. received during sports activities) are minor causes. Recurrent acute pancreatic disease is almost always associated with biliary-tract disease. Other diseases associated with the development of acute pancreatitis include hyperparathyroidism, hyperlipidaemia and mumps.

Symptoms

The primary symptoms are extreme epigastric pain often radiating to the back, abdominal tenderness and, in severe cases, hypovolaemic shock. The abdominal wall may be rigid and there are signs of peritoneal irritation. Nausea and vomiting are common and fever, jaundice and ileus may develop. In severe cases ascites, pleural effusions, hypoxia and adult respiratory distress syndrome may occur. Complications include pseudocysts and abscesses.

Treatment

Treatment should be conservative, with laparotomy performed only if there is diagnostic difficulty or underlying biliary-tract disease. No fluids or solids should be given by mouth and any shock should be treated. Opioid analgesics (BNF 4.7.2) may be required for pain relief. In severe cases, the stomach should be aspirated. A range of treatments has been tested in acute pancreatitis. Aprotinin, a proteolytic enzyme inhibitor (BNF 1.9.3), may reduce the effects of released pancreatic enzymes; and glucagon (BNF 6.1.4) has also been used. The value of any of these treatments is currently unsubstantiated.

Chronic pancreatitis

Definition and aetiology

Chronic pancreatitis is characterised by the progressive destruction and fibrosis of pancreatic glandular tissue, resulting in the failure of endocrine and exocrine pancreatic function. It may arise through chronic alcoholism, chronic protein malnutrition, hyperparathyroidism or hyperlipidaemia.

Symptoms

Recurrent episodes of severe epigastric pain lasting about 24–48 hours commonly occur and these may be aggravated by a heavy meal or by alcohol. Alternatively, the pain may be relatively constant, but aggravated by food. Pain may be accompanied by nausea and vomiting and is not relieved by antacids. Jaundice may occur and pseudocysts are common. Chronic pancreatitis results in a reduction in pancreatic size and a dilatation of the pancreatic ducts. Lack of pancreatic enzyme secretion gives rise to malabsorption from the intestine, characterised by steatorrhoea. Initially the endocrine function of the pancreas may continue, but eventually mild diabetes mellitus may occur.

Treatment

Chronic pancreatitis is treated symptomatically. Acute attacks are treated with analgesics (BNF 4.7). A low-fat high-protein diet should be given, alcohol forbidden and replacement therapy with pancreatin supplements (BNF 1.9.4) provided when required. Insulin (BNF 6.1.1) may be needed for the treatment of diabetes, as oral hypoglycaemic agents are unlikely to be effective. Surgical treatment may be necessary.

1.10 Anatomy and physiology of the digestive system

The digestive system (Figure 1.6) comprises the gastrointestinal tract and associated organs. Its structure is modified along its length to allow the sequential processes of intake, digestion, absorption and excretion. (For a description of the anatomy and physiology of the oropharynx, *see* Section 12.4.)

The oesophagus channels food and liquids downward from the mouth to the stomach, aided by mucus and peristalsis. The contents of the stomach are prevented from regurgitating into the oesophagus by the muscular cardiac sphincter.

The stomach is a muscular reservoir whose convoluted inner surface secretes gastric juice (which includes hydrochloric acid and the proteolytic enzyme precursor pepsinogen) in response to the release of the hormone gastrin from the stomach mucosa. Rennin is also secreted in young children. The internal surface of the stomach is protected from the potentially harmful effects of these secretions by the continual regeneration of epithelial cells, the regulation of output so that food is always present when secretion occurs, and the presence of the glycoprotein mucin, which provides a physical and chemical barrier, particularly to the effects of gastric acid. Retention of ingested material occurs mainly in the fundus, but also to a lesser extent in the body of the stomach. Mixing and homogenisation of ingested material into a suspension (chyme) occurs in the body and distal antrum. When the lower portion of the stomach contracts, small quantities of acidic chyme are propelled through the pyloric sphincter into the small intestine.

The small intestine consists sequentially of the duodenum, jejunum and the ileum. When food enters the duodenum, it is modified by secretions from the intestine wall, the liver and the pancreas. Intestinal mucosal and submucosal cells secrete an alkaline mucus which neutralises the acidic character of the chyme.

The liver (*see also below*) secretes bile which is stored in the gall bladder. In the presence of food in the duodenum, the release of bile is stimulated by the action of pancreozymin. Bile contains steroidal bile salts (e.g. sodium glycocholate) which emulsify fats and lipids; bile pigments (containing the breakdown products of haemoglobin), which colour the faeces; and cholesterol, lecithin, water and electrolytes.

The release of exocrine pancreatic secretions is also controlled by pancreozymin. These secretions include amylase, which digests polysaccharides to

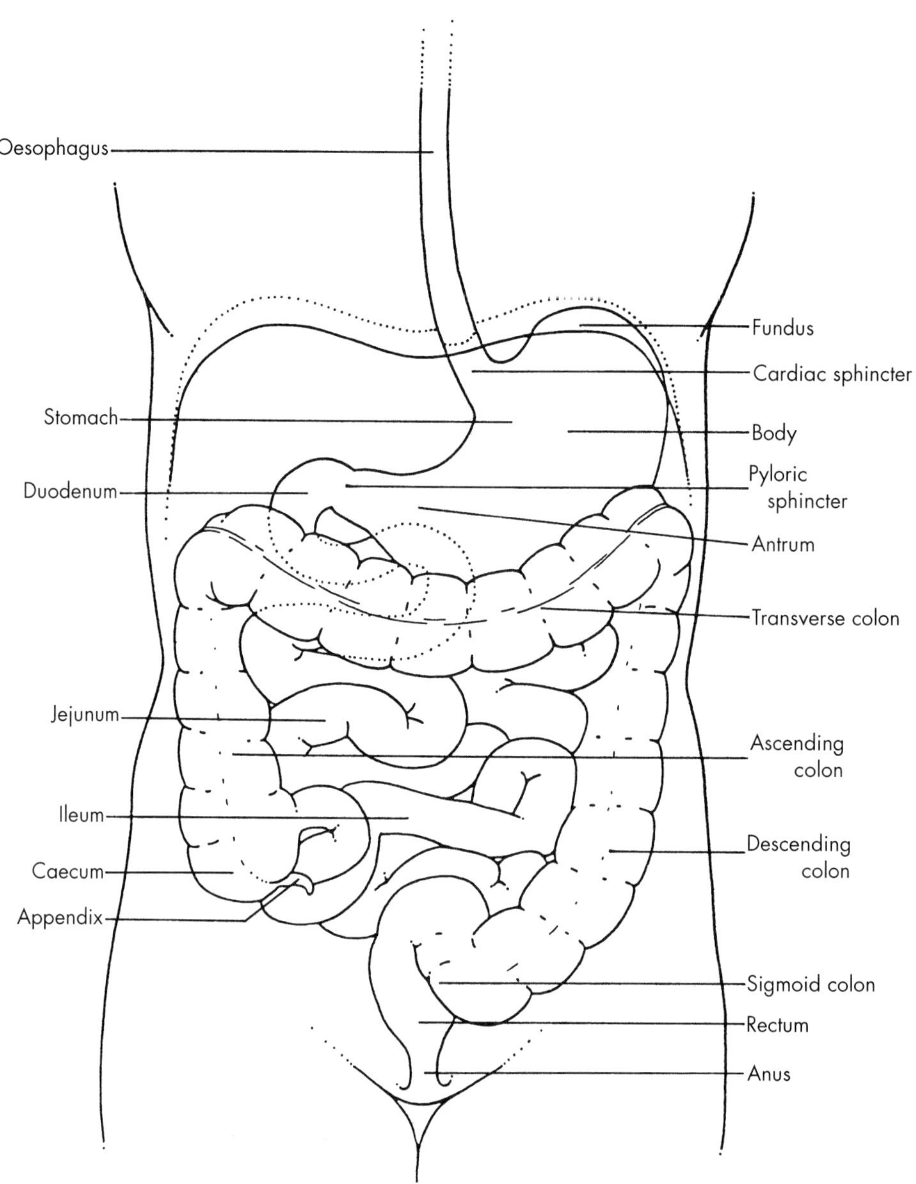

Figure 1.6 Anatomy of the digestive system.

disaccharides; lipase, which converts lipids to fatty acids and glycerol; and the enzyme precursors trypsinogen and chymotrypsinogen, which are converted to active proteolytic enzymes.

The small intestine is the primary site of absorption of the initial products of digestion. The presence of gently oscillating villi (Figure 1.7), tightly packed in the duodenum and jejunum, but more sparsely populating the ileum, greatly enhances the absorptive capacity. These finger-like projections comprise cells which constantly migrate upwards from the base, to be shed within two to three days of formation. As the relatively alkaline luminal emulsion (chyle) is absorbed by the villi, digestion continues within the lining cells. Proteases break

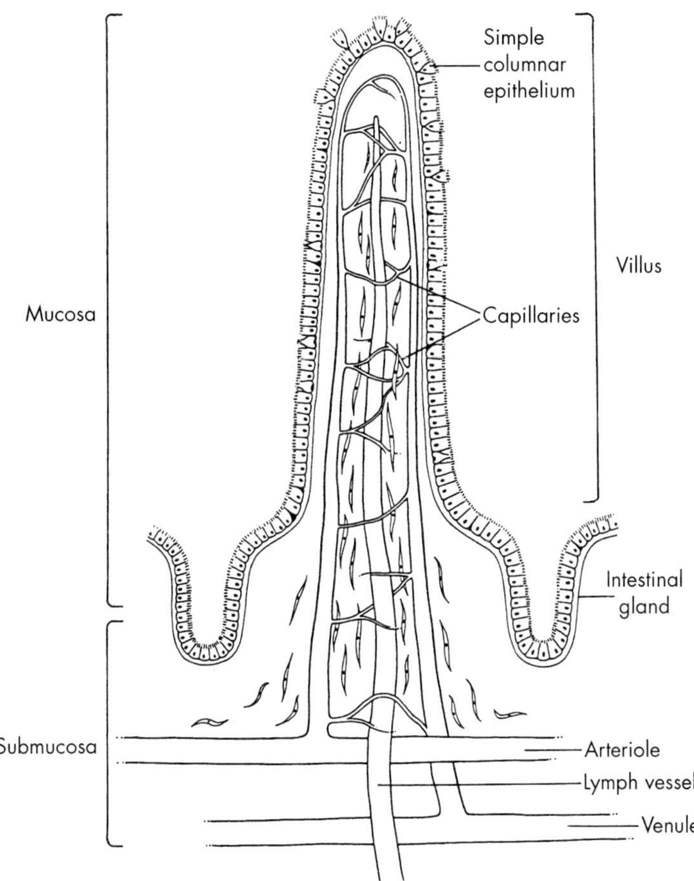

Figure 1.7 Cross-section of a villus.

down peptides to amino acids; lactase, maltase and sucrase break down disaccharides to (mainly) glucose; lipase breaks down the macrostructure of fat droplets to form simple fatty acids and glycerol; and long-chain fatty acids and glycerol, together with phospholipids and proteins, recombine to produce chylomicrons. Water-soluble vitamins, including vitamin B_{12}, iron and folic acid are also absorbed.

The intestinal liquid chyle enters the ascending colon through the ileocaecal valve. The colon acts as the final site of water and electrolyte reabsorption, causing the intestinal mass to become firmer as it passes towards the rectum. The presence of a bulky mass produces stimulation of the stretch receptors in the colon and rectum, inducing peristalsis and initiating the evacuation of the faeces.

The liver lies in the upper portion of the peritoneal cavity, immediately beneath the diaphragm. It is composed of lobules (Figure 1.8) formed of sheets of radiating cells orientated around a central branch of the hepatic vein. The hepatic arteries bring oxygenated blood from the general circulation, and the hepatic portal veins collect nutrients from along the lower gastrointestinal tract. Both supplies drain into sinusoids between the liver cells.

The liver has many diverse functions. It secretes bile into canaliculi between the sheets of liver cells, from where the bile drains into the bile ducts. Excess glucose is removed from the hepatic-portal system and stored as glycogen or fat. In hypoglycaemia, glycogen is reconverted into glucose and released into the circulation. The liver also stores vitamins A, D and B_{12} and

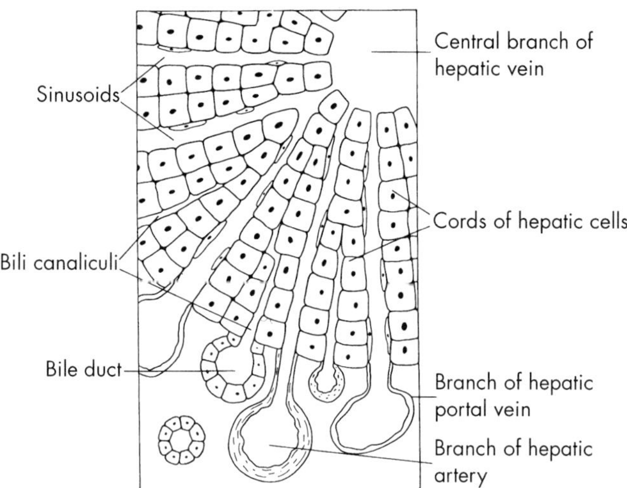

Figure 1.8 Schematic diagram of a portion of a liver lobule.

iron and deaminates amino acids. One fragment of the amino acid is converted into glucose and utilised as energy. The second fragment is converted into ammonia in the liver and excreted via the urea cycle. The synthesis of non-essential amino acids is also carried out by the liver through transamination reactions. It produces plasma proteins and blood coagulation factors. The liver also has an important protective role. Bacteria are removed by phagocytosis, drugs and chemicals are detoxified, and aged erythrocytes and leucocytes are destroyed. Homeostatic regulation is also achieved through the controlled inactivation of endocrine hormones.

2

Cardiovascular system disorders

2.1 General disorders

Cardiac arrest

Definition and aetiology
Cardiac arrest is the sudden cessation of cardiac function and often occurs in conjunction with respiratory failure. Cardiac contraction is absent or inadequate, resulting in the termination of an effective cardiac output. It is a common cause of death. It usually occurs as a result of ventricular fibrillation, heart block or acute circulatory failure.

Symptoms
It is characterised by absent pulse, heart sounds and blood pressure. Apnoea, dilated pupils and unconsciousness also occur.

Treatment
Immediate treatment is essential and initially consists of artificial respiration and external cardiac massage. Normal heart function may be restored by cardioversion. Drug treatment appropriate to the underlying cause may be necessary.

Circulatory failure, acute

Definition and aetiology

Acute circulatory failure, or lack of an adequate blood supply to the tissues and organs, results from arterial hypotension caused by a substantial uncompensated reduction in cardiac output. In transient form this gives rise to syncope, and in more prolonged form to shock.

Syncope

Definition and aetiology

Syncope (faint) is a transient reversible loss of consciousness caused by an acute reduction in blood supply to the brain (cerebral ischaemia), resulting from acute circulatory failure. Reduction in cardiac output may be the consequence of insufficient venous return to the heart caused by peripheral vasodilatation (e.g. in hot weather) or by venous pooling below the heart (e.g. after prolonged standing). It may also be caused by instability of vasomotor control (e.g. orthostatic hypotension caused by ganglion-blocking agents or bilateral sympathectomy). Cardiogenic syncope, caused by transient failure of the diseased heart to provide sufficient cardiac output (e.g. in myocardial infarction), may be followed by shock. Psychogenic factors may also precipitate syncope through vagal overactivity.

Symptoms

Syncope is usually preceded by feelings of lightheadedness, nausea, pallor, sweating and tachypnoea. The hypotensive episode may be accompanied by bradycardia, particularly if due to vagal overactivity.

Treatment

Unconsciousness is brief and recovery may be hastened by laying the patient flat and raising the legs. Further treatment is usually unnecessary.

Shock

Definition and aetiology

Shock is caused by derangement of circulatory control or loss of circulating fluid, resulting in severe reduction in cardiac output. Intense sympathetic vasoconstriction initially maintains the arterial pressure and blood flow to the brain and other vital organs, although at inadequate levels.

Hypovolaemic shock may be caused by massive loss of body fluids arising from haemorrhage, fractures, extensive muscle trauma, burns, vomiting or diarrhoea. It may also be caused by release into the circulation of endotoxins (septic shock) or tissue breakdown products which cause vasodilatation and increased capillary permeability (e.g. in peritonitis, septicaemia and pancreatitis).

Cardiogenic shock results from a marked decrease in cardiac output and may be caused by heart disease (e.g. myocardial infarction and serious arrhythmia) or pulmonary embolism (*see also* Cardiac arrest).

Anaphylactic shock occurs as a result of a specific antigen–antibody reaction, which results in the release of histamine and other chemical mediators. In addition to cardiovascular symptoms, respiratory and skin reactions are common.

Symptoms

All vital activities are depressed, causing weakness, subnormal temperature, sweating and apathy. Consciousness is generally maintained, although syncope (*see above*) may occur if the patient stands up. The skin is pale, cold and cyanotic and the pulse is weak and rapid. There is hypotension, tachypnoea, hypoxia and a reduction in renal blood flow which results in decreased urinary output and fluid and electrolyte retention. Metabolic disturbances result in a metabolic acidosis.

Treatment

The incidence and severity of shock may be minimised by gentle handling of injuries, protection from cold and prevention of further losses of blood and electrolytes. Treatment should be instituted as soon as possible and consists of the administration of opioid analgesics (BNF 4.7.2), fluid and electrolytes (BNF 9.2), correction of blood loss, oxygen therapy (BNF 3.6) and the correction of metabolic acidosis (BNF 9.2.2). In addition, anti-arrhythmic drugs (BNF 2.3) or sympathomimetics with inotropic activity (BNF 2.7.1) may be of value in cardiogenic shock and adrenaline, followed by corticosteroids (BNF 6.3.2), may be given in anaphylactic shock.

Cor pulmonale

Definition and aetiology

Cor pulmonale is pulmonary hypertension complicated by right ventricular hypertrophy and right heart failure, developing as a result of lung diseases (e.g. asthma, chronic bronchitis and emphysema, pulmonary fibrosis or pulmonary embolism).

Symptoms

All symptoms of cor pulmonale are associated with pulmonary hypertension, right ventricular hypertrophy and right heart failure. They include arrhythmias, hepatomegaly, increased venous pressure, oedema and hypercapnia. In severe disease, the nephrotic syndrome may develop.

Treatment

Treatment involves identification and treatment of the underlying lung disorder. Oxygen therapy (BNF 3.6) and respiratory stimulants (BNF 3.5) may be necessary in some patients. Diuretics with potassium salts (BNF 2.2) are used to control heart failure and venesection may be indicated.

Heart failure

Definition and aetiology

Heart failure is an acute or chronic condition in which the heart fails to maintain an adequate blood supply to the tissues despite normal ventricular filling. It may occur in the left heart (left ventricular failure), the right heart (right ventricular failure), or both sides (congestive heart failure). Since coronary arteriosclerosis, hypertension and rheumatic heart disease (arising from rheumatic fever) affect mainly the left heart, left ventricular failure is more common than right. Left ventricular failure, however, is the most common cause of right heart failure.

Causes of heart failure include myocardial disorders and valvular heart disease, anaemia, hyperthyroidism, hypertension and arrhythmias. Right heart failure may be secondary to lung disease (e.g. pulmonary embolism and chronic bronchitis and emphysema) and under such circumstances it is termed cor pulmonale (*see above*).

Symptoms

Failure of one side of the heart leads to congestion and oedema in the tissues from which the venous supply is drained. Thus left heart failure produces pulmonary oedema, pulmonary hypertension and breathlessness (dyspnoea, orthopnoea and paroxysmal nocturnal dyspnoea) caused by pulmonary congestion. Other symptoms are cyanosis, fatigue, haemoptysis and tachycardia. Right heart failure produces peripheral oedema (e.g. of ankles), cyanosis, fatigue, hepatic enlargement and tenderness and sometimes ascites. In addition, the inadequate cardiac output leads to a disproportionate reduction in renal blood-flow, resulting in sodium and water retention. In congestive heart failure the symptoms are a combination of those described above and result in marked physical incapacity, breathlessness and peripheral oedema.

Treatment

Treatment should be directed at the underlying cause and patients should be advised to rest in order to reduce cardiac work. Positive inotropic drugs (BNF 2.1), diuretics with potassium supplements (BNF 2.2), angiotensin-converting enzyme inhibitors (BNF 2.5.5) or vasodilators (BNF 2.6) are used in the treatment of heart failure. Heart transplantation is effective, producing a one- and three-year survival rate of 82% and 75% respectively.

Hypertension

Definition and aetiology

Hypertension is abnormally high arterial blood pressure. The blood pressure of healthy individuals may extend over a wide range of values that tend to increase with age. It can vary on different occasions on which it is measured. The pressure at which blood pressure is described as abnormal is at present controversial. In the young or middle-aged, a resting systolic pressure in excess of 150 mmHg or a diastolic pressure greater than 100 mmHg would warrant treatment by most authorities, although these pressures apparently have no ill-effects in some subjects.

Essential (primary) hypertension is idiopathic and is the most common form of the disease. Age, arteriosclerosis, diet, family history and obesity may be factors in its development.

Secondary hypertension occurs as a result of other underlying disorders. Possible causes include renal disease (e.g. renal artery stenosis and pyelonephritis), endocrine disorders (e.g. Cushing's syndrome, primary aldosteronism and phaeochromocytoma) and drug administration (e.g. oral contraceptives and corticosteroids). Other rarer causes are coarctation of the aorta and eclampsia.

Malignant (accelerated) hypertension is usually characterised by a diastolic pressure greater than 140 mmHg. It is most common in patients over 40 years of age and in those with chronic renal disorders.

Essential hypertension occurs in about one in three males who are between 18 and 74 years of age. By comparison, secondary hypertension caused by renal disease occurs in less than 5% of the population.

Symptoms

Hypertension is usually asymptomatic, although blurred vision, dizziness, dyspnoea and nocturia may occur. Although headaches are commonly thought to be associated with hypertension, they are usually only a symptom of severe hypertension. The main complications of hypertension, which may be fatal, are heart failure, myocardial infarction, renal failure, ruptured aneurysm and stroke. These complications are often the presenting features of hypertension.

Treatment

Thresholds and targets for treatment of hypertension are printed and regularly updated in the *British National Formulary*. An initial approach to treatment of hypertension is the identification and treatment of any underlying cause. If no cause can be found, patients should be encouraged to adjust their lifestyle, lose excess weight, stop smoking and reduce alcohol consumption. Low-salt diets and stress reduction may also be beneficial.

Drug treatment may be necessary. This includes the use of thiazide and related diuretics (BNF 2.2.1), beta-adrenoceptor blocking drugs (BNF 2.4), angiotensin-converting enzyme (ACE) inhibitors (BNF 2.5.5), calcium-channel blockers (BNF 2.6.2), alpha-blockers (BNF 2.5.4) and angiotensin-II receptor antagonists (BNF 2.5.5.2). Periodic examination of heart size and of the retina and testing urine for proteins, are desirable in such subjects to assess deterioration of cardiovascular and renal function. Drug treatment should also take into account the age of the patient and the presence of diabetes, pregnancy or renal disease. Malignant hypertension is a medical emergency and requires immediate hospitalisation.

Orthostatic hypotension

Definition and aetiology

Orthostatic (postural) hypotension is a fall in blood pressure of between 10 and 20 mmHg which occurs upon rising abruptly from the supine to the erect position. It may also occur when standing motionless in a fixed position. It is often caused by drug therapy (e.g. benzodiazepines, levodopa, phenothiazines, thiazides and tricyclic and related antidepressants). It may also occur after prolonged bed rest and as a result of autonomic nervous system disorders (e.g. Shy–Drager syndrome) and is common in the elderly.

Symptoms

Orthostatic hypotension is often asymptomatic. It may, however, result in blurred vision, dizziness and syncope caused by impairment of the cerebral circulation.

Treatment

Treatment consists of withdrawal or dosage reduction of the offending drug. Patients should be advised to stand up slowly and to wear graduated compression hosiery to prevent pooling of blood in the feet and lower limbs. Drug therapies that have been tried include ephedrine, propranolol and midodrine.

Pericarditis

Definition and aetiology

Pericarditis is inflammation of the membranous sac (the pericardium) surrounding the heart. It may be caused by viral, bacterial (including tuberculous) or fungal infection; it can also follow myocardial infarction or heart surgery. Other causes include rheumatic fever, connective tissue disorders, hypothyroidism and malignant disease. It may also arise as a result of irradiation, trauma or the administration of drugs (e.g. hydralazine and procainamide).

Symptoms

Pericarditis is characterised by arrhythmias and a sharp continuous chest pain that is relieved by sitting up. Symptoms may be preceded by a general influenza-like malaise. Breathing may also be painful, resulting in dyspnoea. Pericarditis may result in accumulation of fluid within the pericardium (pericardial effusion), causing cardiac tamponade in which the pressure of accumulated fluid interferes with ventricular filling. Ventricular filling may also be restricted by thickening of the pericardium.

Treatment

Pericarditis may be self-limiting and require only symptomatic treatment. The underlying cause should, however, be treated. Indometacin (BNF 10.1.1) and analgesics may be given to reduce pain and inflammation; corticosteroids (BNF 6.3.2) may be indicated. Antimicrobial drugs (BNF 5.1) may be required. Emergency treatment of cardiac tamponade by pericardial aspiration may be necessary. Surgery may be required in cases of pericardial constriction caused by thickening of the pericardium.

Pulmonary hypertension

Definition and aetiology

Pulmonary hypertension is a very rare condition in which abnormally high blood pressure occurs in the pulmonary circulation. The systolic pressure rises above 30 mmHg or the diastolic pressure rises above 15 mmHg. Lung disease (e.g. chronic bronchitis and emphysema or pulmonary embolism) produces an increase in pulmonary vascular resistance due to chronic hypoxia. The ensuing pulmonary hypertension is followed by right ventricular hypertrophy and subsequent right heart failure (cor pulmonale).

Other causes of pulmonary hypertension include congenital heart disease and mitral stenosis. Increased pulmonary blood pressure of unknown cause is termed primary pulmonary hypertension.

The condition affects five times more women than men. The average age on diagnosis is 35 years of age.

Symptoms

Severe pulmonary hypertension is characterised by fatigue and dyspnoea on effort together with chest pain, haemoptysis, peripheral cyanosis and syncope.

Treatment

Treatment of pulmonary hypertension is directed toward the underlying heart or lung disease. The use of vasodilators (BNF 2.5.1) has been proposed. The course is relentlessly downhill for most patients and heart–lung transplantation offers the only hope of prolonged survival.

Pulmonary oedema

Definition and aetiology

Pulmonary oedema is the abnormal accumulation of fluid in pulmonary tissue and the alveoli. It is often due to left ventricular failure, but may also occur as a result of mitral stenosis, pneumonia or the accidental inhalation of gastric contents.

Symptoms

Pulmonary oedema is characterised by acute worsening dyspnoea. Anxiety and a sensation of suffocation are common symptoms. A cough and the production of pink frothy sputum may also occur. Cyanosis may develop and the condition can be fatal.

Treatment

Early treatment is essential and comprises sitting the patient up and administering oxygen (BNF

3.6), diuretics (BNF 2.2), bronchodilators (BNF 3.1), vasodilators (BNF 2.5.1) and an opioid analgesic (BNF 4.7.2). The underlying disorder must be identified and treated.

Valvular heart disease

Definition

Valvular heart disease is characterised by inadequate functioning of the mitral, aortic and tricuspid valves of the heart. Pulmonary valve disease also occurs but is uncommon.

Mitral stenosis

Definition and aetiology

Mitral stenosis is a narrowing of the orifice of the left atrioventricular (mitral) valve. It is usually caused by rheumatic heart disease (arising from rheumatic fever); it may also develop as a result of congenital abnormalities, infective endocarditis and systemic lupus erythematosus. Disease of rheumatic origin is much more common in women.

Symptoms

Mitral stenosis usually develops insidiously over several years, but may occur abruptly. The most common symptoms are reduced exercise tolerance, followed later in the disease by paroxysmal nocturnal dyspnoea caused by pulmonary oedema. Palpitations may arise through atrial fibrillation. Haemoptysis may be a consequence of bronchial vein rupture, left heart failure and pulmonary embolism. Angina may occasionally occur. Severe cases may be complicated by pulmonary hypertension, which leads to right heart failure.

Treatment

Treatment of atrial fibrillation with anti-arrhythmic drugs (BNF 2.3), fluid retention with diuretics (BNF 2.2), chest infections with antibacterial drugs (BNF 5.1) and anticoagulants (BNF 2.8) for atrial fibrillation and pulmonary embolism should be undertaken. Surgical treatment may be necessary and mitral valve dilatation (valvotomy) or replacement may be performed. Antibacterial prophylaxis (BNF 5.1) is necessary for patients requiring minor surgery (e.g. dental surgery).

Mitral regurgitation

Definition and aetiology

Mitral regurgitation is the backflow of blood from the left ventricle to left atrium, caused by a defective mitral valve. It may be due to rheumatic heart disease. Other causes include a floppy mitral valve, infective endocarditis, ischaemic heart disease, cardiomyopathy and valve calcification. 50% of cases are associated with mitral stenosis (*see above*).

Symptoms

Symptoms are variable, developing gradually or suddenly, and include fatigue, dyspnoea, pulmonary oedema and embolism, congestive heart failure, heart murmurs and conduction defects.

Treatment

Mild mitral regurgitation often requires no treatment, apart from antibacterial prophylaxis (BNF 5.1, table 2) as appropriate, although treatment of the underlying disease may be necessary. In severe disease, surgical repair or replacement of the mitral valve may be indicated.

Aortic stenosis

Definition and aetiology

Aortic stenosis is characterised by a narrowing of the aortic orifice of the heart, reducing the outflow of blood from the left ventricle. There may be a pressure difference of more than 10 mmHg across the obstruction. It may be caused by congenital abnormalities (e.g. an abnormal bicuspid valve) or may result from rheumatic heart disease, valve calcification or infective endocarditis.

Symptoms

Symptoms tend to occur late in the course of the disease and include anginal pain, dyspnoea and syncope on exercise. Sudden death may occur in about half of all cases.

Treatment
Most asymptomatic patients require little treatment, apart from appropriate antibacterial prophylaxis (BNF 5.1, table 2). The symptomatic patient may, however, benefit from bed rest, diuretics (BNF 2.2) and surgical aortic valve replacement. Angina should be treated with beta-adrenoceptor blocking drugs (BNF 2.4) as vasodilators may aggravate symptoms.

Aortic regurgitation

Definition and aetiology
Aortic regurgitation (aortic incompetence or insufficiency) is the backflow of blood from the aorta into the left ventricle caused by a defective aortic valve. It may develop as a result of rheumatic heart disease, rheumatoid arthritis, ankylosing spondylitis, infective endocarditis, trauma, dissecting aneurysm, syphilis, ulcerative colitis or congenital conditions (e.g. Marfan's syndrome or abnormal bicuspid valves).

Symptoms
Aortic regurgitation may be asymptomatic for many years. Dyspnoea, however, is a common symptom, particularly on exercising, and chest pain and heart murmurs may also occur. Palpitations may also be experienced.

Treatment
Antibacterial prophylaxis (BNF 5.1, table 2) against endocarditis is appropriate. Surgical valve replacement may be necessary in severe cases.

Tricuspid stenosis

Definition and aetiology
Tricuspid stenosis is a narrowing of the tricuspid orifice of the heart, which is almost always caused by rheumatic heart disease. As a consequence, flow of blood from the right atrium to the right ventricle is restricted.

Symptoms
Symptoms are similar to those of mitral and aortic valve disease (*see above*), but ascites and peripheral oedema may be prominent in severe stenosis.

Treatment
Treatment includes the administration of diuretics (BNF 2.2). Although valve replacement should be avoided, dilatation (valvotomy) or repair may be necessary in very severe cases.

Tricuspid regurgitation

Definition and aetiology
Tricuspid regurgitation is the backflow of blood from the right ventricle to the right atrium caused by a defective tricuspid valve. It may arise as a result of rheumatic heart disease, infective endocarditis, carcinoid syndrome, pulmonary hypertension or congenital abnormalities.

Symptoms
Symptoms include raised venous blood pressure, oedema, ascites and hepatomegaly with nausea and epigastric pain. Mild jaundice may occur. One characteristic symptom is a pulsing sensation in the neck.

Treatment
Treatment comprises bed rest and the administration of diuretics (BNF 2.2) and vasodilators (BNF 2.5.1). Surgical valve replacement may be beneficial.

2.2 Myocardial disease

Cardiomyopathy

Definition and aetiology
A cardiomyopathy is a disorder of the myocardium. Most cases are of unknown aetiology and cardiomyopathy is a frequent cause of sudden death.

Dilated (congestive) cardiomyopathy, the most common of the cardiomyopathies, is the dilatation of left or right ventricles, or both. It is thought to be due to inflammation of the myocardium, alcohol abuse or hypertension. Hypertrophic cardiomyopathy, which may be familial, consists of hypertrophy of the left, and occasionally right, ventricle. Restrictive cardiomyopathy, the least common of the cardiomyopathies, is due to fibrosis or scarring of the endomyocardium, which becomes rigid.

Symptoms

Dyspnoea on exercise and fatigue are common to each cardiomyopathy. Oedema and embolism may occur in dilated and restrictive cardiomyopathies, whereas angina pectoris and syncope are characteristic of hypertrophic cardiomyopathy. Tachycardia may develop in dilated and hypertrophic forms of the disease, although both may be asymptomatic.

Treatment

The treatment of cardiomyopathies varies according to symptoms and may include the use of anticoagulants (BNF 2.8), diuretics (BNF 2.2), vasodilators (BNF 2.5.1), beta-adrenoceptor blocking drugs (BNF 2.4) and anti-arrhythmic drugs (BNF 2.3). Bed rest, weight loss and avoidance of alcohol are useful measures in the management of dilated cardiomyopathy. Surgery may be carried out in all forms of cardiomyopathy. Heart transplantation may be necessary in severe cases of dilated and restrictive cardiomyopathy. The prognosis for dilated cardiomyopathy and restrictive cardiomyopathy is poor, with 70% mortality within five years. There is a 4% annual mortality rate for hypertrophic cardiomyopathy.

Myocarditis

Definition and aetiology

Myocarditis is inflammation of the myocardium. It is usually caused by viral, bacterial, fungal or parasitic infections, or may be secondary to an underlying systemic disease process (e.g. connective tissue disorders). It may also occur as a side-effect of drug administration (e.g. cytotoxic drugs and chloroquine) and lead poisoning.

Symptoms

Myocarditis may be asymptomatic, or may present with the symptoms of myocardial infarction or angina pectoris. Symptoms include arrhythmias, tachycardia, chest pain, dyspnoea, fatigue, fever, oedema and heart failure. Sudden death may occur.

Treatment

Treatment is directed towards the underlying cause. Heart failure and arrhythmias may also require treatment.

2.3 Ischaemic heart disease

Angina pectoris

Definition and aetiology

Stable angina pectoris arises through cardiac muscle ischaemia, resulting from coronary artery insufficiency and hypertension or, rarely, anaemia and valvular heart disease. Attacks may be precipitated by exertion or emotional disturbances, are relieved by rest, and are most likely in patients whose coronary arteries are partially occluded by arteriosclerotic lesions. Nocturnal or decubitus angina can be considered an intermediate stage between stable and unstable angina. In unstable angina pectoris, symptoms occur more frequently, at rest, and are more severe. It can be caused by coronary vasospasm.

Symptoms

Angina pectoris is characterised by paroxysmal pain (or tightness) in the chest which may extend to the shoulder, arms, throat, back and jaw. Other symptoms are dyspnoea, dizziness, nausea and sweating.

Treatment

Patients should regulate the amount of exercise taken to minimise the occurrence of attacks. Other lifestyle changes should be encouraged: emotional disturbances, temperature extremes and overwork should be avoided; loss of excess weight and abstention from smoking are also necessary. Aspirin (BNF 2.6 and 2.9) is given to patients with both stable and unstable angina. Beta-adrenoceptor blocking drugs (BNF 2.4), nitrates (BNF 2.6.1) or calcium-channel blockers (BNF 2.6.2) may be employed to prevent or relieve attacks. Coronary bypass surgery or angioplasty may be required for failure of medical management and in younger patients with extensive coronary artery disease.

Myocardial infarction

Definition and aetiology

Myocardial infarction is occlusion of a coronary vessel which leads to ischaemia and subsequently destruction (necrosis) of heart muscle. The occlusion is usually caused by coronary artery thrombosis, resulting from coronary atherosclerosis. Occlusion may also be due to coronary artery spasm or stenosis. An increased risk of myocardial infarction has been associated with hypertension, hypercholesterolaemia, smoking, emotional disturbances and lack of exercise.

Coronary heart disease (CHD) is a major cause of death and morbidity, with one in three men and one in four women across all ages dying from CHD. It is the cause of premature death in 1 in 15 men under 65 years of age. Diet, alcohol intake levels, serum cholesterol levels and genetic factors are all important in determining the risk of myocardial infarction. Environmental factors also play a part. People moving from a region with a relatively low incidence of the disease become similarly at risk to others who have lived their whole lives in the higher incidence areas.

There may also be a circadian rhythm to the occurrence of myocardial infarction during the day. Higher rates of occurrence are seen early in the morning (after waking), with another peak around 1700 hours.

Symptoms

If the affected area is localised, the unaffected remainder of the myocardium continues to function, although often with a decreased cardiac ouput which can cause hypotension. This may be accompanied by severe prolonged chest pain, which resembles the pain of angina pectoris. The pain is often described as a tightness, bursting or crushing sensation. However, unlike the pain of stable angina, that associated with myocardial infarction cannot be relieved by rest or the administration of vasodilators. Other symptoms include anxiety, fatigue, dyspnoea, sweating, and nausea and vomiting. Acute myocardial infarction may lead to arrhythmias, heart block and cardiogenic shock.

Treatment

Treatment, which is commonly undertaken in a coronary-care unit, consists initially of complete bed rest. The value of early (within 12 hours, but ideally within one hour of the myocardial infarction) administration of fibrinolytic drugs (BNF 2.10) and aspirin (BNF 2.9) has been demonstrated. A wide range of other drugs may be administered, which include oxygen (BNF 3.6), opioid analgesics (BNF 4.7.2), anti-emetics (BNF 4.6), anxiolytics (BNF 4.1.2), parenteral anticoagulants (BNF 2.8.1), beta-adrenoceptor blocking drugs (BNF 2.4), nitrates (BNF 2.6.1), ACE inhibitors (BNF 2.5.5) and calcium-channel blockers (BNF 2.6.2). For the treatment of complications, *see* Arrhythmias, Heart failure *and* Shock.

Patients may be maintained on aspirin, nitrates, beta-adrenoceptor blocking drugs, oral anticoagulants (BNF 2.8.2), ACE inhibitors, statins (BNF 2.12) or antiplatelet drugs (BNF 2.9). The importance of lifestyle changes should be emphasised: stopping smoking, increased exercise and returning to a full and active life as rapidly as possible.

Self-help organisations

Association for Children with Heart Disorders
British Heart Foundation
British Hypertension Society
Cardiomyopathy Association
Chest Heart and Stroke Association
Coronary Prevention Group
Family Heart Association
National Heart Forum
Northern Ireland Chest, Heart and Stroke Association

2.4 Arrhythmias

Bradycardia

Definition and aetiology

Bradycardia is an unusually slow heart-rate (less than 60 beats per minute), resulting from increased vagal or diminished sympathetic tone. It may occur normally during sleep and in healthy young adults and athletes. Bradycardia also occurs after myocardial infarction and certain infections and in raised intracranial pressure, hypothyroidism and jaundice. Cardiac glycosides, beta-adrenoceptor blocking drugs, opioid analgesics and some centrally acting antihypertensive drugs also slow the heart-rate, leading to bradycardia.

Treatment

Although bradycardia does not normally require treatment, the administration of atropine (BNF 2.3.2) or surgical placement of a pacemaker may be necessary.

Ectopic beats

Definition and aetiology

Ectopic beats (extrasystoles) are cardiac contractions which arise earlier than expected in the cardiac cycle. They are caused by impulse formation at an abnormal focus of electrical activity in the atria or ventricles. Most ectopic beats are followed by a diastolic pause, as the arrhythmia renders the cardiac muscle refractory to the effects of the next normal impulse. This results in coupling of heart beats, followed by a long pause. Ectopic beats may be associated with rheumatic heart disease (arising as a consequence of rheumatic fever), ischaemic heart disease and acute myocardial infarction. They may occasionally occur in the absence of cardiac disease. Large quantities of alcohol, caffeine or tobacco and overdosage with cardiac glycosides may also cause ectopic beats.

Symptoms

Ectopic beats may be asymptomatic, but palpitations may occur.

Treatment

If palpitations occur in the absence of heart disease, patients should be advised to avoid fatigue, emotional disturbances and excessive consumption of alcohol, caffeine or tobacco. Anti-arrhythmic drugs (BNF 2.3) may be needed to prevent the development of more serious arrhythmias.

Fibrillations

Definition

A fibrillation is a small rapid series of uncoordinated contractions of muscle which, in cardiac tissue, produces irregular and ineffective emptying of the heart chambers. A flutter is a less disturbed, more regular, form of a fibrillation.

Atrial fibrillation

Definition and aetiology

Atrial fibrillation is a common and important form of tachycardia. Integrated atrial contractions disappear and are replaced by rapid fibrillary twitching of the atria. This leads to random rapid ventricular contractions, and the pulse is irregular in rhythm and force. Atrial fibrillation is usually associated with rheumatic heart disease (arising as a consequence of rheumatic fever), mitral stenosis, ischaemic heart disease, hyperthyroidism and hypertension. Less commonly, lung cancer, other malignant diseases, congenital heart disease, infective endocarditis and pericarditis may be involved.

In the presence of other serious heart disease, the onset of atrial fibrillation may lead to congestive heart failure. Systemic embolism is a common complication when atrial fibrillation is caused by valvular heart disease. The onset of atrial fibrillation may be precipitated by alcohol and by mental or physical stress.

The incidence of atrial fibrillation increases with age, and may have an incidence of as high as 1 in 20 in the very elderly.

Symptoms

Some patients, especially in the chronic phase of the condition, may be unaware of the arrhythmia. Paradoxically, palpitations may be a significant problem in the early stages of the disease. Attacks of atrial fibrillation may be accompanied by dizziness, syncope and chest pain.

Treatment

Any underlying cause should be treated. When there is tachycardia (*see below*) or any evidence of congestive heart failure, positive inotropic drugs (BNF 2.1) are used to reduce the rapid ventricular rate. If there is no evidence of serious organic disease, atrial fibrillation may be converted to normal (sinus) rhythm by cardioversion (direct-current shock). Anti-arrhythmic drugs (BNF 2.3) may be used to maintain normal rhythm and oral anticoagulants (BNF 2.8.2) to prevent embolism.

Atrial flutter

Definition and aetiology

Atrial flutter is similar to atrial fibrillation. There is coordinated, but rapid, atrial muscle action, slower than in atrial fibrillation, but more rapid than in paroxysmal atrial tachycardia (*see below*). Atrial flutter is almost always associated with organic heart disease, and rapidly progresses to the more commonly encountered atrial fibrillation.

Symptoms

Symptoms are similar to those experienced in atrial fibrillation.

Treatment

The treatment of atrial flutter is the same as for atrial fibrillation.

Ventricular fibrillation

Definition and aetiology

Ventricular fibrillation is a serious condition in which the ventricles fail to contract effectively and cardiac output falls, so that perfusion of vital organs (e.g. the brain) ceases. It often occurs at the end-stage of a number of life-threatening cardiac conditions. Death rapidly follows if ventricular fibrillation is not reversed. The causes are the same as those of ventricular tachycardia (*see below*).

Treatment

Treatment comprises cardioversion or the administration of anti-arrhythmic drugs (BNF 2.3).

Heart block

Definition and aetiology

In heart block (atrioventricular block), there is a defective conduction of the impulse which arises in the sino-atrial (SA) node in the right atrium and passes to the ventricles. This may be due to a defect in the atrioventricular (AV) node or in the bundle of His. In partial heart block, the atrial impulse may be delayed in its conduction from the atria to the ventricles (first degree block). Intermittent failure of atrioventricular conduction may cause beats to be missed (second degree block).

In complete heart block, there may be atrioventricular dissociation, causing the ventricles to beat at their intrinsic rate of about 30–40 beats per minute (third degree block). This rate is completely dissociated from and unaffected by external stimuli. However, because of the slow rate, there is increased ventricular filling which may maintain a normal cardiac output. Heart block is usually due to idiopathic fibrosis or congenital lesions of the conducting system, myocardial infarction or cardiac glycoside toxicity.

Symptoms

First degree block is asymptomatic. Second degree block may be asymptomatic, although it may suddenly become a complete block. In complete heart block, sudden attacks of syncope commonly occur (Stokes–Adams syndrome). The loss of consciousness is abrupt, with few or no warning signs, and is associated with extreme bradycardia. Consciousness returns when the ventricular rate increases.

Treatment

Sympathomimetics with inotropic activity (BNF 2.7.1) may be given to increase the heart-rate and prevent the Stokes–Adams syndrome, although intolerable palpitations or ventricular ectopic beats may prevent their continued use. In established heart block, artificial pacemaking of the heart is indicated.

Tachycardias

Definition and aetiology

In tachycardia, the heart-rate is abnormally rapid (more than 100 beats per minute), usually caused by increased sympathetic or decreased vagal tone. It often occurs in congestive heart failure and as a result of anaemia, anxiety, exercise, haemorrhage, hyperthyroidism, hypotension or infections. It may also be a consequence of excessive consumption of caffeine or tobacco, or be caused by anticholinergic drugs.

Paroxysmal atrial tachycardia

Definition and aetiology
Paroxysmal atrial (supraventricular) tachycardia is characterised by sudden onset and termination of periods of tachycardia. It may be associated with various forms of heart disease.

Treatment
Attacks of paroxysmal atrial tachycardia may be terminated by massage of the carotid sinus. Beta-adrenoceptor blocking drugs (BNF 2.4), anti-arrhythmic drugs (BNF 2.3) or positive inotropic drugs (BNF 2.1) may also be used.

Ventricular tachycardia

Definition and aetiology
In ventricular tachycardia, the rapid beating of the ventricles (120–250 beats per minute) is caused by an abnormal focus of excitation within the ventricles themselves. It is usually caused by ischaemic heart disease, myocardial infarction, mitral valve disease, cardiomyopathy or by overdosage with cardiac glycosides or sympathomimetics. Acute heart failure, ventricular fibrillation and death may follow if the condition is not treated.

Treatment
Treatment comprises cardioversion or administration of anti-arrhythmic drugs (BNF 2.3).

2.5 Vascular disease

Acrocyanosis

Definition and aetiology
Acrocyanosis is characterised by a persistent symmetrical blue discoloration (cyanosis) of the hands and, less commonly, feet. It is thought to arise from excessive vasoconstriction of the arterioles and occurs almost exclusively in women.

Symptoms
The affected extremities are blue, cold, sweat profusely and may become swollen, although the condition is painless. The condition is more severe in cold weather.

Treatment
Treatment is usually unnecessary, but cold conditions should be avoided.

Aneurysm

Definition and aetiology
An aneurysm (Figure 2.1) is a localised dilatation of a blood vessel that affects mainly the aorta or a peripheral artery. Saccular aneurysms usually

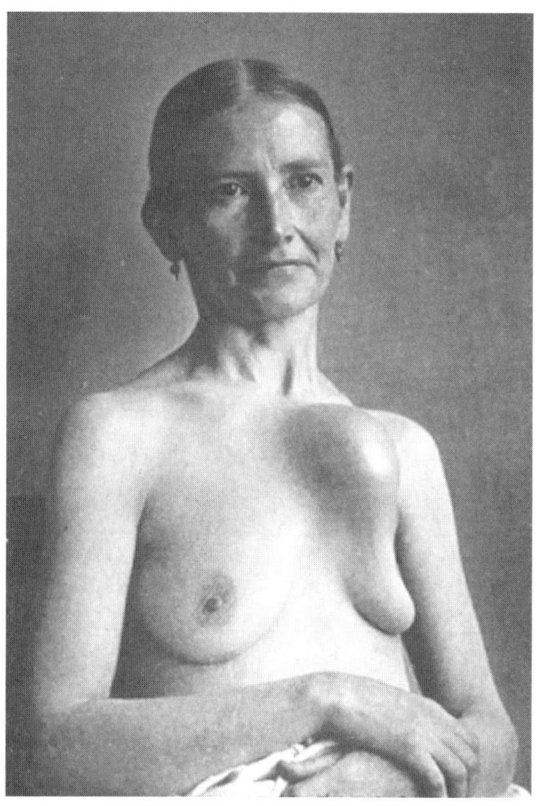

Figure 2.1 Aortic aneurysm. (Reproduced with permission of Stanley B Burns MD & The Burns Archive N.Y./Science Photo Library.)

occur at arterial junctions (e.g. cerebral aneurysm). Longitudinal aneurysms occur along the complete length of a vessel (e.g. aortic aneurysm) due to replacement of the vessel wall with fibrous tissue. The penetration of blood into the vessel wall, causing its layers to separate, is referred to as a dissecting aneurysm. Aneurysms are commonly caused by atherosclerosis (*see below*), but may also arise due to congenital abnormalities, injury or inflammation.

Aortic aneurysm

Definition and aetiology
Abdominal aortic aneurysms are three times more common than those occurring in the thoracic cavity (thoracic aortic aneurysms). Both types can be caused by hypertension, cigarette smoking and atherosclerosis; injury and bacterial or fungal infection are less common causes.

Symptoms
Abdominal aortic aneurysm is characterised by severe abdominal tenderness and pain which may radiate to the back. Equally, however, it may arise asymptomatically and be detected only on rupture, which causes acute circulatory failure, shock and rapid death.

Thoracic aortic aneurysm is often asymptomatic, but chest pain that radiates to the back may occur. Pressure on adjacent organs may produce dysphagia and cough. Rupture may result in sudden death.

Dissecting aneurysm of the thoracic aorta is usually associated with atherosclerosis and hypertension. It produces chest and back pain, which may radiate to the neck or arms and can be difficult to differentiate from the pain of myocardial infarction.

Treatment
Treatment is by surgery. Antihypertensive therapy (BNF 2.5) may be useful in dissecting aneurysms.

Cerebral aneurysm

Definition and aetiology
Cerebral (berry) aneurysms occur in intracranial arteries. They may be caused by congenital abnormalities or may develop as a result of atherosclerosis or hypertension.

Subarachnoid haemorrhage is bleeding into the subarachnoid space (i.e. between the arachnoid membrane and the pia mater), commonly caused by a ruptured cerebral aneurysm. Subarachnoid haemorrhage may also be a consequence of congenital vascular abnormalities, cerebral haemorrhage, head injury or a blood-clotting disorder.

Symptoms
Cerebral aneurysms are often multiple and may be asymptomatic. They can rupture, resulting in subarachnoid haemorrhage. In subarachnoid haemorrhage, the onset of symptoms is usually very sudden and is characterised by severe headache, which may spread into the neck and back by the passage of blood down the spinal cord. Vomiting is common, and confusion, drowsiness, hemiplegia, neck stiffness and, occasionally, convulsions may occur. Patients may subsequently become irritable, drowsy and confused. Consciousness is often impaired and coma may develop. Prolonged coma usually results in death.

Treatment
Treatment consists of hospitalisation and the administration of beta-adrenoceptor blocking drugs (BNF 2.4) or antihypertensive therapy (BNF 2.5). Antifibrinolytic drugs (BNF 2.10) have also been used. Surgery may be indicated, but is hazardous.

Arteriosclerosis

Definition and aetiology
Arteriosclerosis is the term applied to a group of blood vessel diseases in which loss of elasticity and increased thickening occur, caused by the replacement of muscle and elastic tissue by fibrous tissue.

The most common form of arteriosclerosis is atherosclerosis, although arteriolosclerosis (affecting the arterioles) may also occur, usually as a consequence of hypertension.

Arteriosclerosis is the leading cause of morbidity and mortality in most Western nations. The death rate from coronary artery disease in men between 25 and 34 years of age is 1 in 10 000;

between 55 and 64 years of age, this increases to 1 in 100.

Atherosclerosis

Definition and aetiology

Atherosclerosis is characterised by the development of yellowish fatty plaques (atheromas), containing cholesterol and other lipids. The plaques subsequently haemorrhage, calcify and become ulcerated. They are formed within the endothelial lining of the walls of large and medium-sized arteries. They most commonly cause problems when they arise in coronary and cerebral arteries and peripheral arteries of the lower limbs. Their development is part of the natural ageing process, with the disease becoming progressive.

Non-reversible factors which predispose to the development of atherosclerosis are age, being a male, and a family history of the disease. Reversible risk factors include abnormal serum lipid levels, diabetes mellitus, hypertension, obesity, a lack of exercise, cigarette smoking and possibly emotional disturbances.

Symptoms

Atheromas cause narrowing and ultimately occlusion of the arteries, resulting in chronic ischaemia of the structures supplied by the arteries. Atheromas also provide a surface on which thrombosis can occur, producing acute ischaemia and infarction.

The symptoms of ischaemia depend upon the organ supplied by the artery and upon whether occlusion is acute or chronic, as the latter may be offset by the development of a collateral circulation. Atherosclerosis occurring in coronary vessels can give rise to angina pectoris, myocardial infarction and arrhythmias. Its occurrence in cerebral arteries can cause forgetfulness, confusion, personality changes or a stroke. In the arteries of the leg, intermittent claudication of calves and gangrene of toes may develop.

Atherosclerosis may cause hypertension through increased peripheral resistance of the narrowed arteries or because of stenosis of the renal artery. A long-standing atheroma may extend into the wall, with weakening of the artery. Aneurysms are formed when rupture of the lining of the artery wall allows blood to collect beneath the outer fibrous coat, which becomes grossly distended. They produce symptoms by pressing on the surrounding structures or by rupturing.

Treatment

Control of predisposing factors is the most important element of prevention and control of atherosclerosis. Plasma lipid concentrations may be lowered by dietary control and by the administration of lipid-lowering drugs (BNF 2.12). The patency of severely narrowed arteries may sometimes be restored by coronary artery bypass surgery and by transluminal angioplasty using balloon catheters.

Chilblains

Definition and aetiology

Chilblains are local inflammatory lesions, bluish-red in colour, which occur as an abnormal reaction to cold damp weather. They are less common in cold dry conditions.

Their aetiology is unclear, but a possible mechanism involves vasoconstriction of subcutaneous arteries and arterioles and vasodilatation of surface capillaries produced by low temperatures. Arteriolar constriction is less persistent than venule constriction. As a result, re-warming leads to a fluid accumulation in the tissues.

Symptoms

Chilblains appear on dorsal surfaces of fingers, hands or feet, or on the ears or nose. They may also appear on lower parts of the leg. They are often accompanied by tenderness and intense pruritus; more severe cases may blister, ulcerate and blacken due to tissue necrosis. Chronic ulcers may occur on repeated exposure to cold and these can cause atrophy and scarring of the tissue.

Treatment

Treatment is usually unnecessary, as chilblains may be prevented by wearing warm clothing in cold weather and by adequate indoor heating. Peripheral vasodilators (BNF 2.6.4.1) have been used, and topical preparations for circulatory disorders (BNF 13.14) are also available, but are of debatable value.

Raynaud's syndrome and phenomenon

Definition and aetiology
Raynaud's syndrome is vasospasm of arterioles or arteries in the distal areas of limbs and in fingers and toes, and may be triggered by cold or emotional disturbances. Up to 90% of all idiopathic disease occurs in young women. Secondary causes include occlusive arterial disease, connective tissue disorders, trauma or administration of drugs (e.g. beta-adrenoceptor blocking drugs). When the condition is secondary to underlying disease, it is termed Raynaud's phenomenon.

Symptoms
Symptoms include blanching, cyanosis and numbness, followed by reactive hyperaemia which causes redness and throbbing pain. Ischaemia may lead to atrophy of the skin or small painful ulcers on the digital tips. Attacks may last for minutes or hours.

Treatment
Patients should be advised to avoid extreme cold and other factors that may produce vasoconstriction (e.g. smoking). Treatment with nifedipine (BNF 2.6.2) or prazosin (BNF 2.5.4) may be beneficial. Surgery (regional sympathectomy) may be helpful in Raynaud's syndrome.

Varices

Definition
Varices are abnormally dilated tortuous veins, arteries or lymphatic vessels. They commonly occur in veins of the gastrointestinal tract (e.g. oesophageal varices, *see* Section 2.1) and of the legs (varicose veins).

Varicose veins

Definition and aetiology
Varicose veins (Figure 2.2) are varices which usually involve the superficial (saphenous) veins of the leg. They are associated with defective valves, particularly between the superficial and deep veins of the leg. They may be due to congenital valve defects, thrombophlebitis, deep vein thrombosis, pregnancy, ascites, malignant disease and excessive body-weight.

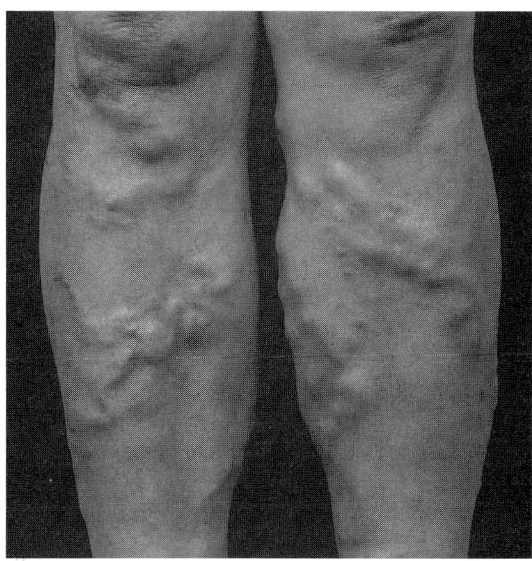

Figure 2.2 Varicose veins. (Reproduced with permission of Alex Bartel/Science Photo Library.)

Symptoms
The affected superficial veins are often visible and symptoms may include local pain and oedema, which may be exacerbated by prolonged standing, but disappear on resting. The calf muscles often become easily fatigued. Varices of the deep veins may result in chronic venous insufficiency, and are characterised by oedema and fibrosis. Local brown pigmentation may develop, together with a pruritic eczematous rash. Ulceration of the skin may occur.

Treatment
Treatment consists of support with graduated compression hosiery or bandages, and elevation of the legs. Local sclerosants (BNF 2.13) may be useful and surgical ligation or stripping may be necessary.

2.6 Anatomy and physiology of the cardiovascular system

The cardiovascular system comprises a pump, the heart and the circulatory system, which may be divided into the systemic (peripheral) and pulmonary branches.

The heart lies behind the sternum and costal cartilages in the mediastinum, and ventral to the oesophagus. The heart and great vessels are enclosed within a sac, the pericardium, which consists of an outer fibrous layer and an inner membranous layer, the epicardium. The epicardium is continuous with the outermost surface of the heart muscle, while the pericardium acts to limit the movement of the heart as it contracts.

The heart is composed of cardiac muscle, the myocardium, which has an inner lining, the endocardium.

Internally, the heart (Figure 2.3) consists of two pairs of chambers, the right pair being separated from the left by a continuous septum. Deoxygenated blood enters the heart at the right atrium via the inferior vena cava (bringing blood from all lower parts of the body) and the superior vena cava (carrying blood from the brain and tissues lying above the plane of the heart). On contraction of the atrium, blood passes through the right atrioventricular (tricuspid) valve into the right ventricle. The valve, as the name implies, consists of three cusps formed from a fold of the endocardium. All valves of the heart open and close passively (i.e. when the forward or backward pressure is sufficient to force them to do so). The tricuspid valve closes on ventricular systole to prevent the backflow of blood into the atrium. Blood leaves the right ventricle through the semi-lunar (pulmonary) valve.

Once the blood has been oxygenated in its passage through the lungs, it returns to the heart via two pulmonary veins from each lung, to re-enter the left atrium. From there, it passes through the left atrioventricular (mitral) valve into the thick-walled left ventricle, from which it is pumped through the semi-lunar (aortic) valve via the aorta to all parts of the body.

The cardiac cycle is the period between two successive heart contractions. The cycle is initiated by the spontaneous generation of an action potential in the sino-atrial node (the pacemaker), which is located in the right atrium near the point of entry of the superior vena cava. The action potential travels rapidly through both atria to depolarise the atrioventricular node.

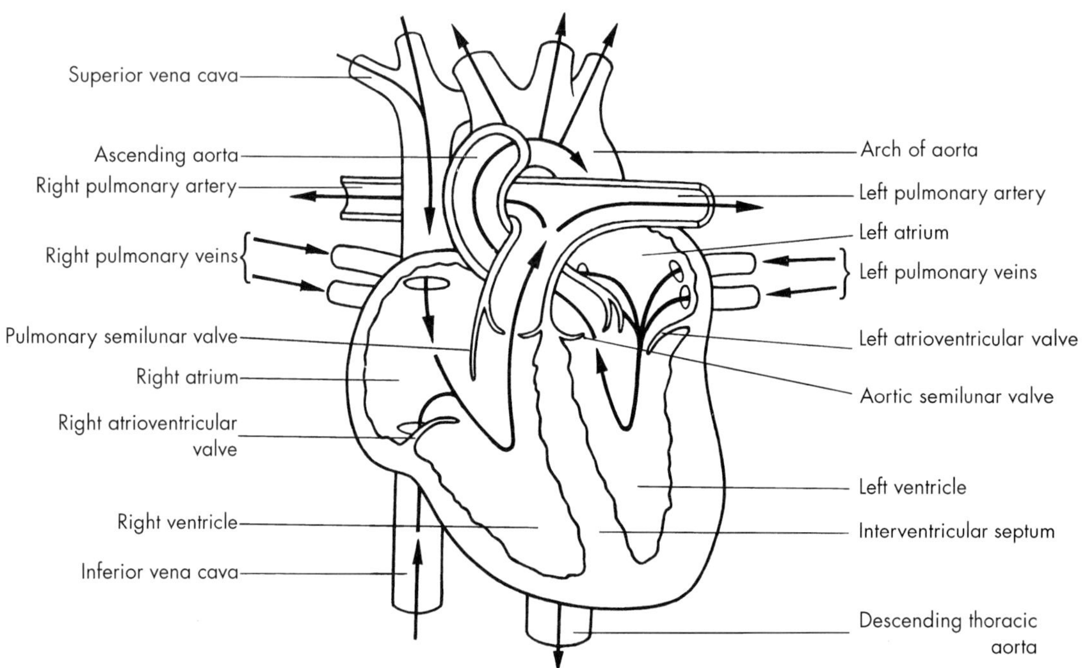

Figure 2.3 Anterior view of the heart.

From here it passes via the atrioventricular bundle (bundle of His) to the furthermost point of the ventricles. Contraction of the atria occurs fractionally ahead of the ventricles, allowing the blood to enter the ventricles from the atria before it is pumped around the body.

The action potential of heart activity may be monitored using an electrocardiogram (ECG). This technique also provides a powerful means of assessing defects in cardiac contractility. The P wave is produced by depolarisation of the atria immediately before contraction. The characteristic QRS complex is caused by depolarisation of the ventricles prior to contraction, and the T wave indicates the period of repolarisation of the ventricles (the repolarisation of the atria is not recorded as it is swamped by the considerably greater QRS complex). The PR interval is about 0.16 seconds and the total duration of the cardiac cycle is about 0.8 seconds.

Heart sounds may also be an important indicator of cardiac disease, particularly disease affecting the valves. Sounds are produced by the closure of the valves, and are commonly described as 'lub' and 'dup'. The resonant 'lub' sound is produced during ventricular systole when the left and right atrioventricular valves close to prevent the backflow of blood into the atria. The more abrupt 'dup' sound indicates the closure of the semi-lunar valves as the ventricles enter a diastolic phase. 'Murmurs' may be produced by diseased valves.

The heart is a thick-walled muscle. The presence of a supply of blood continually bathing its internal surfaces is not sufficient to satisfy the muscle's energy requirements. To allow for this, coronary vessels supply the external layers of the cardiac muscle with oxygenated blood. Two coronary arteries branch off from the aorta almost immediately after its emergence from the left ventricle. These arteries divide rapidly to produce a fine capillary network visible over the heart's external surface. The competence of this network is essential to the viability of cardiac function.

The systemic circulation consists of all blood vessels, except the pulmonary vessels. The arteries transport blood under high pressure to tissues and modulate the beating impulse of blood flow by their inherent elasticity. The wall of an artery consists of three layers (Figure 2.4):

- the outermost layer, the tunica externa (composed of connective tissue)

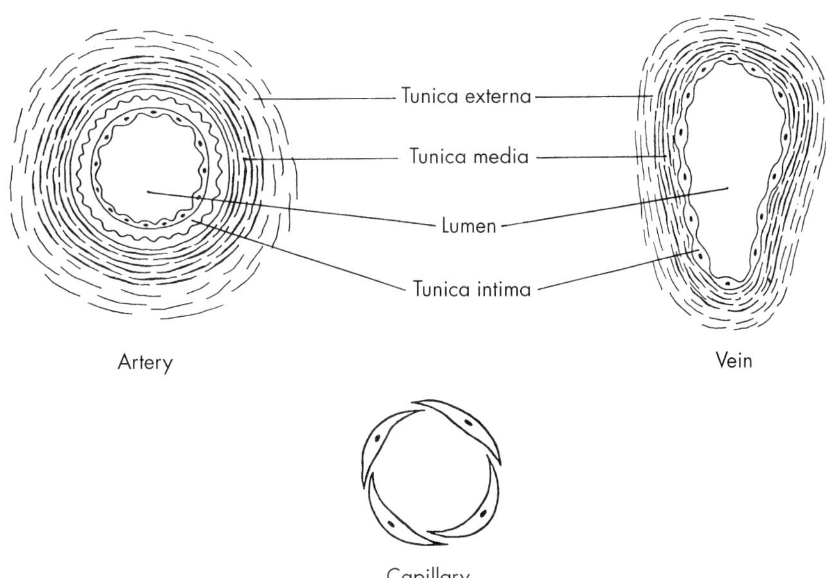

Figure 2.4 Cross-section of blood vessels.

- the tunica media (a mixture of smooth muscle and elastic tissue)
- the innermost layer, the tunica intima (elastic tissue lined by a smooth endothelium).

The arterioles contain a higher proportion of muscle tissue than other vessels, and provide the greatest resistance to the flow of blood. This bottle-neck effect is reflected by a drop in pressure from a mean of 90 mmHg in the smaller arteries to 30 mmHg in the arterioles. The arterioles act as 'control valves', through which blood is released to the capillaries. The return of blood in the venous system occurs via the venules, veins and the venae cavae. The blood is at negligible pressure within these vessels, and from many parts of the body it has to flow against gravity. The return is encouraged by the muscular pump (particularly within the legs); by negative intrathoracic pressure, which effectively draws blood from the lower vessels in the abdomen into thoracic vessels; and by the presence of valves within the veins, which help prevent the back-flow of blood.

The pressure within the cardiovascular system is produced by the pumping action of the heart, the elasticity of the blood vessels, and blood viscosity. It is homeostatically maintained by the stimulation of baroreceptors, which lie in the aorta and carotid arteries. Increased pressure within the system increases the stimulation of the baroreceptors, which transmit an inhibitory response affecting the activity of the sympathetic neurons in the cardiovascular centre in the medulla. As a result, sympathetic tone in the arterioles is decreased and peripheral resistance is reduced.

Average figures are often quoted for blood pressure (e.g. 120 mmHg systole and 80 mmHg diastole). However, these figures do not reflect the wide range of values which may be recorded in a representative cross-section of the healthy population. The residual diastolic resistance is generally taken as the most useful indicator of cardiovascular integrity and health, as it indicates the minimum pressure within the system at all times.

The pulmonary circulation consists only of the blood supply to and from the lungs. Despite receiving a volume of blood equivalent to the aortic output, the blood flow to the lungs is considerably less regulated than that to other parts of the body. Pulmonary vessels offer little resistance to flow and the pressure within the system is consequently much lower (average values of 24 mmHg systole and 9 mmHg diastole).

3

Disorders of the respiratory system

3.1 General disorders

Alveolitis

Definition
Alveolitis is inflammation of the alveoli.

Fibrosing alveolitis

Definition and aetiology
Fibrosing alveolitis is a syndrome characterised by inflammation and fibrosis of the alveoli, and production of exudate. It is idiopathic, although it may be associated with a concurrent connective tissue disorder or exposure to ionising radiation (e.g. X-rays).

Symptoms
Common symptoms include dyspnoea on exertion, dry cough, arthralgia, weight loss and malaise. Bacterial infection is a common complication.

Treatment
See Extrinsic allergic alveolitis *below*.

Extrinsic allergic alveolitis

Definition and aetiology

Extrinsic allergic alveolitis is alveolar inflammation caused by vasculitis and leading to fibrosis. It occurs as a result of a hypersensitivity reaction to prolonged exposure to high concentrations of an allergen (e.g. avian protein causing bird-fancier's lung and mouldy hay, straw or grain causing farmer's lung), which may be encountered in the course of work or leisure pursuits. A wide range of causative organisms have been recognised, including *Faenia rectivirgula* and *Thermoactinomyces vulgaris*. Particle sizes of antigens in the range 0.5–5 μm are required for their deposition in the alveoli.

It has been estimated that extrinsic allergic alveolitis accounts for about 2% of occupational lung diseases in the UK. By comparison, asthma accounts for more than a quarter of such diseases.

Symptoms

It may take weeks or even years for an individual to become sensitised to the antigen. When symptoms do arise, they usually occur 4–8 hours after exposure and subside within 24–48 hours. They include dry cough (which may become productive if the disease becomes chronic), dyspnoea, tightness in the chest, fever with rigors and general malaise. The disease may become chronic on continued allergen exposure and such exposure should be avoided.

Treatment

Prevention of inhalation of antigenic material may be possible with industrial respirators, although they may be uncomfortable to wear, especially during hot weather. Treatment of fibrosing and extrinsic allergic alveolitis includes the administration of corticosteroids (BNF 6.3.2) and oxygen therapy (BNF 3.6).

Bronchiectasis

Definition and aetiology

Bronchiectasis is chronic dilatation of the bronchi. It may develop as a result of infection (e.g. pneumonia, tuberculosis, measles or pertussis), but this has become considerably less common with the advent of antimicrobials. It may also occur as a result of bronchial obstruction, cystic fibrosis or the inhalation of toxins (e.g. from smoking), or it can be congenital (e.g. Kartagener's syndrome).

Death rates have diminished and death occurs at a later age, mainly due to antimicrobial treatment and its role in reducing the incidence of severe sequelae (e.g. amyloidoisis and cor pulmonale).

Symptoms

Repeated respiratory-tract infections, cough and purulent sputum production are the most common symptoms; the cough may be described as 'crackling' or wheezing. There may be no symptoms in between infective bouts. Other symptoms include dyspnoea, haemoptysis and malaise.

Treatment

Drug treatment is directed towards management of airways obstruction and any underlying infection. It includes the systemic and nebulised administration of appropriate antibacterial drugs (BNF 5.1), often in high doses. Postural drainage is a vital daily routine. Surgery may occasionally be useful in persistent and widespread haemoptysis. Bronchodilators (BNF 3.1) may be beneficial in patients with demonstrable reversible airways obstruction; immunosuppressive therapy may also be helpful. Patients should be advised to stop smoking.

Cough

Definition and aetiology

Coughing arises through a defensive reflex mechanism caused by the stimulation of receptors in the upper respiratory tract by irritant substances (e.g. dust, foreign bodies, mucus or smoke). It is characterised by forced expiration against a closed glottis, which suddenly opens to expel air and unwanted substances from the lungs. It is symptomatic of a wide range of underlying disorders (e.g. asthma, bronchiectasis, bronchitis, lung cancer, heart failure, pneumonia, pulmonary fibrosis and tuberculosis). Its most common cause is a minor self-limiting upper respiratory-tract infection.

Symptoms

A dry cough, characterised by the absence of sputum, may be irritating, hacking, short and repetitive; or harsh, hoarse and painful (croup) when associated with laryngitis.

The appearance of sputum (which may be clear to white or yellowish-green and offensive in the presence of infection) is indicative of a 'productive' cough. If coughing is rapidly repetitive, the pressure build-up behind the glottis may impede venous filling of the heart and cough syncope may result from the decreased cardiac output.

Treatment

Treatment involves the administration of cough suppressants (BNF 3.9.1) to control a dry cough, demulcents (BNF 3.9.2) for their soothing action on the pharyngeal mucosa and expectorants (BNF 3.9.2), which may increase bronchial secretions and facilitate expulsion of tenacious mucus. Water is of value in treating dry and productive coughs, taken orally or as inspired humidified air. In the presence of a prolonged cough, the possibility of an underlying disorder should be considered.

Croup

Definition and aetiology

Croup (acute laryngotracheobronchitis) occurs in young children (usually between six months and three years of age) and arises as a result of narrowing of the airway in the region of the larynx. The most common cause is a viral infection (particularly parainfluenza viruses), although bacteria may also be responsible (*see also* Epiglottitis). Rarer causative agents are respiratory syncytial virus (RSV) and influenza viruses. The partial obstruction is due to inflammation and oedema. Other causes include allergic responses or the presence of foreign bodies.

The occurrence of croup is seasonal. Croup caused by parainfluenza viruses tends to develop in the autumn; that caused by RSV and influenza occurs largely in the winter and spring.

Symptoms

Croup is characterised by a paroxysmal 'barking' cough and inspiratory stridor, which may be accompanied by fever, wheezing and tachypnoea. The symptoms often occur at night and, if severe, may cause respiratory distress, leading to cyanosis and exhaustion. Respiratory failure and pneumonia are potentially fatal complications.

Mild cases are self-limiting and symptoms resolve within three to four days. In severe cases, complete obstruction of the airway may occur.

Treatment

There is no specific antiviral therapy, but antibacterials (BNF 5.1) may be indicated if secondary bacterial infection has developed. Mild cases may be treated at home. Bed rest and adequate fluid intake are essential and home humidifiers or vaporisers may prove beneficial. Severe cases should be treated in hospital and may require oxygen therapy (BNF 3.6), intubation or assisted ventilation.

Pneumoconioses

Definition and aetiology

Pneumoconioses are a group of chronic pulmonary conditions resulting from prolonged inhalation of dust. The dust is usually of occupational or environmental origin (e.g. coal dust causing coal-miner's pneumoconiosis; silicon dioxide causing silicosis; and asbestos fibres causing asbestosis). Inhalation results in fibrosis of the lung.

Coal worker's pneumoconiosis has become less common in the UK as the mining workforce has decreased. However, in other countries (e.g. India), it remains very common, affecting between 1% and 2% of miners. Silicosis is also rare in the UK, with less than 100 cases reported annually. The incidence of asbestosis has decreased with the replacement of asbestos in buildings and other environments; between 100 and 150 cases are now notified annually.

Symptoms

Symptoms include cough, dyspnoea and obstructive airways disease (e.g. emphysema). Respiratory failure may occur in severe cases and death may follow. Silicosis is associated with an increased risk of tuberculosis and asbestosis with an increased incidence of malignant disease.

Treatment

Patients should be advised to avoid further exposure to the offending dust and aggravating factors (e.g. cigarette smoke).

Respiratory distress syndrome

Definition

Respiratory distress syndrome is an acute respiratory insufficiency, which may arise in adults with previously normal function or in neonates.

Neonatal respiratory distress syndrome

Definition and aetiology

Neonatal respiratory distress syndrome is one of the most frequent life-threatening disorders in neonates. It occurs most commonly in premature infants, but also occasionally develops in those born to diabetic mothers or by caesarean section. It is thought to be due to hyaline membrane disease in which alveolar surfactant is deficient.

Symptoms

Symptoms develop soon after birth and include dyspnoea and tachypnoea, expiratory grunting and cyanosis. The syndrome may be fatal, although the large majority of infants survive with appropriate treatment.

Treatment

Urgent supportive treatment is essential and consists of assisted ventilation with oxygen (BNF 3.6). The probability of premature infants developing the syndrome may be predicted by amniocentesis.

Adult respiratory distress syndrome

Definition and aetiology

Adult respiratory distress syndrome (ARDS) is a non-specific reaction of the lungs, which commonly follows a clinical crisis (e.g. major trauma, hypovolaemic or septic shock, aspiration pneumonia, burns, smoke inhalation, drug overdose, embolism or surgery). Its development is characterised by pulmonary oedema and fibrosis, and it can be fatal.

It has an incidence of about 6 per 10 000 population and accounts for about 1 in 20 of all admissions to intensive care units and 0.25% of all hospital admissions.

Symptoms

The symptoms of the syndrome occur in a recognised pattern of four stages. The initial stage is characterised by hyperventilation with alkalosis, soon after the precipitating event. Mild tachypnoea may develop within 24–72 hours, although the patient may appear stable. Pulmonary oedema follows, together with dyspnoea, cyanosis and worsening hypoxaemia. Finally, hypoxaemia, hypercapnia and acidosis develop and lead to coma and heart failure.

Treatment

Treatment is directed at preventing the last two stages of the syndrome and comprises assisted ventilation, oxygen therapy (BNF 3.6) and careful fluid management. Corticosteroids (BNF 6.3.2) have been used. The administration of diuretics (BNF 2.2) and sympathomimetics with inotropic activity (BNF 2.7.1) may be necessary. Antibacterial therapy (BNF 5.1) is indicated for any underlying infection.

Respiratory failure

Definition and aetiology

Respiratory failure arises as a result of impaired pulmonary gas exchange. It is characterised by abnormally low arterial oxygen tension (PaO_2) or high arterial carbon dioxide tension ($PaCO_2$). It usually occurs when a chronic illness (e.g. chronic bronchitis and emphysema, myasthenia gravis, pleural effusion or poliomyelitis) undergoes an exacerbation as a result of an acute precipitating illness (e.g. infection, asthma, heart failure or pneumothorax). It may also be precipitated by sedative drugs or following surgery.

Treatment

Treatment consists of controlled oxygen therapy (BNF 3.6) with assisted ventilation, if necessary. The administration of a respiratory stimulant (BNF 3.5) may be helpful. Appropriate antibacterial therapy may be necessary and bronchodilators (BNF 3.1), diuretics (BNF 2.2) and corticosteroids (BNF 6.3.2) may be indicated.

Sudden infant death syndrome

Definition and aetiology
The sudden infant death syndrome (SIDS) or 'cot death' is the unexplained and unexpected death of an otherwise previously healthy baby. It is the most common cause of death (30% of all deaths) in babies under one year of age, with the incidence reaching a peak in the third and fourth month of life. A greater prevalence has been associated with prematurity, social poverty and bottle-feeding.

Almost all deaths occur during sleep between the hours of midnight and 0900 hours. As its definition implies, the aetiology of sudden infant death syndrome is unclear, although various factors appear to culminate in a final disorder of respiratory mechanism.

Chronic hypoxia may occur immediately before death, due to prolonged periods of apnoea. Laryngospasm or nasal obstruction have been implicated in the development of apnoea.

Cardiovascular abnormalities (e.g. arrhythmias, conduction disturbances or an electrolyte imbalance) have been proposed as possible causative factors. Other general aetiological mechanisms suggested include overheating, nitrous fumes from domestic gas burning or the use of drugs such as phenothiazines. The evidence to support these suggestions, however, is limited.

Prevention
Some health authorities have adopted a multifactorial approach to accumulate data from patients in obstetric units and following delivery in an effort to identify those infants thought to be at risk. Certain common factors emerging (e.g. age of parents, similar sibling death, parity, antenatal care, obstetric complications and environmental factors) may allow identified infants to be closely monitored during the high-risk period. Parents should be educated about nutrition (stressing the importance of breast-feeding) and the general care of the infant.

Self-help organisation
Foundation for the Study of Infant Deaths

3.2 Obstructive airways disease

Asthma

Definition and aetiology
Asthma is a reversible obstructive airways disease of varying severity. The symptoms are caused by constriction of bronchial smooth muscle (bronchospasm), oedema of bronchial mucous membranes and blockage of the smaller bronchi with plugs of mucus. Asthma may occur, particularly in children, as a result of identifiable trigger factors or allergens (extrinsic asthma). Immunological mechanisms involving specific allergens (e.g. house-dust mite, pollens and animal danders) may be responsible. Reflux of gastric acid into the oesophagus also causes narrowing of the airways. Non-specific trigger factors that trigger intrinsic asthma include viral infection, exercise, dust and irritants (e.g. cigarette smoke), beta-adrenoceptor blocking drugs, emotional disturbances and non-steroidal anti-inflammatory drugs (e.g. aspirin and indomethacin).

Asthma occurs in many cases before 10 years of age. At this age, it is up to four times more common in boys than in girls. Intrinsic asthma commonly occurs in middle-aged (between 40 and 50 years of age) patients, with both sexes equally affected. As many as 10–15% of the population may suffer from asthma at some stage of life, and about 2000 deaths a year are attributed to asthma.

Symptoms
Symptoms of asthma range from mild to severe and life-threatening. The main symptoms are dyspnoea, wheezing on both inspiration and expiration, and tightness of the chest. Cough, with or without the production of sputum, is common and is often the presenting symptom. Other symptoms include tachycardia, tachypnoea, fatigue and drowsiness.

Treatment
Reassurance and education are important components of treatment. Patients should be advised

to avoid known trigger factors and be encouraged to maintain an active life. Smoking should be discouraged. Drug treatment includes the use of bronchodilators (BNF 3.1). Prophylaxis with inhaled corticosteroids (BNF 3.2) or non-corticosteroid agents (e.g. sodium cromoglicate and nedocromil) (BNF 3.3) is recommended. Oxygen therapy (BNF 3.6) may be necessary and hyposensitisation (BNF 3.4.2) may be considered. Antimuscarinic bronchodilators (BNF 3.1.2) administered by inhalation may be used in the management of chronic asthma for patients already being treated with high-dose inhaled corticosteroids.

Treatment of acute severe asthma requires the administration of selective beta$_2$-adrenoceptor stimulants (BNF 3.1.1) (most commonly via a nebuliser), assisted ventilation and parenteral corticosteroids (BNF 3.1.1). Oxygen therapy (BNF 3.6) may be necessary.

Self-help organisations
Action Against Allergy
British Lung Foundation
National Asthma Campaign

Bronchitis

Definition and aetiology
Bronchitis is characterised by inflammation of the trachea and bronchi and may be acute or chronic (*see* Chronic obstructive pulmonary disease).

Acute bronchitis

Definition and aetiology
Acute bronchitis is a very common condition that is usually self-limiting. It is commonly caused by a viral infection, usually following a cold or influenza. Implicated viruses in adults include adenovirus, rhinovirus or influenza virus; in children and the elderly, it can be caused by respiratory syncytial virus (RSV) and parainfluenza virus. The causative microorganisms of secondary bacterial infection are commonly *Streptococcus pneumoniae* and *Haemophilus influenzae.*

Symptoms
Common symptoms include general malaise and cough, which may be dry or productive. A sore feeling in the chest may be present, with tracheitis and expiratory wheezing, which can be cleared by coughing. A sore throat and runny nose are also common, and indicate an upper respiratory-tract infection.

Treatment
In otherwise healthy patients, treatment is not usually necessary, although antibacterials (BNF 5.1) are often given due to the probability of secondary bacterial infection. A cough suppressant (BNF 3.9.1) may be indicated in the presence of a troublesome dry cough.

Self-help organisations
Age Concern England
British Lung Foundation
Chest Heart and Stroke Association

Chronic obstructive pulmonary disease

Definition and aetiology
Chronic obstructive pulmonary disease (COPD) (a term that has replaced chronic bronchitis and emphysema) is an irreversible obstructive airways disease, which usually results from smoking or prolonged exposure to environmental irritants. It is defined as cough with the production of sputum for at least three months in at least two successive years. Repeated respiratory-tract infections may contribute to its development. It is a definition of exclusion: the presence of infection with *Mycobacterium tuberculosis*, lung cancer or chronic heart failure must have been eliminated.

Emphysema is an irreversible chronic obstructive airways disease, which is characterised by dilatation of the air spaces distal to the terminal bronchioles and destruction of the alveolar walls. The outstanding feature is loss of the elastic tissue of the lungs. It usually develops in association with chronic bronchitis, and is invariably due to smoking. One causative factor in emphysema that has received increasing attention is the absence of an enzyme, alpha-1-antitrypsin (also called alpha-1-proteinase inhibitor). Its absence removes a homeostatic mechanism by which lung tissue is protected from protease enzymes.

In the UK, up to 1 in 5 men and 1 in 12 women have chronic cough and catarrh, classic COPD symptoms. Mortality from COPD has fallen in the past 20 years, largely due to a decrease in cigarette smoking, which is considered to be the primary causative factor. In the USA, nearly 100 000 people die each year from COPD.

Symptoms

Chronic bronchitis and emphysema are characterised by a chronic or recurrent cough and the production of excess sputum, which may be clear or purulent in the presence of concurrent infection. Symptoms tend to be more marked on waking and during the winter months. Other symptoms include dyspnoea and tachypnoea on exercise, and wheezing. In severe disease, drowsiness, headache, weight gain and peripheral oedema may occur.

Treatment

Patients should be advised to stop smoking and avoid exposure to other irritants, and attempts should be made to increase exercise tolerance. Drug treatment comprises the administration of bronchodilators (BNF 3.1). The value of long-term administration of corticosteroids has not been proven. Antibacterial therapy (BNF 5.1) is indicated in the presence of respiratory-tract infection. Oxygen administration (BNF 3.6) may be necessary. Mucolytics (BNF 3.7) and cough suppressants (BNF 3.9.1) are sometimes used, and physiotherapy may be beneficial.

3.3 Pleural disorders

Pleurisy and pleural effusion

Definition and aetiology

Pleurisy is inflammation of the pleura. It may be accompanied by pleural effusion, which is characterised by the presence of fluid (exudate or transudate) in the pleural space. The accumulated fluid may be purulent (empyema) or contain blood (haemothorax). Common causes include heart failure, hepatic or renal impairment, infection (e.g. pneumonia and tuberculosis), malignant disease, pancreatitis, pulmonary infarction or oedema, and physical trauma.

Symptoms

Pleurisy is characterised by sudden sharp chest pain, which is exacerbated by movement and inspiration. This pain may disappear on the development of pleural effusion, which may be asymptomatic. Dyspnoea and dull chest pain may occur as the volume of accumulated fluid increases, and there may be poor expansion of the affected side of the chest.

Treatment

Treatment is directed at the underlying cause. In pleural effusion, surgical aspiration may be necessary and continuous drainage indicated.

Pneumothorax

Definition and aetiology

Pneumothorax is the accumulation of air in the pleural space. It often occurs spontaneously, usually in thin young men. It may also arise as a result of physical trauma, underlying pulmonary disease (e.g. asthma, bronchitis, cystic fibrosis, emphysema and tuberculosis) or malignant disease.

Symptoms

Pneumothorax may be asymptomatic, with only a vague discomfort in the chest, but severe chest pain, dyspnoea and cyanosis may occur.

Treatment

Pneumothorax may resolve without treatment, but underwater seal drainage may be required and thoracic surgery is indicated in resistant or recurring cases.

3.4 Anatomy and physiology of the respiratory system

The respiratory system in humans is responsible for the processes of gas exchange between the atmosphere, the circulation and the cells of the body; for the homeostatic maintenance of blood pH; and for the provision of vocal expression (i.e. speaking and singing).

Air enters the respiratory tree through the nasal passages and the mouth, and is warmed, humidified and partially filtered as it passes over the mucosal membranes and cilia. From the nasal passages, the air passes through the pharynx

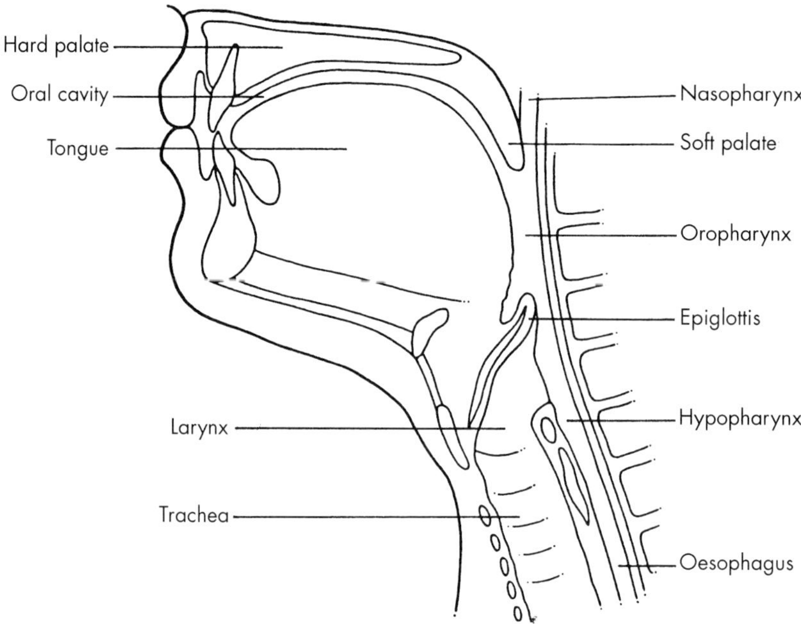

Figure 3.1 Upper respiratory tract.

(Figure 3.1). The upper portion of the pharynx (above the level of the soft palate) is called the nasopharynx, from which the Eustachian tubes branch off. These link the middle ear with the nasopharynx, and assist in the maintenance of atmospheric pressure within the tympanic cavity (*see* Section 12.4). The lower reaches of the pharynx may be subdivided at the upper edge of the epiglottis into theoropharynx and the hypopharynx (laryngopharynx). The entry to the trachea is guarded by the larynx, situated immediately below the pharynx. The larynx also produces vocal sounds through the action of the vocal cords in the glottis. Food and liquids are prevented from entering the larynx by a flap of cartilage, the epiglottis, which closes over the entrance to the larynx on swallowing.

The trachea links the larynx to the right and left bronchi and is prevented from collapsing by the presence of approximately 20 horseshoe-shaped rings of cartilage. The incomplete sections of cartilage are located adjacent to the oesophagus.

On passing through the trachea, air enters the lungs via the bronchi, bronchioles and alveoli (Figure 3.2). The bronchi walls contain rings of cartilage interspersed throughout smooth muscle, and their inner surface is lined by cilia whose roots are in the mucous membrane. The rings of cartilage prevent the collapse of the bronchi when the internal pressure changes, and the beating cilia assist in the upward and outward movement of unwanted fine particles.

The bronchioles are narrower versions of the bronchi, usually of less than 1 mm diameter. However, unlike the bronchi, their walls are not reinforced with cartilage, and they may open and narrow to modify the resistance to the passage of air. Deeper within the lung, the bronchioles repeatedly branch, giving rise to terminal bronchioles. The terminal bronchioles divide further into respiratory bronchioles, which possess end outgrowths, the alveoli (Figure 3.3). The walls of the respiratory bronchioles and alveoli are thin, covered in a network of fine capillaries, and are the sites of gaseous exchange.

An alveolar surfactant is present in the fluid lining the surface of the air sacs. This surfactant, which consists of phospholipids and is secreted by the alveolar cells, reduces surface tension and hence the energy required to keep the alveoli inflated.

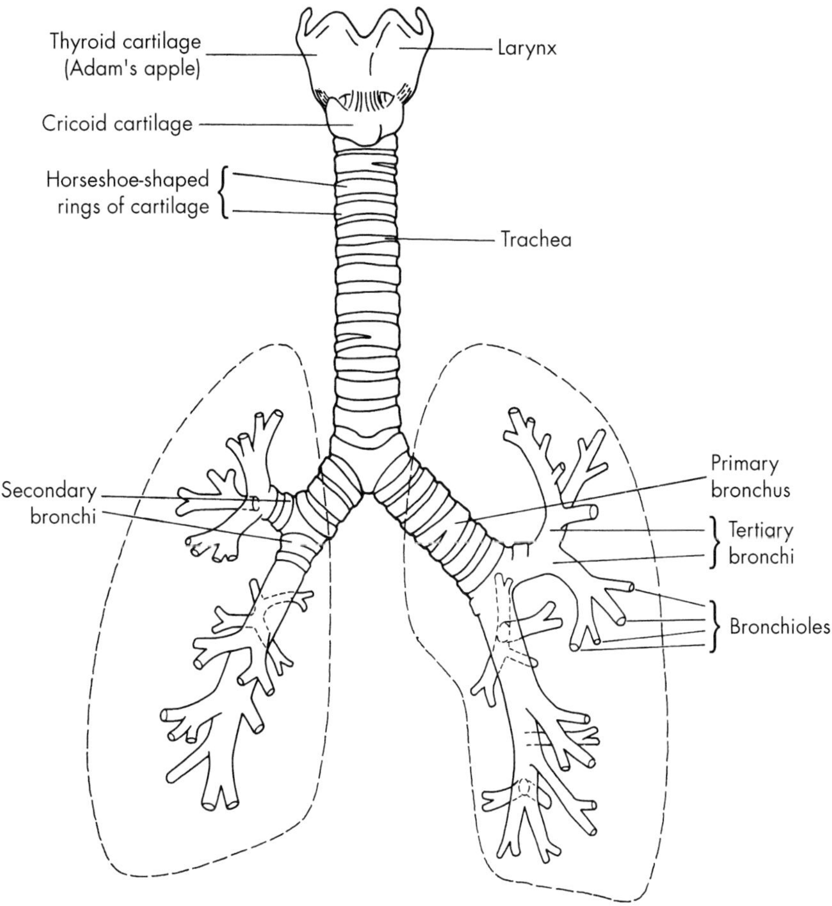

Figure 3.2 Anterior view of bronchial tree.

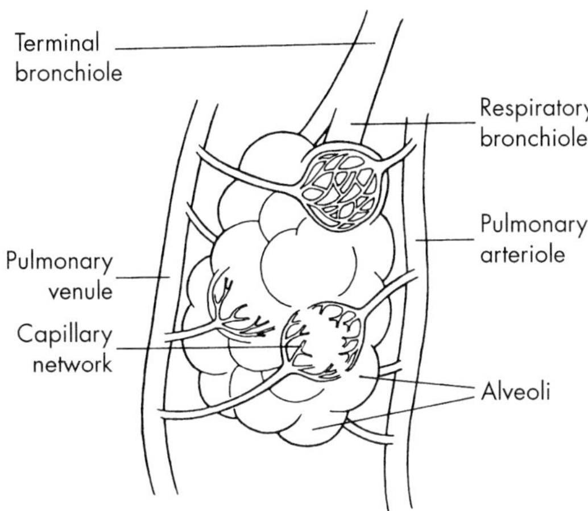

Figure 3.3 Areas of gaseous exchange.

The lungs are located in the thoracic cavity, and the two non-identical lobes are separated by the heart in the mediastinum. The right lung consists of an upper, middle and lower lobe, while the left lung comprises only an upper and lower lobe. Internally, each lobe is further subdivided into two to five segments, which may provide the localised sites of many pulmonary disorders.

Each lung is surrounded by two closely associated membranes, the pleura. The space between the two membranes (the pleural cavity) is filled with fluid (cf. two plates of glass separated by a thin film of water). The outer parietal membrane lines the inner wall of the thoracic cavity, and the inner visceral pleural membrane follows the contours of the outer surfaces of the lungs. The pleura of each lung are not linked.

4

Disorders of the nervous system

4.1 General disorders

Cerebral oedema

Definition and aetiology
Cerebral oedema is the excessive accumulation of fluid in the brain and is accompanied by an increase in intracranial pressure (*see also* Papilloedema, Section 11.1). It is often due to physical trauma or malignant disease, but may also result from hypoxia at high altitude (high-altitude cerebral oedema), poisoning (e.g. with CNS depressants, carbon monoxide or lead) or meningitis.

Symptoms
It is characterised by altered consciousness followed by coma. Other symptoms include slow respiration leading to apnoea, pupillary dilatation and a decerebrate posture. Death may follow.

Treatment
Early treatment is essential, and neurosurgical decompression or assisted ventilation may be necessary. Drug treatment consists of the administration of intravenous osmotic diuretics (BNF 2.2.5); corticosteroids (BNF 6.3.2) are used to treat cerebral oedema due to trauma.

Cerebral palsy

Definition and aetiology
Cerebral palsy constitutes a group of non-progressive neurological motor disorders, resulting from faulty development of the brain or damage sustained in the uterus or in early infancy. Causes include fetal disorders, birth trauma, birth asphyxia, neonatal jaundice, cerebral haemorrhage or infarction or severe systemic disease (e.g. meningitis) in early infancy.

It has an incidence of about 0.1% for full-term babies, increasing to 1% for those born prematurely or of low birth weight.

Symptoms
The characteristics and symptoms of cerebral palsy depend on the cause, extent and location of the brain damage. Spastic syndromes (e.g. hemiplegia, paraplegia, quadriplegia and diplegia) occur most commonly, and are characterised by muscular hypertonicity, weakness and contractures. There may also be auditory and visual impairment, athetosis, ataxia, dysarthria, dysphagia, persistent dribbling, epilepsy and temper tantrums. Mental retardation may occur on its own or in conjunction with any of the above problems.

Treatment
Treatment depends on the severity of physical and mental disability, and is likely to be long term. Physiotherapy, occupational and speech therapy, and educational and social support may be necessary. Orthopaedic surgery may be beneficial in selected cases. Antiepileptics (BNF 4.8) may be required to control seizures.

Self-help organisation
SCOPE

Headache

Definition and aetiology
Headache may be idiopathic or a symptom of a disease process, with its frequency, duration, nature and location depending on the disease. It may arise from systemic infection (e.g. syphilis and tuberculosis), meningitis, osteitis deformans, trigeminal neuralgia (*see below*), vascular disturbances, head injuries, severe hypertension and giant cell arteritis. It may also be caused by disease of the nose, sinuses, eyes, ears or teeth. Headaches are commonly due to muscle tension, which may be associated with anxiety, emotional disturbances and fatigue.

Migraine

Definition and aetiology
Migraine is of unknown aetiology. Disturbances of cranial-blood circulation have been demonstrated and it may be familial. It may be triggered

by agents (e.g. combined oral contraceptives and alcohol) or by hunger, smoking, emotional disturbances, menstruation and specific food intolerance (e.g. to chocolate or tyramine-containing foods).

The condition can affect approximately one in five women and about one in seven men at some time during their lifetime. Nearly all first attacks in both sexes occur before 30 years of age.

Symptoms

Migraine without an aura (common migraine) occurs in three out of four patients with migraine. It has been defined as a succession of five unilateral pulsating headaches lasting 4–72 hours. Their severity restricts normal daily activities and they may be accompanied by nausea or vomiting, or both, and sensitivity to light or noise.

In migraine with an aura (classic migraine), which occurs in about one in five migraine patients, visual disturbances (e.g. flashing lights and blurred vision) occur between 5 and 20 minutes before the headache, but last less than an hour. Paraesthesia in the face, hands and feet can also develop.

Treatment

Treatment of migraine consists of the administration of non-opioid analgesics (BNF 4.7.1) for mild attacks and tolfenamic acid (BNF 4.7.4.1) for an acute attack. Other agents indicated for acute attacks include diclofenac potassium (BNF 10.1.1), sumatriptan and other $5HT_1$ agonists (BNF 4.7.4.1) and ibuprofen (BNF 10.1.1). Anti-emetics (BNF 4.6) and anxiolytics (BNF 4.1) may also be useful.

Prophylactic treatment may be given by pizotifen, clonidine and methysergide (BNF 4.7.4.2), tricyclic antidepressant drugs (BNF 4.3.1), calcium-channel blockers (BNF 2.6.2) and selected beta-adrenoceptor blocking drugs (BNF 2.4). Patients should be advised to avoid known trigger factors.

Self-help organisations

Action Against Allergy
Migraine Action Association
Migraine Trust

Cluster headache

Definition and aetiology

Cluster headache (migrainous neuralgia or histamine headache) consists of paroxysmal acute pain centred around one eye. Cluster headache is more common in men and appears to be due to an abnormality of the autonomic nervous system. Trigger factors include alcohol and sleep.

Symptoms

The attacks last from 15 to 180 minutes. They tend to occur three to four times daily in clusters over a period of several weeks, followed by a prolonged attack-free period. The affected eye may appear bloodshot, with swelling of the eyelids. Pupillary constriction, enophthalmos, ptosis and loss of sweating on the same side of the face may accompany the headache. Vasodilatation and nasal congestion on the same side of the face are common.

Treatment

Non-opioid analgesics (BNF 4.7.1), certain antimigraine drugs (BNF 4.7.4) and verapamil (BNF 2.6.2), the calcium-channel blocker, may be of value. Antimanic drugs (BNF 4.2.3) have also been used in chronic cases.

Tension headache

Definition and aetiology

Tension headache (muscle contraction headache) is due to sustained contraction of skeletal muscle of the scalp, jaw and neck. It is often associated with anxiety and emotional disturbances, and is the most common form of chronic, recurrent headache. Tension headache may be differentiated from migraine as the pain is continuous, not pulsatile, giving the impression of pressure on both sides of the head.

Symptoms

It is characterised by a steady non-pulsatile ache, which may be unilateral or bilateral in the temporal, occipital, parietal or frontal regions. It may last for hours or occur intermittently for years.

Treatment
Treatment consists of the administration of non-opioid analgesics (BNF 4.7.1) or the removal of any underlying stress.

Trigeminal neuralgia

Definition and aetiology
Trigeminal neuralgia (tic douloureux) is a syndrome characterised by brief attacks of severe pain over an area of the face innervated by one or more branches of the trigeminal nerve. The pain may be triggered by touching hypersensitive areas on the skin, by face and jaw movements or exposure to cold draughts on the face. It is generally of unknown aetiology and encountered in people over 50 years of age. In younger patients, it may be due to multiple sclerosis.

Treatment
Treatment consists of the administration of carbamazepine, phenytoin, or both (BNF 4.7.3). If drug therapy is unsuccessful, thermocoagulation of the ganglion may have to be considered.

Hydrocephalus

Definition and aetiology
Hydrocephalus is an increase in the volume of cerebrospinal fluid (CSF) within the skull. It is caused by increased secretion of CSF or by interference with the flow of CSF within the ventricles of the brain. In infants (infantile hydrocephalus), it may be due to congenital brain abnormalities which interfere with CSF circulation. It can also be caused by meningitis, subarachnoid haemorrhage arising from birth trauma, or in association with spina bifida. Hydrocephalus may also occur in adults as a result of malignant disease, meningitis or subarachnoid haemorrhage.

There are about 4 per 10 000 live births of hydrocephalus (excluding those who also present with spina bifida).

Symptoms
Symptoms are due to increased intracranial pressure. In infants, they include head enlargement, bulging of the forehead, and prominent scalp veins. In severe cases, mental retardation may occur, with limb spasticity and visual disturbances. Other symptoms are headache and convulsions.

Treatment
Treatment is by the surgical insertion of a valve or shunt.

Insomnia

Definition and aetiology
Insomnia is the disturbance of normal sleep patterns, which may be manifested by difficulty in falling asleep, early waking, intermittent waking or fitful sleep.

Transient insomnia may occur due to extraneous factors (e.g. noise, room-temperature changes or shift work). Short-term insomnia may be caused by emotional disturbances or medical illness. It usually lasts a few weeks, but can recur. Chronic insomnia may be associated with psychiatric disorders (e.g. depressive disorders and anxiety), daytime sleeping, abuse of drugs and alcohol, pain, cough, pruritus or dyspnoea.

Some patients who complain of insomnia may be found on enquiry to have adequate sleep, and others may sleep better if they avoid excitement or stimulants (e.g. coffee or tea).

It has been estimated that about 10% of the population have chronic insomnia, and that half the population suffers from varying degrees of insomnia at some time during their lives.

Treatment
Patients, especially the elderly, should be advised to avoid alcohol and daytime sleeping. They should try to establish a regular sleeping schedule, improve the comfort of the bed, and to take some form of physical exercise (e.g. walking) during the day to generate physical tiredness. Any underlying disorder should be treated and any causative factor remedied.

Drug treatment consists of the judicious administration of hypnotics (BNF 4.1.1), whose choice depends on the type of insomnia. Non-prescription products have appeared in recent years in which the active ingredient is an antihistamine.

Malignant hyperthermia

Definition and aetiology

Malignant hyperthermia (malignant hyperpyrexia) is a rare, but potentially fatal, disorder characterised by a sudden and dramatic increase in body metabolism and temperature. It occurs in susceptible patients on exposure to anaesthetics (e.g. succinylcholine and halothane), and is due to a hereditary disorder of muscle metabolism. Its incidence is about 1 in 20 000.

Symptoms

The chief symptoms are high fever, acidosis and widespread muscular rigidity. Death may ensue.

Treatment

Treatment consists of the administration of dantrolene sodium (BNF 15.1.8). Offending anaesthetics should be avoided in susceptible patients and their families.

Motion sickness

Definition and aetiology

Motion sickness is caused by repetitive movement (e.g. that experienced when travelling by air, rail, road and sea). Its exact mechanism is unknown, but it is thought to be due to excessive stimulation of the vestibular system.

Symptoms

It is characterised by dizziness, nausea and vomiting. Increased salivation, pallor and cold sweating of the face and hands may also occur. If prolonged, motion sickness can lead to anorexia, apathy, dehydration and depression, and it may have a marked adverse effect on performance.

Treatment

Prevention is more successful than treatment and comprises the administration of hyoscine or an antihistamine (BNF 4.6) before travelling. Visual mechanisms are thought to be significant and, when travelling, subjects should be advised to focus on distant objects or to keep their eyes closed with the head in a fixed position.

Myasthenia gravis

Definition and aetiology

Myasthenia gravis is a neuromuscular disorder characterised by muscle weakness and arising from defective neuromuscular transmission. It is thought to be caused by an autoimmune mechanism involving the production of antibodies to the acetylcholine receptors present in the neuromuscular junction.

Myasthenia gravis affects about 8 per 100 000 population, and can occur at any age.

Symptoms

Symptoms may be episodic, with patients experiencing permanent or temporary remissions. Relapses may occur, however, after months or years.

The primary symptom is muscle weakness affecting most commonly the muscles of the eyes, lips, tongue, throat, neck and shoulders. The weakness worsens on exercise, and causes diplopia and ptosis, chewing and swallowing difficulties, speech disorders and drooping of the head. Limb muscles may also be affected and movement may become restricted. Dyspnoea and respiratory paralysis may arise from involvement of the respiratory muscles and the consequences may be fatal. Symptoms are exacerbated by strenuous exercise, emotional disturbances, fatigue, pregnancy, and by the administration of certain drugs (e.g. aminoglycosides). Myasthenia gravis may be accompanied by thymic enlargement, which may be caused by a thymoma.

Treatment

Treatment is by the administration of an anticholinesterase (BNF 10.2.1). Corticosteroids (BNF 10.2.1) may be beneficial in unresponsive cases. Thymectomy may be beneficial in some patients and plasmapheresis may be indicated in severe cases.

Nausea and vomiting

Definition and aetiology

Nausea and vomiting are common symptoms. Examples of disturbances which can cause nausea and vomiting include gastric irritation, irradiation (radiation sickness) and travel (motion sickness). Nausea and vomiting may also occur during pregnancy (morning sickness) or be due to psychogenic factors. They may also occur post-operatively or following the administration of certain drugs. Haematemesis or 'coffee-ground vomitus' is an indication of serious organic disease. Projectile vomiting is the forceful ejection of vomit without prior retching, and is characteristic of pyloric stenosis.

Treatment

Nausea and vomiting may be prevented or treated by the administration of anticholinergic drugs, phenothiazines or other anti-emetics (BNF 4.6). The most powerful of these drugs may also be effective in the treatment of post-operative vomiting and radiation sickness. Drug treatment for 'morning sickness' should be avoided if possible because of teratogenic risk. Persistent nausea and vomiting may be an indication of serious gastrointestinal, neurological or metabolic disorders, and if this is suspected it may be desirable to withhold treatment until a diagnosis has been made. Complications of persistent vomiting include dehydration (BNF 9.2), hypokalaemia and alkalosis, for which fluid and electrolyte replacement may be necessary.

Pain

Definition and aetiology

Pain may be caused by physical or psychological disturbances, or a combination of both. It may be characteristic of a disease and is sometimes the only presenting symptom. The nature of a particular pain may help in the diagnosis of the underlying condition. The location of a pain may indicate the part of the body affected, although pain felt in one position may sometimes be referred from pathology in another part of the body (e.g. shoulder-tip pain occurs with gall bladder disease). This occurs when pain cannot be felt in the affected area (e.g. the viscera) or when it causes pressure on a nerve. Some forms of pain do not remain localised in one area, but move around. The pain may radiate to a characteristic region where discomfort is felt (e.g. cardiac pain is usually felt as central chest pain, but often radiates to the shoulders and left arm).

Symptoms

Pain varies in severity from mild to severe. It may only appear at certain times of the day or night, or be continuous for many hours. Varied descriptions may be given by the patient (e.g. stabbing, crushing, gnawing, burning or throbbing) and pain may be acute, chronic or intractable.

Treatment

Treatment, which is symptomatic, is usually directed towards the underlying cause. Pain may resolve with reassurance in the absence of treatment, or relief may be obtained by rest, warming, cooling or changing position. Patients should be advised to avoid any aggravating factors. Drug treatment for the relief of pain consists of the administration of analgesics (BNF 4.7). Local anaesthesia (BNF 15.2) may be used for certain types of localised pain. Antidepressant drugs (BNF 4.3), anxiolytics (BNF 4.1) and corticosteroids (BNF 10.1.2) may be used in the treatment of certain types of pain. In various cases of intractable pain, relief may be obtained from surgical section of the afferent sensory pathways.

Self-help organisations

Back Care
Pain Interest Group
Pain Relief Fund
Pain Society

Restless leg syndrome

Definition and aetiology

Restless leg syndrome (Ekbom's syndrome) is characterised by unpleasant sensations in the legs, which only develop at rest. The cause is unknown, although iron-deficiency anaemia, pregnancy and uraemia may be contributory factors.

Symptoms

The symptoms, which may be intolerable, only occur when the legs are at rest and include 'pins and needles', burning sensations, twitching and, sometimes, pain. These sensations, which usually occur between the ankle and knee, may be relieved by movement, but return when movement ceases. Insomnia frequently occurs as a consequence.

Treatment

Many patients do not require drug treatment. Should drug treatment be considered, oral iron (BNF 9.1.1), clonazepam (BNF 4.8), carbamazepine (BNF 4.7.3) and orphenadrine (BNF 4.9.2) have been used, although only clonazepam and carbamazepine have been proven to be clinically effective.

Spina bifida

Definition and aetiology

Spina bifida is an idiopathic congenital neural tube disorder characterised by defective closure of the spinal column. The defect occurs most commonly in the lower thoracic, lumbar and sacral regions. In spina bifida occulta, there is no outward sign of a spinal defect. In spina bifida cystica, the meninges and cerebrospinal fluid (CSF), and more commonly also the nerves and part of the spinal cord, protrude in a sac through the vertebral defect (Figure 4.1). It is the most common defect present at birth in the UK, affecting 15 per 100 000 births, although the incidence has fallen drastically during the 1970s and 1980s.

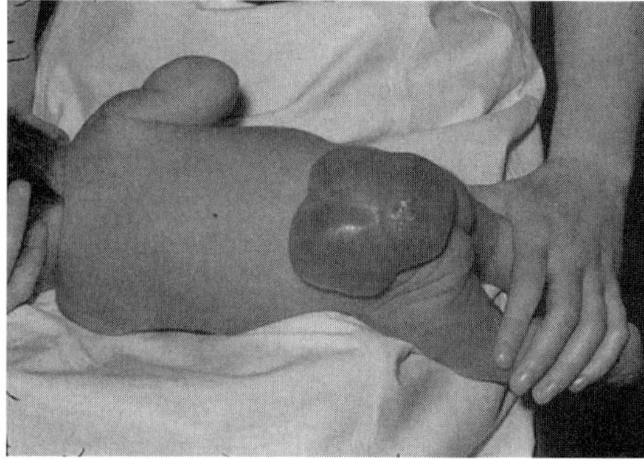

Figure 4.1 Spina bifida. (Reproduced with permission of Biophoto Associates/Science Photo Library.)

Symptoms

The severity of the disorder varies according to the type and location of the defect. Varying degrees of paralysis and sensory loss may occur. The lower limbs may be affected and incontinence may be caused by paralysis of the rectal and bladder sphincters. In spina bifida cystica, the sac containing the protruding cord and meninges may rupture, resulting in leakage of CSF and an increased risk of meningitis. Hydrocephalus and multiple congenital defects may accompany spina bifida at birth.

Treatment

Treatment consists of surgical closure of the defect, although the patient will often remain paraplegic and incontinent. Surgery may also be necessary if hydrocephalus is present, and appropriate antibacterial therapy (BNF 5.1) is indicated if meningitis develops. In many cases, long-term medical and nursing care is necessary.

Self-help organisations

Association for Spina Bifida and Hydrocephalus
Urostomy Association

Vertigo

Definition and aetiology

Vertigo is the sensation of movement, particularly of rotation. It may occur normally in response to certain stimuli (e.g. motion sickness), but may be the symptom of labyrinthine disorders (e.g. Ménière's disease or vestibular neuronitis). Vertigo may also arise as a result of central disorders (e.g. epilepsy, migraine and multiple sclerosis) or as a side-effect of administration of drugs (e.g. aminoglycosides).

Symptoms

Vertigo, which is often described as dizziness, is frequently accompanied by nausea and vomiting, and nystagmus.

Treatment

Treatment varies according to the underlying disorder, but may include the administration of antihistamines or phenothiazines (BNF 4.6), both for their anticholinergic activity.

Vestibular neuronitis

Definition and aetiology
Vestibular neuronitis is a labyrinthine disorder in which vestibular function is disturbed in the absence of deafness. It usually occurs between 30 and 50 years of age. It often follows a febrile illness and, although its cause is unknown, it may be associated with viral infection.

Symptoms
It is characterised by severe vertigo, which may be precipitated by the adoption of certain positions of the head, but may also be exacerbated by movement. The vertigo decreases in severity over a period of days, although occasional attacks may occur for weeks or even months.

Treatment
Treatment is symptomatic, and antihistamines and phenothiazines (BNF 4.6) may be helpful.

4.2 Cerebrovascular disorders

Stroke

Definition and aetiology
A stroke (cerebrovascular accident) is caused by an acute vascular lesion in the brain and is characterised by an area of ischaemic infarction. It is usually due to cerebral embolism or thrombosis, and less commonly due to cerebral haemorrhage. These in turn may be caused by aneurysm, atherosclerosis, heart disease, hypertension, diabetes mellitus, alcohol and smoking. Stroke may follow a transient ischaemic attack.

The incidence of stroke is about 5 per 1000. As the incidence increases with age, the number affected by stroke is growing due to a larger elderly population.

Symptoms
Symptoms vary according to the area and site of brain tissue affected. The onset of symptoms may be sudden, particularly if stroke is due to cerebral embolism or haemorrhage. Alternatively, there may be a short prodromal or warning phase prior to actual onset, particularly when cerebral thrombosis is the cause. Symptoms are usually limited to the side of the body opposite to the half of the brain in which the stroke occurs (i.e. stroke in the left half of the brain produces right-sided symptoms).

Common symptoms, which by definition last more than 24 hours (*see also* Transient ischaemic attacks), include hemiplegia, hemiparesis, sensory loss, speech disorders and visual disturbances. A sudden loss of consciousness may occur which, although often regained, can deepen and lead to death. Surviving patients may suffer permanent neurological damage, resulting in marked suffering and loss of dignity through disability (e.g. incontinence, amnesia, paralysis and speech disorders). Some patients become 'locked-in' and, although conscious, are unable to move, speak or swallow. Cerebral oedema is an important local complication of stroke, and other general complications associated with paralysis are decubitus ulcers, pneumonia and urinary-tract infections.

Treatment
Treatment depends on the severity of the symptoms and aims to overcome any resultant disability. Any underlying cause should be treated to prevent further attack. The use of tissue plasminogen activator given within 3 hours of the stroke can be beneficial. Low-dose aspirin (BNF 2.9) has been advocated in all stroke victims. Long-term nursing care and physiotherapy are often necessary.

Prevention of stroke is a primary healthcare objective in many western countries. Detection and treatment of hypertension, stopping smoking, increased exercise, reduced bodyweight and decreased salt intake are all measures that can influence the occurrence of stroke.

Self-help organisations
Action for Dysphasic Adults
British Heart Foundation
Stroke Association

Subdural and extradural haemorrhage

Definition and aetiology
Subdural haemorrhage is bleeding into the subdural space (i.e. between the dura mater and

arachnoid membrane). It is usually due to trauma, and elderly, alcoholic or epileptic patients are particularly at risk.

Extradural haemorrhage is a consequence of a tear in a middle meningeal artery. It is commonly caused by a skull fracture, which can follow a direct blow to the temple.

Symptoms

The onset of symptoms in subdural episodes is usually insidious, and they may not develop until several weeks after the trauma. Symptoms often mimic those of a slowly developing stroke and include a changing level of consciousness, headache, muscle weakness, personality changes, spasticity and unequal-sized pupils.

In extradural haemorrhage, the patient may report a minor head injury that produced brief unconsciousness. Subsequently, a full recovery appears to take place, but within a few hours there is a rapid deterioration into confusion, hemiparesis and unequal-sized pupils.

Treatment

Treatment consists of prompt surgery (craniotomy), following which complete recovery is likely.

Transient ischaemic attacks

Definition and aetiology

Transient ischaemic attacks (TIAs) are brief cerebral disturbances of vascular origin whose effects, by definition, last less than 24 hours (*see also* Stroke). They have the same causes as stroke, but are often associated with occlusion of the carotid artery. They may also be due to anaemia, epilepsy, hypotension, hypoglycaemia or migraine. Smoking and hypertension are particularly high-risk factors in patients who have had a stroke.

There is a ratio of TIA to stroke of about 1 to 10; the incidence of TIA is about 0.5 per 1000 population. About one in eight cases of TIA develop further to stroke within one year; 1 in 15 may develop stroke after the first year.

Symptoms

Attacks may be single or multiple. The onset is usually abrupt, and common symptoms include hemiparesis, sensory loss, speech disorders and visual disturbances. Ataxia, deafness, dysphagia, nausea and vomiting, and vertigo may also occur. Each attack usually lasts only a few minutes, and never longer than 24 hours. Unlike stroke, there is no permanent neurological damage, but an attack may warn of an impending stroke.

Treatment

Treatment comprises the administration of oral anticoagulants (BNF 2.8.2). Long-term aspirin (BNF 2.9) may be of value in some patients. Corrective surgery of the carotid artery (carotid endarterectomy) may be beneficial. Patients should be advised to avoid smoking following an attack.

4.3 Disorders of higher function

Amnesia

Definition and aetiology

Amnesia is characterised by an inability to remember information, and is a common sign of many central nervous system pathologies (e.g. Alzheimer's disease). If the lesions in brain tissue are localised, memory impairment may be limited. Severe amnesia involves much more generalised pathology and may be due to thiamine deficiency, tumours around the third ventricles, meningitis, Alzheimer's disease and severe head injuries which produce prolonged unconsciousness.

Symptoms

Impairment of short-term memory involves difficulty in remembering recent conversation, names, messages and recently read material. Severe amnesia produces extreme problems in retaining material for more than a few seconds, and even this may be lost if the patient is distracted. Severe cases commonly produce retrograde amnesia, in which memory loss of events prior to the cerebral pathology may also occur.

Treatment

Treatment consists of the management of the underlying condition. Although amnesia may resolve spontaneously, there is no recognised treatment.

Anxiety

Definition and aetiology

Anxiety is a normal response to stress or anticipated danger, and is characterised by feelings of apprehension and fear. It is considered abnormal when it is excessive, inappropriate, or without obvious cause. If anxiety occurs in response to everyday problems, it tends to become chronic with acute exacerbations. Acute anxiety to specific stimuli (e.g. spiders) is classed as a phobic state.

Anxiety is more common in women and typically occurs in early adulthood. Family history and current environmental circumstances are possible contributory factors. It is often a symptom of depressive or other psychiatric disorders (e.g. delirium, dementia and schizophrenia).

Panic attacks are acute bouts of anxiety with marked physical symptoms, usually associated with chronic anxiety. The precipitating factor can be an emotional stress (e.g. bereavement), but it may be a more trivial distressing event in the presence of chronic anxiety. The attacks can occur irregularly and unpredictably, each lasting up to several hours.

Symptoms

Central symptoms include irritability, poor memory, loss of concentration, insomnia and nightmares. These are accompanied by physical symptoms, which include tension headache, tremor, chest pain, dizziness, dyspnoea, palpitations, dry mouth, difficulty in swallowing, urinary frequency, back pain and a general feeling of weakness. The prognosis is good, provided the precipitating factor is self-limiting.

Treatment

Reassurance and explanation may be sufficient for many patients, and relaxation techniques may be beneficial. Anxiolytics (BNF 4.1.2), beta-adrenoceptor blocking drugs (BNF 4.1.2) and antidepressant drugs (BNF 4.3) have been used with varying degrees of success. Short-term treatment with antipsychotic drugs may be used in severe anxiety.

Autism

Definition

Autism is a syndrome of deviant and delayed development that usually occurs from birth; occasionally, it may develop in the second year after a period of apparently normal development. It has an incidence of 2 to 4 per 10 000 live births, and occurs more frequently in boys.

Symptoms

It is characterised by the failure to develop social relationships (e.g. lack of attachment to parents and avoidance of eye contact), by resistance to change (e.g. rituals, attachment to familiar objects, and repetitive acts), and by language and speech disorders (e.g. delayed onset of speech, total muteness and idiosyncratic use of language). In addition, there is usually mental retardation.

Treatment

Treatment consists of behaviour therapy for very severe cases and psychotherapy and special schooling for less severe cases.

Dementia

Definition and aetiology

The latest definition of dementia has eliminated the phrase 'global impairment in intellectual function'.

Dementia is 'a syndrome of progressive impairment in two or more areas of cognition . . . sufficient to interfere with work, social function or relationships in the absence of delirium or major non-organic psychiatric disorders.' It is usually chronic and progressive, and the majority of cases are irreversible. Dementia is primarily a disease of the elderly. Its incidence doubles for every five years of increased age over 65 years of age. Twenty per cent of those over 80 years of age suffer from dementia. Senile dementia usually occurs in patients over 70 years of age, is more common in women, and consists of a gradual (though sometimes rapid) and progressive decline.

It often accompanies other irreversible degenerative processes in the brain (e.g. Alzheimer's disease, arteriosclerosis, Pick's disease, multiple sclerosis or Huntington's chorea). Reversible causes include megaloblastic anaemia, hypothyroidism, heart block, alcohol and normal pressure hydrocephalus.

Pre-senile dementia is a syndrome with a slowly progressive decline, usually occurring under 60 years of age. It occurs without apparent cause, although a family history may exist. Alzheimer's disease is the most common cause of pre-senile dementia, but other causes include Pick's disease and Huntington's chorea.

Alzheimer's disease is the commonest cause of the progressive dementias and affects both men and women. Rarely, it may begin as early as the late teens or twenties. The frequency increases progressively with age, affecting about 5% of people over 65 years of age and 20% of people over 80 years of age. Formerly, patients under 65 years of age were classified as having pre-senile dementia and older patients as having senile dementia, as they were thought to be different illnesses. Clinically and pathologically, however, Alzheimer's disease and senile dementia are identical. The disease may, however, progress more rapidly in older patients, and the onset may be abrupt and associated with minor illnesses or operations.

Arteriosclerotic dementia usually occurs in the middle-aged or elderly. It is more common in men, and consists of repeated episodes of cerebral function impairment leading to a fluctuating decline. There may be evidence of arterial disease, hypertension or a history of cerebrovascular disease.

Symptoms

The onset of dementia is insidious. Initial symptoms include a decreasing ability to concentrate, memory impairment and an inability to cope with intellectual demands. This may progress to further memory loss, with thoughts becoming few and disconnected. The personality may deteriorate, leading to self-neglect, rigidity, depressive disorders and unpredictable behaviour. Emotions may become blunted, shallow or labile and incontinence may occur. There may also be symptoms of brain damage (e.g. aphasia, apraxia, agnosia or convulsions).

Treatment

Treatment consists of the management of underlying or associated conditions (e.g. depressive disorders), together with psychological and social support. Patients with potentially reversible causes of dementia require prompt treatment if permanent damage is to be avoided. Social contact with friends and relatives should be encouraged, and occupational therapy may be beneficial. In severe cases, hospitalisation may be necessary. Acetylcholinesterase drugs are used in some patients with Alzheimer's disease (BNF 4.11). Cerebral vasodilators (BNF 2.6.4) have been used in the treatment of dementia.

Self-help organisations

Alzheimer's Disease Society

Depressive disorders

Definition and aetiology

Depressive disorders are affective conditions characterised by an abnormal experience of sadness and misery, accompanied by loss of interest, a decreased capacity for enjoyment or productive work and a feeling of dejection and unworthiness. They should be distinguished from a normal response to unhappy events, physical illness or environmental stresses, which lessen with the passage of time.

Previously, depressive disorders were classified as reactive or endogenous, but this classification has now been superseded by reference to the severity of symptoms (i.e. mild, moderate or severe).

Aetiological factors in depressive disorders are varied, and include genetic predisposition, adverse childhood experiences, personality and persistent socio-economic difficulties (e.g. single parents). These factors may operate through abnormal biochemistry in brain tissue, which affects neurotransmitters (e.g. serotonin and noradrenaline).

The condition is common, with an incidence of about 2 per 1000 in men and 6 per 1000 in women. The incidence in patients experiencing physical discomfort is considerably higher, but tends to be overlooked.

Symptoms

Mild depressive disorders are characterised by apathy, low mood, lack of interest and irritability. Sleep disruption may occur through early waking or difficulty in falling asleep. Mild disorders may be characterised by anxiety, phobic states and obsession, which are commonly classified as neurotic symptoms.

Moderate depressive disorders have similar, but worsened, symptoms of lack of energy, disinterest and irritability. Speech is drone-like and slowed. The patient becomes withdrawn, and feels that everyday tasks are major obstacles. Somatic features include loss of appetite and weight, malaise, reduced libido and, in women, amenorrhoea. These symptoms may antagonise the depressive state, as patients worry that they have a serious illness.

Depressive disorders of a severe nature present with all the above symptoms, but to a greater degree. Additionally, delusions and hallucinations may occur (commonly classified as psychotic symptoms) in which guilt and persecution may be prominent. Such patients present a high risk of suicide.

Treatment

Mild cases of depressive disorders usually require only supportive treatment and behaviour therapy. Moderate to severe manifestations may require additional antidepressant drugs (BNF 4.3). Anxiolytics (BNF 4.1.2) may be used with caution in depressive states associated with agitation. Hospitalisation can be helpful in moderate cases and is often essential in severe conditions. In severe cases, electroconvulsive therapy may be indicated.

Drug dependence

Definition and aetiology

Drug dependence is a psychic, and sometimes physical, state characterised by behavioural and other responses. It always includes a compulsion to take a drug or other substance on a continuous or periodic basis in order to experience its psychic effects, and sometimes to avoid the discomfort of its absence (i.e. withdrawal symptoms).

Psychic dependence is characterised by an intense craving and compulsive need to take a drug in order to produce its pleasurable psychic effects or to avoid withdrawal symptoms. Physical dependence is an adaptive state, characterised by intense physical trauma on withdrawal of the drug, which can only be relieved by the administration of the same drug or another with similar pharmacological action. Tolerance, which may or may not be present, is the requirement to increase the dose to maintain the desired effect. Cross-tolerance between drugs may also occur, and dependence is often not restricted to one drug.

Symptoms

The psychic and physical characteristics of drug dependence vary with the type of drug, amount used, frequency of use and the route of administration.

Treatment

General measures used in the treatment of drug dependence are described below.

Alcohol-type drug dependence

Definition

Drug dependence of the alcohol-type is characterised by mild to marked psychic and physical dependence, with some tolerance to its effects. There is mutual, but incomplete, cross-tolerance between alcohol and barbiturates.

Symptoms

Alcohol-dependent patients may experience impairment of judgement, thought and psychomotor coordination, which may result in deterioration of work performance and in accidents, exhibitionism, aggressive behaviour and violence. Patients may be predisposed to physical illness, which may also arise through personal neglect. The intensity of the withdrawal symptoms, which include delirium tremens and convulsions, vary with the duration and amount of alcohol taken. They may be mild, but life-threatening symptoms may occur.

Self-help organisations

Accept Services
Al-Anon
Alcohol Concern
Alcoholics Anonymous
Alateen
Medical Council on Alcoholism
Scottish Council on Alcohol
Turning Point

Amphetamine-type drug dependence

Definition
Dependence of the amphetamine-type occurs with the amphetamines and other central nervous stimulants. It is characterised by mild to marked psychic dependence, little (if any) physical dependence and by marked tolerance.

Symptoms
Persons dependent on these drugs may be prone to accidents, aggressive behaviour and, particularly after intravenous use, to psychotic episodes involving hallucinations and delusions. There are no characteristic withdrawal symptoms, but mental and physical depression may occur.

Barbiturate-type drug dependence

Definition
Dependence of the barbiturate-type occurs with barbiturates and other sedative drugs (e.g. chloral hydrate, meprobamate and the benzodiazepines). It is characterised by mild to marked psychic and physical dependence, and substantial tolerance. There is mutual, but incomplete, cross-tolerance between these drugs and alcohol.

Symptoms
Persons dependent on these drugs may show impaired mental function, confusion, increased emotional instability and a distorted perception of time. They may also be accident-prone and violent. There may be a risk of sudden overdosage and relatively limited tolerance to the lethal dose. The intensity of the withdrawal symptoms, which include anxiety, headache, vomiting, insomnia and tachycardia, varies with the type of drug, dose, duration and method of use. They may only be mild but life-threatening symptoms (e.g. convulsions) may develop.

Cannabis-type drug dependence

Definition
Dependence of the cannabis-type is characterised by mild to moderate psychic dependence, with little (if any) physical dependence. There may be some tolerance at higher doses and acute psychotic episodes may occur. Cannabis is unusual in that it induces both hallucinogenic (at high doses) and depressant properties (at lower doses).

Symptoms
On long-term regular use, persons dependent on cannabis may show impaired psychomotor coordination and perception. There are no characteristic withdrawal symptoms.

Cocaine-type drug dependence

Definition
Cocaine-type dependence is characterised by mild to marked psychic dependence (with a strong tendency to continue administration) and no physical dependence or tolerance.

Symptoms
On long-term use, persons dependent on cocaine may show personality deterioration, unreliability and loss of self-control. High doses may precipitate a psychotic state with hallucinations and delusions, which may result in aggressive and violent behaviour. There are no characteristic withdrawal symptoms, but depressive disorders and delusions may occur.

Hallucinogen-type drug dependence

Definition
Dependence of the hallucinogen-type occurs with lysergide (LSD) and other hallucinogens (e.g. dimethyltryptamine, mescaline and psilocybin). It is characterised by mild to moderate psychic dependence and no physical dependence. The degree of tolerance (which may be marked) varies according to the drug used and cross-tolerance occurs within the group.

Symptoms
Persons dependent on hallucinogens may suffer from serious impairment of judgement. Reactions, including panic reactions to the hallucinations and delusions, may lead to accidents. There are no characteristic withdrawal symptoms, but agitation or psychotic episodes may occur.

Opiate-type drug dependence

Definition
Dependence of the opiate-type occurs with opium, morphine, diamorphine, codeine and synthetic opioid drugs (e.g. methadone and pethidine). It is characterised by moderate to marked psychic dependence and marked physical dependence and tolerance, each of which develop readily with low doses and produce cross-tolerance within the group.

Symptoms
Persons dependent on these drugs may be prone to physical neglect, malnutrition and infection. There may also be apathy, lethargy and a disruption of interpersonal relationships. These drugs produce characteristic withdrawal symptoms, which include yawning, lachrymation, rhinorrhoea, sneezing, muscle tremor, agitation and diarrhoea. The intensity of withdrawal symptoms depends on the drug, dose and method of use.

Volatile solvent-type drug dependence

Definition
Dependence of the volatile solvent-type (inhalant-type) occurs with volatile solvents (e.g. acetone or toluene, as found in some types of glue, butane and petrol) and anaesthetic agents (e.g. ether and chloroform). It is characterised by mild to moderate psychic dependence with little, if any, physical dependence. Tolerance may develop with some agents (e.g. toluene), and there is cross-tolerance between alcohol and some anaesthetic agents.

Symptoms
Persons dependent on these agents may show aggressive and violent behaviour, impaired psychomotor coordination, and may be prone to physical illness. Reactions to the hallucinations caused by the agents may lead to accidents. There are no characteristic withdrawal symptoms, but acute psychotic episodes may occur.

Treatment of drug dependence
Treatment, which is usually long term, depends on the type of dependence and includes identification of predisposing factors, drug or agent withdrawal and, in some cases, substitution. If withdrawal symptoms occur, symptomatic drug treatment may be necessary. Psychotherapy and supportive counselling may be helpful.

Self-help organisations
Alcoholics Anonymous
DrugScope
Families Anonymous
Narcotics Anonymous
Northern Ireland Community Addiction Service
Release
Re-Solv
Standing Conference on Drug Abuse
Terrence Higgins Trust
Turning Point

Epilepsy

Definition and aetiology
Epilepsy is characterised by seizures caused by recurrent paroxysmal disturbances in the electrical activity of the brain. An epileptic seizure may be defined as more than one non-febrile transitory disorder of cerebral function (seizure), usually associated with a disturbance of consciousness and accompanied by sudden excessive electrical changes in the cerebral neurons. It may be idiopathic or precipitated by an underlying disease (e.g. infection, metabolic disorders or an intracranial tumour). It may also be due to head injury or the administration of some drugs (e.g. phenothiazines) or abrupt withdrawal of antiepileptics or benzodiazepines.

The incidence of epilepsy is much higher in children under 16 years of age (700 per 100 000) than in adults (330 per 100 000). It has been estimated that there are about 50 per 100 000 new cases of epilepsy each year. Overall, it affects about 1 in 30 of the population at some time during their lives.

Treatment
Measures used in the treatment of the various forms of epilepsy are described below.

Generalised seizures

Definition and aetiology
Generalised seizures are usually characterised by a loss of, or alteration to, consciousness. This

accompanies generalised symmetrical electrical changes, which spread rapidly to all parts of the brain.

Tonic-clonic (grand mal) seizures, absence (petit mal) seizures and myoclonic seizures are examples of generalised attacks. Other types of seizure, which are generalised at the outset, include tonic seizures, clonic seizures, atonic or akinetic seizures, atypical absence seizures and infantile spasms.

Symptoms

Tonic-clonic seizures are characterised by a loss of consciousness, followed by a tonic phase in which the muscles become rigid. A characteristic cry may be heard, and there may be tongue biting and incontinence. Cyanosis may develop due to interrupted respiration. The tonic phase is followed by a clonic phase, which produces rhythmic contraction and relaxation of the limbs and trunk. A period of deep stupor and confusion precedes regaining consciousness. Headache and muscle soreness are common post-seizure symptoms. The seizures may last several minutes and can occur at any age.

Absence seizures usually begin in childhood, but rarely persist into adult life. They are characterised by very brief lapses of consciousness, which begin and end abruptly and may go unnoticed. Occasionally, there is clonic jerking of the arms, although a blank expression or fluttering of the eyelids may be the only signs.

Myoclonic seizures occur as random involuntary movements, usually involving the limbs and are frequently provoked by noise or other sensory stimuli. They may be associated with tonic-clonic or absence seizures.

Partial seizures

Definition and aetiology

Partial (focal) seizures are usually caused by a disturbance in electrical activity in a localised area (the focus) of the brain, which does not spread. Partial seizures can become generalised, and the symptoms of the partial seizure appear as an aura prior to rapid generalisation. Types of partial seizures include psychomotor (temporal lobe) epilepsy, jacksonian epilepsy and sensory epilepsy.

Psychomotor seizures may develop at any age, and are usually associated with structural lesions, often in the temporal lobe of the brain.

Symptoms

Partial seizures are characterised by a dream-like state and amnesia. Consciousness is not usually lost, and the location of the focus determines the symptoms.

Symptoms of psychomotor seizures depend on the site of the lesion. A very common initial symptom is a vague feeling of discomfort in the upper abdomen and a sense of fullness in the head. These symptoms constitute the aura, which may be experienced if the seizure becomes secondarily generalised. Other symptoms may include memory loss, disorientation, feeling of re-experiencing the environment (déjà-vu) and a sense of unreality. Initially motor activity ceases, to be replaced by simple movements (e.g. swallowing and chewing). Fear, dizziness and hallucinations may occur.

Status epilepticus

Definition and aetiology

Status epilepticus can occur with tonic-clonic seizures (tonic-clonic status), absence seizures (absence status) and psychomotor seizures (psychomotor status). It is characterised by a rapid succession of seizures without a recovery period, and may consequently be fatal unless rapidly controlled. It may be precipitated by alcohol or abrupt withdrawal of antiepileptic drugs.

Treatment of epilepsy

Treatment of all types of epilepsy consists of the administration of antiepileptics (BNF 4.8). The choice of drug is governed by the type of seizure, which is usually confirmed by reference to an electroencephalogram (EEG). Drug combinations may be needed where different types of seizure coexist, although the use of more than two antiepileptics is rarely justified. Care is required, however, in avoiding the large number of interactions that occur between individual antiepileptic drugs.

Patients should be advised to avoid any causative factors, and underlying disorders (e.g.

metabolic disorders) should be treated. Children with seizures unresponsive to antiepileptics may benefit from a ketogenic diet, and some types of seizure and refractory cases may benefit from surgery.

Withdrawal of antiepileptic drugs needs to be carried out with caution, to prevent the risk of rebound seizures. In patients receiving more than one antiepileptic drug, only one drug should be withdrawn at a time.

Status epilepticus requires immediate control with parenteral antiepileptics, and steps may be necessary to maintain the airway.

Self-help organisations

British Epilepsy Association
Epilepsy Association of Scotland
National Society for Epilepsy

Mania and manic-depressive illness

Definition and aetiology

Mania is an uncommon affective disorder, which is characterised by elation, hyperactivity, hyperirritability and delusions. Mild forms of mania are referred to as hypomania. Mania may occur as an uncomplicated disorder, but may also exist in combination with depressive disorders as a bipolar manic-depressive illness. The exact cause of mania and manic-depressive illness is unclear, but several theories exist as to their aetiology. They may arise as a result of disordered brain biochemistry, or electrolyte or endocrine disturbances. Childhood experiences or life events may also have some bearing.

Manic-depressive illness has an incidence of up to 15 per 100 000 in men and up to 30 per 100 000 in women.

Symptoms

The onset of mania is often gradual with only mild symptoms (hypomania), which may include early waking, excitement and restlessness, and loss of concentration. The patient may indulge in irrational behaviour and become sexually promiscuous. This may be followed by more severe symptoms characteristic of true mania. These include hyperactivity and hyperirritability, wild illogical speech, marked elation and delusions of grandeur. The patient may lose weight as a result of a failure to eat and may become exhausted.

In manic-depressive illness, a period of depression follows the manic phase, and this is characterised by the gradual onset of depressive symptoms.

Treatment

Antipsychotic drugs (BNF 4.2.1) may be administered for the short-term treatment of acute mania, and antimanic drugs may also be useful. Antimanic drugs (BNF 4.2.3) are also given as prophylaxis for manic-depressive illness, and electroconvulsive therapy (ECT) may be beneficial. In severe cases of mania and manic-depressive illness, hospitalisation may be necessary, and psychotherapy and occupational therapy are often employed.

Mental retardation

Definition and aetiology

Mental retardation is a state of permanent impaired intelligence, which may be present at birth or appear during the first two years of life. As a consequence of the abnormality, special care and training is required, which in severe cases must be continuous.

Prenatal causes of mental retardation include chromosome disorders (e.g. phenylketonuria), congenital infections (e.g. rubella), drugs and alcohol, maternal illness and radiation. Children born to very young mothers present a high risk of cerebral palsy, whereas children produced late in the mother's reproductive life are particularly prone to Down's syndrome.

Complications that arise at birth may also cause mental retardation. Premature and underweight babies have an increased risk, and trauma during birth (e.g. breech or high-forceps delivery) increases the likelihood of impaired mental development.

After birth, encephalitis and meningitis, lead poisoning and physical injury or asphyxiation are possible causes of mental retardation.

Children are educationally classified as having either a severe or moderate learning disability, the boundary of which form is determined by assessment of the intelligence quotient

(IQ). The incidence of moderate learning disability is up to 25 per 1000; severe learning disability occurs in between 3 and 4 per 1000. Moderately subnormal and severely subnormal children possess an IQ of 50–69 and below 50 respectively. Profound retardation is indicated by an IQ of less than 30.

Symptoms

The outward signs of mental retardation may vary significantly according to the cause of the condition. Stature and unusual head growth may be indicative of certain types of prenatal lesions. Metabolic disorders may present as a failure to thrive, lethargy, vomiting, convulsions and external manifestations (e.g. coarse facial features).

Developmental tests are used to assess children who produce no outward signs of illness, but who are apparently slow to develop. Developmental milestones (see Section 15.4) may be missed, and this may be the only outward indication of retardation.

Treatment

Most cases of mental retardation are not treatable, although the causes may be treatable to prevent their worsening. Those that are amenable to treatment often have fluctuating symptoms, and include phenylketonuria, galactosaemia, hydrocephalus and some epileptic syndromes.

Self-help organisations

Down's Syndrome Association
Leonard Cheshire Foundation
MENCAP
National Autistic Society

Phobic states

Definition

A phobic state is characterised by the emergence of inappropriate anxiety or panic attacks and morbid fear of certain objects or situations. It is usually a chronic condition, which may begin in early adulthood, with various degrees of remission and relapse. It results in the avoidance of the phobic stimulus, and anticipatory anxiety may be present before subsequent exposure to the stimulus. The condition can become disabling if the stimulus cannot be easily avoided.

Simple phobias are characterised by the presence of abnormal fear or common fears (e.g. of injections or of heights). Agoraphobia is a phobic state due to open and public places or crowds. Claustrophobia is due to confined or enclosed spaces. Other types of phobia include those of objects (e.g. spiders) or social phobias (e.g. the presence of other people or eating in public places).

Treatment

Treatment consists of behaviour therapy to condition the patient to the phobic stimulus and hypnotherapy. Drug treatment with anxiolytics (BNF 4.1.2) may be used to alleviate anticipatory anxiety and antidepressant drugs (BNF 4.3) to prevent panic attacks.

Schizophrenia

Definition and aetiology

Schizophrenia, a functional mental disorder, is the most severe form of a psychotic state with disturbance of mind and personality, but without impairment of consciousness. It may be caused by a combination of environmental and genetic factors.

Schizophrenia has an incidence of between 1 and 2 per 10 000 which, because many cases become chronic, gives an annual prevalence of about 30 per 10 000 population.

Symptoms

Two main forms of schizophrenia are recognised: acute and chronic. Symptoms of the acute form include auditory hallucinations (in which patients hear their own thoughts spoken aloud or others talking about them), thought disorders, and persecution and grandiose delusions ('positive' symptoms). Chronic episodes tend to feature 'negative' symptoms: apathy, slowness and social withdrawal. The two forms are not exclusive, and remissions and relapses commonly occur.

The diagnostic symptoms of schizophrenia are termed 'first-rank symptoms'. The occurrence of any one of these symptoms in the absence of other physical disease is strongly suggestive of schizophrenia. 'First-rank symptoms' include auditory hallucinations.

Treatment
Treatment consists of the long-term administration of antipsychotic drugs (BNF 4.2.1). In certain cases, electroconvulsive therapy (ECT) may be useful. Psychotherapy, counselling, occupational therapy and social rehabilitation and support may also be necessary.

Self-help organisations
National Schizophrenia Fellowship (NSF)
National Schizophrenia Fellowship (Scotland)
Schizophrenia Association of Great Britain

Speech disorders

Definition and aetiology
Disorders of speech indicate a derangement of higher nervous function caused by lesions at specific sites within the cerebral cortex.

Aphasia

Definition and aetiology
Aphasia (dysphasia) is the disturbance of language function caused by damage to the language centres, which are located primarily in the left cerebral hemisphere of most people, whether right- or left-handed. It is due to transient ischaemic attacks or to intracranial tumours, and may occur in children or adults.

Symptoms
Disturbances to the delivery of speech may range from complete loss to speech that is non-fluent, ungrammatical and difficult to comprehend. The presence of aphasia is frequently accompanied by writing disorders of a similar degree.

Treatment
Spontaneous recovery from aphasia may occur over a period of months. However, this happens less frequently in affected adults than in children.

Dysarthria

Definition and aetiology
Dysarthria is a disorder of speech that arises through disruption of the mechanical production of speech. The muscles that generate speech may themselves be damaged, or they may malfunction secondary to cerebral cortex damage.

Symptoms
Speech in dysarthria often contains the correct words, but they may not be understandable.

Stuttering

Definition and aetiology
Speech production may be impaired due to the disturbance of the normal sequence of muscular function in the larynx. It may be of psychogenic origin and occurs occasionally in conjunction with aphasic symptoms.

Symptoms
Stuttering is characterised by hesitation and repetition in speech delivery, which produces disjointed conversation in which words or syllables may be missing altogether.

Self-help organisations
Action for Dysphasic Adults
Association for Stammerers
British Dyslexia Association
Chest Heart and Stroke Association
Motor Neurone Disease Association

4.4 Degenerative disorders

Bell's palsy

Definition and aetiology
Bell's palsy is facial paralysis due to a lesion of the seventh cranial nerve within the facial canal. It is of unknown aetiology, of rapid onset and usually

occurs unilaterally. The nerve is inflamed, and compression within the facial canal may contribute to axonal damage. Mild cases are due to a local conduction block within the facial canal, which may be due to demyelination without axonal degeneration. In more severe cases, there may be total paralysis and axonal degeneration.

Symptoms

Paralysis usually reaches its maximum in one to two days, and may be accompanied by transient pain below the ear or in the mastoid region. Other symptoms may include dysarthria, difficulty in eating, dribbling, impairment of taste, intolerance of noise and sagging of the face. Voluntary eye closure is usually impossible, and the eye may water or be dry. Ectropion may also be present, especially in the elderly. Patients with no axonal degeneration usually recover within a few weeks. If axonal degeneration is present, recovery usually begins after about three months with regeneration, but may be incomplete or fail to occur.

Treatment

In the early stages of the condition, treatment is directed towards preventing axonal damage, and corticosteroids may be administered. Preparations for tear deficiency (BNF 11.8.1) should be used if the eye is dry, and patients are advised to protect the eye from light.

Carpal tunnel syndrome

Definition and aetiology

Carpal tunnel syndrome is compression of the median nerve within the wrist. It most commonly occurs in middle-aged women who are overweight, and is usually idiopathic. It may, however, be due to tenosynovitis of the flexor tendons after excessive or unaccustomed use of the hand or due to rheumatoid arthritis or osteoarthritis. Other predisposing factors include hypothyroidism, acromegaly, pregnancy, the menopause, oral contraceptive use and diabetic neuropathy.

Symptoms

Numbness and tingling (paraesthesia) and a burning pain in the hand, thumb, fingers and occasionally the forearm, commonly occur at night. The hand may feel useless on waking. There may also be weakness and wasting of the muscles involved and sensory loss over the tips of the affected fingers (acroparaesthesia).

Treatment

Treatment depends on the severity of the symptoms. If acroparaesthesia is the only symptom, reduced use of the hand may be all that is required. Splinting of the wrist and local corticosteroid injections may help. If symptoms persist, or if muscle weakness and wasting are present, surgical decompression of the nerve may be indicated.

Diabetic neuropathy

Definition and aetiology

Diabetic neuropathy is a peripheral neuropathy, which occurs as a complication of diabetes mellitus in up to one in six diabetics. Contributory factors include the age of the diabetic, the duration of the condition, poor diabetic control and nerve damage due to ischaemia or compression. It affects the legs and feet predominantly, but the arms and hands may also be affected.

Symptoms

Symmetrical polyneuropathy may occur, ranging from numbness to total loss of sensation, together with loss of joint-position sense, muscular pain and weakness. Dysaesthesia may occur and include feelings of numbness, compression, warm or cold, tingling, pricking or diffuse irritation. Motor neuropathy may occur, causing sudden knee and hip weakness with pain and wasting of the thigh muscles. Autonomic neuropathy involving the sympathetic ganglia may occur and result in orthostatic hypotension, diarrhoea, impotence, urinary retention and sweating at the start of a meal (gustatory sweating). Mononeuropathy may also occur (e.g. carpal tunnel syndrome).

Treatment

Drug treatment of diabetic neuropathy (BNF 6.1.5) is symptomatic. Close diabetic control may be beneficial. Patients with sensory loss should be advised about their vulnerability to injury, which may predispose the patient to infection, ulceration and gangrene.

Encephalopathy

Definition
Encephalopathy is any degenerative disease of the brain.

Dialysis encephalopathy

Definition and aetiology
Dialysis encephalopathy may occur after prolonged repeated haemodialysis, possibly as a result of high aluminium concentrations in haemodialysis solutions.

Symptoms
Symptoms include amnesia, convulsions, dementia, somnolence and speech disorders.

Treatment
Treatment consists of reducing the aluminium concentration of haemodialysis solutions, withdrawing oral aluminium preparations, or both.

Hepatic encephalopathy

Definition and aetiology
Hepatic encephalopathy is a neurological syndrome, which occurs as a result of advanced liver disease. It may be due to the toxic effects of substances (e.g. ammonia) normally metabolised by the liver.

Symptoms
It is characterised by altered consciousness and may result in coma (hepatic coma). Other symptoms include anxiety, ataxia, mania, speech disorders, somnolence, tremor and rigidity.

Treatment
Treatment comprises the withdrawal of dietary protein and the administration of lactulose (BNF 1.6.4) and neomycin (BNF 5.1.4).

Hypertensive encephalopathy

Definition and aetiology
Hypertensive encephalopathy consists of a group of neurological symptoms associated with severe hypertension.

Symptoms
It is characterised by severe headache, convulsions, and nausea and vomiting. Stupor and coma may follow.

Treatment
Urgent treatment is essential, and involves the reduction of blood pressure. Antiepileptic drugs (BNF 4.8) may be required.

Guillain-Barré syndrome

Definition and aetiology
Guillain-Barré syndrome (acute idiopathic inflammatory polyneuropathy) is characterised by proximal, distal or generalised polyneuropathy, with inflammation, oedema and demyelination of the affected nerves. It is idiopathic, but many cases follow viral infection or surgery.

Symptoms
Motor nerves are predominantly affected, usually starting distally and slowly ascending, resulting in paralysis of all limbs and loss of tendon reflexes. In severe cases facial, trunk and respiratory muscles may be involved. Sensory nerve involvement may result in touch, vibratory and postural sensory loss. There may also be autonomic involvement.

Treatment
Treatment is supportive and may include assisted ventilation. Patients usually recover within weeks or months, but recovery may be prolonged in severe cases and muscle weakness may remain.

Motor neuron disease

Definition and aetiology
Motor neuron disease is a rare, progressive, degenerative disorder of the motor neurons, which occurs most commonly in middle-age. Its cause is unknown.

Symptoms
Symptoms include muscle wasting and weakness in the hands and arms, and spasticity of the legs. Muscle cramps, occasionally with pain, may

occur. Dysphagia and speech disorders are also common. There is no sensory loss. The disease is always fatal and death usually occurs within three to five years of the onset.

Treatment

No treatment is known.

Self-help organisations

Motor Neurone Disease Association
Scottish Motor Neurone Disease Association

Multiple sclerosis

Definition and aetiology

Multiple sclerosis (disseminated sclerosis) is characterised by patches of demyelination of nerves within the central nervous system, including the optic nerves. The axons are initially unaffected, but in later stages axonal degeneration occurs. The peripheral nervous system is not affected. It is of unknown aetiology, has a peak onset around 30 years of age, and is usually chronic.

Its course is highly variable and unpredictable, and remissions and relapses are common. After an initial attack there may be complete recovery, but subsequent relapses may lead to a progressive decline. It may also be chronically progressive from onset, especially in older patients.

Symptoms

The presence and severity of symptoms is variable and depends on the sites of the lesions. Initial symptoms may include weakness in one or both legs, dysarthria, loss of coordination and sensory loss, visual disturbances due to retrobulbar neuritis and vertigo. Other symptoms include nystagmus, ataxia, tremor, facial twitching, dementia, muscle spasms of the limbs, urgency of micturition, incontinence and impotence. Trigeminal neuralgia may occur in younger patients. Symptoms tend to worsen with small increases in body temperature (e.g. during fever and hot baths), fatigue or exertion. In advanced stages, and in conjunction with a variety of other disabilities, patients may become confined to a wheelchair or require full nursing care, or both. Complications (e.g. urinary-tract infection, decubitus ulcers and coma) may be fatal.

Treatment

No special treatment exists. Corticosteroids (BNF 6.3.2), corticotrophin (BNF 6.5.1) and immunosuppressants (BNF 8.2) have been used to treat acute relapses and delay progression. Skeletal muscle relaxants (BNF 10.2.2) are used to treat muscular spasm. Interferon beta is approved for relapsing, remitting multiple sclerosis in those patients who are able to walk unaided. Its objective is to reduce the frequency and severity of clinical relapses.

Patients should be advised to avoid fatigue, and physiotherapy may be beneficial early in the course of the disease. Incontinence aids may benefit some patients.

Syringomyelia and syringobulbia

Definition and aetiology

Syringomyelia is the occurrence of a tubular fluid-filled cavity (the syrinx) in the spinal cord, often in the cervical region. It is termed syringobulbia when the brain stem is involved. It is thought to be a congenital disorder, although symptoms do not usually develop until early adulthood.

Symptoms

Symptoms of syringomyelia include sensory loss in the hands (which also become wasted) and lower limb spasticity. Syringobulbia is characterised by atrophy of the tongue, dysphagia, speech disorders, deafness, vertigo, nystagmus and sensory loss over the face. Sensory loss may become widespread. Symptoms may be mild and stable, but may become progressive and rapidly deteriorate.

Treatment

Treatment is by surgical decompression.

4.5 Extrapyramidal disorders

Chorea

Definition and aetiology

Chorea is characterised by brief involuntary muscle contractions. It results in a continuous series of irregular jerky movements, which move rapidly from one part of the body to another at random. It may be due to an underlying disorder or to certain drugs (e.g. antipsychotic drugs and phenytoin). Hemichorea affects only one side of the body.

Huntington's chorea

Definition and aetiology
Huntington's chorea is a rare (incidence of 1 in 20 000), dominantly inherited, progressive disease characterised by chorea and dementia.

Symptoms
There is general brain damage and atrophy, with extensive neuronal loss. Onset is insidious and usually occurs between 30 and 50 years of age. Initial symptoms include personality disorders (e.g. loss of drive and irritability), followed by progressive dementia and chorea. Severe depression is common. In advanced stages, the chorea may be slowed due to the development of rigidity and akinesia. The patient finally becomes bedridden and death eventually follows.

Treatment
No specific treatment exists. Antipsychotic drugs (BNF 4.2.1) administered in doses that are increased until the chorea is controlled or drug-induced parkinsonism is disabling. Permanent hospitalisation is almost inevitable, and family support may be required.

Sydenham's chorea

Definition and aetiology
Sydenham's chorea (St. Vitus' dance) is a rare disease characterised by chorea and psychological disturbances and accompanied by inflammatory encephalitis. As it commonly occurs up to six months after rheumatic fever, the decline in rheumatic fever has led to a corresponding decline in Sydenham's chorea.

Symptoms
Onset is frequently insidious and usually occurs between 7 and 12 years of age. It may recur in later life, especially in pregnant women and in those taking oral contraceptives. Initial symptoms include psychological disturbances (e.g. irritability, agitation and inattentiveness), followed by a generalised chorea resulting in difficulty in walking and handling objects, and impaired speech. In severe cases, flaccidity and weakness may also be present.

Treatment
The condition is self-limiting, but drug treatment for chorea (BNF 4.9.3) may be necessary, in conjunction with bed rest. Antibacterial prophylaxis may be necessary to prevent recurrence of rheumatic fever.

Parkinsonism

Definition and aetiology
Parkinsonism is a syndrome commonly caused by Parkinson's disease (paralysis agitans), a progressive disorder of insidious onset which usually begins between 50 and 65 years of age. In the majority of cases, there is no definable cause (idiopathic parkinsonism), although it may be due to poisoning with carbon monoxide, manganese or other metals, brain tumours in the basal ganglia, cerebral trauma, degenerative diseases, or following encephalitis (post-encephalitic parkinsonism). Drug-induced parkinsonism may also occur (e.g. following administration of antipsychotic drugs).

In Parkinson's disease, there are degenerative changes with loss of cells in the substantia nigra and basal ganglia. There may also be degenerative changes in the brain stem or cranial nerve nuclei, or atrophy of the cerebral cortex. Depletion of the neurotransmitter dopamine results in an imbalance between the cholinergic and dopaminergic neurons in the extrapyramidal system.

It is a common disorder, with an incidence of 1 in 1000, which increases with increasing age to 1 in 200 in the elderly.

Symptoms
Parkinsonism is characterised by tremor, muscular rigidity, loss of postural reflexes and akinesia (with hypokinesia and bradykinesia). The patient has a mask-like expression and a monotonous voice, and may experience fatigue, drooling of saliva, dysphagia, constipation and excessive sweating. Speech disorders and depressive disorders are common.

Treatment

Treatment consists of the administration of dopaminergic drugs (BNF 4.9.1), antimuscarinic drugs (BNF 4.9.2), or both. Drug-induced parkinsonism, however, may only be treated with antimuscarinic drugs, and remission often occurs on withdrawal of the causative drug. Physical therapy and aids may also be useful.

A high level of physical activity is recommended to prevent the worsening of rigidity and akinesia.

Tardive dyskinesia

Definition and aetiology

Tardive dyskinesia is a chronic movement disorder usually associated with antipsychotic drug treatment. It is characterised by repetitive uncontrollable movements, occurring most noticeably on the face and upper trunk.

It occurs most commonly in women, the elderly, and in those with brain injury. Although it is usually precipitated by antipsychotic therapy, symptoms may persist after treatment has stopped. It is thought to be associated with increased sensitivity of dopaminergic receptors as a consequence of their constant blockade by antipsychotics.

Symptoms

Symptoms appear usually after at least six months dosage with antipsychotics, and their onset may be associated with a reduction or cessation of dosage. The most apparent signs are continuous chewing movements, lip smacking and continual darting of the tongue from the mouth. Body-rocking and incessant movement of the fingers and toes also occur. 'Marching in place' may appear as a result of repetitive movement of the legs. The most distressing symptom described is the feeling that the person is about to jump out of his skin. Anticholinergic drug administration aggravates the symptoms.

Treatment

Re-introduction of the antipsychotic drug (BNF 4.2.1) may ameliorate symptoms, although in some cases paradoxical worsening of the condition may occur. Reserpine and clonazepam have been found useful in some patients.

Tics

Definition and aetiology

A simple tic is a rapid, involuntary, twitching movement which is repetitive and occurs at the same site, usually the face or shoulders. They commonly occur in childhood and are usually self-limiting (transient tics of childhood) but may persist into adult life. Such tics are rarely considered abnormal (chronic simple tics), but may become severe and be associated with a psychological disorder (complex tics).

Gilles de la Tourette syndrome

Definition and aetiology

Gilles de la Tourette syndrome is a chronic disorder characterised by multiple tics and involuntary verbal manifestations. It is idiopathic, but may be due to organic disease of the central nervous system.

Symptoms

Typical onset is before 15 years of age. Initial symptoms include blinking, nodding, sniffing or stuttering, but other tics may appear. Involuntary noises (e.g. grunting or barking) subsequently develop and are commonly transformed into swear-words (coprolalia). Patients may also repeat words spoken to them (echolalia), words spoken by them (palilalia), and may indulge in obscene gesturing (copropraxia) or imitation of the movement of others (echopraxia).

Treatment

Treatment consists of the administration of antipsychotic drugs (BNF 4.2.1) to control the symptoms.

4.6 Anatomy and physiology of the nervous system

Introduction

The nervous system is the medium through which the body experiences changes in the internal and external environments, and coordinates the responses made to these changes. It may be classified anatomically into two major components. The central nervous system (CNS) comprises the brain and spinal cord, and the peripheral nervous system is made up of the nerves and ganglia throughout the rest of the body.

Functionally, the nervous system may also be classified as the somatic (voluntary) nervous system, which receives impulses from skeletal muscles, ligaments, bone, eye, ear and skin and returns impulses to skeletal muscles; and the autonomic (involuntary) nervous system (ANS), which coordinates the activities of heart muscle, smooth muscle and glands and therefore the major organs of the body. The autonomic nervous system comprises the sympathetic and parasympathetic divisions. Most visceral organs are innervated by both components. In general, stimulation of the sympathetic division produces responses that prepare the body for an emergency (e.g. increased cardiac output, increased blood pressure and bronchodilatation), while stimulation of the parasympathetic division produces opposing actions. Autonomic nervous system function is regulated by the relative activity of the two divisions.

The brain is the highly developed outgrowth of the spinal cord, which is contained within and protected by the cranium. The brain stem connects the spinal cord to the two cerebral hemispheres, and is divided into the medulla, midbrain and pons. The cerebellum is closely linked anatomically to the brain stem. It consists of two hemispheres connected by a central mass, the vermis.

The cerebral hemispheres

The two cerebral hemispheres develop as the enlarged outgrowths of the brain stem. On continued evolutionary development, the outermost surfaces of the two hemispheres have become highly convoluted, and this distinguishes gross human brain structure from that in other animals. The folds (gyri) in the outer surface of the cerebral hemispheres produce deep fissures and more shallow sulci. In the hemispheres, the grey matter containing cell bodies overlies white matter formed of tracts of nervous tissue, whereas in the brain stem and spinal cord, the reverse is true. The two cerebral hemispheres are connected by a tract of white matter, the corpus callosum.

The cortical surfaces of the cerebral hemispheres are divided into four main regions, and each region has distinct sensory or motor functions. The sensory cortex comprises the parietal lobe (e.g. concerned with sensations of touch) and the occipital lobe (which contains the visual cortex). The temporal lobe is also largely concerned with sensory input, converting and interpreting the information received. The frontal lobe of the cerebral cortex is the main site of motor control (e.g. affecting the movements of the hands and facial muscles) (Figure 4.2).

The cranial nerves

Information is transmitted to and from the brain via the spinal cord and the 12 pairs of cranial nerves. Ten pairs of cranial nerves originate in the underside of the brain stem, and innervate primarily the head and neck. They are numbered with Roman numerals according to the order in which they arise from brain tissue. The nerves may be sensory (e.g. the optic (II) nerve); exhibit a mixture of sensory and motor functions (e.g. the vagus (X) nerve and the trigeminal (V) nerve); or mixed, but primarily motor (e.g. the oculomotor (III) nerve).

Cerebrospinal fluid

Brain tissue is very soft and easily traumatised. In order to reduce potential damage, it floats in cerebrospinal fluid (CSF) located between two of the three membranes (the meninges), which encase the brain and spinal cord. CSF is also found in the spaces, the ventricles, within the brain. The outermost meningeal membrane (the dura mater) lies immediately inside the cranium and acts as the main buffer against movement of the brain within the skull. It also protects the delicate brain tissue from the comparatively rough inner surface of the skullbone. Immediately inside the dura mater is the arachnoid membrane. The space between the arachnoid membrane and the third membrane (the pia mater) is termed the subarachnoid space, and contains CSF. The pia mater is a thin highly vascularised membrane,

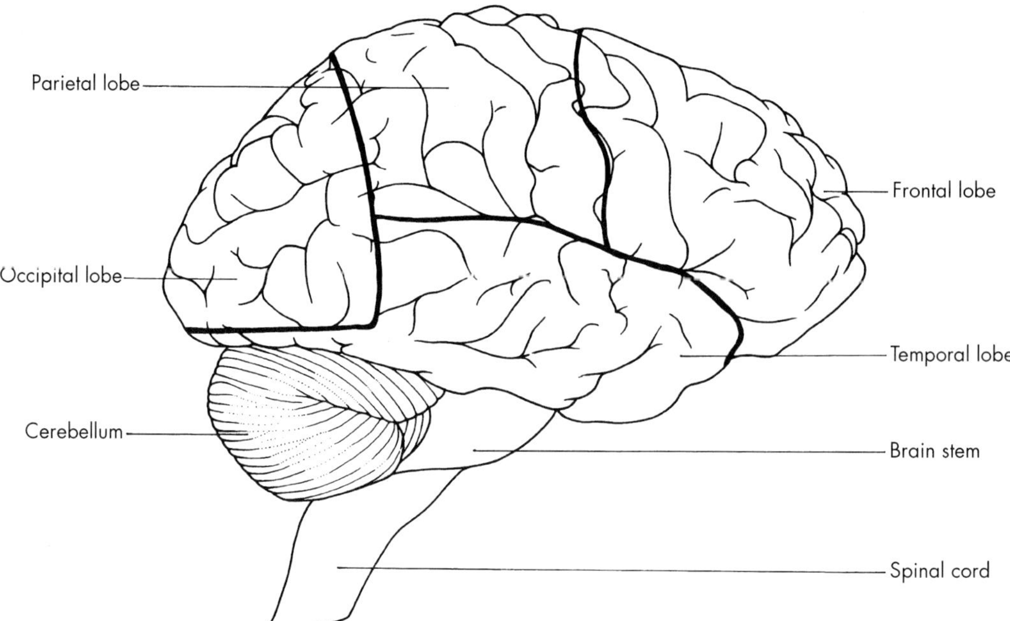

Figure 4.2 Brain (lateral view).

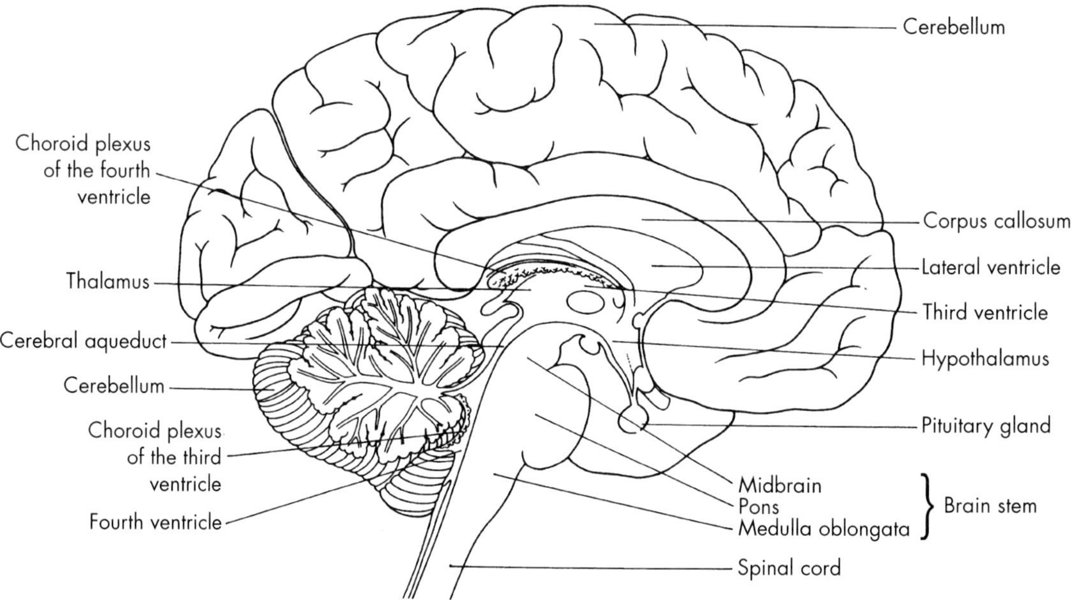

Figure 4.3 Brain (sagittal section).

which closely follows all the contours of the convoluted brain surface.

CSF is produced by projections of the pia mater (the choroid plexuses) within the hemispheres, which are located on the ventricles (Figure 4.3). From here, it passes sequentially to the third and fourth ventricles. The CSF reaches the subarachnoid space through small holes in the roof of the fourth ventricle, and is distributed around the brain and spinal cord.

The extrapyramidal system

The extrapyramidal system is one of the functional components involved in the control of movement in the body initiated by the motor cortex. The system comprises the basal ganglia, which lie deep within the cerebral hemispheres, and the upper portion of the brain stem. These interconnected masses of grey matter include the substantia nigra, the putamen, globus pallidus and the caudate nucleus. Information received by these centres is passed to the extrapyramidal tract, from where it proceeds down the spinal cord to the effector muscle.

The blood supply to the brain

The brain is a prolific metabolic organ, which uses a disproportionate amount of oxygen and glucose in relation to its size. The maintenance of an adequate blood supply to the brain to provide these nutrients is vital. Deficiencies for periods of as short as one or two minutes may result in unconsciousness, and permanent brain damage may result from an interruption of four minutes or longer.

Blood reaches the brain from the aorta via the brachiocephalic artery and the carotid artery. On the underside of the brain surface, the left and right carotid arteries join the basilar artery to form a circular arterial network called the circle of Willis, from which the arteries supplying the brain arise. The circle of Willis also equalises the pressure of blood supplied to the brain from different arteries, and enables alternative blood supply pathways to be adopted in the event of arterial damage.

5

Infections

5.1 Infections of non-specific origin

Dysentery

Definition and aetiology

Dysentery is a serious form of diarrhoea accompanied by the passage of blood and mucus. It is due to infection and inflammation of the colonic mucous membranes, resulting in ulceration. It is commonly caused by amoebiasis (amoebic dysentery), in which the infecting organism is *Entamoeba histolytica*, or shigellosis (bacillary dysentery), which is caused by *Shigella dysenteriae* (*see* Section 5.2). Amoebic dysentery is common in the tropics but rare in temperate climates.

Symptoms

Common symptoms include abdominal pain, colic, tenesmus, and the frequent passage of soft or watery stools containing blood and mucus. Vomiting may occur, and there may be a slight fever. In severe prolonged cases, patients may become emaciated and debilitated. Dehydration may be life-threatening, particularly in infants, the elderly and malnourished individuals, and perforation and peritonitis may occasionally occur.

Treatment

Dehydration should be prevented or treated by administration of oral or intravenous fluids (BNF 9.2.1). All patients with amoebiasis should be treated by administration of amoebicides (BNF 5.4.2), but only severe cases of shigellosis require specific antibacterial therapy (BNF 5.1, table 1).

Infective arthritis

Definition and aetiology

Infective arthritis (septic arthritis) is arthritis which occurs as a result of infection of a joint and associated tissues. It may occur in a previously healthy or already diseased joint. The involvement of only one or a limited number of joints (and in particular if only one joint is affected) suggests an infective cause. Patients with existing rheumatoid arthritis, especially those receiving corticosteroid therapy, are particularly at risk. Infective arthritis is often transmitted via the circulation from some primary infection, but it may also occur following joint surgery or an intra-articular injection. The infection is commonly caused by *Staphylococcus aureus*, but other microorganisms (e.g. *Haemophilus influenzae*) may be responsible, especially in children under two years of age.

Symptoms

The onset is usually marked by an acutely painful joint, which becomes hot, stiff and swollen. The infection can affect weight-bearing joints, especially the knee in adults. Fever and rigors can develop and, in the absence of treatment, joint destruction may occur.

Treatment

Treatment consists of the prompt administration of an appropriate antibacterial drug (BNF 5.1, table 1). Aspiration or surgical drainage of the joint may be indicated, and immobilisation (i.e. splinting) may be necessary. Physiotherapy is often beneficial in restoring joint function after recovery.

Infective endocarditis

Definition and aetiology

Infective endocarditis is a rare infection of the endocardium, with between 1000 and 2000 cases each year in the UK. The condition commonly occurs in the elderly. It causes vegetation and inflammation of the heart chambers or, more commonly, the heart valves. It may be acute or subacute. It usually occurs as a result of bacterial infection, with streptococci or staphylococci accounting for more than 80% of all cases. Streptococcal infection commonly derives from dental procedures (e.g. extraction and de-scaling). Fungi may also be responsible. It may arise in the presence of existing cardiac lesions (e.g. rheumatic or congenital heart disease or mitral valve prolapse) or of prosthetic heart valves; or it may occur in the absence of underlying heart disease. It may also develop as a consequence of the intravenous abuse of drugs.

Symptoms

The symptoms of acute infective endocarditis are severe and rapid in onset. The subacute form commonly develops insidiously, usually in patients with acquired or congenital heart disease. Such patients may suffer non-specific chronic ill-health. The symptoms are, however, similar for both forms of the disease and both may be fatal if untreated. Characteristic symptoms are fever, embolisms and heart murmurs. Other symptoms may include malaise, arthralgia, congestive heart failure, petechial and ophthalmic haemorrhages, renal impairment with haematuria, and splenomegaly. Meningitis is a possible complication. Confusion and memory loss may occur, particularly in the elderly.

Treatment

Treatment comprises the intravenous administration of antibacterial drugs (BNF 5.1, table 1). Surgery may be necessary in unresponsive cases. Antibacterial prophylaxis (BNF 5.1, table 2) is indicated in susceptible patients undergoing dental, gastrointestinal or genito-urinary procedures.

Meningitis

Definition and aetiology

Meningitis is inflammation of the meninges, which comprise the dura mater, pia mater and arachnoid membranes. It may be caused by bacterial, fungal or viral infection, cerebral abscess, demyelinating disorders and malignant diseases.

Pyogenic meningitis

Definition and aetiology

Pyogenic meningitis is caused by pyogenic microorganisms and usually results from bacterial infection of the upper respiratory tract, lungs, middle ear or nasopharynx. Microorganisms commonly involved include *Streptococcus pneumoniae* (pneumococcus), *Neisseria meningitidis* (meningococcus, *see* Meningococcal infections, Section 5.2) and *Haemophilus influenzae* type B.

Symptoms

Onset is usually rapid and characterised by fever, headache, vomiting, neck stiffness, rigors and delirium. Other symptoms may include sensorineural deafness, facial palsy and loss of consciousness. In meningococcal infections, there is usually an associated rash.

Treatment
Treatment consists of the identification of the infecting microorganism and appropriate parenteral antibacterial therapy (BNF 5.1, table 1). Fluid and electrolytes may be necessary (BNF 9.2). Symptomatic treatment may be necessary for headache, restlessness or convulsions.

Tuberculous meningitis

Definition and aetiology
Tuberculous meningitis is a secondary infection of the meninges resulting from infection elsewhere, usually the chest, by *Mycobacterium tuberculosis* (*see also* Tuberculosis, Section 5.2). The disease is a major problem in developing countries, but its incidence has fallen in developed nations in line with the decline in the incidence of tuberculosis. Most cases are in young children. The spread of human immunodeficiency virus has recently led to an increase in the occurrence of tuberculosis and consequently tuberculous meningitis.

Symptoms
It is usually insidious in onset with a prodrome of mild fever, general malaise and loss of appetite that can last from two to eight weeks. This is followed by headache, vomiting and stiff neck, and more severe symptoms which may include ocular and facial palsy, deafness, stupor and coma. Convulsions may occur in later stages. Raised intracranial pressure manifests itself by increased headache, vomiting and impairment of consciousness. Hydrocephalus may also develop.

Treatment
If untreated, death is inevitable. Antituberculous drugs (BNF 5.1.9), fluid and electrolytes (BNF 9.2), and symptomatic treatment of convulsions is necessary.

Viral meningitis

Definition and aetiology
Viral meningitis is commonly due to enteroviruses or mumps virus.

Symptoms
Symptoms of viral meningitis start suddenly, with headache and neck stiffness. Other symptoms may include back pain, myalgia, retro-orbital pain, pain on lateral movement of the eyes, fever, vomiting, anorexia, lassitude and photophobia.

Treatment
There is no specific treatment, but symptomatic treatment for headache, pain and fever may be required. Viral meningitis is self-limiting and usually results in complete recovery. Lumbar puncture is required to differentiate viral from bacterial infection.

Paronychia

Definition and aetiology
Paronychia is an infection of the nail fold and may be acute or chronic. *Staphylococcus aureus*, usually the offending microorganism in the acute form, penetrates the skin at a site of local trauma. The chronic condition is generally of fungal origin, most often due to *Candida albicans*. Chronic infection occurs in people whose hands are frequently or for prolonged periods immersed in water, as the microorganism gains entry through the macerated and damaged cuticle. Absent or poor nail manicuring, and nail-biting are also frequent causes.

Symptoms
The symptoms of acute paronychia are usually more severe than in the chronic form. It is characterised by a painful red swelling of the nail fold, and in some cases a purulent exudate. A similar, although less painful, lesion occurs in chronic paronychia, and may spread to other fingers with loss of the cuticle. If the condition persists untreated, the nail matrix may become infected, resulting in a deformed and discoloured nail body. Occasionally, the microorganism may directly attack the nail body. The condition may be complicated by acute attacks due to secondary bacterial infection.

Treatment
The hands should be kept dry for as long as is possible. Treatment consists of the local application of an appropriate anti-infective skin preparation (BNF 13.10), or a skin disinfectant and cleanser (BNF 13.11). A systemic antibacterial

drug (BNF 5.1) or antifungal drug (BNF 5.2) may be indicated. Surgical removal of the nail body is occasionally necessary in chronic cases where it has become directly infected.

Pneumonia

Definition and aetiology

Pneumonia is inflammation of the lungs with the production of exudate, which enters the alveoli, causing consolidation. The lesions may be localised and confined to a complete lobe (lobar) or lobule (segmented or lobular). Diffuse lesions affect the bronchi and bronchioles (bronchopneumonia) causing consolidation in adjacent lobules. The distribution may be unilateral or bilateral. Most cases of pneumonia are due to infection with bacteria. Some bacteria are capable of invading normal lung, whereas others can only invade the lung when resistance to infection is lowered (opportunistic infection). Common microorganisms which cause pneumonia include *Streptococcus pneumoniae* (the pneumococcus), *Staphylococcus pyogenes* and *Klebsiella pneumoniae*. Infections due to *Mycoplasma* and *Chlamydia* species and *Legionella pneumophila* are less common. Pneumonia may also be caused by viruses, fungi, protozoa (e.g. *Pneumocystis carinii*), chemical or physical irritants, or allergic reactions in the lung.

Pneumonia is one of the leading causes of death in the community, with 30 000 fatalities in England and Wales in 1991. There is a high mortality rate for those admitted to hospital with pneumonia, with up to a 50% rate for the bacterial form of the disease. Pneumonia affects up to three times as many men as women.

Symptoms

Common symptoms include cough, dyspnoea with tachypnoea, chest pain, purulent sputum production (initially scanty), haemoptysis and diminished chest movements on the affected side. There is fever with rigors, and other symptoms of systemic infection (e.g. insomnia, headache, delirium and weakness). Complications of pneumonia include pleural effusion, empyema, lung abscess, spontaneous pneumothorax, pericarditis and meningitis.

Non-respiratory symptoms can be the presenting feature: abdominal pain, rigidity and ileus may all occur. There is also mental confusion in advanced cases of pneumonia.

Treatment

Treatment consists of bed rest, and the administration of oral (BNF 9.2.1) or intravenous fluids (BNF 9.2.2) and appropriate antibacterial drugs. Oxygen therapy and regular physiotherapy may be necessary. A vaccine is available to provide protection against pneumococcal pneumonia. The outlook for treatment depends upon the causative organism and the general state of health of the patient. Bacteraemia is a particularly bad sign, with a death rate of up to one in three.

Salpingitis

Definition and aetiology

Salpingitis is infection of the Fallopian tubes. It is usually bilateral and occurs predominantly in young, sexually active women. It may be gonococcal, or due to infection with a non-gonococcal microorganism (e.g. *Chlamydia trachomatis* or *Mycoplasma hominis*), enteric anaerobic microorganisms, or viruses. Rarely, salpingitis may result from tuberculosis. Non-gonococcal salpingitis may be associated with minor gynaecological procedures, abortion, childbirth, previous pelvic inflammatory disease or intra-uterine contraceptive devices, but frequently no factors are found.

Symptoms

Salpingitis is characterised by constant lower abdominal pain and tenderness. Vomiting, low back pain and profuse vaginal discharge may also be present. Symptoms are usually more severe and abrupt when the infection is gonococcal and fever is often present. Complications include generalised pelvic inflammatory disease (e.g. peritonitis), pyosalpinx, tubal abscess, hydrosalpinx, pelvic abscess, infertility or reduced fertility, increased incidence of ectopic pregnancy, dyspareunia and perihepatitis. Recurrent cases may also occur. These complications are more common in patients with non-gonococcal salpingitis.

Treatment

Treatment consists of bed rest, hospitalisation in severe cases, and administration of high doses of penicillins (BNF 5.1.1) for gonococcal infections or oral tetracyclines (BNF 5.1.3) for non-gonococcal salpingitis. Fluid and electrolytes (BNF 9.2) may be necessary.

Septicaemia

Definition and aetiology

Septicaemia (blood poisoning) is an acute and serious clinical condition arising as a result of the presence in the bloodstream of pathogenic microorganisms or their toxins. Any microorganism may be responsible, either singly or with others, and will have originated from an existing focus of infection (e.g. appendicitis, cellulitis, cholecystitis, infection of the gastrointestinal or genito-urinary tracts, pelvic inflammatory disease, pneumonia, or decubitus ulceration). Indwelling urinary catheters, intravenous lines and surgical wounds may also provide points of entry in hospitalised patients.

Individuals most at risk of developing septicaemia are the elderly, malnourished, alcoholics, and those suffering from severe burns and with debilitating diseases (e.g. cirrhosis of the liver or diabetes mellitus).

Symptoms

The onset is abrupt (particularly if due to Gram-negative microorganisms) and is marked by chills, fever, diarrhoea, and nausea and vomiting. There may be prior warning signs, which include apprehension, diminished consciousness, lethargy and tachypnoea; further symptoms are hypotension and prostration. Secondary infections may arise in any organ and hypotension may cause heart failure, jaundice, or renal complications due to inadequate perfusion of vital organs. Death due to septic shock (*see below*) may be the final outcome.

Treatment

The prognosis is dependent on the virulence of the infecting microorganism, the age of the patient, other predisposing factors, and the speed with which treatment is started. The source of sepsis should be removed or drained where possible, and high-dose, intravenous, 'blind' antibacterial therapy (BNF 5.1, table 1) initiated until the causative microorganism(s) has been identified. Large volume intravenous infusions may be required to restore normal blood pressure. Additional supportive measures may be necessary to manage underlying disorders and organ failure.

Septicaemia may be prevented in hospitals by strictly adhering to the rules for aseptic procedure at all times and closely monitoring those most at risk.

Septic shock

Definition and aetiology

Septic shock is acute circulatory failure arising as a result of septicaemia (*see above*). It is most often caused by endotoxin-releasing Gram-negative bacteria, although Gram-positive infections are more likely to produce complications at sites distant from the causative infection.

It occurs most frequently in hospitalised patients, particularly in the newborn, elderly, or those with an underlying debilitating disorder. Patients receiving antimicrobials, corticosteroids or cytotoxic drugs are also at risk.

Symptoms

The initial symptoms are as for septicaemia, with progression to shock as toxins in the blood activate a series of reactions, which include the complement and blood clotting systems. Disseminated intravascular coagulation, metabolic acidosis, and poor perfusion may all contribute to end organ damage. Complications (e.g. adult respiratory distress syndrome, heart failure and renal failure) may occur.

Treatment

The prognosis is poor once shock has developed, and mortality may be as high as 50–90% if early therapy is not available. Antimicrobial therapy and preventive measures are as for septicaemia; supportive measures are described under shock (*see* Circulatory failure, Section 2.1).

Tonsillitis

Definition and aetiology

Tonsillitis is inflammation of the tonsils, which may be due to streptococcal or viral infection. It is most common in children and young adults and is usually transmitted by droplets or dust, especially in crowded or poorly ventilated conditions. It may be acute or chronic.

Symptoms

Acute tonsillitis, which is sudden in onset, is characterised by marked soreness of the throat, with pain and difficulty on swallowing. It may also be accompanied by pharyngitis. The tonsils become red and swollen and a purulent tonsillar exudate may be present. Fever, headache and malaise are common, and arthralgia and myalgia may develop. Rare complications include acute glomerulonephritis and rheumatic fever. A peritonsillar abscess (quinsy) may develop and is characterised by a marked increase in pain and fever. Repeated acute attacks may result in the development of chronic tonsillitis.

Treatment

Treatment includes bed rest and the administration of plenty of fluids. If a virus is responsible, treatment is symptomatic. A penicillin (BNF 5.1.1), given for about 10 days, may be beneficial in the presence of streptococcal infection. If an abscess forms, surgical drainage is essential. In chronic cases, tonsillectomy may be necessary, especially when the symptoms are removed only temporarily by antibiotic treatment.

Urinary-tract infections

Definition and aetiology

Urinary-tract infection (UTI) may be present at any level of the urinary tract, i.e. urethra (urethritis), bladder (cystitis), prostate (prostatitis), ureters or the kidney (pyelonephritis). The infection is usually characterised by bacteriuria with symptoms of urinary-tract inflammation, although these symptoms are not a reliable guide to the exact location of the infection. The infection may be acute, chronic or recurrent. Most UTIs are caused by Gram-negative bacteria, and common infecting microorganisms include *Escherichia coli*, and species of *Proteus* (especially *P. mirabilis*) and *Pseudomonas*. Occasionally *Klebsiella* spp. are involved. Gram-positive microorganisms include *Staphylococcus* and *Streptococcus* spp.; infection with *Staph. saprophyticus* is especially common in women.

Urinary-tract infection is common in women, particularly following sexual intercourse, and in both sexes on urinary catheterisation. Any increase in the residual bladder urine volume predisposes to the development of UTI.

Symptoms

Symptoms are usually confined to the lower urinary tract. They include urinary frequency and urgency, dysuria, and occasionally haematuria. Asymptomatic infection may also occur, especially in pregnancy.

Urethritis

Definition and aetiology

Urethritis is an inflammation of the urethra, and can be gonococcal or non-specific (non-gonococcal). In both cases, transmission is by sexual intercourse. Although no infecting microorganism can be detected, it is commonly attributed to species of *Chlamydia*, *Trichomonas*, *Corynebacterium*, and rarely *Mycobacterium*. Herpes simplex virus may also be responsible. An attack of non-specific urethritis may be precipitated by a large intake of alcohol.

Symptoms

Urethritis is characterised by dysuria and frequency, and accompanied by a mucopurulent urethral or vaginal discharge, or both. Inflammation of the urinary meatus may occur in men, and cervicitis or vaginitis in women. Complications include cystitis, epididymitis, prostatitis, salpingitis and urethral stricture. Reiter's disease, in which urethritis is accompanied by arthritis and conjunctivitis, may develop in a few patients.

Treatment

Treatment is by the avoidance of sexual intercourse and alcohol, and the administration of a tetracycline (BNF 5.1.3) or other appropriate antimicrobial.

Cystitis

Definition and aetiology
Cystitis is inflammation of the bladder and may be acute or chronic. Acute attacks may occur in isolation with no indication of the underlying cause; alternatively they may be the precursors of chronic infection.

Symptoms
Symptoms include dysuria and frequency, fever, haematuria, malaise and suprapubic pain.

Treatment
Treatment is similar to that described under Pyelonephritis (*see below*).

Pyelonephritis

Acute pyelonephritis is an acute, sometimes pyogenic, infection resulting in inflammation of the pelvis and parenchyma of one or both kidneys. It may be associated with urinary-tract obstruction.

Symptoms
The onset of symptoms may be rapid, with dysuria, fever and rigors, and loin pain and tenderness. It may, however, be insidious with anorexia and lethargy. Repeated attacks may result in chronic pyelonephritis, which is characterised by persistent inflammation and may eventually culminate in renal failure.

Treatment
Treatment consists of bed rest and the administration of appropriate antibacterial drugs (BNF 5.1, table 1). Drugs to increase urinary pH (BNF 7.4.3) may relieve some symptoms, but will not eliminate the underlying infection. Patients should be encouraged to increase fluid intake. Sexual intercourse should be avoided for the duration of the infection. Surgery may be required for urinary-tract obstruction.

Vincent's infection

Definition and aetiology
Vincent's infection (acute ulcerative gingivitis, acute necrotising ulcerative gingivitis, trench mouth or Vincent's disease) is an acute or chronic infection of the gums. It usually begins in the gingival papillae between the teeth, but may extend throughout the gums. The microorganisms responsible are often fusiform bacilli and spirochaetes. The most common cause is the presence of dental plaque arising from poor oral hygiene. Other precipitating factors include emotional disturbances, systemic disease and smoking.

Symptoms
The onset is usually abrupt and is characterised by general malaise, marked gingival bleeding, inflammation and swelling. Fever is generally absent, but pain may be so severe as to render eating and talking impossible. Halitosis and excessive salivation are also common. Characteristic 'punched-out' gingival ulcers often develop. These ulcers, which bleed readily, may develop a membranous covering.

Treatment
Patients should be advised to avoid precipitating factors. Proper oral hygiene and regular dental treatment should be encouraged. A non-opioid analgesic (BNF 4.7.1) may be necessary, and an appropriate systemic oropharyngeal anti-infective drug (BNF 12.3.2) may be indicated. Minor surgery (i.e. gingivectomy) may be beneficial.

5.2 Bacterial infections

Actinomycosis

Definition and aetiology
Actinomycosis is a chronic infection caused by *Actinomyces* spp., particularly *A. israelii*, or *Propionibacterium* spp., which are Gram-positive, anaerobic or microaerophilic, filamentous bacteria.

The genera *Actinomyces* and *Propionibacterium* are present as part of the normal oral and gastrointestinal flora, and actinomycosis usually arises endogenously. It is rarely transmitted from person to person. The microorganism is present commensally on gums, teeth and tonsils. It invades through breaks in mucous membranes and multiplies in anaerobic conditions (e.g.

created by poor vascular supply or the presence of necrotic tissue.

About 60% of cases are in the cervicofacial region (lumpy jaw), often associated with dental caries or gingivitis. Abdominal actinomycosis accounts for approximately 20% of cases and may be associated with appendicitis, gastrectomy or other trauma. Pulmonary actinomycosis is usually associated with an underlying lung disorder. It results from inhalation of the microorganism into the lungs, or contiguous spread from cervicofacial or abdominal actinomycosis. Pelvic actinomycosis is most commonly due to colonisation of intra-uterine contraceptive devices, but may also spread from an abdominal ulcer.

Symptoms

Actinomycosis is characterised by multiple small abscesses that are surrounded by granulation tissue. Draining sinuses and fibrosis are also present. Common systemic symptoms may include anorexia, fever, wasting and leucocytosis. In addition, there are specific symptoms related to the site of the abscesses. Cervicofacial actinomycosis may involve the salivary glands, tongue, pharynx and larynx. It occurs more commonly in males and symptoms include painful swellings, trismus and a purulent discharge with yellowish-white granules (containing sulfur).

Abdominal actinomycosis is characterised by an inflammatory mass on the abdominal wall, and may result in anaemia. The most commonly affected areas are the caecum and appendix.

Symptoms of pulmonary actinomycosis may be productive cough and haemoptysis. Pelvic actinomycosis may cause cervicitis, endometritis or salpingitis, and common symptoms include vaginal discharge, irregular bleeding, abdominal pain and, in severe cases, vomiting.

Treatment

Actinomycosis is a progressive disease and may be fatal. With prompt treatment, however, the prognosis is good.

Treatment comprises prolonged administration of an antimicrobial, usually amoxicillin and clavulanic acid (BNF 5.1.1.3), and surgical drainage or excision of abscesses.

Anthrax

Definition and aetiology

Anthrax is a rare zoonotic infection caused by *Bacillus anthracis*, a Gram-positive, aerobic, rod-shaped spore-forming bacterium. It occurs worldwide, although it is no longer endemic in developed countries.

Spores, which may remain viable for years under the right conditions, are formed from bacilli excreted into the external environment in faeces, urine, saliva and other discharges from infected animals (particularly cattle, goats and sheep). Alternatively, spores may form when an animal dies from anthrax, and they can contaminate animal products (e.g. bones, hair, hide, wool and meat). Animals contract the infection by ingestion or inhalation of spores present in their immediate environment. Transmission of infection to humans is mainly by inoculation of spores into wounds or abraded skin (cutaneous anthrax), although inhalation (pulmonary anthrax) and ingestion (gastrointestinal anthrax) may also occur.

It is primarily a disease of workers engaged in the processing of animal-derived products, particularly those imported from endemic areas. Shepherds and cattle rearers in developing countries are also at risk. Human-to-human transmission has not been known to occur.

Symptoms

The incubation period of cutaneous anthrax is five to seven days, of pulmonary anthrax (which is less common) three to four days, and of gastrointestinal anthrax (the least common and occurring mainly in endemic areas) two to five days.

Cutaneous anthrax is marked by a small pruritic papule at the inoculation site, which develops into a vesicle surrounded by a ring of erythema and, in some cases, further vesicles. The central area ulcerates and finally develops into a dry, black, adherent scab. This characteristic anthrax sore is called a 'malignant pustule', although it is neither malignant nor does it contain pus. Oedema may spread out from the sore into surrounding tissues, and local lymph nodes may become enlarged. General symptoms include anorexia, chills, headache, nausea and, in some cases, fever. Mild cases may recover without treatment, but in severe cases septicaemia may occur and result in collapse and death within three to five days. Healing of the sore in surviving patients is slow and may leave a scar.

The onset of pulmonary anthrax is abrupt and common symptoms include non-productive cough, mild fever, malaise and myalgia. Severe respiratory distress may follow an apparent improvement and can be rapidly fatal if untreated.

Gastrointestinal anthrax initially resembles an acute case of gastroenteritis, with rapid progression to toxaemia, shock and death.

Anthrax meningitis may occur as a secondary complication of all types of anthrax as a result of bacteraemia. Death is usually inevitable.

Treatment

Anthrax responds readily to treatment, which comprises administration of benzylpenicillin (BNF 5.1.1.1) or other broad-spectrum antibiotics, and antimicrobial resistance is rare. Anthrax sores may be covered with clean dressings, but require no further attention. Intensive supportive measures may be necessary in severe cases, particularly for pulmonary and gastrointestinal anthrax, and when complicated by septicaemia.

Anthrax may be prevented in endemic areas by improvements in animal husbandry. Dead infected animals should be burned or buried deeply, their stalls disinfected, and bedding and straw burned. Stringent precautions are necessary in factories to prevent infection of workers. These include decontaminating raw materials by autoclaving, gamma irradiation and using oxidising agents, and providing protective clothing and respirators where necessary. Anthrax vaccine is also available for active immunisation of humans at risk.

Botulism

Definition and aetiology

Botulism is a severe disease caused by various highly potent exotoxins produced by *Clostridium botulinum*, a Gram-positive, spore-forming, anaerobic bacillus. It is rare in the UK, with less than 50 people affected by localised outbreaks over the last 80 years.

In most cases, the disease is caused by the ingestion of preformed toxin in poorly prepared canned, fermented or smoked food, rather than by ingestion of spores, which are regularly consumed without causing illness. Spores, which are widely distributed in the environment, are highly resistant and able to withstand prolonged boiling at 100°C. They are able to germinate, multiply and produce toxin in the anaerobic environment created by some methods of food preservation. Infants under nine months of age can, however, develop botulism on ingestion of spores, which germinate and produce toxin in the gastrointestinal tract. One source of infant botulism has been traced to spore-contaminated honey. Wound botulism is a rare form of the disease caused by bacilli producing toxin within a wound.

Symptoms

The incubation period varies from 2 hours to eight days, although in most cases it is within 12–72 hours.

The toxin is absorbed through the mucous membrane and spreads in the bloodstream. It irreversibly binds to receptors at cholinergic neuromuscular junctions, blocking the release of acetylcholine. Symptoms vary in severity, ranging from mild illness to severe, flaccid, and often bilateral paralysis, commencing with the cranial nerves and progressively descending. Initial neurological symptoms include dry mouth, dysphagia, diplopia, diminished acuity, loss of accommodation, speech difficulties and dizziness. They may be preceded in some cases by symptoms of gastrointestinal disturbance (e.g. nausea and vomiting, diarrhoea and abdominal pain). As the disease progresses, there may be constipation, urinary hesitancy, hypotension, difficulty in holding up the head, and finally paralysis of respiratory muscles.

Very severe cases usually have a short incubation period and can progress to death within a day. Surviving patients generally show a complete recovery, as new nerve terminals may form from axons.

Wound botulism has a longer incubation period (ranging from 4 to 17 days) and shows fewer gastrointestinal symptoms.

Treatment

The prognosis is good, with less than 10% mortality if there is adequate intensive respiratory support, which may be necessary for several weeks. Gastric lavage, enemas or purgatives may be of value early in the course to eliminate toxin from the gastrointestinal tract. Botulism antitoxin may be administered at any time to neutralise toxin present in the bloodstream. It prevents further progress of the disease, but is unable to dislodge toxin already bound to receptor sites and is of little value in infant botulism. Guanidine has been used to increase acetylcholine release, although its efficacy remains unproven.

Botulism may be prevented by ensuring high standards of food preservation. Irradiation or exposure to moist heat for 30 minutes at 120°C will kill spores. Any toxin already formed may be destroyed by heating food for 30 minutes at 80°C. Germination of spores may be prevented by a low pH, drying, refrigeration, freezing, or use of salt, sugar and sodium nitrite as preservatives. Honey should not be given to infants under one year of age.

Brucellosis

Definition and aetiology

Brucellosis (Malta fever, Mediterranean fever or undulant fever) is an infection of animals caused by species of the genus *Brucella*, which are Gram-negative, aerobic, non-sporing, pleomorphic coccobacilli. *Brucella abortus* affects mainly cattle and the disease occurs worldwide, although it has been eradicated in 17 developed countries (which includes the UK and the Channel Islands). *Br. melitensis* causes disease primarily in goats and sheep, particularly in the Mediterranean basin, Asia, Africa, and Central and South America. *Br. suis* infects pigs, caribou and reindeer in the Americas, South East Asia and arctic Russia.

The disease in humans is contracted from infected animals by ingestion of untreated milk products or close contact with blood or secretions. Invasion occurs through the gastrointestinal mucosa, conjunctiva and skin abrasions. It is an occupational disease of abattoir workers, farmers and veterinary surgeons.

Symptoms

Brucellosis may be acute with an incubation period of two weeks (range one to three weeks) or several months may elapse before symptoms present.

In acute cases, initial symptoms include headache, low back pain and myalgia accompanied by fluctuating (undulant) fever, drenching sweats, rigors and prostration. There may also be hepatosplenomegaly, palpitations, gastrointestinal disturbances and weight loss. The symptoms of chronic disease, which may be insidious in onset or follow an untreated acute attack, are similar, although the patient's temperature is very often normal.

Granulomatous nodules arising from phagocytosed microorganisms may deposit in the bone marrow, liver and spleen. They may suppurate in untreated cases, resulting in bacteraemia and spread to other organs. Complications include arthritis, pneumonia, cholecystitis, endocarditis, epididymo-orchitis, meningo-encephalitis and sciatica. Abortion, which is the most common symptom in infected animals, does not appear to occur in humans.

The course is variable and many cases resolve spontaneously, although relapses may occur for up to two years, especially if untreated. Infections with *Br. suis* and *Br. melitensis* are generally more serious than *Br. abortus*. One attack of brucellosis usually confers life-long immunity.

Treatment

All cases of brucellosis must be treated to prevent relapses and possible complications. Appropriate antibacterials include tetracyclines (BNF 5.1.3) and an aminoglycoside antibiotic (BNF 5.1.4).

Brucellosis may be prevented by heat-treating all milk and milk products, and ensuring adequate protection for those in high-risk occupations. The microorganism may be eradicated in farm stock by active immunisation of calves, destruction of infected animals, and effective controls over the sale of livestock.

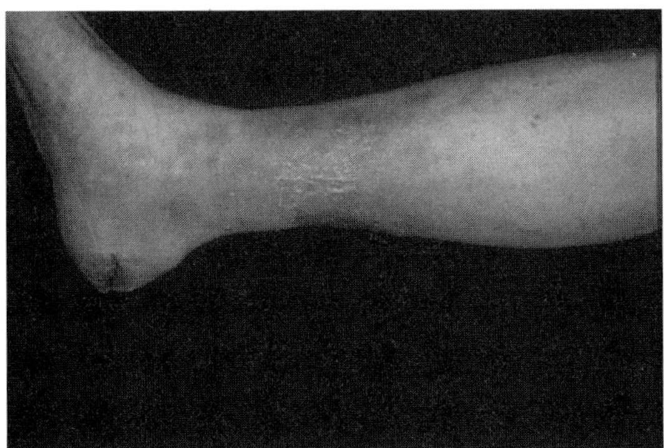

Figure 5.1 Cellulitis. (Reproduced with permission of Mike Wyndham.)

Cellulitis

Definition and aetiology

Cellulitis (Figure 5.1) is a diffuse inflammatory condition affecting subcutaneous tissues (*see also* Erysipelas). It is most commonly caused by group A β-haemolytic streptococci or occasionally by *Staphylococcus aureus*. It may arise at a site of existing trauma or infection, or can develop in previously healthy skin.

Symptoms

Cellulitis most commonly affects the arms and legs and is characterised by red, hot, oedematous areas with ill-defined margins. Vesicles and bullae may be present. In severe cases, other symptoms may include fever, malaise and headache. The condition frequently results in lymphangitis and lymphadenopathy.

Treatment

Treatment consists of bed rest and the oral, or if necessary intravenous, administration of an appropriate antibacterial drug (BNF 5.1). Elevation of the affected area may facilitate drainage.

Cholera

Definition and aetiology

Cholera is an acute infection of the bowel caused by *Vibrio cholerae*, a Gram-negative, aerobic rod. It is endemic in the Ganges delta and Bangladesh, and is responsible for epidemics throughout India. Pandemics also occur periodically: the latest one started in 1991 in South America, occurring first in Peru and rapidly spreading to other South and Central American countries.

Humans are the only known reservoir of infection, and transmission occurs via faecal-contaminated drinking water. Food washed with contaminated water, or shellfish harvested from contaminated seawater, may also be the source. Flies can also transfer bacteria from faeces to food.

Achlorhydria, antacid therapy and gastric surgery render individuals particularly susceptible to developing cholera, as vibrios are very sensitive to gastric acid. Children and adults are equally at risk, except in endemic areas where repeated ingestion of vibrios confers some degree of immunity in adults. One attack does not, however, always produce immunity.

Symptoms

The number of microorganisms necessary to produce clinical symptoms in previously healthy individuals is very large, and the degree of severity varies from an asymptomatic carrier state to severe, fulminating and fatal disease. The incubation period is usually 12–72 hours (range 12 hours to six days).

Symptoms, of which diarrhoea is often the first, are caused by an enterotoxin, which disrupts intracellular transport mechanisms responsible for maintaining the optimum fluid and electrolyte balance. The onset is rapid, and characterised by large volumes of white, mucoid, odourless, isotonic stools ('rice-water' stools), which may be followed by vomiting and muscle cramps (especially in the calf muscles). Mild cases may start to resolve after 3–12 hours, but in severe cases further symptoms may include intense thirst, cyanosis, exhaustion, hypothermia, hypotension, tachycardia and reduced skin turgor. Children also develop hypoglycaemia, a consequence of which may be CNS complications (e.g. stupor, convulsions or coma). Progressive fluid losses (exceeding one litre per hour in some cases) result in severe dehydration, hypovolaemia and metabolic acidosis, and may prove rapidly fatal in about 50% of untreated cases. Convalescent patients continue to excrete vibrios in their faeces for one to three weeks.

Treatment
There is complete recovery in almost all patients receiving adequate oral (BNF 9.2.1) or intravenous electrolyte (BNF 9.2.2) and water replacement therapy. The use of tetracycline may be indicated as an adjunct in severe cases to reduce the volume of diarrhoea, duration of illness and carrier state. The emergence of resistant strains, however, precludes indiscriminate use.

Cholera may be prevented in endemic areas by improving sanitation and providing a clean water supply. Where this is not available, drinking water should be boiled and consumption of raw unpeeled fruit and vegetables avoided. A vaccine is available (BNF 14.4), which confers immunity for three to six months in about 50% of individuals. It does not, however, prevent excretion of vibrios and is thus of no value in curbing the spread during an outbreak.

Diphtheria

Definition and aetiology
Diphtheria is an infection caused by *Corynebacterium diphtheriae*, a Gram-positive, aerobic, nonsporing bacillus. It occurs worldwide, particularly in temperate and cold climates in early winter, although active immunisation programmes in recent years have reduced the incidence and mortality. It has been virtually eliminated from the UK.

It is directly transmitted from person to person by droplets. The reservoir of infection is maintained by asymptomatic nasal carriers and individuals suffering from chronic cutaneous diphtheria (a condition existing mainly in the tropics).

Children between one and five years of age are most susceptible to developing clinical illness, although non-immune adults are also at risk.

Symptoms
Diphtheria may be asymptomatic or symptoms may vary in severity from mild, to fulminating and life-threatening. The incubation period is short, usually two days, extending in some cases to five days.

The bacilli colonise the fauces, nose, larynx, pharynx, tonsils and skin, and produce an exotoxin which can spread via the circulation to other organs and cause serious complications. A characteristic greyish-white membrane, composed of dead epithelial cells, fibrin, leucocytes and red blood cells is produced in most forms of diphtheria as a response to the inflammatory process induced by the multiplying bacteria. It changes colour as the disease progresses and eventually sloughs off during recovery.

Anterior nasal diphtheria is a mild condition with few, if any, constitutional symptoms as the toxin is not absorbed from this site. It is characterised by the production of a nasal discharge, which becomes progressively thick, purulent and blood-stained. A thin membrane develops in the nose, and there may be irritation of the nares and upper lips.

Tonsillar (faucial) diphtheria has a slow onset and is marked by a membrane which grows to cover the tonsils. Other symptoms caused by mild toxaemia may include fever, headache, malaise, fatigue, dysphagia, and nausea and vomiting. Local lymph nodes may become enlarged. The membrane may spread to the uvula, palate, pharynx and nasal mucosa (nasopharyngeal diphtheria), becoming severe and life-threatening due to extreme toxaemia. Oedema and enlarged lymph nodes may result in a characteristic 'bull-neck', and breathing difficulties due to obstruction.

Symptoms of laryngeal diphtheria, which usually occur in conjunction with tonsillar diphtheria, are due to the presence of a membrane involving the larynx and extending in some cases to the trachea and bronchi. Symptoms include hoarseness, non-productive cough or croup, stridor, dyspnoea and cyanosis. The condition may be fatal if breathing is obstructed, but there are generally no toxaemic complications.

Cutaneous diphtheria is usually a chronic condition marked by painless slow-growing ulcers, often on the legs. Constitutional symptoms are usually absent because little toxin is absorbed from the skin.

Common complications of toxaemia are myocarditis and neuritis, which may be fatal, but usually resolve completely in adequately treated patients.

Treatment

Treatment of cases and carriers comprises administration of an appropriate antibacterial preparation such as benzylpenicillin (BNF 5.1.1.1) or erythromycin (BNF 5.1.5) to destroy the bacteria. Symptomatic patients additionally require diphtheria antitoxin (BNF 14.4) to neutralise the toxin. Bed rest is also necessary. Intensive care, assisted ventilation or tracheostomy may be necessary in the management of complications.

Diphtheria may be prevented by active immunisation of all infants (*see also* Section 15.5). Spread of infection during an outbreak may be curbed by isolating patients and carriers until three consecutive negative nose and throat swabs have been obtained. Contacts may be protected by administration of diphtheria antitoxin, but should be closely observed for signs of developing infection.

Epididymitis

Definition and aetiology

Epididymitis is inflammation of the epididymis and is usually due to bacterial infection, which often results from a primary urinary-tract infection. The infection may be gonococcal, but other microorganisms (e.g. *Escherichia coli* and *Pseudomonas* spp.) may be responsible. Most cases in men under 35 years of age are due to a sexually transmitted microorganism.

Symptoms

The onset of symptoms may be sudden or insidious. The infection is usually unilateral and is characterised by acute pain, swelling and scrotal redness. It is often accompanied by malaise and mild fever. Fibrosis may persist after recovery.

Treatment

Treatment comprises bed rest and the administration of an appropriate antimicrobial drug, usually a tetracycline (BNF 5.1.3). A non-opioid analgesic (BNF 4.7.1) may be required and the patient may find it helpful to wear a scrotal support. If the condition becomes chronic, surgery (epididymectomy) may be necessary.

Epiglottitis

Definition and aetiology

Epiglottitis is characterised by inflammation and oedema of the epiglottis. It is due to infection with *Haemophilus influenzae, Staphylococcus pneumoniae* or *Staph. aureus* and is most common in children between two and four years of age. Its incidence has decreased significantly over the past 10 years.

Symptoms

It is usually preceded by an upper respiratory-tract infection, which suddenly worsens. The child becomes severely ill due to septicaemia and acute dyspnoea with stridor. Other symptoms include hoarseness, pain on swallowing with excessive drooling, muffling of the voice, and swelling of the neck. Epiglottitis may be fatal due to airway obstruction. The condition should be distinguished from the milder condition, croup (*see* Section 3.1).

Treatment

Immediate hospital treatment is essential. An adequate airway must be maintained and it may be necessary to insert an endotracheal tube or perform a tracheostomy. Appropriate antibacterial therapy, usually a third-generation cephalosporin (BNF 5.1.2) or chloramphenicol (BNF 5.1.7), is indicated.

Erysipelas

Definition and aetiology

Erysipelas is an infection of the dermis (*see also* Cellulitis), most frequently caused by group A β-haemolytic streptococci, which are Gram-positive facultative anaerobes. It may arise at a site of existing trauma or skin infection (e.g. impetigo or via a sore between the toes). However, in many cases, there is no obvious point of entry, and the offending microorganism may be present in the eye, nose, or throat. It most commonly affects the face, arms and legs.

Symptoms

Erysipelas has an abrupt onset after an incubation period of two to five days. It is characterised by a tender, red, oedematous area with well-defined borders. Vesicles and bullae are often present. The skin lesions are frequently preceded by headache, fever, malaise and vomiting. The condition, if untreated, may result in nephritis and septicaemia, especially in infants and the elderly, and may even prove fatal. Recurrent attacks may cause lymphoedema.

Treatment

Treatment consists of the oral administration of an appropriate penicillin (BNF 5.1.1) or erythromycin (BNF 5.1.5). A non-opioid analgesic (BNF 4.7.1) may provide pain relief.

Furunculosis

Definition and aetiology

Furunculosis is the recurrence of furuncles over weeks or months, or the coincidental occurrence of several furuncles.

Furuncles

Definition and aetiology

Furuncles (boils) are acute inflammatory nodules arising from infection of the hair follicles. The microorganism responsible is usually *Staphylococcus aureus*, a Gram-positive, facultatively anaerobic coccus, which is carried as part of the normal skin flora of many individuals. The nares and perineum are the most common reservoirs of the microorganism. Furuncles occur more commonly in males and are generally found in the axillae, anogenital region and on the back of the neck. The predisposing factors are largely unknown, although seborrhoea, malnutrition, diabetes mellitus and leukaemia may precipitate the appearance of furuncles. Anaemia, fatigue and stress have also been implicated as causative factors.

Symptoms

Furuncles may occur as single or multiple lesions, which are tender and painful, and become pustular with a single head. Those occurring on the nose, ears or fingers can be especially painful. There is a blood-stained, purulent exudate as the necrotic core is discharged, and scarring may ensue. Fever, pyaemia and septicaemia may occur in severe cases.

Treatment

Treatment consists of cleansing the affected area with suitable skin disinfecting and cleansing agents (BNF 13.11) and the application of an appropriate anti-infective skin preparation (BNF 13.10). The application of moist heat and magnesium sulfate paste (BNF 13.10.5) may also be beneficial, and patients should be discouraged from squeezing lesions. Penicillinase-resistant penicillins (BNF 5.1.1.2) and surgical drainage may be indicated in severe or recurrent cases. The nares and perianal skin should also be treated in an effort to prevent further infection.

Carbuncles

Definition and aetiology

Carbuncles (Figure 5.2) are formed by the confluence of several furuncles, or by the spread of infection, in the subcutaneous tissues. They tend to occur on the shoulders, hips, thighs and back of the neck and are most common in middle-aged or elderly men. Predisposing factors may include diabetes mellitus, nephritis, debilitating disease and prolonged corticosteroid therapy.

Symptoms

Carbuncles are painful and tender with multiple heads. Purulent ulcers are formed with extensive

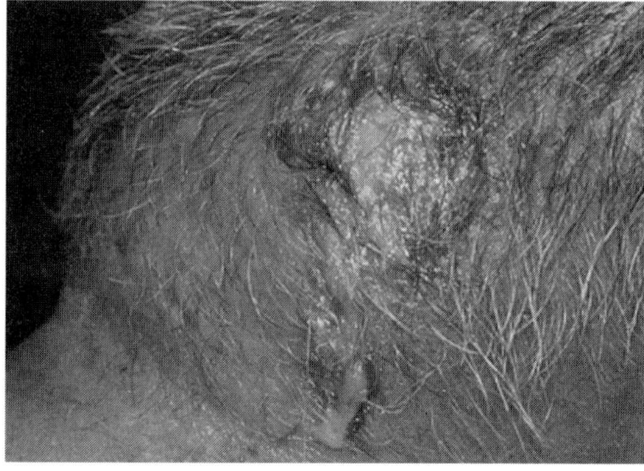

Figure 5.2 Carbuncles. (Reproduced with permission of Science Photo Library.)

areas of necrotic tissue, which separates as a slough. There may be malaise and fever, and in severe cases, septicaemia. Healing is often slow and generally results in scar formation.

Treatment

Treatment is the same as for furuncles (*see above*).

Gas gangrene

Definition and aetiology

Gas gangrene (clostridial myonecrosis) is a serious infection of muscle tissue. It is caused by exotoxins produced by various species of *Clostridium* (particularly *C. perfringens*), which are Gram-positive, anaerobic, spore-forming bacilli.

Clostridial species naturally inhabit the soil and gastrointestinal tract of mammals. They may become pathogenic in the presence of penetrating surgical or traumatic wounds (e.g. after hip or colonic surgery, gunshot wounds, crush injuries, burns or open fractures). Clostridial growth is facilitated by the hypoxic conditions generated in such wounds by ischaemia, and the presence of necrotic tissue and foreign bodies (e.g. dirt, shrapnel or pieces of clothing). Very rarely, gas gangrene may occur in an extremity due to secondary spread from an intestinal neoplasm, or as a primary infection in the absence of trauma, usually in the perineum or scrotum.

Symptoms

The incubation period is usually less than four days, but can vary from a few hours to several weeks.

The onset is sudden and characterised by severe pain. The wound becomes oedematous and may ooze a thin serous exudate with a sweet odour. The skin becomes bronze-coloured, and haemorrhagic bullae and necrosis may develop. Subsequently the traumatised area may become extremely tender. In some cases, gas may be present within the tissues as a late symptom. Accompanying constitutional symptoms include fever, sweats, tachycardia and anxiety. Septicaemia, hypotension, renal failure and haemolytic anaemia may arise as complications and, if untreated, can be rapidly fatal.

Treatment

Prompt treatment is essential as the mortality may be up to 30%. Complete surgical removal of all affected muscle is necessary and in severe cases involves amputation of a limb. Adjunctive measures include administration of benzylpenicillin (BNF 5.1.1.1) and the use of hyperbaric oxygen. Supportive treatment (e.g. fluid and electrolyte replacement and blood transfusions) may be required in the event of complications.

Gas gangrene may be prevented by antibacterial prophylaxis (BNF 5.1, table 2) prior to and following surgical operations carrying an associated risk. In the case of traumatic wounds, patients should be evacuated from the accident site and treated as soon as possible. All damaged muscle and skin should be completely excised and wound closure delayed until it is absolutely certain that no infection is present.

Impetigo

Definition and aetiology

Impetigo (Figure 5.3) , which occurs most often in children, is a contagious superficial infection (pyoderma) of the epidermis. It is caused most frequently by *Staphylococcus aureus*, less commonly by group A β-haemolytic streptococci, and in some cases, by the two microorganisms together.

It may arise as a secondary infection in the presence of eczema, fungal infections, insect bites, pediculosis or skin trauma. In many cases, however, it occurs in previously healthy skin. Overcrowded and unhygienic conditions may predispose an individual to develop the infection.

Symptoms

The arms, legs and face, especially around the nose and mouth, are sites most commonly affected. Vesicles appear initially, rupturing rapidly to release an exudate which dries to form yellow or light brown crusts. Other symptoms include erythema, pruritus, and in some cases, bullae. The lesions spread quickly and, if untreated, the condition may result in further complications (e.g. cellulitis, furunculosis, urticaria or acute glomerulonephritis). In less severe cases, impetigo may resolve spontaneously in two to three weeks.

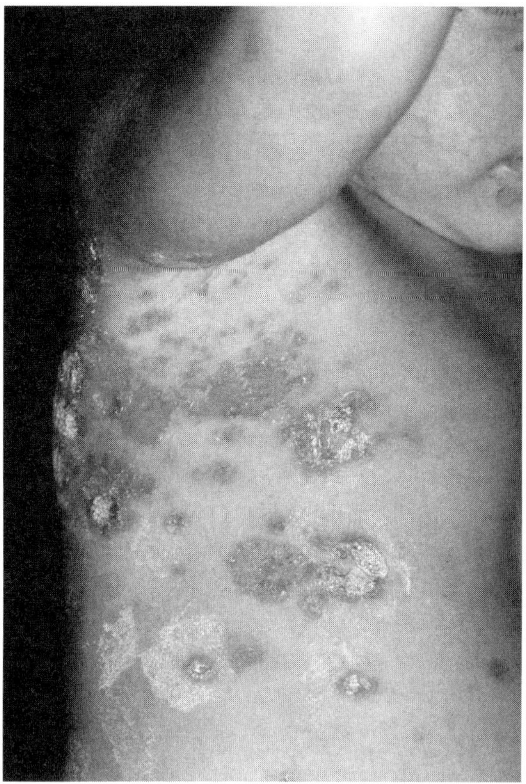

Figure 5.3 Impetigo. (Reproduced with permission of Dr P Marazzi/Science Photo Library.)

Treatment

Treatment comprises the removal of crusts with soap and water or mild skin disinfecting and cleansing agents (BNF 13.11). Topical administration of an appropriate antibacterial preparation (e.g. mupirocin) (BNF 13.10.1.1) may be effective in many cases, although a systemic antimicrobial (BNF 5.1) may be necessary for more severe infections. The nares and perianal skin, which may act as reservoirs of *S. aureus*, should also be treated. Patients should be counselled on personal hygiene to prevent contagion and further attacks.

Legionellosis

Definition and aetiology

Legionellosis is an acute respiratory-tract infection occurring worldwide. It is caused by Gram-negative, aerobic, non-sporing bacilli of the genus *Legionella*. Legionnaires' disease, which was first recognised in 1976, is the most serious form of legionellosis. It is caused by *Legionella pneumophila* and often occurs as outbreaks in hospitals (i.e. a nosocomial disease), hotels or office blocks. Pontiac fever is a much milder form.

The microorganism has been isolated from water in air-conditioning cooling towers and hot-water systems, and is known to be transmitted by inhalation of water droplets. It is uncertain if infection occurs through the gastrointestinal tract, and it appears not to be spread from person to person. Legionella occur naturally in fresh-water ponds, lakes and in moist soil, particularly when temperatures exceed 25°C, the optimum range for growth being 30–38°C. It is possible that the presence of other microorganisms in water (e.g. algae, amoebae and other bacteria) facilitate the growth of legionella.

Individuals most susceptible to developing legionellosis are males between 40 and 70 years of age who smoke or consume excessive quantities of alcohol, those with an underlying disorder (e.g. chronic cardiac, pulmonary or renal disorders, and diabetes mellitus), or immunosuppressed patients.

Symptoms

About half of those infected develop clinical symptoms. The incubation period is usually 36 hours (range 5–66 hours) for Pontiac fever and five to seven days (range 2–10 days) for Legionnaires' disease.

Pontiac fever resembles an acute attack of influenza, with common symptoms including fever, headache, myalgia, cough, and nausea and vomiting. Sore throat, diarrhoea, chest pain and confusion may also occur. It is self-limiting, and patients generally recover within one week. No fatalities have been recorded to date.

Legionnaires' disease is characterised by the development of pneumonia and, in severe cases, the involvement of other organs (e.g. liver, kidney, gastrointestinal tract and central nervous system). Initial symptoms include malaise, myalgia, headache, fever, weakness, anorexia and dry cough. These are followed a few days later by chest pain, dyspnoea, tachypnoea, abdominal pain and watery diarrhoea. Neurological disturbances which may occur include amnesia, ataxia, slurred speech and hallucinations. Mild cases may resolve spontaneously after five to seven days, but severe pneumonia or renal failure may be fatal.

Treatment

Pontiac fever is mild and self-limiting and requires no treatment. Erythromycin (BNF 5.1.5) is always indicated in Legionnaires' disease and gives a good prognosis if started early. Ciprofloxacin and azithromycin have also been used. Premature cessation may precipitate potentially fatal relapses. Supportive treatment may be necessary in severe cases, and includes assisted ventilation and maintenance of adequate fluid and electrolyte levels.

The exact source of the microorganism in air-conditioning and hot-water systems must be located during outbreaks, and eradication attempted by chlorination or raising the water temperature to at least 55°C. It is uncertain whether chemicals are an effective means of prevention.

Leprosy

Definition and aetiology

Leprosy (Hansen's disease) is a chronic infectious disease caused by *Mycobacterium leprae,* an acid-fast bacillus. It occurs mainly in tropical climates (e.g. Asia and Africa), but may also occur in some temperate regions (e.g. Japan, Korea, southern Europe, and some southern states of the USA).

The microorganism is an obligate intracellular parasite, which may be transmitted to new hosts via the nasal secretions from untreated patients. It is also present in the breast milk of infected mothers. The exact mode of entry into the host is, however, unknown.

The prevalence of leprosy is associated with conditions of overcrowding and poor standards of living, and it occurs most commonly between 10 and 30 years of age.

Symptoms

The incubation period is from 3 to 10 years, or even longer in some cases.

Leprosy is characterised by lesions of the skin and peripheral nerves, with the severity of symptoms dependent on the host's resistance.

Indeterminate leprosy occurs most often in children and is marked by one to four hypopigmented macules with ill-defined margins. There may be reduced sensation and sweating within the macular area. The condition is often self-limiting, although 25% of cases may progress to one of the other forms of determinate leprosy.

Tuberculoid leprosy develops in people with some degree of resistance and is consequently localised in the skin or peripheral nerves. There may be one to three asymmetric, well-defined, annular lesions showing a hypopigmented flattened centre and an erythematous raised border. There is reduced sensation and sweating, and the nerves supplying the area become thickened. Caseation necrosis may occur within the nerves causing paralysis of extremities. Spontaneous recovery may occur.

Lepromatous leprosy develops in those with low resistance and is a generalised bacteraemic infection. The lesions are small, widespread, ill-defined, symmetric macules or papules; plaques and nodules may also develop. The nasal mucosa thickens, resulting in blockage, production of a discharge and progressive destruction of nasal cartilage. The skin becomes coarse and thickened, and eyebrows and eyelashes fall out, which combine to cause a change in facial expression. Iritis and keratitis frequently occur and other organs may become involved (e.g. the larynx, pharynx, tongue and testes). Destruction of dermal nerves leads to loss of sensation of pain, temperature and touch. As a result, patients are at risk of repeated trauma, secondary infection and tissue damage.

Borderline leprosy has characteristics of both the tuberculoid and lepromatous forms. The effects of treatment or improvements in the patient's resistance, or both, can cause a regression to the tuberculoid state or, conversely, it may worsen and become lepromatous.

Treatment

Untreated lepromatous leprosy is progressive and, in come cases, fatal, while the other forms often resolve spontaneously.

Treatment of all forms is by the long-term administration of antileprotic drugs (BNF 5.1.10) undertaken in specialist centres. Supportive help includes physiotherapy for patients with paralysed hands or feet; reconstructive surgery may be beneficial in some cases. Patients should be encouraged to examine anaesthetic limbs regularly for signs of injury or developing infection.

Leprosy may be prevented by identifying and treating infected patients, and isolating lepromatous cases during the active infectious stages.

Leptospirosis

Definition and aetiology

Leptospirosis is an enzootic infection that occurs worldwide and is caused by *Leptospira interrogans*, an aerobic spirochaete. The microorganism is a parasite of many different species, including cattle, dogs, foxes, goats, hedgehogs and pigs. The main reservoir of infection, however, exists in rodents, particularly rats, who are able to harbour leptospires permanently without any adverse effects. The bacteria are mainly transmitted in the urine of infected animals and humans, although direct contact with infected blood and tissues may also be responsible. Leptospires may survive for weeks in the external environment in moist conditions. They gain entry into a new host via skin abrasions or mucous membranes. Ingestion of contaminated food or penetration of intact macerated skin are also possible mechanisms.

Symptoms

The incubation period is usually from 7 to 14 days (range 2–20 days). The duration does not affect the severity of the symptoms or the prognosis, which are dependent on inoculum size.

Symptoms vary from a mild, self-limiting condition to severe illness involving the liver and kidneys. The onset is sudden and characterised in the majority of cases by fever, chills, myalgia and severe headache. In addition, there may be abdominal pain, vomiting, injection of the conjunctiva, pharyngitis, non-productive cough and haemoptysis. Weil's disease is a severe form of leptospirosis marked by jaundice, hepatomegaly, proteinuria, haematuria and, in some cases, renal failure.

Mild cases resolve within four to nine days and recovery is usually complete. Mortality is generally as a result of hepatic or renal failure and is greatest in the elderly.

Treatment

Appropriate antibacterial treatment must be started within four days of onset of symptoms to be effective and includes the administration of penicillin, chloramphenicol, erythromycin, streptomycin or tetracycline. The fluid and electrolyte balance should be maintained, and dialysis may be necessary in the event of renal failure.

Leptospirosis may be prevented by controlling the rat population. Penicillin injections should be administered prophylactically to individuals who fall into water containing leptospires.

Listeriosis

Definition and aetiology

Listeriosis is caused by a Gram-positive, facultatively anaerobic, non-sporing bacillus, *Listeria monocytogenes*, and occurs worldwide.

The microorganism is widely distributed in the environment in water, soil, sewage and animal fodder (e.g. silage), and colonises many species of mammals, birds and fish. The exact source of human infection is unclear, but may be from food, which can be contaminated at any stage during agricultural production or during processing. Contamination may also occur via an asymptomatic carrier harbouring microorganisms in the gastrointestinal tract. A small inoculum may multiply to form a significant population in food stored in a refrigerator at 4–6°C. Some cases may be sexually transmitted, as *L. monocytogenes* also colonises the genital tract. Transmission from mother to fetus may occur across the placenta, or at birth during passage along an infected birth canal.

Individuals most susceptible to developing listeriosis are neonates, the elderly, those with an underlying disorder (e.g. cirrhosis, diabetes mellitus and malignant disease), and immunosuppressed patients.

Symptoms

The exact incubation period is unknown, but may vary between 7 and 30 days. The severity of symptoms ranges from subclinical to mild to fatal. Listeriosis is characterised by formation of micro-abscesses in tissues, which may result in a variety of disorders (e.g. arthritis, cholecystitis, conjunctivitis, endocarditis, lymph node enlargement, peritonitis, osteomyelitis, skin rashes and chronic urethritis). Meningitis and septicaemia commonly occur in severe cases.

Listeriosis in pregnancy often results in influenza-like symptoms in the mother, with abortion in early infections or prematurity or stillbirth in late infections. Other symptoms experienced by the mother may include diarrhoea, a rash and convulsions. Surviving neonates may develop septicaemia and pneumonia up to two days after birth. Infection derived from the birth canal usually gives rise to meningitis and, in some cases, hydrocephalus, commencing five to seven days after birth.

Treatment

The prognosis of listeriosis depends on the presence of underlying disease or state of immunosuppression. Prompt treatment significantly reduces the mortality, although in neonates this may still be as high as 50% (compared with 90% in untreated cases).

Effective antibacterial drugs are ampicillin or penicillin, combined with an aminoglycoside (e.g. gentamicin or streptomycin) in severe cases.

Listeriosis may be prevented by adopting stringent controls of hygiene in the preparation and storage of food. Prepared food should not be stored for long periods of time prior to consumption.

Lyme disease

Definition and aetiology

Lyme disease was named after the cluster of cases that occurred in Lyme, Connecticut, USA in 1975. It is a zoonotic infection caused by *Borrelia burgdorferi*, a Gram-negative spirochaete. Cases have been identified in Europe (including the UK and the Republic of Ireland), the USA and Australia, particularly in forested areas.

The infection is transmitted by ticks, *Ixodes dammini* and *I. pacificus* in the USA, and *I. ricinus* in Europe. Other blood-sucking arthropods (e.g. horseflies and mosquitoes) have also been implicated as vectors. Deer are the most likely reservoir of infection, although smaller mammals (e.g. dogs and raccoons) and passerine birds may also be involved. There is evidence that transmission to the fetus may occur *in utero*.

Symptoms

The exact incubation period is uncertain, but may vary from days to weeks after the initial tick bite. Some patients appear to have no history of a bite.

The majority of patients present with erythema chronicum migrans, which is characterised by a small, erythematous, pruritic, painful, papular or macular lesion at the inoculation site. It has indurated borders and gradually spreads outwards, clearing in the centre. It may be followed by secondary, non migrating, annular lesions. Accompanying symptoms at this stage may include fever, malaise, headache, fatigue, arthralgia, myalgia, neck stiffness, nausea and vomiting, and lymphadenopathy. Neurological or cardiac complications may arise weeks or months later in some patients and include Bell's palsy, encephalitis, meningitis, an enlarged heart or atrioventricular block. More than half of all patients develop arthritis, which usually involves the large joints, particularly the knees. It may last for weeks or months and is often recurrent. It may become chronic in some cases and progressively destroy bone and cartilage.

Fetal infection is serious and has resulted in fetal or neonatal death, prematurity, latent development, and blindness.

Treatment

The course of the disease in adults may be halted by prompt treatment with amoxicillin (BNF 5.1.1.3), doxycycline (BNF 5.1.3), or azithromycin (BNF 5.1.5).

Lymphangitis

Definition and aetiology

Lymphangitis is an inflammation of the lymphatic vessels. It usually arises as a result of infection with *Streptococcus pyogenes* (a Gram-positive aerobe) via an abrasion or wound, often of an extremity.

Symptoms

Lymphangitis is characterised by swelling and tenderness of regional lymph nodes, fever and rigors, headache, and tachycardia. Red streaks along the course of the lymphatic vessels may be visible through the skin. Septicaemia may develop.

Treatment

Treatment consists of the administration of an appropriate antibacterial drug (BNF 5.1, table 1).

Mastitis

Definition and aetiology

Mastitis is inflammation of the breast. Acute mastitis usually occurs in lactating females during the first few weeks of nursing a first-born child, and is due to bacterial infection with *Staphylococcus aureus*.

Treatment

Treatment consists of antibacterial drugs (BNF 5.1, table 1). Surgical drainage may be necessary if an abscess develops.

Meningococcal infections

Definition and aetiology

Meningococcal infections are caused by *Neisseria meningitidis*, a Gram-negative, aerobic diplococcus. Epidemics can occur, and outbreaks are not uncommon in Europe and America, particularly amongst young people living in overcrowded conditions (e.g. hostels and military camps).

Humans are the only reservoir of infection, and transmission is by inhalation of airborne water droplets from a carrier.

Children under five years of age are most susceptible to developing clinical illness, although during epidemics, older children and adults are also at risk.

Symptoms

Meningococcal infections may result in mild nasopharyngeal symptoms or potentially fatal meningeal infections. The more serious forms may produce meningitis or acute meningococcaemia, although the two forms are not exclusive.

Nasopharyngeal infection may give rise to an asymptomatic carrier state, which may persist for months, or produce clinical symptoms in susceptible individuals following a short incubation period (one to five days).

Meningitis is produced when the meningococcal microorganism invades the meninges via the circulation. Initial symptoms include headache, fever, rigors, malaise, vomiting and neck stiffness. Convulsions may occur in the young, and infants may experience feeding difficulties. A rash may appear after a week, and approximately half of all patients show petechiae in the conjunctiva, skin or oral mucosa. The condition is fatal in less than 10% of cases, usually the very young. Most patients make a complete recovery, although complications which may occur include arthritis (not usually chronic), permanent deafness, pericarditis and occasionally pneumonia. Abnormalities may show on the electrocardiogram. Herpes simplex lesions may arise in some cases during the recovery period.

Acute fulminating meningococcaemia without meningitis may be fatal within hours due to peripheral circulatory collapse. The onset is rapid and non-specific, with initial symptoms of fever, malaise, headache, diarrhoea and vomiting making diagnosis difficult. A rash may appear locally which rapidly spreads. Occasionally a chronic form persists, characterised by periods of fever, headache, rashes, arthralgia, myalgia, arthritis, and splenomegaly, which may develop into meningitis if untreated.

Treatment

Early administration of an appropriate antibacterial drug (BNF 5.1, table 1) is essential for meningococcal meningitis as most deaths occur during the initial stages. Rehydration (BNF 9.2), analgesics (BNF 4.7) and antiepileptics (BNF 4.8) may also be necessary.

Acute meningococcaemia is an emergency. Treatment comprises immediate antimicrobial therapy and supportive measures, preferably in an intensive-care unit. These include maintenance of fluid and electrolyte levels and acid-base balance, and regular monitoring of blood pressure and the electrocardiogram. Corticosteroids (BNF 6.3.2) given early in the course of the disease and in large doses may be of value to prevent shock.

Patients should be isolated and antibacterial prophylaxis (BNF 5.1, table 2) administered to close contacts to prevent the spread of infection. Contacts should also be closely monitored during the incubation period for signs of developing disease. A meningococcal polysaccharide vaccine is available against some serotypes of *N. meningitidis*, and mass immunisation may curb an epidemic, although it is not very effective in young children. Living conditions should be improved and overcrowding reduced in institutions to prevent outbreaks.

Ophthalmia neonatorum

Definition and aetiology

Ophthalmia neonatorum is an acute purulent inflammation of the eyes in the newborn. It arises from maternal infection transmitted to the infant as it passes through the birth canal. The most common infecting microorganisms are *Chlamydia oculogenitalis* and *Streptococcus pneumoniae*, although gonococci may also be responsible.

Symptoms

Both eyes are usually affected. Symptoms may include copious discharge with local inflammation and swelling. Corneal ulceration may develop in the presence of untreated gonococcal infection.

Treatment

Prevention is of prime importance and any relevant maternal infection should be treated prior to delivery. Maintenance of an aseptic delivery procedure is essential. Nevertheless, if infection is transmitted, prompt administration of an anti-infective preparation (BNF 11.3) is indicated.

Osteomyelitis

Definition and aetiology

Osteomyelitis, which may be acute or chronic, is an infection of bone. It may arise as a result of bone injury or following an acute infection (e.g. otitis media or pneumonia). The most common infecting microorganism is *Staphylococcus aureus*, but a variety of other microorganisms may be responsible. Osteomyelitis may be confined to a localised area of bone marrow, although it may spread to affect the whole bone shaft. The tibia or fibula are the most common sites of osteomyelitis. The acute condition primarily affects children between 5 and 14 years of age, with a greater incidence in boys. It may also occur as a sequel to drug abuse.

Symptoms

Acute osteomyelitis is characterised by marked bone pain with tenderness, fever and restricted mobility of the affected part. Local swelling may develop and adjacent joints can be affected. In some cases, abscess formation may occur and septicaemia can develop. Chronic osteomyelitis arising from the introduction of a prosthetic device may not become symptomatic for many years, although extensive bone destruction may proceed in the intervening period.

Treatment

Treatment comprises the prolonged administration of an appropriate antibacterial drug (BNF 5.1, table 1), usually a penicillinase-resistant semi-synthetic penicillin (e.g. naficillin or oxacillin). Immobilisation (e.g. splinting) of the affected part may be indicated, and surgical removal of any dead bone or prosthetic device may be necessary in chronic disease.

Pertussis

Definition and aetiology

Pertussis (whooping cough) is an infection of the respiratory tract caused by *Bordetella pertussis*, a Gram-negative, aerobic, non-sporing coccobacillus. It occurs worldwide, particularly in temperate climates during the winter months, and epidemics are common in regions where active immunisation is not practised. A decrease in the take-up of vaccination in the late 1970s led to an increase in the incidence of the disease in the UK.

Humans are the only known host, and transmission occurs by droplet-spread from an infected patient. Asymptomatic carriers are rare and are not thought to be significant reservoirs of infection.

The infection may occur at any age, but most frequently affects children under six years of age. It is particularly serious in infants and the elderly.

Symptoms

An incubation period of 7 to 10 days is followed by the catarrhal stage, which is the most infectious period of pertussis and lasts from one to two weeks. Non-specific symptoms resembling a viral upper respiratory-tract infection are common, accompanied by a dry 'hacking' cough, which gradually worsens. The paroxysmal stage follows and is marked by the characteristic inspiratory 'whoop' (which may be absent in infants) terminating a succession of short coughs, during the course of which the patient may become cyanosed. A plug of mucus is often expelled and vomiting frequently occurs. The patient is usually exhausted by the end of an attack, although appears well between attacks.

The interval between paroxysms may be as brief as 30 minutes, and they can cause complications (e.g. epistaxis, hernia, rectal prolapse and conjunctival haemorrhage) due to the effects of increased pressure. Convulsions are common in infants and may arise as a result of cerebral haemorrhage or severe anoxia.

Bronchial obstruction by mucus plugs may cause atelectasis; otitis media and pneumonia may result from secondary infection.

The condition resolves slowly over many weeks or even months, although mild respiratory-tract infections may cause a relapse of the paroxysmal cough until recovery is complete. Complications, particularly in the very young, carry a risk of fatality. One attack often confers life-long immunity.

Treatment

Infants and severe cases should be treated in hospital where effective supportive treatment (e.g. maintenance of adequate fluid and electrolyte levels, and oxygenation) may be carried out. Antibacterial therapy comprises the administration of erythromycin (BNF 5.1.5), tetracycline (BNF 5.1.3) and chloramphenicol (BNF 5.1.7). These are only effective in shortening the course of the infection if treatment is started during the catarrhal stage. Secondary infections may also require treatment. Antibacterial treatment commenced during the paroxysmal stage will not shorten the course of the infection, but will render the patient non-infectious, and may be administered prophylactically to close contacts.

Pertussis may be prevented by active immunisation of infants, which carries a very small risk of causing convulsions and encephalopathy (*see also* Section 15.5). This, however, is much less than the risks of complications associated with pertussis. Infants in whom vaccination may be contraindicated (i.e. those with brain damage or a familial history of convulsions) may be identified and parents counselled accordingly.

Plague

Definition and aetiology

Plague is a zoonotic infection caused by *Yersinia pestis*, a Gram-negative, aerobic, non-sporing bacillus. The disease is endemic in parts of Asia, Africa and the Americas (including the south-western states of the USA), and has occurred historically as worldwide pandemics (e.g. the Black Death).

The reservoir of infection exists in wild rodents (particularly rats), with their associated fleas acting as the vector; humans are an incidental host. Transmission from nasal droplets or from bites of domestic pets (e.g. cats) has also occurred. Direct transmission may occasionally occur by inhalation of airborne droplets from a patient with pneumonic plague.

Symptoms

The incubation period is two to eight days.

Bubonic plague is the most common form of plague and is characterised by a sudden onset of fever, chills, headache, prostration and lethargy. Lymph nodes, particularly in the groin and axillae, become swollen, tender, hard and painful (buboes), and surrounded by oedema. Spread of bacilli to the lungs may cause chest pain, cough and haemoptysis (secondary pneumonic plague). Infection contracted directly from such patients by droplet-inhalation is termed primary pneumonic plague, and may be fatal within 48 hours of onset. Meningitis is a less common but serious complication of plague.

Mild cases may resolve spontaneously before bacilli enter the circulation, whereas severe cases may be fatal in three to six days if untreated.

Treatment

Prompt treatment significantly reduces the mortality of plague, from 60% if untreated to less than 5%. Treatment comprises the parenteral administration of streptomycin, tetracycline, sulphonamides or chloramphenicol (which is particularly useful for meningitis).

Patients with pneumonic plague should be isolated to curb the spread to others, and antibacterial prophylaxis administered to close contacts. Mass immunisation should be undertaken during an epidemic. Plague may be prevented in endemic areas by rat-proofing buildings, using insecticides and wearing protective clothing to minimise the chance of being bitten.

Prostatitis

Definition and aetiology

Prostatitis is inflammation of the prostate gland. It may be acute or chronic and is usually due to bacterial infection. Common infecting micro-organisms include *Escherichia coli*, and *Klebsiella* and *Proteus* species.

Symptoms

Acute prostatitis is characterised by marked fever, chills, severe perineal pain and back pain, together with symptoms of urinary-tract infection. Chronic prostatitis is often asymptomatic, although recurrent urinary-tract infection is common and dysuria and urethral discharge may occur.

Treatment

Treatment consists of the administration of an appropriate antibacterial drug (BNF 5.1, Table 1 and 5.1.13), sometimes for long-term therapy. In severe cases, surgical drainage may be necessary.

Pseudomembranous colitis

Definition and aetiology

Pseudomembranous colitis is an inflammatory bowel condition caused by *Clostridium difficile*, a Gram-positive, anaerobic, spore-forming bacillus.

Exotoxins produced by the bacilli elicit an inflammatory response in the intestinal walls, which results in the formation of adherent exudative plaques. It is an opportunistic infection and 90% of cases occur in association with the use of antibacterials, particularly ampicillin, cephalosporins, clindamycin and lincomycin. No age group is exempt, although the condition occurs more commonly in the elderly. It may also infrequently arise secondary to other conditions (e.g. colorectal cancer, colonic obstruction, Hirschprung's disease, ischaemic gastrointestinal disorders, shigellosis or uraemia). Cases are usually sporadic, although small outbreaks may occur in institutions or hospitals if the environment becomes contaminated with clostridial spores (which can survive for weeks or months).

Symptoms

Pseudomembranous colitis may present during the course of antibacterial therapy or up to six weeks following cessation.

Symptoms, which vary in severity from mild and self-limiting to severe and fulminating, include chills, fever, abdominal pain, leucocytosis, hypoalbuminaemia and watery or 'porridge-like' diarrhoea. Severe cases may be complicated by fluid and electrolyte imbalance, dehydration, toxic megacolon and perforation

Mild cases resolve spontaneously, although symptoms in severe cases may persist for months and prove fatal.

Treatment

Withdrawal of the offending antibacterial may allow the condition to resolve. Vancomycin (BNF 5.1.7), metronidazole or tinidazole (BNF 5.1.11) may be of value in eradication of the bacilli. Fluid and electrolytes (BNF 9.2) may be required in cases of excessive depletion. Colectomy may be necessary in severe cases.

Pseudomembranous colitis may be prevented by avoiding the indiscriminate use in susceptible patients of those antibacterials most often implicated in causing the condition. Patients in institutions should be isolated to prevent spread to others.

Psittacosis

Definition and aetiology

Psittacosis is an infection of the lungs caused by *Chlamydia psittaci*, a weakly Gram-negative, obligate, intracellular parasite. It is mainly a disease of birds (e.g. gulls, pigeons, poultry and psittacine birds such as parrots), that is transmitted to humans by inhalation of dried infected excreta.

Symptoms

The incubation period is 7–14 days with a rapid or insidious onset. Common symptoms include high fever, severe headache, chills, anorexia, malaise, nausea and vomiting, myalgia, cough and haemoptysis. In severe cases, there may be anoxia, dyspnoea, cyanosis, tachycardia, delirium and stupor.

In untreated psittacosis, the fever may last for seven days in mild cases and up to 21 days in more severe forms. It slowly abates and is followed by a long convalescence, but relapses may occur even after treatment. Pulmonary complications account for up to 20% of deaths.

Treatment

The prognosis is good with prompt therapy, which reduces the mortality rate to between 1% and 5%.

Treatment is by the administration of tetracycline or doxycycline (BNF 5.1.3), which must be continued for at least 10 days after the fever has subsided to prevent recurrences.

Psittacosis may be prevented by the control and quarantine of imported birds, and the eradication of disease in breeding stock by supplementing food with antibacterials and vitamins. High standards of hygiene should be maintained in areas where birds are kept. Diseased birds should be isolated and adequately treated or destroyed.

Rheumatic fever

Definition and aetiology

Rheumatic fever is an acute or subacute inflammatory connective tissue disease which follows an upper respiratory-tract infection (usually pharyngitis or tonsillitis). The microorganism responsible for the initial infection is a group A β-haemolytic streptococcus (a Gram-positive facultative anaerobe). An abnormal immune reaction may be responsible for initiating the inflammatory response, although the precise mechanism is unknown.

Overcrowded unhygienic living conditions predispose an individual to developing rheumatic fever and there may be a familial tendency. The disease affects predominantly children and young adults. The first attack usually occurs between 5 and 15 years of age, with the possibility of recurrent attacks and chronic complications throughout adult life. Improvements in living conditions and the advent of antibacterials have reduced the UK incidence from 10% of children in the 1920s to current levels of 0.01%. In developing countries, however, it remains common.

Symptoms

The onset of rheumatic fever, which may be abrupt or insidious, is usually one to six weeks after the initial throat infection.

Intermittent fever, arthralgia and migratory polyarthritis are the earliest symptoms of the acute phase in the majority of patients, affecting the large joints most commonly. The lesions heal in approximately four weeks without any permanent damage.

Carditis, which occurs in up to 40% of patients, may be insidious in onset or even asymptomatic. It is the most serious symptom, as up to 50% may develop rheumatic heart disease in which the valves of the heart become permanently damaged. Endocarditis, myocarditis and pericarditis may also occur, contributing to the development of heart failure.

Painless subcutaneous nodules may arise over bony surfaces or tendons about three weeks after the onset in a small minority of patients. Their appearance usually accompanies carditis, but they generally disappear within two weeks.

Erythema marginatum often accompanies carditis and subcutaneous nodules. It is an evanescent, non-pruritic, macular or papular rash characterised by spreading erythema with loss of colour from the centre of the lesions.

Sydenham's chorea may develop in a small minority of patients up to six months after the onset. In some cases, this may be the only manifestation of rheumatic fever.

Relapses are common following further group A streptococcal infections, and tend to resemble the symptoms of the first attack. Several streptococcal strains exist as part of the body's normal flora (notably in the mouth), and may be responsible for endocarditis in patients with pre-existing rheumatic heart disease who have recently undergone dental or surgical procedures.

Treatment

An untreated attack of rheumatic fever may last up to three months or in the presence of severe carditis, up to six months. Treatment consists primarily of bed rest, with the administration of non-steroidal anti-inflammatory analgesics (BNF 10.1.1) and corticosteroids (BNF 6.3.2) to suppress the inflammatory processes. Heart failure may require further specific therapy, and haloperidol (BNF 4.9.3) is only rarely necessary in severe cases of chorea. Antibacterials (BNF 5.1) may be necessary to eradicate any residual streptococcal infection.

Long-term antibacterial prophylaxis (BNF 5.1, table 2) is necessary to prevent recurrences of rheumatic fever. Additional chemoprophylaxis is indicated in patients with rheumatic heart disease prior to and following surgery.

Salmonellal infections

Definition and aetiology

Salmonellal infections are caused by bacteria of the genus *Salmonella*, which are Gram-negative, facultatively anaerobic bacilli. They are responsible for typhoid and the paratyphoid fevers (collectively known as enteric fever), which are systemic infections with widespread tissue involvement, and salmonellosis (food poisoning), an acute gastroenteritis.

Typhoid fever

Definition and aetiology

Typhoid fever is caused by *Salmonella typhi*, which occurs worldwide and is endemic in regions where poor standards of sewage disposal exist. Cases may be sporadic, or epidemics may occur if local water supplies become contaminated. It is uncommon in developed countries, where most infections are imported by returning travellers or immigrants from endemic areas. The most seriously affected countries include Chile, Indonesia, Nepal and South Africa.

S. typhi bacilli are excreted in faeces and, to a lesser extent, urine. They are transmitted via contaminated drinking water and food. They can withstand freezing and drying, and even remain viable for long periods on soiled clothing or bedding.

Humans are the only reservoir of infection. Older children and young adults are most frequently affected, although no age is excluded.

Symptoms

The incubation period varies from 5 to 23 days, and is inversely related to the inoculum size (i.e. large dose, short incubation period). The inoculum size does not, however, determine the severity of subsequent symptoms, which is related to the patient's previous general health, nutritional state and presence of any concurrent disease.

Typhoid fever is marked by phases of approximately one week's duration. The initial phase starts insidiously with a headache, fluctuating fever and abdominal pain, which coincides with bacterial invasion of the bloodstream. Initially, constipation occurs more frequently than diarrhoea; in later stages, the reverse may apply.

Accompanying symptoms may include anorexia, non-productive cough, epistaxis, furred tongue and, in many cases, a characteristic, rose-coloured, macular rash on the abdomen. During the second week, the fever becomes persistent, toxaemia may develop, and there may be signs of mental deterioration leading, in severe cases, to delirium and coma. Re-entry of bacilli into the gastrointestinal tract results in ulceration and necrosis, which may cause greenish diarrhoea (resembling pea soup) and melaena. The fever may start to abate after the third week, although intestinal haemorrhage (causing anaemia if severe) or perforation and peritonitis may delay convalescence. Severe cases may be complicated by invasion of other organs, resulting in cholecystitis or pneumonia.

The infection usually resolves after a debilitating course lasting five to six weeks, or longer if severe. There may be relapses or recrudescences and, in a few cases, complications may be fatal. Convalescent patients remain carriers of the disease for several weeks. Some individuals (who may not have had acute symptoms) exist as chronic carriers. One attack will often confer lifelong immunity.

Treatment

Treatment is directed towards eliminating the infection, restoring fluid and nutritional defects, and guarding against a potentially wide range of clinical complications. Treatment with an appropriate antibacterial drug (BNF 5.1, table 1) is essential for all patients and carriers. Corticosteroids (BNF 6.3.2) may also be indicated in severe cases of toxaemia. Supportive treatment includes maintenance of adequate fluid and electrolyte levels, and blood transfusions in severe anaemia. Surgery may be necessary to repair perforations.

Typhoid fever may be prevented in endemic areas by improving sanitation, hygiene and health education. Transmission may be prevented by isolation or barrier nursing of symptomatic patients, and excluding carriers from food-handling processes. At least three consecutive stool samples negative for *S. typhi* are required before an individual may be declared free from infection. Travellers may be partially protected by active immunisation (BNF 14.4), but should also boil drinking water and avoid the consumption of raw unpeeled fruit and vegetables.

Paratyphoid fever

Definition and aetiology

Paratyphoid fever is caused by *Salmonella paratyphi* A, B or C. Paratyphoid B occurs worldwide. Paratyphoid A occurs mainly in Asia and Africa; paratyphoid C mainly in Asia and the Middle East. Paratyphoid is transmitted in a similar way to typhoid fever.

Symptoms

Paratyphoid fever resembles typhoid fever, but with a more abrupt onset, milder symptoms, and a shorter course. Complications, relapses and fatalities occur less frequently.

Treatment

The treatment is essentially the same as for typhoid fever, although only supportive treatment may be required for mild infections restricted to the gastrointestinal tract.

Salmonellosis

Definition and aetiology

Salmonellosis is an acute enteritis caused by many species of *Salmonella*, which are enzootic amongst mammals and birds. It is often referred to as food poisoning, but this may also be caused by other bacteria (e.g. *Campylobacter* spp., *Clostridium* spp., *Staphylococcus aureus*, *Vibrio parahaemolyticus* and *Escherichia coli* (*see* Gastroenteritis, Section 1.1).

Salmonellae are excreted in faeces. The most important source of human infection is animal-derived products (e.g. meat, particularly poultry, and eggs and milk). Contamination is facilitated by the intensive and crowded farming methods practised in developed countries. Other modes of transmission include direct contact with an infected animal, contamination of food by rodent faeces, or food prepared by an infected person; chronic human carriers are rare. Contaminated food is most likely to cause salmonellosis if it is left for long periods in warm temperatures prior to consumption, allowing multiplication of salmonella.

Achlorhydria, antacid therapy and gastric surgery render affected individuals particularly susceptible to infection, as salmonella are normally killed by gastric acid. The old, young and severely debilitated are also at risk.

Symptoms

The number of salmonellae needed to produce clinical symptoms is large. The incubation period reflects the time required for salmonella to multiply further within the gastrointestinal tract. It is usually 12–24 hours, but may vary (i.e. 6–48 hours) and is inversely related to the inoculum size. The onset is sudden with symptoms of acute gastroenteritis, which may be accompanied by headache, chills, muscle cramps, and syncope. In severe cases, mucus and blood may be passed in the stools. Occasionally, septicaemia and symptoms resembling typhoid fever may arise if the bloodstream is invaded.

Salmonellosis is usually self-limiting with a rapid recovery after two to five days. It may, however, be fatal in severe cases, particularly in infants, the elderly, and dehydrated patients. Convalescent patients excrete salmonellae for a few weeks, but rarely longer than six months.

Treatment

Treatment is as for gastroenteritis. An appropriate antibacterial drug (BNF 5.1, table 1) may be necessary in severely ill patients, but is not recommended in uncomplicated cases as it prolongs salmonella excretion.

Salmonellosis may be prevented by observing strict hygeine in the processing, preparation and storage of food. Large frozen joints should be completely thawed before cooking, all food should be thoroughly cooked, and cooked meat should be adequately refrigerated. Milk should be pasteurised, reheating of cooked foods must be thorough and carried out once only, and contact between raw meat and cooked foods should be prevented.

Scarlet fever

Definition and aetiology

Scarlet fever (scarlatina) follows an attack of pharyngitis caused by erythrogenic toxin-producing strains of group A β-haemolytic streptococci (which are Gram-positive facultative anaerobes). It is endemic in temperate climates and occurs mainly during the summer and early autumn, although the incidence and mortality has decreased significantly in recent years. It is transmitted via droplets from an infected person (including carriers) or via contaminated fomites.

Children are most susceptible to developing scarlet fever, the majority of cases occurring in those under five years of age.

Symptoms

The incubation period is usually two to three days (range 12 hours to six days).

The onset is sudden, and is marked by a sore throat with pain on swallowing, chills, fever, malaise, vomiting, rapid pulse, dry skin, flushed face and furred tongue with protruding red papillae ('strawberry tongue'). A symmetrical non-pruritic rash appears after 24–36 hours, initially on the arms, neck, back and chest, and later spreads to the remainder of the body. It is characterised by red spots appearing against a background of erythema which blanches on application of pressure. Petechiae may be visible as striations in the skin folds (Pastia's sign), and the face is often flushed with a paler region around the mouth. All symptoms worsen for two to three days before gradually resolving. During convalescence, desquamation of the skin may occur.

Complications of scarlet fever include bronchitis (which may be fatal) and otitis media in children, arthritis in adults, and adenitis, rhinitis or nephritis in any age group.

One attack usually confers life-long immunity which is strain-specific, although relapses do occur in approximately 1% of patients.

Treatment

Treatment consists of the administration of pencillins (BNF 5.1.1). Tepid sponging may be of value to reduce fever.

Scarlet fever may be prevented by improvements in living standards and prompt antimicrobial treatment for streptococcal sore throats. Patients should be isolated until at least one negative throat swab has been obtained.

Shigellosis

Definition and aetiology

Shigellosis (bacillary dysentery) is an acute colitis caused by Gram-negative, facultatively anaerobic, non-sporing bacilli of the genus *Shigella*. *Sh. dysenteriae* is the most virulent species and is responsible for epidemic dysentery in developing countries, where overcrowded conditions exist alongside inadequate sewage disposal. *Sh. flexneri* and *Sh. boydii* infections are of moderate severity, occurring mainly in tropical regions. *Sh. sonnei* causes a mild form of shigellosis, which is endemic in developed countries. Outbreaks occur most frequently in schools and other institutions housing young people.

The only natural reservoirs of infection are humans and higher primates. Transmission occurs by the faecal–oral route, usually by ingestion of contaminated food and water. Shigella may survive for several hours on fingers or even days on fomites (e.g. lavatory seats, door handles and towels) in cold damp conditions. Flies also act as an effective means of transferring bacteria from faeces to food.

Symptoms

The inoculum size required to cause disease is small. The incubation period is short (usually less than three days), although occasionally it may last a week.

The onset of symptoms is generally abrupt, commencing with abdominal pain, headache, tenesmus, vomiting and watery diarrhoea, which may be almost continuous. In severe cases, there may be passage of pus and blood-stained mucus ('redcurrant jelly'), and dehydration may become severe, particularly in infants and the elderly. Other symptoms include anorexia and weight loss. In some, the infection may be very mild or even asymptomatic. After a few days the patient gradually recovers, although shigella continue to be passed in the faeces for several weeks. Serious infections may follow a protracted course which may be fatal in infants, the elderly, and previously debilitated or malnourished individuals.

Complications that can occur with any form of shigellosis include arthritis and haemorrhoids, and in severe cases, peritonitis. Convulsions may occur in children during the early stages.

Treatment

Rehydration is very important and comprises the administration of oral (BNF 9.2.1) or intravenous fluids (BNF 9.2.2). An appropriate antibacterial drug (BNF 5.1, table 1) may be necessary in severe cases. It is, however, not recommended in milder self-limiting forms, particularly during epidemics, as antibacterial-resistant strains rapidly emerge. Drugs which reduce intestinal motility should be avoided, as they prolong the course of the infection and excretion of shigella.

Shigellosis may be prevented in endemic areas by improving sanitation and excluding flies from food-preparation areas. Spread during an outbreak in institutions may be controlled by isolating infected individuals, thoroughly cleansing the hands after defecation, regularly disinfecting lavatories, flush handles, door knobs and taps, and using disposable hand-towels. Infected food handlers should not be allowed to return to work until at least three consecutive stool samples negative to shigella have been passed.

Stye

Definition and aetiology

A stye (hordeolum) (Figure 5.4) is a local pyogenic infection involving the follicle or sebaceous gland of an eyelash, or both. It arises on the outer surface of the eyelid through inflammation of the glands of Zeis or Moll's glands. Its presence on the inner surface caused by inflammation of the Meibomian glands is termed a chalazion. It is most commonly due to staphylococci.

Symptoms

Symptoms of an external stye include painful swelling and inflammation of the edge of the affected eyelid. The swelling 'points' to a head within a few days, and then ruptures, producing a discharge of pus and the relief of pain. Recurrence is common.

For symptoms of an internal stye (which is very rare), *see* Chalazion, Section 11.1.

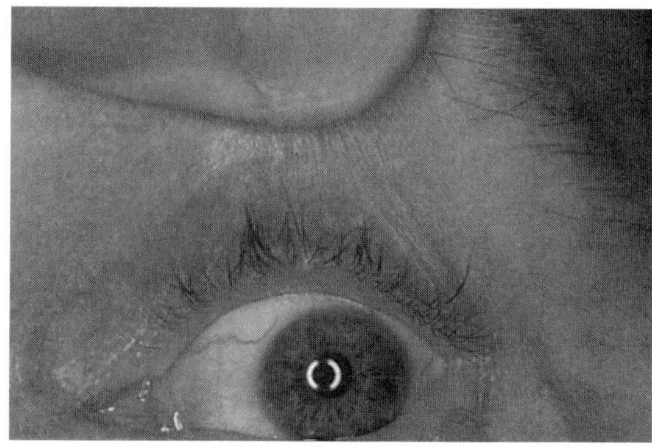

Figure 5.4 Stye on upper eyelid. (Reproduced with permission of Mike Wyndham.)

Treatment

Treatment consists of the application of hot compresses. An appropriate topical anti-infective preparation (BNF 11.3) may be indicated in recurrent cases, or to prevent the spread of infection.

Sycosis barbae

Definition and aetiology

Sycosis barbae is an inflammatory infection of the hair follicles in the bearded region caused by *Staphylococcus aureus*. There may be a correlation of incidence with a greasy skin, and recurrence may be caused by emotional disturbances and fatigue.

Symptoms

The condition occurs in males generally between 30 and 40 years of age. It is characterised by red oedematous papules or pustules at the point of emergence of the hair. In chronic forms, larger raised lesions may arise from several confluent infected follicles. Complete follicles may be destroyed, resulting in scarring.

Treatment

Treatment is as for Folliculitis (*see* Section 13.1), although systemic antibacterial drugs (BNF 5.1) may be necessary in unresponsive cases. The nares, which in some individuals are a possible reservoir of infection, should also be treated.

Tetanus

Definition and aetiology

Tetanus (lockjaw) is caused by a potent exotoxin, tetanospasmin, produced by *Clostridium tetani*, a Gram-positive, anaerobic, spore-forming bacillus. The disease occurs worldwide, although the incidence in developed countries is low due to active immunisation programmes and good standards of hygiene and healthcare.

The spores are present in soil and in the faeces of many mammals (including humans). They are highly resistant, remaining viable for years under dry conditions and able to withstand boiling for hours. Spores contaminating a wound germinate if anaerobic conditions prevail (e.g. in deep punctures or in the presence of necrotic tissue or foreign bodies). The infected wound may be minor and ignored by the patient. The toxin produced by vegetative bacilli is carried in the bloodstream and nerve fibres to the central nervous system, where it acts at the presynaptic terminal of inhibitory spinal neurons to prevent the release of inhibitory transmitter. Sensory and autonomic nerves take up some toxin, but the major effect is hyperactivity of motor neurons, which results in muscular rigidity and spasm.

Neonatal tetanus occurs predominantly in developing countries, and is caused by infection of the umbilicus due to use of contaminated instruments or dressings. In developed countries, the elderly are most at risk of contracting tetanus, although no age group is exempt. Drug abusers are also susceptible due to contamination of some samples of crude heroin with spores.

Globally, tetanus is responsible for 50 000 deaths each year; about 800 000 deaths are caused by neonatal tetanus. It is relatively rare in western countries, with about 80 cases reported each year in the USA.

Symptoms

The incubation period varies from 1 to 14 days, with an average of seven days, although some spores may remain dormant for several months.

Tetanus is characterised by muscular rigidity, which may commence with the muscles of the jaw (lockjaw or trismus), and contraction of facial muscles, causing a 'sneering' expression (*risus sardonicus*). Pain and stiffness in the muscles of the neck and back may cause a 'ramrod' posture, or backward curvature of the spine (opisthotonos) if there is excessive contraction of the long muscles. The muscles of the abdomen are also rigid. In moderately severe cases, the pharyngeal muscles may be involved and this results in dysphagia.

Reflex spasms may arise, usually as a result of external stimuli (e.g. movement, injections, sudden noise or passing a nasogastric tube), which intensify the underlying hypertonia. The spasms become spontaneous in severe tetanus, and increase in intensity and frequency. Complications include spinal fractures due to extreme opisthotonos, and respiratory failure due to respiratory-muscle spasm. Other respiratory complications include atelectasis and bronchopneumonia. The autonomic nervous system is also frequently involved in severe cases, causing a fluctuating blood pressure, high fever, peripheral vasoconstriction, increased cardiac output, arrhythmias and, if persistent, cardiac arrest.

Most deaths are due to cardiac or pulmonary complications and occur during the first eight days. Surviving patients usually show a gradual but complete recovery in four to six weeks.

Treatment

The prognosis is poor in severe tetanus, with 50% mortality rising to 90% in neonatal tetanus. Less than 10% of milder cases are fatal.

Treatment comprises the administration of a benzylpenicillin (BNF 5.1.1.1) to eliminate bacteria, passive immunisation with tetanus immunoglobulin of human origin (HTIG) (BNF 14.5) to neutralise toxin circulating in the bloodstream, and a skeletal muscle relaxant (BNF 10.2.2). Thorough cleansing and debridement of the wound after administration of the antitoxin may also be of value in eradicating a known focus of infection. Intensive supportive measures are necessary in moderate and severe cases until the disease has run its course, as toxin cannot be removed from the CNS. These include endotracheal intubation, tracheostomy, and enteral (BNF 9.4.2) and intravenous (BNF 9.3) nutrition. Respiratory complications may require assisted ventilation in conjunction with peripheral neuromuscular blockade. A beta-adrenoceptor blocking drug with alpha-blocking activity (BNF 2.4) or an opioid analgesic (e.g. morphine, BNF 4.7.2) may be indicated for cardiovascular complications. It may also be necessary to monitor the fluid and electrolyte balance.

The most effective means of preventing tetanus is by active immunisation with tetanus vaccine (BNF 14.4) in infancy, followed by regular booster doses throughout adult life (*see also* Section 15.5). Adsorbed tetanus toxin is usually given in combination with diphtheria and pertussis vaccines. Any wound contaminated with soil or faeces should be treated promptly, and HTIG administered if the patient's immunity is in doubt. A course of adsorbed tetanus toxin should also be administered to all patients with tetanus as an attack does not confer immunity. Neonatal tetanus may be prevented by immunisation of pregnant women and use of sterile equipment and dressings at delivery.

Toxic shock syndrome

Definition and aetiology

Toxic shock syndrome (TSS) is due to the effects of a toxin produced, in the majority of cases, by *Staphylococcus aureus*. It is rarely the result of bacteraemia.

It occurs most frequently in association with the use of highly-absorbent tampons by menstruating women. The synthetic material contained in these tampons is broken down by specific enzymes produced by host and bacterial cells, which may be found in the vagina under normal circumstances. The end-product of degradation is glucose, providing an ideal source of nutrient for toxin-producing strains of *S. aureus*, which may be present in up to 17% of women.

Less than 10% of cases have been reported as occurring in men, children, and non-menstruating women. In these cases, the primary focus of infection may be an abscess or empyema, or colonisation of surgical sutures or contraceptive diaphragms and sponges.

Symptoms

TSS has an abrupt onset and is characterised by high fever, myalgia, nausea and vomiting, and watery diarrhoea. Other symptoms may include conjunctivitis, headache, lethargy, sore throat and intermittent confusion. A rash resembling sunburn appears, which desquamates, particularly on the palms of the hands and soles of the feet, after three to seven days. The condition may rapidly progress to hypotension and shock, which may be fatal if untreated. Complications involving any organ may occur due to the effects of shock (e.g. acute renal failure and adult respiratory distress syndrome). Recurrences are common for up to six months in 10% of patients continuing to use tampons.

Treatment

The treatment is supportive, as described under shock (*see* Circulatory failure, acute, Section 2.1). Antibacterial drugs (BNF 5.1) will not modify the course of the syndrome, but may be of value in removing the primary focus of infection and preventing recurrences.

TSS may be prevented in menstruating women by avoiding the continual use of tampons, particularly those with high absorbency.

Trachoma

Definition and aetiology

Trachoma (granular conjunctivitis) is a chronic inflammatory disease of the conjunctiva and cornea due to infection with *Chlamydia trachomatis*, a weakly Gram-negative, obligate, intracellular parasite. It is endemic in many developing parts of the world (e.g. in rural areas of Africa, Asia, the Middle East, and South and Central America), and is the most common worldwide cause of blindness.

The infection is transmitted by contact with infected conjunctival secretions via fingers, fomites (e.g. handkerchiefs and eye makeup applicators) and flies. It may also be transmitted sexually, the main reservoir of infection being the cervix in the female genital tract. The sexually transmitted form is a common cause of trachoma in urban areas of developed countries. Neonatal trachoma arises as a result of passage through an infected birth canal.

Symptoms

The exact incubation period is unknown, but may be between one and three weeks. Neonatal trachoma usually arises between 5 and 14 days after birth; sexually transmitted infections may present with symptoms in less than two weeks.

Trachoma usually affects both eyes and is characterised by local inflammation, lachrymation, pain, discharge, erythematous and swollen eyelids, ptosis and photophobia. As the disease progresses, follicles develop in the conjunctiva and papillary hyperplasia occurs. Eventually, vascularisation of the cornea (i.e. pannus formation) occurs, resulting in ulceration and scarring. The degree of visual impairment may vary, but in severe cases, blindness may occur. Reinfection is common, as is secondary bacterial infection.

The symptoms of neonatal trachoma are similar, although the cornea may be unaffected. Adult sexually transmitted trachoma is often unilateral.

Treatment

Treatment includes the topical (BNF 11.3.1) or systemic (BNF 5.1.3) administration of a tetracycline, or both. A systemic sulphonamide (BNF 5.1.8) may also be effective. Erythromycin (BNF 5.1.5) should be used in children. Surgery may be necessary in severe cases.

Trachoma may be prevented in endemic areas by mass therapy using topical anti-infective preparations (BNF 11.3.1), and improvements in living standards and encouragement of scrupulous hygiene. Topical erythromycin administered prophylactically may be of value in preventing neonatal trachoma.

Tuberculosis

Definition and aetiology

Tuberculosis is a chronic infectious disease usually caused by *Mycobacterium tuberculosis*, an acid-fast bacillus. Other species (e.g. *M. bovis*) may also be responsible. It is prevalent in developing countries, particularly where conditions of poor housing, overcrowding, poverty, poor nutrition and inadequate medical care prevail.

The microorganism is an obligate parasite, which is transmitted from person to person by inhalation of airborne droplets. Ingestion of unpasteurised milk from infected cows is a mode of transmission which is of historic interest only in developed countries, but accidental skin inoculation in laboratory personnel is a possibility. Disease develops in only 5% to 15% of infected people and is dependent on various factors (e.g. inoculum size, virulence of infecting strain, the host's age, inherent resistance, and state of health and nutrition). It most commonly affects the respiratory tract (pulmonary tuberculosis) and may be primary or post-primary. It is characterised by inflammatory infiltrations, tubercle formation, caseation, fibrosis and calcification. In up to one-third of patients, the microorganism may spread in the blood circulation and lymphatics to other organs (e.g. lymph nodes, heart, gastrointestinal or genito-urinary tracts, meninges, bones, joints and skin), and several organs may be affected simultaneously (miliary tuberculosis).

The incidence of tuberculosis had been relatively stable up to the middle of the 1980s. However, from that time, an increase in the incidence of the disease occurred, not only in developing but also in developed countries. Whilst some of this increase could be attributed to social conditions and migration of people in the developing world, most has been caused by the occurrence of human immunodeficiency virus (HIV). Tuberculosis has been quick to capitalise on the immunocompromised state of these patients. In developing countries, tuberculosis has become a disease primarily of young adults.

Primary pulmonary tuberculosis

Definition and aetiology

Primary pulmonary tuberculosis occurs in previously uninfected subjects and is most common in children. It is usually caused by droplet inhalation and it results in pulmonary inflammation and exudate production. Although necrosis and cavitation of the lungs do not frequently occur, calcification is common.

Symptoms

It is usually a mild disease and is often asymptomatic. Nevertheless, common symptoms include cough (usually non-productive), fever, malaise, wheezing, anorexia with weight loss, and occasionally erythema nodosum. In severe cases, respiratory distress may occur. The primary disease usually resolves spontaneously within a few weeks, although it may occasionally become progressive and affect other organs.

Treatment

See Post-primary pulmonary tuberculosis *below*.

Post-primary pulmonary tuberculosis

Definition and aetiology

Post-primary pulmonary tuberculosis occurs as a result of reactivation of latent primary infection and is more common in the elderly. Other contributory factors include diabetes mellitus, administration of drugs affecting the immune response, and poor nutrition. It results in pulmonary caseation, with extensive necrosis and cavitation followed by fibrosis. It may be acute or chronic and may become progressive.

Symptoms

Post-primary disease has an insidious, often asymptomatic, onset. Early symptoms, however, include anorexia with weight loss, fever and malaise. Other common symptoms are cough with the production of purulent sputum, chest pain, haemoptysis, night sweats, anxiety, depressive disorders, resistant pneumonia and chronic ill-health.

Treatment

The treatment of both primary and post-primary tuberculosis consists of the long-term administration of antituberculous drugs (BNF 5.1.9). Bronchoscopy may occasionally be required to clear diseased airways, and surgical drainage, excision of lesions, or reconstruction may be necessary in rare cases.

The spread of tuberculosis may be prevented by the identification, using the Mantoux test, and treatment of all infected individuals. Close contacts of patients should receive antibacterial prophylaxis (BNF 5.1, table 2), and all tuberculin-negative children should be actively immunised with the bacillus Calmette-Guérin (BCG) vaccine (BNF 14.4). Host resistance in endemic areas may be increased by improvements in living conditions, nutrition and medical care.

Typhus fevers

Definition and aetiology

Typhus fevers are caused by species of *Rickettsia*, which are Gram-negative, pleomorphic, obligate intracellular parasites. These fevers are now uncommon in developed countries, although they have been associated historically with periods of famine, mass poverty or war.

R. prowazekii is responsible for classical epidemic typhus, which is transmitted to people in the faeces of the human body louse (*Pediculus humanus corporis*). The microorganism gains entry via skin abrasions (including the louse-bite site), or the respiratory tract if dried faeces are inhaled. The louse acquires the infection during a blood meal on a patient with typhus. Brill-Zinsser disease is a milder form of epidemic typhus occurring as a recrudescence of the primary infection due to the persistence of bacteria within the tissues. The milder form may occur many years after the primary infection.

Murine (endemic) typhus and scrub typhus are zoonotic infections involving rodents (e.g. rats) as the reservoir of infection, and fleas or mites respectively as vectors, with humans an incidental host.

Symptoms

The incubation period of epidemic typhus fever is between 5 and 14 days.

The onset is sudden and is characterised by sustained fever, rigors, severe and persistent headache, facial flushing, myalgia (particularly in the back and legs), prostration and a dulled mental state. A macular rash may become petechial in severe cases. Later symptoms include deafness, incontinence, restlessness, delirium, profound prostration and stupor.

Mortality is greatest in untreated patients over 40 years of age. Death is usually due to peripheral vascular collapse, renal failure or pulmonary complications. Surviving patients start to recover after approximately two weeks of fever.

The symptoms of murine typhus are similar but milder; the course is shorter and the mortality rate lower. Lymph nodes become enlarged and other constitutional symptoms similar to those of epidemic typhus fever develop.

Treatment

Treatment is effective and can dramatically reduce the mortality rate.

Tetracyclines (BNF 5.1.3) are appropriate antibacterial drugs used in the treatment of rickettsial diseases. Chloramphenicol (BNF 5.1.7) and corticosteroids (BNF 6.3.2) may be used in severely ill patients.

Patients should be deloused and all clothes and bedding decontaminated to curb further spread. Wider measures to prevent typhus fevers include the control of rat and flea populations, and wearing clothes treated with insect repellents in endemic areas. A vaccine (BNF 14.4) is available for travellers likely to be at risk of contracting epidemic (not scrub) typhus (e.g. those coming into close contact with the indigenous population).

5.3 Viral infections

Acquired immune deficiency syndrome

Definition and aetiology

Acquired immune deficiency syndrome (AIDS) arises as an end-stage manifestation of infection by human immunodeficiency virus type 1 (HIV-1), and is prevalent worldwide. Human immunodeficiency virus type 2 (HIV-2) will also cause AIDS, and is largely confined to West Africa. HIV infection results in the reduction of the number of T-cells, particularly helper T-cells, although other leucocytes are also susceptible (e.g. B-cells, monocytes, and macrophages).

Primary manifestations of HIV infection are progressive immunodeficiency (particularly affecting cell-mediated immunity), diminished immunosurveillance and the direct effects of HIV on tissues (e.g. the central nervous system and gastrointestinal tract). Secondary manifestations of HIV infection occur as a result of impaired immunity and include malignant disease and infections.

In the absence of other causes of immunodeficiency, diagnosis of HIV infection is based upon the presence of circulating HIV antibodies. HIV infection can be transmitted if the virus gains entry into the blood circulation. This can occur through sexual intercourse (heterosexual and homosexual), transplantation of infected organs and tissues, transfusion of infected blood or blood products, contaminated equipment (e.g. during parenteral drug abuse), and from an infected mother to child *in utero*, during childbirth, or possibly during breast feeding.

There has been no accurate assessment of the number of AIDS patients globally. Estimates suggest infection of 40 million people worldwide in the year 2000. Most of these live in developing countries: in Africa, South and South East Asia, Latin America and the Caribbean.

Three distinct patterns of the epidemic have been suggested. In developed countries, the disease occurs predominantly in young homosexual men and intravenous drug users, with the latter group becoming increasingly dominant. Heterosexual transmission is also increasing. The second group occurs in sub-Saharan Africa and the Caribbean, where transmission occurs mainly by heterosexual and perinatal routes. Roughly equal numbers of females and males are affected in this group. The third group exists in those countries in which AIDS became a problem relatively late in its spread. These include North Africa, the Middle East and Asia. Although still relatively small in numbers affected, these areas have seen a great increase in the cases within closely defined groups (e.g. intravenous drug users).

Symptoms

Symptoms of HIV infection depend upon the clinical stage of the infection. Progression from infection by HIV to development of AIDS may take months or years. It is unpredictable and patients may remain asymptomatic for many years. Following infection there is a latent period of between 4 and 12 weeks which, on rare occasions, can be longer. During this time, there is no immune response, and the infection cannot, therefore, be detected. This period is followed by acute HIV infection, with the formation of HIV antibodies (seroconversion). Most patients are asymptomatic, but non-specific symptoms can occur and are generally self-limiting. These include arthropathy, diarrhoea, fever, headache, malaise, myalgia, nausea and vomiting, and photophobia. Transient lymphadenopathy, rashes, convulsions and coma may also occur.

Progression to chronic HIV infection may be asymptomatic, or may result in persistent generalised lymphadenopathy. During the later stages the patient may develop the AIDS-related complex (ARC), which is characterised by fever, lethargy, malaise, night sweats, persistent diarrhoea and weight loss. Minor opportunistic infections may also occur, including folliculitis, herpesvirus infections, oral candidiasis, oral hairy leucoplakia, tinea infections and warts.

Further progression to AIDS (end-stage disease or full-blown AIDS) occurs when immunity is severely impaired. Patients usually develop life-threatening opportunistic infections or malignant disease. These most commonly include *Pneumocystis carinii* pneumonia or Kaposi's sarcoma, which may occur together. Other opportunistic infections may also occur, including cerebral toxoplasmosis, cytomegalovirus infection, meningitis and pulmonary tuberculosis. Other malignant disease may be present (e.g. non-Hodgkin's lymphoma and cerebral lymphoma).

Neurological disease associated with HIV infection may occur with varying severity and at any stage. It includes dementia, encephalopathy and neuropathy, and is thought to be caused by the direct effect of the virus.

Treatment

There is no effective treatment or prophylaxis of HIV infection. Patients usually require counselling and regular monitoring of health. Antiviral drugs (BNF 5.3) have been developed that slow or halt the disease progression and increase life expectancy.

Prevention of further transmission comprises the primary basis of management of HIV infection. This includes screening donor blood, organs and tissues; heat-treatment of blood products; adoption of safer sexual activities; and avoidance of contaminated equipment. In addition, women within high-risk groups (e.g. drug abusers) who are pregnant or who may be planning a pregnancy should be screened and counselled.

Common cold

Definition and aetiology

The common cold (acute coryza or infective rhinitis) is caused by infection of the nose, nasopharynx and upper respiratory tract, mainly by rhinoviruses. However, a wide variety of other viruses including coronaviruses, adenoviruses and myxoviruses are also responsible. The infection occurs worldwide, particularly during the autumn and winter months in temperate climates. Infection spreads rapidly (especially in crowded conditions) via nasopharyngeal droplets, which may be inhaled directly or passed indirectly on fingers. The latter mode of transmission may be more significant than formerly thought; saliva does not appear to be an important means of viral transmission. The major portals of entry are the nasal mucosa and conjunctiva.

Children are particularly susceptible and may have several colds each year, although physical resistance in any age group may be lowered by physical or emotional disturbances or ill-health. Exposure to low temperatures does not cause the common cold and appears to have little effect on lowering host resistance.

Symptoms
The incubation period is one to four days, with the period of greatest infectivity starting about 24 hours before and, lasting for up to five days, after the onset of symptoms.

The onset is abrupt and is characterised by discomfort in the eyes, nose and throat, with nasal congestion and discharge. There may also be sore throat and cough. Mild fever occasionally occurs in children, but is uncommon in adults, and this is an important means of differentiating a common cold from influenza. There is usually complete recovery within 4–10 days of onset, although complications (e.g. laryngitis, sinusitis and otitis media) may develop, and secondary bacterial infection may follow.

Treatment
Treatment is symptomatic and may include the administration of non-opioid analgesics (BNF 4.7.1), systemic (BNF 3.10) or topical nasal decongestants (BNF 12.2.2), and antitussives (BNF 3.9). Aromatic inhalations (BNF 3.8) may be useful.

Production of an effective vaccine is unlikely, as many strains of different viruses are responsible. Spread of the common cold within households may be prevented by regular handwashing, avoiding hand-to-face contact, and taking measures to curtail droplet spread.

Encephalitis

Definition and aetiology
Encephalitis is inflammation of the brain, usually arising from a viral infection. A wide variety of viruses may be responsible, but paramyxoviruses (e.g. measles and mumps viruses) are commonly implicated, together with arboviruses and herpesviruses. The infecting virus may vary according to geographical location.

Symptoms
The onset may be sudden or insidious and is characterised by an alteration in consciousness, which may vary from lethargy to coma and headache. Other symptoms include convulsions, fever, neck stiffness, raised intracranial pressure, and motor and sensory disturbances. Confusion and behavioural disturbances may occur. Encephalitis may be fatal, and surviving patients may suffer permanent disability (e.g. epilepsy or intellectual impairment).

Treatment
Treatment is supportive with the administration of analgesics (BNF 4.7) for headache, tepid sponging for fever, and the maintenance of an adequate fluid intake. Corticosteroids (BNF 6.3.2) and antiviral drugs (BNF 5.3) have been used. Antiepileptics (BNF 4.8) may be necessary. Neurosurgical decompression may be indicated.

Subacute sclerosing panencephalitis

Definition and aetiology
Subacute sclerosing panencephalitis is a rare form of encephalitis found in children and young adults, and is due to a persistent measles virus infection, first contracted at an early age.

Symptoms
The onset of symptoms is insidious, usually occurs around six years after primary infection with the measles virus, and is initially characterised by general lethargy. Weeks or months later, clumsiness and involuntary movements develop. Visual disturbances are common and, as the disease progresses, intellectual impairment, spasticity and rigidity occur. Death usually follows within two years.

Treatment
No effective treatment exists.

Herpesvirus infections

Definition and aetiology

Herpesviruses are widely distributed throughout the animal kingdom, although some (e.g. cytomegalovirus) are highly specific for a particular host. It is common for the virus to become latent after the primary infection, with reactivation of disease occurring in response to a variety of stimuli despite the presence of circulating antibodies. Most infections are mild and non-life-threatening, although serious and fatal disease may occur in infants or immunocompromised hosts and by viruses not normally specific for humans.

Herpes simplex virus infections

Definition and aetiology

Herpes simplex virus (HSV) infections are transmitted directly from person to person via oral secretions (usually HSV type 1) or genital secretions (usually HSV type 2). Transmission does not always take place in the presence of active lesions, and asymptomatic carriers may represent an important reservoir of infection. In some cases, auto-infection may occur.

Herpes labialis (cold sore or fever blister) occurs as a recurrence of an HSV 1 infection. The latent virus, present in ganglia of the trigeminal nerve, may be reactivated by emotional disturbances, fever, menstruation, sunlight or local trauma.

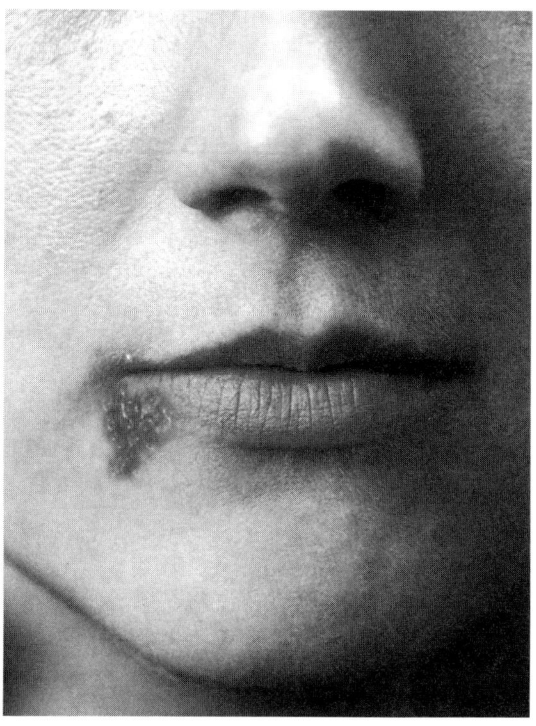

Figure 5.5 Herpes labialis (cold sore). (Reproduced with permission from *Pharmaceutical Journal*.)

Symptoms

The incubation period is from 2 to 12 days for HSV 1 infections and 2–7 days for HSV 2 infections.

Primary infection with HSV 1 may be asymptomatic or can present with prodromal symptoms that include fever, malaise, gingivitis, pharyngitis and generalised adenopathy (especially in the cervical region). Vesicles appear within the mouth and on the lips, rupturing to form painful ulcers. Accompanying symptoms in some are excessive salivation and halitosis. The condition is self-limiting and untreated ulcers heal without scarring within 14 days.

Herpes labialis is characterised by the appearance of vesicular eruptions on the edges of the lips (Figure 5.5), preceded by a prodromal phase during which the patient experiences localised burning and itching sensations. Eruptions develop singly or in crops and persist for up to 10 days, during which time they rupture and become encrusted. Local inflammation often occurs and secondary bacterial infection may develop. Recurrence may occur, usually at the same site, over a period of many years.

HSV 2 infections are characterised by painful vesicular lesions appearing in the anogenital region. Accompanying constitutional symptoms include anorexia, fever, malaise and lymphadenopathy. Dysuria or urinary retention may occur in females and the infection may be transferred to neonates during delivery. Lesions may take several weeks to heal. Recurrent infections are generally less severe and extensive, and the lesions may be preceded by burning or itching sensations.

Other sites may be involved in primary infections with both types of virus. Herpetic whitlows occur on fingers and are often seen in medical and dental personnel. Infections of the eye result in keratoconjunctivitis, which may be recurrent. Encephalitis is an uncommon, but potentially fatal, complication, particularly in neonates.

Treatment

Herpes simplex virus infections respond well to systemic antiviral drugs (BNF 5.3). Additional local measures include ophthalmic anti-infective preparations (BNF 11.3.1), antiviral skin preparations (BNF 13.10.3), or an oropharyngeal anti-infective mouthwash (BNF 12.3.2).

Spread of infection may be prevented by avoiding contact with active lesions. Caesarean delivery may be necessary for babies born to infected mothers, and chemoprophylaxis with antiviral drugs may be administered to immunocompromised hosts.

Varicella-zoster virus infections

Definition and aetiology

The primary infection in non-immune individuals caused by the varicella-zoster virus is chickenpox (varicella), an acute, highly contagious disease. Following recovery, the virus remains latent within sensory root ganglia and may be reactivated by stimuli (e.g. malignancy, irradiation with X-rays or ultraviolet light, immunosuppressant therapy or trauma), resulting in herpes zoster shingles (Figure 5.6). In many cases, there appears to be no obvious stimulus.

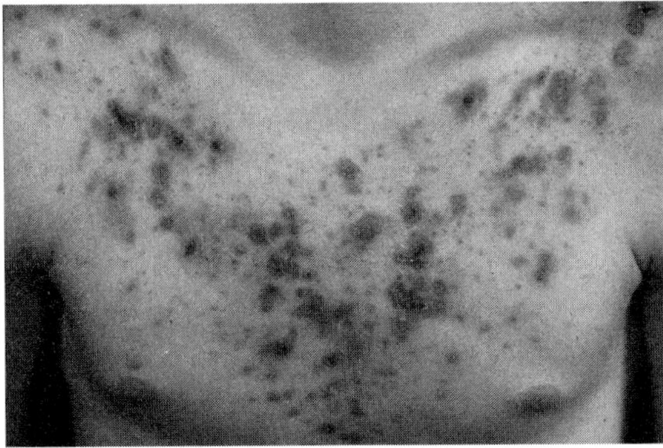

Figure 5.6 Herpes zoster. (Reproduced with permission from *Pharmaceutical Journal*.)

Chickenpox is transmitted between individuals via airborne droplets or by contact with active lesions. Contrary to popular belief, it is unlikely that herpes zoster arises as a result of contact with a chickenpox sufferer (i.e. it is not a re-infection). However, a non-immune subject may develop chickenpox following contact with a herpes zoster patient.

Chickenpox is primarily a disease of the young and is most prevalent in children between two and eight years of age. Herpes zoster may occur at any age, although the greatest incidence is in the elderly. Second attacks of either disease are uncommon.

Symptoms

The incubation period of chickenpox is usually between 14 and 16 days, although the range may extend from 10 to 23 days. The infection is most contagious during the period immediately before the rash starts, and infectivity lasts until the vesicles have formed crusts. Prodromal symptoms, which may be absent or only mild in the very young, include fever, malaise and anorexia. These symptoms are more severe in adults, who may also suffer with headache, back pain, myalgia, chills and vomiting. The lesions, which commonly appear on the trunk and scalp, are macular, develop rapidly into vesicles, and finally become pustular and encrusted. Successive crops appear over several days, but rarely spread to the limbs.

Accompanying pruritus may allow development of secondary infections, particularly with staphylococci, through scratching. Mucous membranes (e.g. conjunctiva, the buccal mucosa, pharynx and vagina) may also be involved. Pneumonitis is a potentially fatal complication, and occurs in up to one-third of adult patients. Encephalitis may occur in any age group, but is uncommon. Herpes zoster is characterised by a unilateral rash, which generally follows the course of sensory nerves innervating those areas where the chickenpox rash is most commonly seen (i.e. the trunk and along the trigeminal nerve). The lesions are similar in nature to those seen in chickenpox, although they are usually accompanied by paraesthesia, neuralgia, and in some cases lymphadenopathy. Paralysis of motor nerves may occasionally occur, although this is not permanent in the majority of cases. Ophthalmic zoster (involving the eye) is a serious complication, which may cause blindness if untreated. Some patients, particularly the elderly, suffer persistent pain (post-herpetic neuralgia) for many months or years after the lesions disappear.

Treatment

Treatment of chickenpox is usually symptomatic, comprising the administration of antipruritic preparations (BNF 13.3) and non-opioid analgesics other than aspirin (BNF 4.7.1). Specific antiviral therapy (BNF 5.3) is usually reserved for those at risk of developing serious disease (e.g. immunocompromised patients). Herpes zoster may be treated with a combination of systemic antivirals (BNF 5.3), antiviral skin preparations (BNF 13.10.3) and analgesics (BNF 4.7). Institution of early therapy is essential and may help to reduce the incidence of post-herpetic neuralgia. Antiviral ophthalmic ointments (BNF 11.3.1) are indicated for eye infections, for which patients are referred to a specialist. All patients should be discouraged from scratching lesions, to reduce the chance of secondary bacterial infection and scarring on healing. Spread of infection may be prevented by avoiding contact with active lesions. Anti-varicella-zoster immunoglobulin injection (BNF 14.5) is also available as prophylaxis for highly susceptible groups.

Cytomegalovirus infection

Definition and aetiology

Cytomegaloviruses are widely distributed throughout the animal kingdom, although individual members of this group are host-specific. Human cytomegalovirus, which is found worldwide, is transmitted by close contact with body tissues and fluids. As with other herpesviruses, latent infections may be reactivated after the primary infection. In adults, the infection is common and, in most cases, trivial. Neonates with congenital infections and immunocompromised patients (e.g. those with AIDS) are most susceptible to developing serious disease.

Symptoms

Acquired infections in otherwise healthy individuals are often asymptomatic or present with mild, non-specific, self-limiting symptoms. More serious symptoms may include hepatosplenomegaly, lymphadenopathy, pneumonia, ulcerative colitis and encephalitis. Some patients may present with a syndrome resembling infectious mononucleosis (*see below*). Congenital infections may cause cerebral palsy, hepatosplenomegaly, jaundice, microcephaly and purpura and, to a lesser extent, chorioretinitis, sensorineural deafness and epilepsy. In some cases, there may be no detectable symptoms at birth, although available data indicate that such infants may later have learning and developmental difficulties.

Treatment

The prognosis for immunocompromised hosts varies considerably from complete recovery to death. There is as yet no effective antiviral agent available to treat cytomegalovirus infections, although ganciclovir (BNF 5.3) may be used in immunocompromised patients. Reduction in the level of immunosuppressants may be of value in reducing the severity of infection in graft patients.

Infectious mononucleosis

Definition and aetiology

Infectious mononucleosis (glandular fever) is caused by the Epstein–Barr virus, which is distributed worldwide. Infection with the virus is associated with conditions of overcrowding and poor hygiene, and is almost universal amongst children in developing countries. It is less prevalent in developed countries, although more likely to cause clinical illness, especially amongst young people living together in groups (e.g. military recruits and college students). The exact mode of transmission is unknown, but is likely to be via oropharyngeal secretions. Infected individuals may excrete the virus for up to a year.

Symptoms

Many cases are asymptomatic, but in those that do develop symptoms the incubation period is from five to seven weeks. There may be a prodromal period of four to five days with symptoms of headache, fatigue and malaise followed by fever, sore throat and cervical adenopathy. Additional symptoms may include oedema of the oronasopharyngeal region, resulting in dysphagia, periorbital oedema, and petechiae and vesicles on the palate. There may be a non-pruritic maculopapular rash in a few cases. Splenomegaly frequently occurs and in rare cases may lead to rupture. Other complications include jaundice, myocarditis, pneumonitis, meningo-encephalitis, Bell's palsy, Guillain-Barré syndrome, and aplastic or haemolytic anaemia. The acute phase generally lasts for four to six weeks, although fatigue and lethargy often persist during convalescence and may continue for many months afterwards. One attack usually confers lifelong immunity, although immunosuppression at a later date may initiate reactivation.

Treatment

There is no specific treatment for infectious mononucleosis. Patients should be advised to rest and be reassured that the illness is self-limiting. Antipyretics (BNF 4.7.1) may be of value in alleviating fever. Corticosteroids (BNF 6.3.2) have been used in cases where complications become life-threatening.

Influenza

Definition and aetiology

Influenza is an acute infection of the respiratory tract caused by influenza viruses A, B and C, which occur worldwide and are responsible for causing epidemics and pandemics. The highest incidence in the UK is between December and May, with a peak during February and March. Influenza virus A is the least stable antigenically and is usually responsible for epidemics and pandemics. Type B also causes epidemics, but they are less frequent and more localised as the virus is more stable. Type C is the most stable and least pathogenic serotype, and generally produces mild or subclinical infections.

Influenza is highly contagious and is transmitted by droplet inhalation. Elderly and debilitated individuals are particularly susceptible, and infection may be life-threatening in such patients.

Symptoms

The incubation period is one to three days. The patient is most infectious from the day preceding symptoms until three to seven days after onset. Influenza may be differentiated from the common cold by fever and a sudden onset of symptoms, which may include rigors, headache, myalgia, vertigo and back pain. Dry cough, nasal congestion and sore throat are common respiratory symptoms, and anorexia, depression, and nausea and vomiting may also occur. In mild cases, symptoms may last for only 24 hours. However, the more usual course for uncomplicated influenza is a gradual improvement after four to five days, with full recovery 7–10 days from onset. In some, cough and malaise may persist for longer. Secondary bacterial invasion may cause more serious respiratory-tract infections (e.g. pneumonia), and is a common cause of death, particularly in elderly patients. There may also be cardiac complications (e.g. myocarditis) and a worsening of other chronic conditions (e.g. diabetes mellitus). Convulsions and croup may occur in young children, and Reye's syndrome is a rare but serious complication.

Treatment

Treatment consists of bed rest and the administration of adequate fluids and antipyretic non-opioid analgesics (BNF 4.7.1). Oxygen therapy (BNF 3.6) and assisted ventilation may be required in severe cases of pneumonia. An influenza vaccine (BNF 14.4) is available for prophylaxis in susceptible individuals, and amantadine and rimantadine have also been used.

Lassa fever

Definition and aetiology

Lassa fever, caused by the Lassa virus, was first identified in 1969 in Nigeria, and subsequent outbreaks have occurred in Liberia and Sierra Leone and other countries of West Africa.

Mastomys natalensis, a rat commonly found in regions south of the Sahara, acts as the reservoir of infection. The rodent is unaffected by the infection, but passes the virus in urine and other body fluids throughout life. Humans primarily become infected as a result of contact with infected rat urine, although the exact portal of entry is unknown. Lassa fever is highly contagious. Viral transmission usually occurs via the patient's body fluids, and contacts (including attendant medical staff) may become secondarily infected. Many of the outbreaks have been nosocomial, and fatal infections in laboratory personnel have also occurred.

It is estimated that there are about 100 000 cases of Lassa fever each year in the endemic area, with several thousand deaths. Antibody detection may be as high as 60% of the population of some villages in the affected areas.

Symptoms

The incubation period is between 3 and 16 days. Subclinical infections may occur or symptoms can vary in severity from mild to fulminating and fatal. The onset is usually insidious, with non-specific symptoms of malaise, myalgia and chills followed by fever, headache and sore throat. Symptoms gradually worsen as fever and prostration increase. Exudative pharyngitis is characteristic and other symptoms may include diarrhoea, dysphagia, nausea and vomiting, infection of the conjunctiva, chest pain and cough. Capillaries become damaged, resulting in increased permeability, which causes haemorrhage, hypotension and hypovolaemic shock. Severe cases show a sudden worsening of symptoms during the second week, and death due to cardiac arrest, respiratory insufficiency or shock may follow. Vertigo and deafness can occur, and the latter may be permanent. Excretion of the virus may continue for up to five or six weeks after recovery.

Treatment

Patients must be barrier-nursed in isolation, taking stringent precautions against contagion. Supportive therapy, including maintenance of fluid and electrolyte levels and other measures to control shock, is necessary. Lassa-immune plasma taken from convalescent patients and administered to others early in the course of infection has been of value. It may, however, exacerbate some cases, as it is believed symptoms may be caused in part by antigen–antibody complexes. Ribavarin has been successful in some cases as an antiviral agent. There is as yet no vaccine available, and the only means of control are rapid identification and isolation of patients and control of the rat population in endemic areas.

Marburg disease and Ebola fever

Definition and aetiology

Marburg disease (green monkey or vervet monkey disease) and Ebola fever are very rare haemorrhagic fevers caused by the Marburg and Ebola viruses respectively. These filoviruses are morphologically identical, but differ antigenically. The first cases of Marburg disease were reported in 1967 amongst laboratory personnel in Europe, who contracted the infection from imported vervet monkeys (*Cercopithecus aethiops*). Subsequent outbreaks have originated in the equatorial belt of Africa, although it is unclear exactly where the reservoir of primary infection lies. Person-to-person transmission occurs mainly by contact with infected blood, although sexual transmission has also been documented.

The first cases of Ebola fever were reported in the Sudan and Zaire in 1976. Both viruses cause pathological changes in the liver, lymph nodes and spleen, while the Ebola virus has a predilection for the gastrointestinal tract, lungs and genitalia. All ages are susceptible to contracting the infection, although there appears to be a greater likelihood in adults.

Symptoms

The incubation period for the Marburg virus is three to nine days, and 4–16 days for the Ebola virus. Both viruses produce a similar clinical illness in humans and monkeys. The onset may be abrupt or insidious, usually commencing with a severe headache and fever. Myalgia and especially back pain, prostration, watery diarrhoea, and nausea and vomiting are also common. A non-pruritic maculopapular rash (which is less obvious on black skins) may develop, followed by desquamation after three to four days. In addition, chest pain, cough, sore throat, and scrotal and labial inflammation are common in Ebola fever. Severe internal bleeding usually starts within five to seven days, characterised by haematemesis, melaena, epistaxis, subconjunctival haemorrhage and petechiae. There may also be bleeding from the gums, vagina and needle-puncture sites. In some cases, disseminated intravascular coagulation and renal failure may develop. Severe blood loss results in death due to shock within 16 days, particularly in primary infections. Patients with secondary infections are more likely to survive, although recovery is slow.

Treatment

The mortality may be as high as 90% in rural areas of developing countries where modern methods of intensive supportive care are not available. There is no specific antiviral therapy, but administration of plasma obtained from convalescent patients has been of value in some cases. Disseminated intravascular coagulation may be prevented by the early administration of heparin (BNF 2.8.1) under strict supervision.

Spread of the infection may be prevented by barrier-nursing patients in isolation and decontamination of all excreta and fomites.

Measles

Definition and aetiology

Measles (morbilli or rubeola) is an acute infection caused by the measles virus. It occurs worldwide, although the morbidity and mortality are greater in developing countries where overcrowded and poor socio-economic conditions prevail (e.g. West Africa). The disease is epidemic every three to five years in remote rural villages of developing countries, but has become endemic in urban areas. In the northern hemisphere, it has traditionally occurred as a biennual epidemic lasting three to four months during the winter and spring, although immunisation programmes have modified this picture in some countries.

The measles virus is transmitted from person to person in airborne droplets (e.g. by coughing or sneezing), and gains entry via the respiratory tract or the conjunctiva. It is highly contagious, infecting up to 90% of close contacts. Those most susceptible in developed countries are children starting school. Maternal antibodies protect infants under six months of age and the majority of adults have acquired immunity through active immunisation or previous infection. In developing countries, younger children are most at risk.

Symptoms

The incubation period is usually about 10 days, although it may range from 8 to 14 days or even be up to three weeks in adults. The onset is often abrupt, with prodromal symptoms of fever, sneezes, cough, nasal discharge, conjunctivitis, photophobia, and myalgia. This catarrhal stage is the most infectious. Characteristic white spots surrounded by a red ring (Koplik's spots) appear on the buccal mucosa in the region of the lower molars. After about four days, the fever abates and the Koplik's spots disappear as a maculopapular rash erupts. The rash starts on the neck and face and spreads to the rest of the body. Initially, the lesions are reddish-brown and blanch on pressure, but finally become coalescent and non-blanching. The disappearance of the rash after about five days is marked by desquamation.

Further symptoms include bronchitis, laryngitis and occasionally diarrhoea. Convalescence is rapid in uncomplicated measles. In severe cases, secondary infections may give rise to otitis media, enteritis, ulcerative herpes simplex lesions and bronchopneumonia (the most common cause of death). Corneal ulceration in vitamin A-deficient children may result in impaired vision. Encephalitis is a rare but serious complication. Subacute sclerosing panencephalitis is a rare but fatal disorder caused by persistence of the measles virus in the brain.

Treatment

There is no specific antiviral therapy for measles. Appropriate antibacterial drugs should be administered for secondary infections, while symptomatic treatment may include administration of non-opioid analgesics and antipyretics (BNF 4.7.1). Patients should be confined to bed, preferably in a darkened room if suffering with photophobia.

A measles vaccine (BNF 14.4) is available for active immunisation and is thought to confer life-long immunity with a single dose (*see also* Section 15.5). Passive immunisation using normal immunoglobulin (BNF 14.5) may be offered to contacts most at risk (e.g. pregnant women, immunocompromised individuals and tuberculosis patients).

Mumps

Definition and aetiology

Mumps (epidemic parotitis) is an acute infection caused by the mumps paramyxovirus, and occurs worldwide with a peak incidence in winter and spring. The infection is endemic in urban areas and also gives rise to epidemics. Mumps virus is transmitted in airborne droplets and enters a new host via the respiratory tract. The infection occurs most commonly in children between 5 and 15 years of age, only rarely affecting infants.

Symptoms

The incubation period is 14–18 days, and the patient becomes infectious about four days before symptoms develop. Many infected individuals are asymptomatic, although still infectious. The onset of mumps is marked in most cases by pain and swelling of the salivary glands (most commonly the parotid), which occur unilaterally or bilaterally. The patient may have a dry mouth as a result of blockage of saliva flow, and other symptoms include malaise, fever and chills. Mumps virus frequently penetrates the central nervous system and can cause mild meningitis, which does not usually leave any permanent sequelae. Encephalitis is less common, but more serious, and may cause convulsions. Orchitis may develop in males infected after puberty and is characterised by headache, fever, chills, lower abdominal pain, and a swollen and tender scrotum. One or both testes may be affected, causing varied degrees of testicular atrophy on recovery which, contrary to popular belief, only rarely leads to infertility. Other complications can include pancreatitis, oophoritis, vertigo and deafness, which may be permanent.

Mumps is rarely fatal. In most cases, there is complete recovery and life-long immunity.

Treatment

There is no specific antiviral therapy, but symptomatic treatment may include administration of analgesics except aspirin in children (BNF 4.7). The patient should be confined to bed and may appreciate a diet of soft or semi-solid foods. Inflamed testes should be well-supported, but not encased in tight bandages.

A mumps vaccine (BNF 14.4) is available for active immunisation as part of the mumps, measles and rubella vaccine.

Poliomyelitis

Definition and aetiology

Strains of poliovirus are responsible for causing poliomyelitis (infantile paralysis, polioencephalitis or paralytic poliomyelitis syndrome). They occur worldwide with a peak incidence during the summer and autumn. In areas where conditions of overcrowding and poor sanitation prevail, individuals become infected in early childhood and generally suffer only mild illness. A large proportion of the adult population is thus immune to further infection, although the immunity is strain-specific. As living conditions are improved, the age of first exposure rises and this usually results in more serious infections and epidemics. This situation has been brought under control in developed countries by the introduction of routine active immunisation programmes, but epidemics still occur in developing countries.

Poliovirus type 1 is often responsible for endemic and epidemic cases; type 3 is usually the cause of the sporadic cases in a vaccinated population. Type 2 is the least virulent strain.

The virus is transmitted from person to person via nasopharyngeal secretions and the faecal–oral route.

Symptoms

The incubation period varies from 4 to 12 days, and may even be as long as 35 days. The most infectious stage commences about five days before the onset of symptoms and lasts about 10 days. Many infected individuals remain asymptomatic, although still capable of transmitting the virus.

Initial symptoms are non-specific and include fever, sore throat, diarrhoea, anorexia, and nausea and vomiting. Some patients may recover after a few days; others may progress (in some cases, following a period of remission) to show signs of neurological involvement. These include headache, anxiety, irritability, neck and back stiffness, and drowsiness. About two-thirds of these patients do not recover at this stage and progress to develop flaccid paralysis. There may be varying degrees of improvement over weeks or months in some patients, while in others the paralysis is permanent. Complete recovery from this stage is unusual.

Paralysis of muscles involved in respiration is life-threatening, and bronchopneumonia is a common cause of death. Paralysed muscles in growing children may result in shortened limbs and other deformities.

Treatment

There is no specific antiviral therapy, but antipyretics and non-opioid analgesics (BNF 4.7.1) may be administered symptomatically. Paralysed muscles should be kept warm and prevented from being stretched. Strenuous exercise, injection of vaccines and tonsillectomy (or other surgery) during the course of the disease should be avoided as they have been linked to exacerbations of the extent of paralysis.

A vaccine is available for active immunisation (*see also* Section 15.5), and should be included in the vaccination programme for all children. Travellers to endemic areas should also be immunised. Patients in vaccinated communities should be isolated during the infectious period, and all body discharges handled with care to prevent the spread of infection. Isolation is not an effective means of control in endemic areas.

Postviral fatigue syndrome

Definition and aetiology

Postviral fatigue syndrome (myalgic encephalomyelitis) is an ill-defined condition that occurs predominantly following a viral infection. It affects mainly adults, with a greater proportion of women reporting symptoms. Although a wide range of causes and aetiological factors have been postulated, the chronic presence of enteroviruses in muscle and gut is the most likely cause, but has not been conclusively demonstrated.

Symptoms

Symptoms often appear after an upper respiratory-tract infection and may last for months or years. The dominant features of the syndrome are muscular fatigue and emotional disturbances. Fatigue is aggravated by exercise, even to the extent that it may last for weeks following a single session of activity. Emotional disturbances may be apparent in the presence of disturbed sleep patterns, inability to concentrate, anxiety and depressive disorders. A wide range of other symptoms have also been associated with the syndrome (e.g. headache, neck pain, paraesthesia, cold extremities, muscle weakness and blurred vision).

Treatment

There is no proven treatment for the condition other than complete rest. Symptomatic treatment may be beneficial and includes non-opioid analgesics (BNF 4.7.1). In cases of underlying emotional disturbances and with appropriate professional support, anxiolytics (BNF 4.1.2) and antidepressant drugs (BNF 4.3) may be useful.

Rabies

Definition and aetiology

Rabies (hydrophobia) is a zoonotic infection of warm-blooded animals caused by the rabies virus. The disease occurs worldwide, except in Australia and Antarctica, but has been successfully eliminated from some geographically isolated countries as a result of eradication programmes (e.g. Japan and the UK).

The virus is present in saliva and other body fluids and is transmitted to humans in most cases via bites. In developed countries, rabies control measures have confined the reservoir of infection to wild animals, the species involved varying between regions (e.g. skunks, raccoons and foxes in the USA, vampire bats in Latin America, and foxes in Europe). In these areas, people contract the infection in 90% of cases from domestic animals who have had contact with wild animals. Rabies has also been transmitted by inhalation of infected secretions in bat caves. Human-to-human transmission rarely occurs, although rabies has been reported in patients receiving infected corneal transplants. In developing countries, rabies is endemic in urban areas and thus poses a greater threat to humans.

Symptoms

The incubation period is usually between one and two months, although longer periods have been reported. Only about one in six humans bitten by rabid animals develop the disease. The risks are greater the closer the location of the bite to the head, which also tends to shorten the incubation period.

The onset is marked by a prodrome of non-specific symptoms, which include anorexia, malaise, fatigue, fever, myalgia and headache. The bitten area, which may already have healed, becomes painful and irritable. As the virus enters the nervous system, there may be behavioural changes (e.g. a wish to be alone) and feelings of apprehension, anxiety, depression or agitation. Further symptoms include hallucinations, convulsions, paralysis and short periods of aggressive behaviour (e.g. thrashing or biting). These symptoms may arise as a reaction to various stimuli (e.g. noise, water or air draughts). Between attacks, the patient is lucid. Hydrophobia is a characteristic symptom of rabies, marked by laryngeal spasm in response to sight, sound or feel of water. The patient may die of cardiac arrest or respiratory failure during a spasm, or progress to paralysis, coma and death. This sequence of events is termed furious rabies and is the most common form in humans.

Paralytic (dumb) rabies occurs in less than 20% of cases, and is particularly associated with infection contracted from vampire bats or in patients who have received post-exposure rabies vaccine. Hydrophobia does not usually occur following the prodromal period, but flaccid paralysis dominates the course, and is terminated by coma and death.

Treatment

Rabies is invariably fatal once the virus enters the nervous system. There is no specific antiviral therapy and only a very small number of patients have survived as a result of intensive supportive care.

Rabies may be prevented from developing by thorough cleansing and careful management of the wound, commenced as soon as possible after the bite. Rabies vaccine (BNF 14.4) may be administered during the incubation period as post-exposure treatment, together with antirabies immunoglobulin (BNF 14.5). Rabies vaccine may be offered as pre-exposure prophylaxis to individuals at risk (e.g. veterinary surgeons, employees in quarantine stations, wild animal collectors and dog catchers). In endemic areas, spread of rabies may be prevented by vaccination of domestic animals and destruction of strays. Control of wild animal reservoirs is more difficult. In rabies-free areas, strict regulations governing import and quarantine of animals is required.

Rubella

Definition and aetiology

Rubella (German measles) is caused by the rubella virus, and occurs worldwide with a peak incidence in spring and early summer in temperate climates.

The virus resides in the upper respiratory tract and is transmitted from person to person by droplets. Rubella occurs most commonly in children, particularly those under nine years of age, although non-immune young adults living together in groups (e.g. college students and military recruits) are also susceptible.

Symptoms

The incubation period is usually 17 days, although it can range from 14 to 21 days. The most infectious period commences about one week before the rash appears and lasts about 11 days.

Rubella is a mild self-limiting infection characterised by a rose-coloured, evanescent, papular rash spreading from the face to the trunk and finally the limbs. It may be accompanied by mild constitutional symptoms of malaise, slight fever, headache, conjunctivitis and lymphadenopathy. Arthritis occurs frequently in adults (particularly women), but is rarely permanent.

The rash usually lasts for a maximum of three days. It is followed by a rapid and complete recovery, with lifelong immunity against subsequent attacks. In some cases, rubella may occur without the rash, making accurate diagnosis difficult.

Rubella occurring during pregnancy (particularly the first trimester) poses a threat to the fetus, and may result in abortion, stillbirth or congenital malformations, some of which may not present until later in life. Cataracts, heart defects and deafness are common disorders. Hepatitis and hepatosplenomegaly, visual defects, meningo-encephalitis, microcephaly and osteopathy may also occur.

Treatment

There is no specific antiviral therapy and symptomatic treatment is rarely required. Women contracting rubella early in pregnancy may wish to consider therapeutic abortion. Alternatively, passive immunisation with normal immunoglobulin (BNF 14.5) may afford some protection to the fetus.

Rubella vaccine (BNF 14.4) is available for active immunisation of non-immune females to prevent congenital rubella infections in subsequent pregnancies (*see also* Section 15.5). It is a component of mumps, measles and rubella (MMR) vaccine.

Smallpox

Definition and aetiology

The world was officially declared free from smallpox in 1980, more than two years after the last reported endemic case in Somalia in 1977.

Smallpox was caused by the variola virus and, before eradication, was endemic in parts of Africa, South East Asia and Brazil, although no country was free from the risk of imported cases.

Transmission of infection occurred from person to person via the respiratory tract. There was no known animal reservoir, the infection did not become latent in surviving patients, and there were no chronic carriers. Spread of infection was slow and resulted in highly localised incidence. The combination of these factors made eradication possible.

Symptoms

The incubation period was about 12 days, during which time the patient was not infectious.

The onset was abrupt with symptoms of fever, prostration, headache, aching, and nausea and vomiting. A characteristic maculopapular rash appeared after three to five days as the fever abated. The lesions became vesicular and then pustular, forming scales, and finally separating after about three weeks, leaving hypopigmented areas. Smallpox lesions were all at the same stage of development, unlike those of chickenpox, which appear in crops. The patient was infectious until the rash subsided. The severity of symptoms depended to a great extent on the host's resistance, and varied from subclinical non-infectious cases to haemorrhagic smallpox, which was invariably fatal.

Death generally occurred during the second week of the rash. Surviving patients were usually marked by dermal pits and scars and many suffered loss of vision.

Treatment

There was no specific treatment for smallpox. Early administration of smallpox vaccine or immunoglobulins or methisazone to contacts prevented development of the disease or converted it to a milder form.

Routine active immunisation against smallpox (BNF 14.4) is no longer practised in any country. The vaccine is held in selected centres and only deemed necessary for laboratory personnel working with orthopoxviruses.

Eradication of the disease was effected by a worldwide campaign begun in 1967. Mass immunisation in endemic areas was undertaken, and the chain of transmission broken by seeking and isolating infected patients and vaccinating contacts. The search continued for two years after the last reported case in each area to ensure complete eradication.

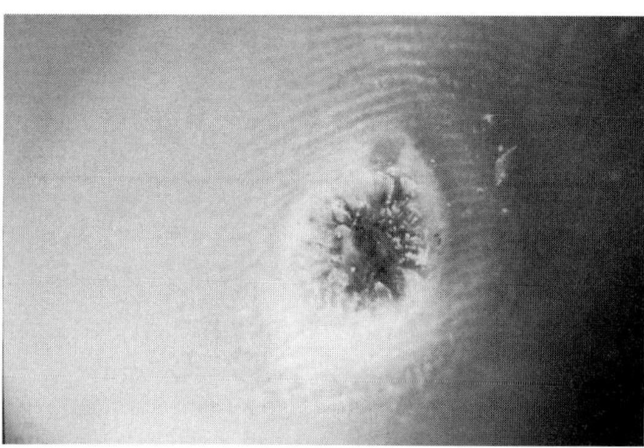

Figure 5.7 Verucca. (Reproduced with permission from *Pharmaceutical Journal*.)

Warts

Definition and aetiology

Warts (verrucae) (Figure 5.7) are circumscribed, benign, contagious, epithelial growths induced by human papillomavirus. Viral entry is effected through damaged or moist skin.

Symptoms

Warts occur most frequently in older children and are generally uncommon in infants and the elderly. The lesions are firm and may be single or multiple, flesh-coloured, brown, grey, yellow or black. They often regress spontaneously within 6–24 months.

Common warts (verruca vulgaris) occur most frequently. They are usually located on the hands and fingers, less commonly on the elbows and knees. They may be irregularly shaped or round with a rough surface. Peri-ungual warts occur around the nails, are usually associated with nail-biting, and are often painful. Verruca plana are warts occurring on the face. Plantar warts (verruca plantaris) are commonly referred to as verrucae, and occur on the soles of the feet, usually in the weight-bearing regions. They are flattened by pressure and are often tender and painful. Small black pinpoints representing thrombosed blood vessels may be seen on paring away the surface. Mosaic warts are groups of plantar warts occurring close together or becoming confluent. Condylomata acuminata (anogenital warts) are sexually transmitted warts and are usually moist and soft.

Treatment

In most cases, warts will disappear spontaneously. Where indicated, treatment may involve the use of a keratolytic preparation for warts and calluses (BNF 13.7). For common and plantar warts, this may be followed by careful removal of dead tissue (debridement). Soaking the affected foot in a solution of formaldehyde may be of value in treating mosaic warts. Physical means of removal (e.g. cauterisation, curettage, electrodesiccation, liquid nitrogen and solid CO_2), may be necessary in resistant cases.

Prevention of transmission of warts can be encouraged by avoiding barefooted communal activities (e.g. swimming in public baths) and ensuring only personal use of towels and bath mats. An occlusive dressing may also minimise the risks of transmission.

Yellow fever

Definition and aetiology

Yellow fever is a haemorrhagic fever, endemic in tropical areas of Africa and South and Central America (but not Asia) and caused by the yellow fever virus. Epidemics do still occur, the most recent in West Africa between 1986 and 1991, in which 100 000 cases were identified.

The vector of the infection is a mosquito (*Aedes* spp.), which maintains a cycle with humans in urban areas. In forested regions, yellow fever is a zoonotic infection involving monkeys, mosquitoes and humans.

Symptoms

The incubation period is three to six days. The severity of symptoms varies from mild to fulminating and fatal, often being more severe in travellers than in the indigenous population. Yellow fever has an abrupt onset with fever, headache, rigors, myalgia, back pain, and nausea and vomiting. The face is often flushed and oedematous, with swollen lips and gums and injection of the conjunctiva. Bleeding from the nose and gums may also occur. A period of remission usually occurs after one to three days, during which time the fever and other symptoms subside. Mild cases may start to recover at this stage, but in severe cases the symptoms reappear in a more exaggerated form. Jaundice may become obvious, and more serious bleeding results in melaena, haematemesis ('coffee grounds' or black vomit), petechiae and ecchymoses. Renal damage may occur, causing albuminuria and a reduction in urine output.

The overall mortality rate of yellow fever is 5%, although 50% of severe cases may be fatal with death almost always occurring before the tenth day. Relapses in surviving patients are uncommon.

Treatment

There is no specific treatment for yellow fever; symptomatic treatment is required.

Supportive treatment includes maintenance of fluid and electrolyte levels, blood transfusion, dialysis, and intensive monitoring of all vital functions.

An effective and safe vaccine (BNF 14.4), which confers long-term immunity, is available and mandatory for travellers to many countries. Spread of yellow fever in endemic areas may be controlled by the use of nets and screens to prevent mosquitoes from gaining access to patients. Mass immunisation and control of the mosquito population using insecticides should be undertaken during epidemics.

5.4 Fungal infections

Aspergillosis

Definition and aetiology

Aspergillosis is an opportunistic fungal infection caused by *Aspergillus* species, which may be found worldwide in a variety of habitats including soil, vegetation, grain and materials used for construction. The most common pathogenic species is *A. fumigatus*, although *A. flavus* is often a cause of infections of the upper respiratory tract and *A. niger* a cause of infections involving the external ear.

Inhaled airborne spores colonise lung tissue which has been damaged by other chronic respiratory disease (e.g. bronchitis or tuberculosis). Antimicrobial therapy predisposes susceptible hosts to developing the disease, and immunocompromised patients are also at risk. Transmission of infection from animals or person-to-person is unlikely.

An allergic reaction to spores or fungi in the respiratory tract (allergic bronchopulmonary aspergillosis) may also occur, particularly in asthma patients.

Symptoms

An aspergilloma (fungal ball) consisting of tangled hyphae and other debris may develop in lung cavities previously created by an unrelated disorder (e.g. tuberculosis or bronchiectasis). They rarely invade and may spontaneously resolve or be expectorated. The only symptoms may be cough and occasionally haemoptysis. Invasion of tissues may occur in transplant patients and other immunocompromised individuals, and can be fatal. In most instances, the fungus remains confined to the lungs, although spread to other sites via the circulation (e.g. to the brain, liver, skin or gastrointestinal tract) is a possibility. The infected tissue becomes necrotic and suppurative. Symptoms of invasive chronic pulmonary aspergillosis include fever and productive cough.

Patients with allergic reactions may have symptoms of wheezing, dyspnoea and productive cough, and may develop permanent pulmonary fibrosis and bronchiectasis. The condition can be recurrent.

Treatment

Surgery may be necessary for serious life-threatening aspergillomas. Invasive aspergillosis requires prompt treatment, usually by the parenteral administration of amphotericin B (BNF 5.2). Treatment of allergic bronchopulmonary aspergillosis consists of corticosteroids (BNF 6.3.2), which may be required indefinitely for recurrent cases. Bronchodilators (BNF 3.1) may also be of value.

Candidiasis

Definition and aetiology

Candidiasis (moniliasis or thrush) is an acute or chronic fungal infection caused by species of *Candida*, particularly *C. albicans*. It occurs worldwide and is the most common opportunistic mycosis.

The microorganism is a yeast-like fungus, which exists as part of the normal human flora of the mouth, gastrointestinal tract and vagina. Species other than *C. albicans* may also colonise the skin. Certain factors (e.g. antimicrobial therapy, pregnancy and diabetes mellitus) increase the number of microorganisms present, predisposing the host to the condition. Debilitated and immunocompromised individuals are also susceptible. Trauma and maceration allow development of infections of the nails (*see* Paronychia, Section 5.1) and skin. The latter commonly occur in moist areas, especially folds and other apposed surfaces (e.g. axillae, groin, under the breasts and napkin area). Trauma due to ill-fitting dentures may result in oral candidiasis. Most infections arise endogenously, but transmission can occur to humans from animals or from person to person. Oral candidiasis is common in neonates and arises as a result of passage along an infected birth canal. Inhaled corticosteroids may cause infection of the mouth, pharynx or oesophagus.

Systemic candidiasis occurs in seriously ill hospitalised patients receiving antimicrobial therapy. It may occur in the presence of indwelling catheters or intravascular lines, or following gastrointestinal surgery. Chronic mucocutaneous candidiasis is an uncommon condition characterised by persistent infection at several sites. Susceptibility can be inherited, or cases can be associated with an underlying endocrine disorder (e.g. hypothyroidism or diabetes mellitus). There appears to be an immunological abnormality.

Symptoms

Oral candidiasis is characterised by the appearance of creamy white raised patches on the oral mucosa. These patches may be painful and often bleed if removed. It is most common in young children and often recurs. The infection can be an early symptom of AIDS.

Vaginitis is characterised by a thick, creamy white discharge, pruritus and an inflamed mucosa with white plaques. The irritation may be exacerbated by sexual intercourse, urination or hot baths. Male genital infection may be asymptomatic or result in balanitis, but it does not occur as frequently as vaginitis in women.

Initial symptoms of skin candidiasis are erythema and pruritus, which may become intense. Wet pustular or dry scaly lesions with well-defined edges and satellite vesicles may develop.

Infections involving the gastrointestinal tract are often asymptomatic, but represent an important source for systemic invasion in immunosuppressed patients.

Systemic candidiasis is rare, but serious and often fatal. Organs which may become involved include the kidneys, brain, liver, bone and joints, spleen, thyroid, lungs and heart. Blindness may develop as a result of systemic spread to the eye.

Treatment

Any underlying condition should be corrected, in addition to the administration of appropriate antifungal drugs (BNF 5.2).

Oral candidiasis may be treated with oropharyngeal antifungal preparations (BNF 12.3.2), and good oral hygiene should be encouraged to prevent further attacks. Vaginal candidiasis is usually treated with an antifungal pessary or cream (BNF 7.2.2). Washing the affected area with warm water may provide relief during an attack of vaginitis, although overwashing and the use of irritant toiletries (e.g. soap, talcum powder or deodorants) should be avoided. It may be necessary to treat sexual partners concurrently to prevent re-infection. Vaginitis may be prevented by good personal hygiene to avoid contamination of the genital area with faecal matter. Tight-fitting garments made from synthetic fabrics should be avoided.

Chronic mucocutaneous candidiasis can rarely be cured, but may respond to antifungal therapy. However, relapses are common if therapy is stopped.

Cryptococcosis

Definition and aetiology

Cryptococcosis is caused by the yeast *Cryptococcus neoformans*. It occurs worldwide, but particularly in the USA and Australia.

The most common source of the microorganism is pigeon excreta, although the birds themselves do not suffer from the infection. Humans become infected by inhalation of microorganisms, but it is not infectious to others. Immunosuppressed patients or those with pre-existing pulmonary disease are particularly at risk of developing cryptococcosis.

Symptoms

The initial site of infection is the lung, and common symptoms include fever, malaise, cough, haemoptysis and chest pain. Cavitation may occur and the condition frequently becomes chronic. Some cases, however, resolve spontaneously.

The infection may spread from the lungs, most commonly to the meninges, although other sites (e.g. kidney, liver, bone, skin and spleen) may be involved. Cryptococcal meningitis is characterised by headache. Accompanying symptoms may include lethargy, confusion, agitation, behavioural changes, blurred vision, photophobia, and nausea and vomiting. The course may be chronic and progressive. Most cases prove fatal within two years if untreated.

Treatment

Treatment, consisting of systemic antifungal drugs (BNF 5.2), is only required for progressive cases of pulmonary cryptococcosis or in the presence of underlying disorders or immunosuppression. Meningitis and any other signs of extrapulmonary infection always require therapy.

Pityriasis versicolor

Definition and aetiology

Pityriasis versicolor (tinea versicolor) is a chronic skin infection caused by *Malassezia furfur* (*Pityrosporum orbiculare*), which is a commensal yeast found on skin. The condition occurs more commonly in tropical regions. In temperate zones, cases occur most frequently during the warmer months. The infection may affect any age group, although it is most commonly seen in young adults.

Symptoms

Pityriasis versicolor is characterised by oval, slightly wrinkled, well-defined macules, which may coalesce. They may be pink, white or brown and do not tan on exposure to ultraviolet radiation. They occur most frequently on the upper part of the trunk, although spread may occur to the neck, upper arms and abdomen. There may be mild irritation, and fine scales are shed on scratching. Spontaneous resolution occasionally occurs in cooler climates, but the infection is more likely to persist for years if untreated. In some cases, non-scaly depigmented areas may remain for some months after treatment. Relapse is not uncommon, particularly in tropical climates.

Treatment

Topical application of suspensions containing selenium sulfide, sodium hyposulfate or pyrithione zinc may be effective (BNF 13.9). Topical antifungal drugs (BNF 13.10.2) may also be beneficial. In resistant or recurrent cases, an appropriate systemic antifungal drug (BNF 5.2) may be indicated.

Sporotrichosis

Definition and aetiology

Sporotrichosis is a fungal infection of the skin and lymphatics caused by *Sporothrix schenkii*. It frequently occurs in Central America and Brazil, but is no longer common in Europe.

The microorganism is present in soil, plants and bark and represents a source of infection for those whose occupation brings them into close contact with timber and vegetation (e.g. wood cutters, farmers or horticulturists). The portal of entry is likely to be an abrasion, scratch or insect bite. Inhalation of spores may cause pulmonary infection, although this is uncommon.

Symptoms

Sporotrichosis occurs most commonly as a subcutaneous infection. Ulceration of the primary nodule at the inoculation site is followed days or weeks later by secondary nodules, which appear along the course of the lymph channels draining the region. These may also ulcerate through the skin. 'Fixed' infections are confined to the inoculation site only, and are characterised by a single lesion, which may ulcerate. Sporotrichosis may be progressive or resolves spontaneously. Remissions and relapses over a period of years are, however, the common course.

Pulmonary sporotrichosis is usually chronic and symptoms may resemble pulmonary tuberculosis. It is often fatal if untreated. Dissemination to other sites is rare, but usually involves bone and joints.

Treatment

Cutaneous and pulmonary sporotrichosis may be treated by the oral administration of a saturated solution of potassium iodide. Itraconazole is an alternative treatment. Amphotericin B (BNF 5.2) may be of value for pulmonary and disseminated infections, but surgery may be necessary for cases of pulmonary cavitation.

Tinea infections

Definition and aetiology

Tinea infections (dermatophyte infections or ringworm) are common fungal infections of the skin, hair and nails caused by species belonging to the genera *Trichophyton*, *Epidermophyton* and *Microsporum*. The infections occur worldwide, although the species responsible may vary from region to region.

The microorganisms have a variety of habitats. Geophilic infections are transmitted to humans from soil, zoophilic infections from animals (e.g. dogs, cats or cattle), and anthropophilic infections from other humans. Human infections derived from animals are generally more inflammatory than those from other humans.

The microorganisms colonise keratin and invasion is facilitated by heat, moisture and occlusion.

Tinea capitis

Definition and aetiology

Tinea capitis (scalp ringworm) is an infection of the scalp, which is rare in adults but occurs most frequently in children. The most common causative microorganism in the UK is *Microsporum canis*, derived from dogs and cats. *M. audouinii* is spread from child to child, giving rise to epidemics in schools, mainly in tropical regions. (*M. audouinii* used to be a common cause of infection in the UK.) *Trichophyton* species (e.g. *T. tonsurans* and *T. violaceum*) are also responsible for scalp infections. Transmission of microorganisms may occur by direct contact, or indirectly by means of shared towels, combs, brushes and hats.

Symptoms

Symptoms of tinea capitis may include patchy alopecia, pruritus and scaling, which can progress to involve the whole scalp. The hair breaks off above the scalp to leave stumps, rather than total loss of the hair follicle. Some species of fungi cause the hair to break at scalp level (black dot ringworm). *M. canis* may produce inflammation and kerions. The infection may resolve spontaneously at puberty.

Treatment

Treatment of tinea capitis consists of the administration of systemic antifungal drugs (BNF 5.2). Infected patients should not share towels or hairdressing implements with others, and in severe cases it may be necessary to cover the head.

Tinea corporis

Definition and aetiology

Tinea corporis (body ringworm) (Figure 5.8) is caused most frequently by *Trichophyton rubrum*. It is transmitted from humans or animals directly by contact with infected lesions or indirectly by skin or scalp scales.

Symptoms

The characteristic ring-shaped lesion is initially flat, round and red, clearing from the centre as it expands. The borders are often raised and may be scaly or blistered. There is seldom more than one lesion, which may occur at any non-hairy site on the trunk, limbs or face. There may be pruritus, especially in animal-derived infections, and this can be further complicated by kerions.

Treatment

Tinea corporis may be treated with topical antifungal preparations (BNF 13.10.2), although refractory cases may require systemic antifungal drugs (BNF 5.2). Patients should be particularly careful about personal hygiene to prevent passing the infection to others.

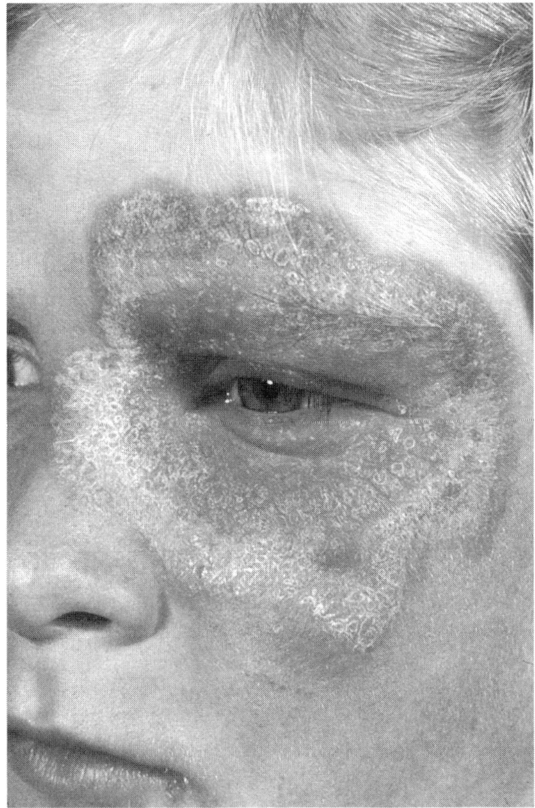

Figure 5.8 Tinea corporis. (Reproduced with permission from *Pharmaceutical Journal*.)

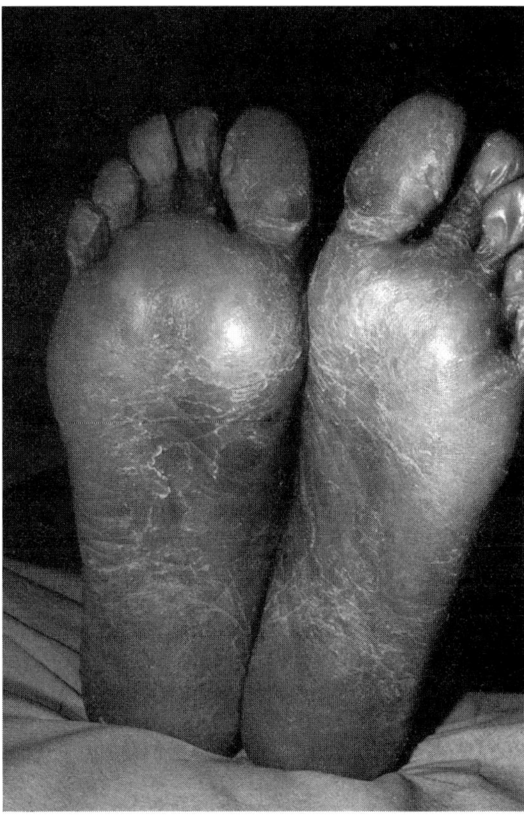

Figure 5.9 Tinea pedis. (Reproduced with permission from *Pharmaceutical Journal*.)

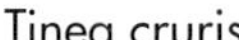

Tinea cruris

Definition and aetiology

Tinea cruris (dhobie itch) is ringworm of the groin, frequently caused by *Trichophyton rubrum* or *Epidermophyton floccosum*. It is common in all climates, although in Europe it affects men more often than women.

Symptoms

Tinea cruris is characterised by ring-like erythematous lesions with raised edges. Pruritus is often a problem and there may be inflammation, maceration or scaling. Both groins are typically affected and the infection may spread to the upper thighs and buttocks. In tropical regions, it may be more extensive and involve the waist. Secondary bacterial infections or candidiasis may develop. Recurrences commonly occur, particularly during the summer.

Treatment

Treatment consists of the application of topical antifungal preparations (BNF 13.10.2), although in refractory cases systemic antifungal drugs (BNF 5.2) may be required. The affected area should be kept as dry as possible, and this may be facilitated by applying a non-perfumed talcum powder. Tight clothing should be avoided.

Tinea pedis

Definition and aetiology

Tinea pedis (athlete's foot) (Figure 5.9) the most common form of dermatophytosis seen in the UK. It is a common infection of the feet, most often caused by *Trichophyton rubrum* and *T. interdigitale*, and to a lesser extent by *Epidermophyton floccosum*. It occurs worldwide, with a greater frequency and severity during the warmer months of the year. A similar infection affects the hands (tinea manuum) and often develops in the presence of existing foot infection. It occurs more commonly in adult men, especially in the presence of excessive perspiration and occlusive footwear.

Transmission may be direct from person to person or indirect via infected skin scales on towels, shoes, socks or floors, particularly in communal washing areas.

Symptoms

Tinea pedis usually starts in the fourth toe cleft, and the skin initially appears cracked and scaly. It may become white and macerated, with developing blisters. Pruritus is often a problem and the skin may become inflamed. Blisters may ooze, forming crusts, and there may be secondary bacterial infection. Spread of infection may involve the rest of the foot, and in severe cases, the nail becomes distorted and thickened (tinea unguium). Recurrences are common.

Treatment

Treatment comprises the application of topical antifungal preparations (BNF 13.10.2) and attention to foot care. Patients should wash feet daily, drying thoroughly. Socks (preferably cotton) should be changed daily and occlusive footwear avoided. Dusting footwear with an antifungal powder may be beneficial. Systemic antifungal drugs (BNF 5.2) may be necessary in severe or chronic cases, and are always indicated if the nails are infected.

Spread of infection may be prevented by regular and thorough cleansing of floors in communal changing rooms. Patients should take care not to contaminate areas used by other people.

5.5 Protozoal infections

Amoebiasis

Definition and aetiology

Amoebiasis (amoebic dysentery) is a protozoal intestinal infection caused by *Entamoeba histolytica*. It occurs worldwide, although most commonly in warm humid climates (e.g. Mexico, South America and southern Africa). It is thought to cause the death of between 40 000 and 110 000 people globally each year.

The source of the infection is faecal matter containing the encysted form of the parasite, and transmission occurs by ingestion of contaminated food or water. Direct transmission during sexual activity may also occur. The ingested cysts release trophozoites, which feed on bacteria in the colon. As they pass along the colon, they develop into cysts, which are excreted in the faeces to continue the cycle. Under certain conditions (e.g. a change in the resistance of the host, malnutrition or immunodeficiency), the commensal relationship between parasite and host is disturbed and tissue invasion occurs, resulting in amoebic colitis.

Symptoms

Symptoms of amoebiasis may arise at any time from a few days to several years after infection, although they occur most commonly during the first four months. Onset may be sudden or insidious and symptoms vary in severity from mild diarrhoea to dysentery. Spread to other organs may occur via the circulation, particularly to the liver, causing amoebic liver abscesses.

Complications of chronic infection include anaemia, emaciation, peritonitis, fibrous strictures (leading to obstruction) and irritable bowel syndrome. The infection resolves spontaneously in some; others experience relapses over several years. Many infected individuals are asymptomatic, although they excrete cysts, which are the infective form of the parasite. Patients with diarrhoea are non-infectious, since they excrete only trophozoites which do not survive in the external environment.

Treatment

The prognosis is good if the infection is uncomplicated and is treated early in its course. Treatment of amoebiasis (BNF 5.4.2) comprises the administration of amoebicides. Asymptomatic cyst carriers should also be treated to control spread of the infection. Supportive treatment (e.g. fluid and electrolyte replacement, or blood transfusion) may be necessary in patients with complications. Aspiration of large liver abscesses may be indicated.

Amoebiasis may be prevented by improving sanitation and observing strict standards of hygiene in food handling. In endemic areas, drinking water should be boiled, and only peeled fruit and vegetables or cooked food consumed.

Giardiasis

Definition and aetiology

Giardiasis is a protozoal intestinal infection caused by *Giardia lamblia*. It occurs worldwide, most commonly in the tropics and subtropics, although endemic giardiasis is also found in some industrialised areas (e.g. St Petersburg and south and eastern Europe).

The source of the infection is human faeces containing the encysted form (the infective form) of the parasite. Ingested cysts release trophozoites which colonise the small intestine. They encyst on passing into the colon and are excreted in the faeces to continue the cycle. It is possible that humans may also be susceptible to *Giardia* species harboured by other mammals. Transmission usually occurs by ingestion of food or water contaminated with faecal matter, although direct transmission from person to person may also occur. Those particularly susceptible to infection include children (especially if malnourished), immunodeficient individuals and travellers to endemic areas.

Symptoms

The incubation period varies from a few days to several weeks. Giardiasis may be acute or chronic and symptoms vary in severity from asymptomatic to marked diarrhoea accompanied by malabsorption and weight loss. There may be abdominal pain and distension, flatulence, anorexia, steatorrhoea, nausea and lethargy. Stools are usually yellow, frothy and malodorous. Children often fail to thrive. Acute giardiasis may resolve spontaneously after two to three weeks (some individuals, however, continue to excrete cysts) or it may become chronic. Many infected individuals are asymptomatic and pass cysts from the onset of infection.

Treatment

Treatment comprises the administration of antigiardial drugs (BNF 5.4.4). It is essential that asymptomatic cyst carriers (pregnant women excluded) are also treated to curb spread of the infection.

Giardiasis may be prevented by improving standards of sanitation and hygiene, particularly with respect to food preparation. In endemic areas, drinking water should be boiled and only cooked food consumed where possible. Raw vegetables and fruit should always be peeled.

Leishmaniasis

Definition and aetiology

Leishmaniasis is a zoonotic infection caused by protozoa of the genus *Leishmania*. It occurs in the semi-arid and desert regions of Africa, central Asia, China, India, the Mediterranean basin, and the Middle East (Old World leishmaniasis), and the tropical forests of central and South America (New World leishmaniasis).

Vertebrate reservoirs of infection include wild and domestic canines, hyraxes, rodents and sloths; humans are generally an incidental host. Transmission is effected by sandflies (*Phlebotomus* spp. in the Old World, and *Lutzomyia* and *Psychodopygus* spp. in the New World) during a blood meal. There are 12 species known to infect humans, the target cells being those within the reticulo-endothelial system. Infection may occasionally be acquired as a result of sexual or congenital transmission, or blood transfusion.

Cutaneous leishmaniasis

Definition and aetiology

Cutaneous leishmaniasis (oriental sore or tropical sore) is due to infection with *L. major*, *L. tropica* and *L. aethiopica* in the Old World, and *L. mexicana* and *L. brasiliensis* in the New World.

Symptoms

The incubation period varies from days to many months. Papular lesions, which may be single or multiple, appear at the inoculation site, usually on exposed parts of the body. They slowly develop into encrusted nodules and finally into ulcers, which may be wet or dry. The lesions heal spontaneously within 18 months, leaving a depressed depigmented scar. New World leishmaniasis tends to be more ulcerative and destructive than the Old World variety. Infections caused by *L. brasiliensis* may, after some years, involve the oro-nasopharynx, resulting in gross deformity (mucocutaneous leishmaniasis). Infection with *L. tropica major* results in immunity, and deliberate infection of the leg with local live strains of *L. tropica major* has been practised as a means of preventing unsightly lesions on the face.

Treatment

Treatment is essential in areas where *L. brasiliensis* occurs. This prevents mucocutaneous complications that may result in death due to aspiration pneumonia or obstruction. Old World cutaneous leishmaniasis is self-limiting and usually requires no treatment unless the ulcers are potentially disfiguring or disabling (e.g. a large ulcer sited over a joint or invasion of cartilage occurs). Treatment consists of the systemic administration of leishmaniacides (BNF 5.4.5). Ulcers may also be treated locally by cryotherapy, curettage or surgery.

Prevention may be effected by using insecticides to control the sandfly population and wearing protective clothing.

Visceral leishmaniasis

Definition and aetiology

Visceral leishmaniasis (kala-azar) is caused by *L. donovani* and affects mainly the bone marrow, liver and spleen. Children and young adults are particularly susceptible.

Symptoms

The incubation period varies from 10 days to more than a year. The onset is usually insidious in endemic areas and characterised by intermittent fever, weakness, sweats, diarrhoea, weight loss, non-productive cough, and discomfort due to an enlarging spleen. Occasionally, there may be spontaneous recovery early in the disease. The usual course, however, is a chronic progression over several years marked by anaemia and leucopenia, hepatosplenomegaly, bleeding from mucous membranes, and emaciation leading to a final cachectic state. Intercurrent infections (e.g. dysentery, pneumonia and septicaemia) are common and a frequent cause of death. Visitors to endemic areas often experience an abrupt onset of symptoms which may include high fever, weakness, dyspnoea, acute anaemia and septiciaemia, with rapid progression of the disease.

Some patients in certain geographical locations (e.g. India) develop subcutaneous nodules containing large numbers of parasites following recovery from visceral disease (post kala-azar dermal leishmaniasis). It may lead to a relapse of the visceral infection. These patients possibly act as the main reservoir of infection in local areas.

Treatment

Visceral leishmaniasis is invariably fatal if untreated. Treatment comprises bed rest and the administration of leishmaniacides (BNF 5.4.5). Intercurrent infections should also be treated with an appropriate antibacterial drug (BNF 5.1). Patients benefit from a protein-rich diet and correction of other nutritional deficiencies. Further supportive treatment (e.g. correction of fluid and electrolyte balance and blood transfusion) may be indicated. There is no effective chemoprophylaxis and the only means of prevention is eradication of reservoir hosts, and vectors where possible. This may be achieved by detection and treatment of human hosts, destruction of infected dogs, and use of insecticides. Individuals in endemic areas should wear protective clothing and sleep under nets.

Malaria

Definition and aetiology

Malaria (ague or jungle fever) is a protozoal infection caused by four species of *Plasmodium* pathogenic to humans: *P. falciparum*, *P. malariae*, *P. ovale*, and *P. vivax*. It is widespead in the tropical areas of Africa, India, northern South America and South East Asia.

Natural transmission in humans occurs by inoculation with sporozoites from the salivary glands of female anopheline mosquitoes during a blood meal. The sporozoites migrate almost immediately to the liver where they undergo asexual division to form merozoites. These leave the liver and infect erythrocytes, and undergo further asexual division. When lysis of erythrocytes occurs, merozoites are released and infect new host cells. Some merozoites develop into gametocytes, which can be ingested by mosquitoes. Sexual reproduction takes place within the vector, producing sporozoites which continue the cycle. Infection may also be acquired as a result of congenital transmission, transfusion of blood from an infected donor, or sharing syringes and needles.

Symptoms

The incubation period varies from 10 days to many months and is determined by species of parasite and chemoprophylaxis, which may mask the initial phase.

The clinical symptoms are entirely due to the asexual blood forms, with the synchronous lysis of erythrocytes causing characteristic periodic paroxysms. There is a prodromal phase marked by influenza-type symptoms. These include anorexia, headache, malaise, myalgia and mild fever. The first paroxysm follows and is characterised by violent shivering and feelings of intense cold, which may be accompanied by nausea, vomiting and diarrhoea. After 1–2 hours, the patient suffers a throbbing headache, hot flushes, palpitations, tachypnoea, postural syncope, vomiting and prostration. A high fever culminates in a drenching sweat, after which the exhausted patient sleeps.

Following an initial phase of irregular fever, regular paroxysms occur every 48 hours with *P. ovale* and *P. vivax* infections and every 72 hours with *P. malariae*. The patient generally feels well between attacks. Periodic paroxysms are unusual with *P. falciparum*. *P. ovale* and *P. vivax* cause relapses over two to eight years due to dormant sporozoites residing in the liver. *P. falciparum* and *P. malariae* cause recrudescent infections, which may persist for years, or in the case of *P. malariae* for decades. Possible complications, particularly with falciparum malaria, include cerebral malaria, anaemia, jaundice, hypoglycaemia, hepatosplenomegaly, acute renal failure and blackwater fever (haemolytic anaemia and haemoglobinuria).

Immunity, which is species specific, may develop in endemic areas following prolonged or repeated infections. It usually renders an infected host asymptomatic rather than preventing the disease, and such individuals continue to act as reservoirs of the infection.

Treatment

Falciparum malaria (malignant malaria) is the most serious form and should be treated as an emergency; cerebral complications account for most fatalities. Treatment of all forms of malaria comprises administration of antimalarials (BNF 5.4.1), bed rest, temperature control, and appropriate management of complications. Drug resistance is a major problem, however, in the management of the disease.

Malaria may be prevented by chemoprophylaxis (BNF 5.4.1), and must be continued for an adequate interval after departing from the endemic area. The changing patterns of drug resistance demand that all advice is completely up-to-date. The spread of the disease may be controlled by destroying mosquito breeding sites, using residual insecticides in buildings, wearing protective clothing, sleeping under nets, and detecting and treating hosts.

Pneumocystis carinii **pneumonia**

Definition and aetiology

This is an uncommon infection caused by *Pneumocystis carinii*, a microorganism of uncertain classification but thought to be protozoan. It has become more common in recent years due to its association with immunocompromised patients, and in particular those with human immunodeficiency virus.

Pneumocystis spp. are harboured by many mammals (e.g. dogs, goats, horses, rodents, rabbits, sheep and humans). However, there does not appear to be any evidence that animals act as reservoirs for human infections. Transmission between humans is possibly by an airborne route or may occur from mother to fetus. The lungs represent the major target organ, although the microorganisms have been found in rare cases in lymph nodes, bone marrow and the spleen. Others who are most susceptible to developing disease are malnourished or premature infants.

Symptoms

A large proportion of healthy individuals are infected with *P. carinii* without showing any clinical signs. *P. carinii* pneumonia is characterised by dyspnoea, tachypnoea and a non-productive cough, often accompanied by fever and cyanosis, and culminating in respiratory insufficiency and death. The course is variable, arising insidiously over weeks or months (characteristic of AIDS patients and children suffering with congenital immunodeficient disorders) or progressing rapidly.

Treatment

The disease is always fatal if untreated. Treatment is usually successful, especially if started early, although some recurrences do occur, particularly with AIDS patients. It consists of the administration of co-trimoxazole (the drug of choice) (BNF 5.1.8), which may also be used as chemoprophylaxis in patients with a high risk of developing active disease. Other more recently introduced agents include pentamidine isetionate, atavaquone and trimetrexate (BNF 5.4.8).

Primary amoebic meningo-encephalitis

Definition and aetiology

Primary amoebic meningo-encephalitis is a rare protozoal infection of the brain and meninges caused by some species of free-living amoebae.

Naegleria fowleri infection appears to be contracted during swimming in contaminated freshwater lakes or pools. The microorganism enters via the nose and crosses the cribriform plate of the ethmoid bone to invade the central nervous system. *Acanthamoeba* and *Hartmannella* spp. are associated with subacute infections in immunocompromised individuals. The pathogenesis is unknown, although it is possible that *Acanthamoeba* spp. gain entry via abrasions on the skin or cornea. They may also be inhaled or swallowed, as they exist as windborne cysts.

Symptoms

Both forms of the infection give rise to fever, meningitis and haemorrhagic encephalitis. *N. fowleri* infections are more fulminant and result in death in a few days.

Treatment

Early treatment is essential, especially for *N. fowleri* infections, and consists of the intravenous and intrathecal administration of amphotericin B.

Toxoplasmosis

Definition and aetiology

Toxoplasmosis is a common protozoal infection caused by *Toxoplasma gondii*. It is a worldwide zoonosis involving birds and mammals (including humans), with the domestic cat as the definitive host.

Sexual reproduction takes place in the intestinal epithelial cells of the cat forming oocysts, which are excreted and may remain viable for many months in warm moist soil (Figure 5.10). The infection is acquired by ingestion of oocysts, present in cat faeces only, or tissue cysts in undercooked meat. Trophozoites are released, invade the intestinal mucosa, and spread to other organs via the circulation. They reproduce asexually until the host develops immunity and cysts are formed within the tissues, particularly in cardiac and skeletal muscle, lymph nodes, the retina and brain. Insects may play a role in transferring oocysts to food. Transmission may also occur from mother to fetus and in organ transplants from infected donors. Children are particularly at risk of becoming infected when playing in soil or sand contaminated with cat faeces.

Symptoms

The majority of patients infected with *T. gondii* are asymptomatic, although cysts may lie dormant in living tissues for years and only cause active disease if the host's immunity is compromised (e.g. those taking immunosuppressant drugs or suffering from AIDS or Hodgkin's disease). Commonly occurring symptoms in mild infections include fever, malaise and lymphadenopathy, and may be accompanied by fatigue, myalgia, and a maculopapular rash. There is usually complete recovery after several weeks or months. Fulminating disseminated toxoplasmosis, which may be fatal, occurs in immunodeficient hosts. Symptoms include hepatitis, hepatosplenomegaly, meningo-encephalitis, myocarditis and pneumonitis.

Congenital transmission only occurs if the mother (who may remain asymptomatic) acquires the infection immediately prior to or after conception. The consequences for the fetus are most severe if the disease is contracted during the first trimester, and may result in abortion or

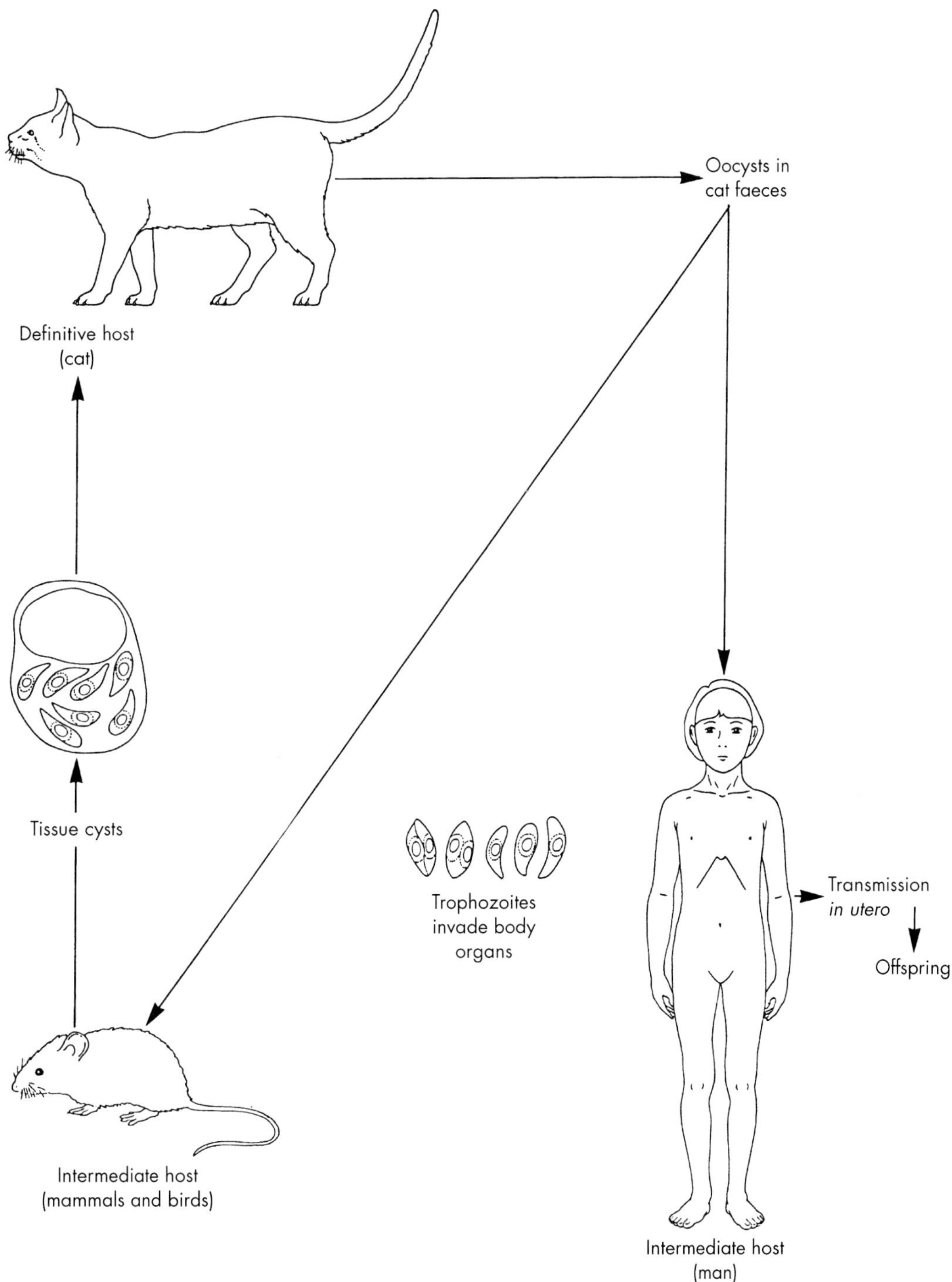

Figure 5.10 Life cycle of *Toxoplasma gondii*.

stillbirth. Symptoms of varying severity which arise at birth or later include hepatosplenomegaly, hydrocephalus, microcephaly, convulsions, mental retardation, spasticity and deafness. Chorioretinitis develops in adulthood and, if recurrent, may lead to loss of vision.

Treatment

Treatment (BNF 5.4.7) is only necessary in the presence of complications and for immunodeficient patients. Treatment of pregnant women is complicated by the risk of teratogenesis. There is no drug available to eradicate tissue cysts. Toxoplasmosis may be prevented by avoiding the consumption of rare meat, especially pork and lamb. Children should be discouraged from sucking their fingers, particularly when playing outside, and instructed to always wash their hands before eating. Cat-litter trays should be cleansed daily and sterilised with boiling water.

Trichomoniasis

Definition and aetiology

Trichomoniasis is a common protozoal infection of the genital tract caused by *Trichomonas vaginalis*. It is sexually transmitted in the majority of cases and occurs most commonly in females during the reproductive years. Males are often asymptomatic carriers of the microorganism.

Symptoms

Symptoms in females vary from mild to severe vaginitis, with a scanty or profuse, frothy, yellow discharge with an offensive odour. Accompanying symptoms include pruritus vulvae, vulval swelling, cystitis and dyspareunia. Males may develop urethritis, cystitis and prostatitis. Trichomoniasis is often associated with other sexually transmitted diseases (e.g. gonorrhoea) because *T. vaginalis* may carry pathogenic bacteria on its surface.

Treatment

Trichomoniasis should be treated promptly and investigations undertaken to detect any other sexually transmitted disease. Treatment consists of the administration of trichomonacides (BNF 5.4.7).

It may be prevented from further spread by concurrent treatment of sexual partners and refraining from sexual intercourse until cured.

Trypanosomiasis

Definition and aetiology

Trypanosomiasis is an infection caused by protozoa of the genus *Trypanosoma*. There are two different forms of the disease: African trypanosomiasis (sleeping sickness) and American trypanosomiasis (Chagas' disease).

African trypanosomiasis

Definition and aetiology

African trypanosomiasis occurs in the tropical regions of Africa and is caused by two subspecies of *T. brucei* pathogenic to humans: *T. b. gambiense* (Gambian sleeping sickness, occurring in West and Central Africa); and *T. b. rhodesiense* (Rhodesian or East African sleeping sickness).

The infection is transmitted as a zoonosis between various mammalian hosts by flies of the genus *Glossina* (tsetse flies). Trypanosomes ingested by a fly during a blood meal from an infected host develop within the vector for two to five weeks, and are then passed on to a new host in the fly's saliva. Humans are the natural host for Gambian sleeping sickness, although animals (e.g. pigs and sheep) may also enter the cycle. Wild game (e.g. antelopes) are the main reservoirs of *T. b. rhodesiense* infection, which is transmitted to humans entering endemic areas. Infection may also arise as a result of laboratory accidents with infected specimens, blood transfusion, and occasionally by congenital transmission.

Symptoms

Gambian sleeping sickness is a chronic disease and develops slowly over two to three years. There is an initial nodular lesion (chancre) at the inoculation site, which may remain unnoticed. Spread to lymph nodes and the bloodstream occurs some weeks or months later and may give rise to intermittent fever, malaise, headache, lymphadenopathy, urticaria and anaemia. An asymptomatic period lasting months or years may follow before invasion of the central nervous system. Once invasion does occur, progressive neurological degeneration results, characterised by personality changes, delusions, hallucinations, mania, drowsiness and convulsions. Severe pruritus, headache and back pain may also occur. A deterioration in the level of consciousness leads to coma. Death is often brought about by a secondary infection (e.g. pneumonia).

The symptoms of Rhodesian sleeping sickness are similar to those of Gambian, but proceed with a more rapid and severe course and less clearly defined stages. Death often occurs within a year due to heart failure, before invasion of the central nervous system has occurred. Patients do not develop immunity to African trypanosomiasis.

Treatment

Once invasion of the CNS has occurred, death is inevitable unless the disease is treated. Most cases respond well to treatment, especially in the early stages. Treatment (BNF 5.4.6) should be undertaken by specialists. Any underlying nutritional deficiencies should be corrected and complications (e.g. anaemia and intercurrent infection) treated. Preventive measures include reducing the human reservoir of infection by detecting and treating infected individuals early.

American trypanosomiasis

Definition and aetiology

American trypanosomiasis is a protozoal infection caused by *Trypanosoma cruzi* and is endemic in remote rural areas of Central and South America.

Reservoirs of infection include the cat, dog, armadillo, opossum, rodents and humans. The vectors are bugs of the family *Reduviidae*, several species of which have adapted to cohabit with humans, living in cracks in the walls of poorly constructed houses. The bug ingests trypanosomes during a blood meal from an infected host. The trypanosomes multiply within the vector and are passed on to a new host during defecation after feeding. The parasite gains entry into the new host through skin abrasions, mucous membranes or the conjunctiva and multiplies in myocardial cells and smooth muscle cells of the gastrointestinal tract.

Symptoms

The incubation period is 4–12 days, although many patients show no detectable signs of disease. The majority of those presenting with an acute phase illness are children, approximately half of whom develop a visible lesion at the inoculation site. Subsequent symptoms, which persist for two to four months, include fever, weakness, facial oedema, lymphadenopathy and hepatosplenomegaly. The ensuing intermediate phase may last for decades in some individuals before signs of chronic disease become apparent. The usual manifestations of chronic disease are cardiomyopathy or dilatation of the oesophagus or colon (mega syndromes). The course of the disease and prognosis are variable. A small proportion of patients die of myocarditis or acute meningo-encephalitis in the acute phase, although some individuals never develop chronic complications. If chronic organ damage does occur, it is irreversible.

Treatment

All acute cases should be treated, as this stage determines the subsequent course of the disease. Treatment (BNF 5.4.6) should be undertaken by specialists and comprises the administration of nifurtimox and benznidazole, which are of value in the acute phase only. Chronic cardiomyopathy requires symptomatic treatment and surgery may be necessary for the mega syndromes. Infected adults showing no abnormalities on the electrocardiogram should be reassured that they may not necessarily develop chronic complications.

American trypanosomiasis may be prevented by improving housing conditions, health education, using insecticides in homes, and detecting and treating infected individuals early in an effort to eliminate the reservoir of infection.

5.6 Helminthic infections

Cestode infections

Definition and aetiology

Dwarf tapeworm infection is caused by *Hymenolepis nana* and occurs in warm, dry climates (e.g. Africa, the Middle East, South America, and south and east Europe). It occurs most commonly in children, as host resistance improves with age and the adult tapeworm survives for only a few months. No intermediate host is required and the infection may be passed from person to person by faecal contamination of food and water. Auto-infection may also occur, internally or by hand-to-mouth transmission.

Fish tapeworm infection is caused by *Diphyllobothrium latum*, which is the largest tapeworm infecting humans (up to 10 m long). It is prevalent in areas where raw or undercooked freshwater fish are consumed (e.g. Alaska, Finland, Japan, Siberia, and Sweden). The first intermediate host is a copepod (a minute aquatic arthropod), which is ingested by freshwater fish (e.g. perch, pike, turbot and salmon). The adult tapeworm may survive for up to 20 years.

Hydatid disease is an infection with larval forms of *Echinococcus granulosus*, which occurs worldwide, particularly in sheep-rearing areas. The definitive host is the domestic or wild dog, with sheep acting as the main intermediate host. Humans are an incidental host and contract the infection by ingesting eggs present in contaminated food and water or by close contact with infected dogs.

Taeniasis is caused by *Taenia saginata* (beef tapeworm) or *T. solium* (pork tapeworm) and occurs worldwide in areas where poor standards of sewage disposal exist. Humans are the only definitive host, contracting the infection by ingesting raw or undercooked beef or pork containing cysticerci (Figure 5.11). The adult tapeworm can survive for years in the small intestine, reaching a length of 2–4 m (*T. solium*) or 4–10 m (*T. saginata*). Cysticercosis occurs if humans ingest eggs and thus become infected with larval forms of *T. solium*, which may migrate to any body tissue but particularly muscle, subcutaneous tissue and the central nervous system. The infection is contracted by consumption of contaminated food or water. It may also be due to auto-infection with eggs in an individual already harbouring an adult tapeworm, either by the hand-to-mouth route or by the passage of eggs to the stomach by reverse peristalsis (e.g. vomiting).

Symptoms

Infections with adult tapeworms are often asymptomatic. However, if the worm load is heavy, mucosal irritation may lead to gastrointestinal disturbances (e.g. abdominal discomfort, diarrhoea, and nausea and vomiting). Other symptoms include weight loss, nervousness, dizziness, fatigue, urticaria, allergic reactions and pruritus ani. Patients suffering with taeniasis are often aware of a 'crawling' sensation as gravid proglottides are shed from the anus. The fish tapeworm may cause pernicious anaemia.

Infections with larval forms (i.e. hydatid disease and cysticercosis) are generally more serious, and symptoms, which may not appear for several years, are due to the effects of enlarging cysts on surrounding tissue (e.g. atrophy, compression or obstruction). Hydatid cysts occur most commonly in the liver and lungs. Symptoms of cysticercosis usually occur when the cysts die and calcify, and are most severe if the brain is involved, resulting in some cases in epilepsy and psychotic changes.

Treatment

Treatment of most cestode infections comprises the administration of taenicides (BNF 5.5.3), while surgical aspiration or excision may be necessary for hydatid cysts. Symptomatic treatment may be required for allergic reactions or epilepsy.

Prevention and control may be effected by ensuring high standards of sewage disposal and general hygiene, and by deep-freezing or thoroughly cooking fish and meat. Dogs should be prevented from gaining access to uncooked sheep meat in areas endemic for hydatid disease.

Nematode infections

Ascariasis

Definition and aetiology

Ascariasis (roundworm infection) is caused by the common roundworm *Ascaris lumbricoides* and occurs worldwide, particularly in warm climates.

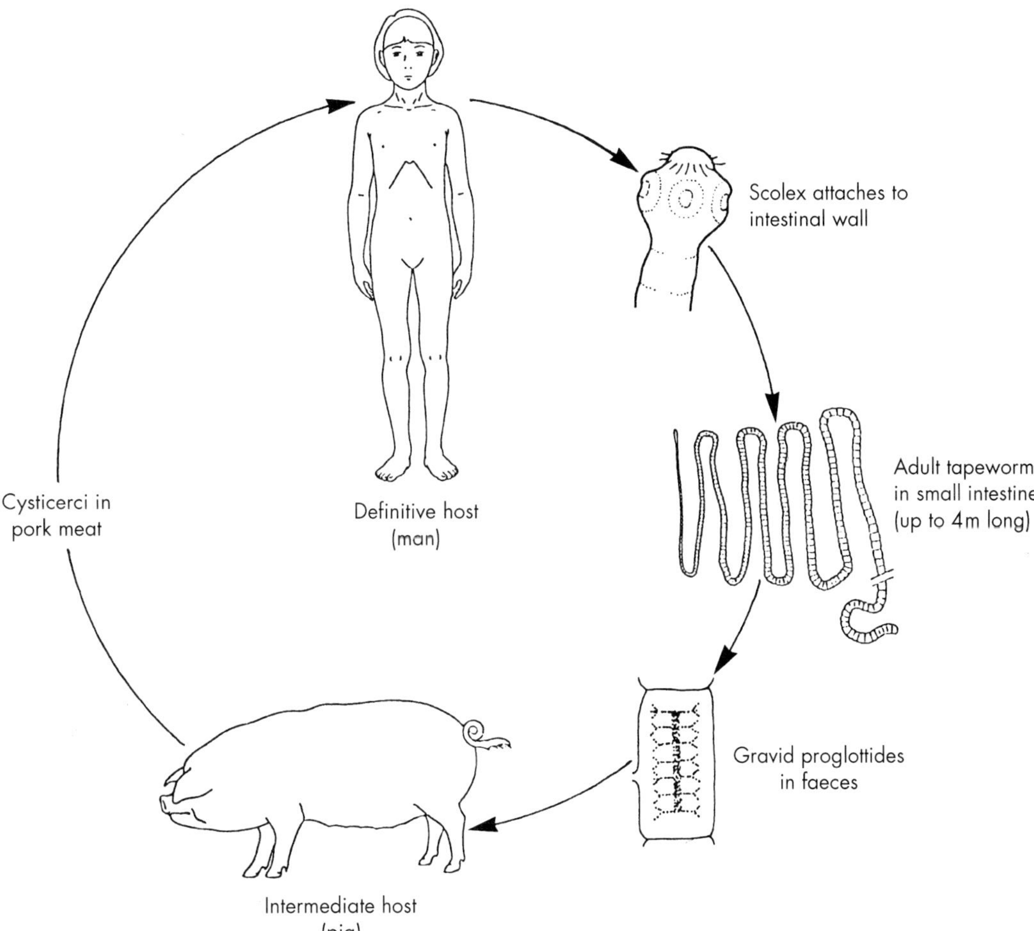

Figure 5.11 Life cycle of *Taenia solium*.

Eggs ingested in faecal-contaminated food and water hatch in the intestine. The larvae pass into the lymphatics and the bloodstream, and migrate to the small intestine via the liver, lungs, trachea and oesophagus. Mature female worms, which may be up to 30 cm long, produce eggs which are passed in the faeces and may remain viable in the soil for several years.

Symptoms

Ascariasis occurs more frequently in children than adults. Symptoms caused by migration of larval forms may include fever, cough, dyspnoea, eosinophilia and urticaria, particularly if they die *en route*, and set up foreign-tissue reactions. Light intestinal infections with adult worms are usually asymptomatic, but large worm loads may lead to colic, diarrhoea, melaena and intestinal obstruction. Worms may occasionally be vomited. Development in children may be retarded. The disease may be fatal if ectopic migration of worms occurs to the appendix, common bile duct and pancreatic duct.

Treatment

Treatment of ascariasis is essential to prevent the possible occurrence of ectopic migration, and consists of the administration of ascaricides (e.g. levamisole, mebendazole, and piperazine) (BNF 5.5.2). Surgery may be necessary to relieve intestinal obstruction.

Transmission of the infection may be prevented by improving sanitation, avoiding the use of human faeces as fertiliser, boiling drinking water, and consuming only cooked food in endemic areas. Regular mass chemotherapy may help to break the cycle.

Dracontiasis

Definition and aetiology

Dracontiasis occurs in rural areas of India and West Africa and is caused by *Dracunculus medinensis* (guinea worm).

A minute aquatic crustacean (*Cyclops* spp.) acts as an intermediate host. Infected cyclops, present in drinking water, release larval forms in the intestinal tract of the definitive host, which migrate to subcutaneous tissues (usually of the leg or scrotum) where they mature into adult worms. The adult female, which may be up to 1 m in length, protrudes a little way through the skin and discharges embryos when the skin is cooled. Those emerging in fresh water enter cyclops and develop into infective larvae.

Symptoms

Generalised symptoms include diarrhoea, eosinophilia, urticaria and vomiting. A painful ulcer often develops at the site of protrusion and can be complicated by secondary infection (e.g. tetanus). Dead worms may calcify under the skin if not removed.

Treatment

The worm must be extracted by surgery or by slowly and carefully winding it out, which is facilitated by first killing it (BNF 5.5.7). Antibacterial drugs (BNF 5.1) may be required to treat secondary infection. (For treatment of ulcers, *see* Section 13.1.)

Transmission of infection may be prevented by filtering or boiling drinking water in endemic areas, and preventing contamination of water supplies by people with guinea-worm ulcers.

Enterobiasis

Definition and aetiology

Enterobiasis (threadworm infection) is a common infection caused by *Enterobius vermicularis* (pinworm or threadworm), occurring worldwide in urban and rural areas.

No intermediate host is required and person-to-person transmission or auto-infection occurs. Eggs, which are ingested in contaminated food or from fingers, hatch and mature in the small intestine. After copulation, the female worms migrate to the caecum and colon, and travel to the anus at night to lay eggs in the perianal region. Their presence results in intense irritation, causing the patient to scratch and pick up eggs on the fingers. Some eggs hatch *in situ* and the larvae return to the rectum to mature.

Symptoms

Children are affected more frequently than adults. The principal symptom is pruritus ani, and intense scratching may lead to secondary infection. Other symptoms include anorexia, emotional disturbances, insomnia, and weight loss. Occasionally, ectopic migration may cause appendicitis and in females, salpingitis. Female worms (8–13 mm in length) may be observed moving in faeces.

Treatment

Treatment of enterobiasis consists of the administration of drugs for threadworms (BNF 5.5.1), combined with measures to break the cycle of auto-infection. These include wearing close-fitting undergarments in bed to reduce the number of eggs shed onto bedding; a bath on rising to wash away eggs deposited during the night; daily changing of bedding and night clothes until the infection is cleared; keeping nails trimmed and well-scrubbed; and always washing hands after using the toilet and before eating or handling food. All the members of a household should be treated at the same time.

Filariasis

Definition and aetiology

Filariasis is a disease caused by filarial worms, eight species being responsible for infection in humans. They all rely on arthropods as intermediate hosts and vectors. Larvae are transferred to people during a blood meal. They mature into adult forms that inhabit the lymphatic system, subcutaneous tissues or connective tissues, depending on the species. After fertilisation, the female continuously produces microfilariae (motile prelarval forms), which circulate in the bloodstream or skin. When ingested by a suitable arthropod, they undergo further development to the infective larval stage. Adult worms of some species may survive for as long as 15 years.

Wuchereria bancrofti and *Brugia malayi* are lymphatic dwelling filariids. The infection is transmitted by mosquitoes in tropical and subtropical regions.

Onchocerca volvulus relies on the female blackfly (*Simulium* spp.) as an intermediate host (Figure 5.12) and causes onchocerciasis (river blindness), a subcutaneous infection occurring in tropical regions of Africa, Mexico and parts of South America.

Loa loa (eye worm) causes loiasis, which is transmitted by deerflies or red-flies (*Chrysops* spp.) in the rain-forest regions of Africa. The adult worms move freely in the subcutaneous tissues and the conjunctiva.

Symptoms

Initial symptoms of lymphatic filariasis, which may not appear until up to two years after infection, include fever, malaise, chyluria, lymphangitis and back pain. Lymphatic blockage causing

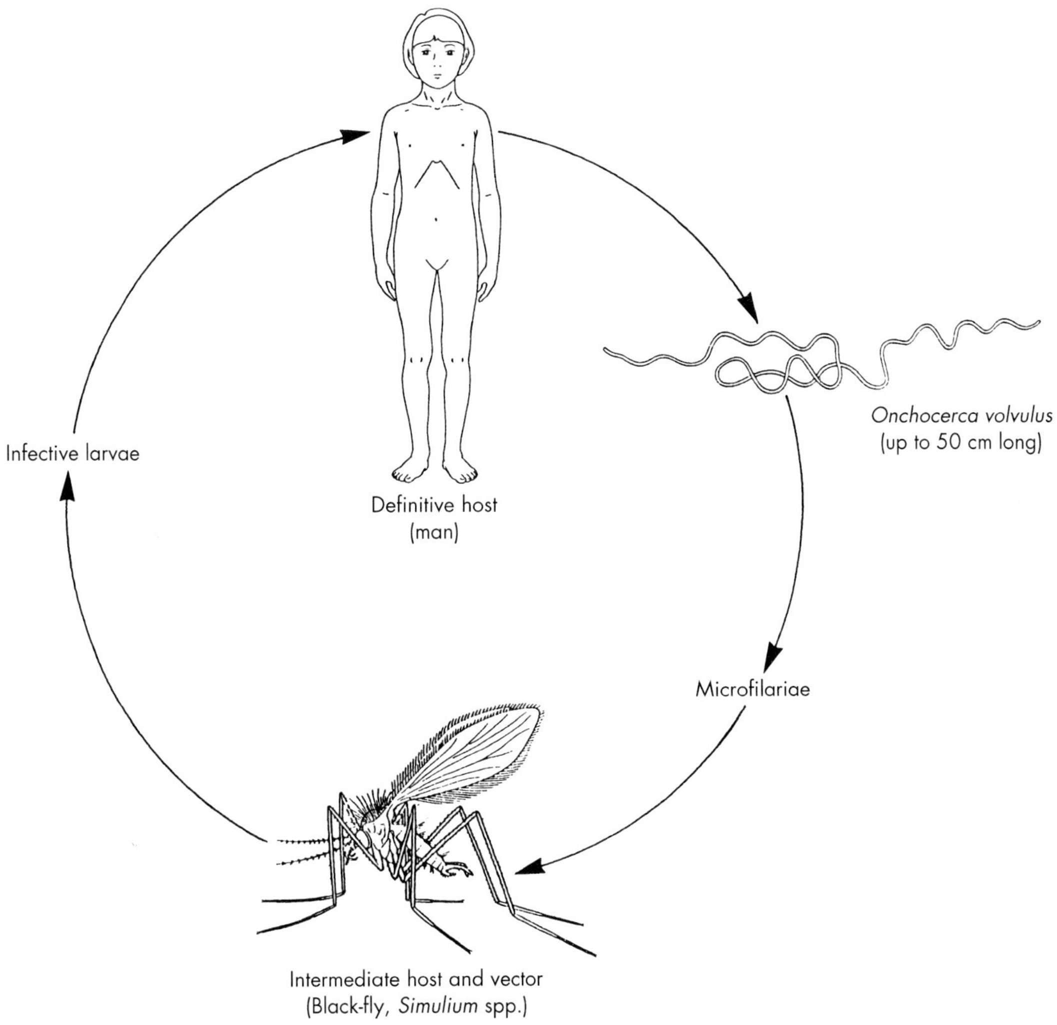

Figure 5.12 Life cycle of *Onchocerca volvulus*.

distension of distal lymph vessels and subsequent inflammation (elephantiasis) may also occur, with the legs and male genital tract most frequently affected. Light infections may be asymptomatic.

In onchocerciasis, the adult worms inhabit subcutaneous fibrous nodules or occasionally deeper nodules in the muscles or joint capsules. Their presence rarely causes symptoms, unlike the skin-inhabiting microfilariae. The incubation period may be as long as 18 months before the initial symptoms of pruritus and maculopapular rash appear. Heavy infection leads to depigmentation, scarring, and loss of elastic tissue. Ocular involvement causes keratitis, which leads to loss of vision if untreated.

The characteristic symptom of loiasis is the Calabar swelling, which develops at least three months after infection. The swelling often develops on the face, particularly close to the eye, and over medium-sized joints. It lasts for two to three days and may be associated with fever, malaise and eosinophilia. The adult worms may be seen migrating through the skin or across the conjunctiva, and felt as a prickling sensation under the skin, or as deeper aches with paraesthesia.

Treatment

Treatment of all types of filariasis comprises the administration of filaricides (BNF 5.5.6). Antihistamines (BNF 3.4.1) and, in severe cases, corticosteroids may be necessary to control the allergic reaction and the initial exacerbation of symptoms caused by destruction of microfilariae.

Prevention of infection may be effected by wearing protective clothing and by sleeping under nets in endemic areas.

Hookworm infection

Definition and aetiology

Hookworm infection is an intestinal infection caused by *Ancylostoma duodenale* (Old World hookworm), occurring in warm, humid, temperate and tropical climates, and *Necator americanus* (New World hookworm), occurring in the tropics.

No intermediate host is required. Larvae present in soil penetrate the host's skin (usually the feet), enter the circulation, and migrate to the intestines via the heart, lungs, trachea and oesophagus. Infection may also be contracted by ingestion of larvae in contaminated drinking water. Mature female worms produce eggs for many years: these are passed in the faeces and hatch in warm, moist soil.

Symptoms

There may be an initial reaction at the site of entry (ground itch). The adult worm feeds upon blood and interstitial fluid in the intestinal wall. Heavy infections produce serious symptoms, including anaemia, abdominal pain, gastrointestinal disturbances, hypoalbuminaemia, oedema, palpitations and retarded growth in children; light infections are usually asymptomatic. Larvae migrating through the lungs in sufficient numbers may result in symptoms of bronchitis.

Treatment

Treatment comprises the administration of drugs for hookworms (BNF 5.5.4). It may also be necessary to treat severe anaemia.

The cycle of transmission may be broken by improving standards of sanitation, boiling drinking water and always wearing shoes outdoors in endemic areas.

Strongyloidiasis

Definition and aetiology

Strongyloidiasis is an intestinal infection caused by *Strongyloides stercoralis*, which occurs in humid tropical climates.

Infective larval forms present in faecal-contaminated soil penetrate a person's skin (usually the feet) and migrate to the small intestine via the lungs, trachea, and oesophagus. They mature into adult worms, which inhabit the mucosa and submucosa. Eggs produced by the female worms hatch within the host, the non-infective larvae passing in the faeces to the external environment where they develop into infective forms. Occasionally, their development may take place in the bowel, thus allowing auto-infection and a build-up of large numbers of worms. The infection may persist for more than 30 years.

Symptoms

Strongyloidiasis is usually asymptomatic if worm loads are light, although there may be an initial reaction (ground itch) at the site of entry. Heavy infection may result in abdominal pain, diarrhoea and, in severe cases, malabsorption. Larvae migrating through the lungs may cause cough, pneumonitis, and sometimes death due to alveolar haemorrhage. Occasionally, larvae may migrate through the skin (cutaneous larva migrans) and cause pruritus and urticaria.

Treatment

Treatment is by the administration of drugs for strongyloidiasis (BNF 5.5.8). Vitamin supplements and iron with folic acid (BNF 9.1.1) may be indicated in patients with chronic disease.

The infection may be prevented by avoiding skin contact with soil in endemic areas and improving standards of sewage disposal.

Toxocariasis

Definition and aetiology

Toxocara canis and less commonly *T. cati* are roundworms of dogs (mainly puppies) and cats respectively. They cause toxocariasis in humans.

The infection is contracted mainly by children ingesting eggs in faecal-contaminated soil. It is also possible to pick up eggs from the coat of an infected dog or from food to which eggs have been transferred by flies. The eggs hatch in the intestine, releasing larvae that can pass to any body tissue via blood and lymph (visceral larva migrans).

Symptoms

Toxocariasis is often asymptomatic. However, if the larvae penetrate vital organs, even light infections are potentially serious. General symptoms may include cough, eosinophilia, fever and malaise; specific symptoms caused by burrowing larvae and granulomatous reactions to dead larvae depend on the site involved. These may include asthma, bronchitis, epilepsy, hepatomegaly and loss of vision. The larvae survive for one year only and the infection resolves spontaneously in the absence of re-infection. Irreparable damage may, however, occur within that time.

Treatment

Diethylcarbamazine is used in the treatment of toxocariasis, but treatment must be started early to prevent permanent damage. Relapses may occur.

The disease may be controlled by prohibiting dog-owners from allowing their pets to foul public parks and children's playgrounds. All dogs (and especially puppies) should be routinely wormed and puppy faeces incinerated. Disinfectants are of little value in destroying the eggs. Children should be encouraged to wash their hands before eating, and discouraged from sucking their fingers or ingesting soil when playing outside.

Trichiniasis

Definition and aetiology

Trichiniasis (trichinosis) is an intestinal infection caused by a small roundworm, *Trichinella spiralis*, which occurs worldwide, particularly in temperate zones.

There are many definitive hosts, including humans. The infection is contracted by ingestion of undercooked infected meat (e.g. pork); no intermediate host is required. Larvae within cysts are released in the small intestine and mature into adult worms. These in turn produce larvae, which are carried in blood and lymph to striated muscle (particularly abdominal muscles, the diaphragm, tongue, larynx and larger voluntary muscles) where they encyst and remain viable for years.

Symptoms

Light infections are often asymptomatic; heavy infections produce symptoms which depend on the parasite's stage of development and the site involved.

Young adult worms burrowing into the intestinal wall may cause abdominal pain, diarrhoea, fever, and nausea and vomiting during the first week. Later symptoms are due to larvae migrating to the muscles, and include eosinophilia, fever, facial oedema and myositis. Invasion of the diaphragm may cause dyspnoea, while involvement of the tongue or larynx may lead to aphonia. Larvae may invade myocardial muscle and cause arrhythmias. After about three weeks, the patient usually starts to recover as cyst formation commences, although fatal complications may arise due to involvement of myocardial tissue, the lungs and the central nervous system.

Treatment

Treatment comprises the administration of tiabendazole (BNF 5.5.8) and symptomatic relief for complications.

The spread of infection may be prevented by thoroughly cooking pork, freezing raw meat at –18°C, and improving the standards of pig-rearing (e.g. by carefully controlling their diet).

Trichuriasis

Definition and aetiology

Trichuriasis is an infection of the large intestine caused by the whipworm, *Trichuris trichiura*, and occurs in warm humid regions (e.g. South East Asia).

No intermediate host is necessary. Infection is contracted by ingestion of contaminated food and water containing eggs, which hatch in the small intestine. Mature worms inhabit the caecum or colon and pass eggs in the host's faeces. The eggs become infective after three weeks in appropriate soil conditions.

Symptoms

Light infections are usually asymptomatic; heavy infections may cause abdominal pain, anaemia (due to intestinal bleeding), colitis, diarrhoea, melaena and weight loss. Occasionally, worms in the appendix may cause appendicitis, and rectal prolapse is a common complication in children.

Treatment

The infection is difficult to eradicate. Drugs in use include mebendazole (BNF 5.5.1) and tiabendazole (BNF 5.5.8).

Prevention may be effected by improving sanitation, avoiding the use of human faeces as fertiliser, and consuming only boiled water and cooked foods in endemic areas.

Trematode infections

Definition and aetiology

Schistosomiasis (bilharziasis) is a chronic blood fluke infection caused by *Schistosoma haematobium*, *S. japonicum* and *S. mansoni*, and occurs in Africa, Asia, and South America. The primary definitive hosts are humans, who contract the infection by contact with contaminated fresh water and pass eggs in urine and faeces.

Intestinal fluke disease occurs in South East Asia and the Far East. The largest intestinal fluke is *Fasciolopsis buski*, whose main definitive host is the pig. Humans may contract the infection in endemic areas by consumption of raw contaminated aquatic vegetation (e.g. water chestnuts). Eggs are passed in the faeces.

Liver fluke disease is caused by several species, the most important being *Clonorchis sinensis* (Chinese liver fluke), prevalent in China and South East Asia. The infection is contracted by the consumption of raw or undercooked freshwater fish (e.g. carp or salmon). *Fasciola hepatica* is a common parasite of sheep in areas of wet pasture, but humans may also contract the infection by ingestion of contaminated aquatic plants (e.g. watercress). The eggs of both species of helminth are passed in faeces.

Lung fluke disease is most commonly due to *Paragonimus westermani* (Oriental lung fluke) and is widespread in Asia. The infection is contracted by the ingestion of raw freshwater crustaceans. The eggs are passed by coughing up and spitting out sputum, or in the faeces if the sputum is swallowed.

Symptoms

The onset of schistosomiasis is usually insidious, although some individuals may present with early symptoms of 'swimmer's itch', a papular pruritic rash caused by cercariae burrowing into the skin. There may be acute symptoms several weeks after infection (Katayama fever), which include anorexia, diarrhoea, hepatosplenomegaly, fever, cough and urticaria. Chronic manifestations may not appear until several years later and are related to the site of the veins infected, which is species specific. Usually those of the intestines or urinary bladder are involved. Symptoms are caused by formation of granulomas around eggs trapped in tissues, and include portal hypertension, cirrhosis of the liver, splenomegaly, melaena and obstruction of urine outflow. Some patients with light infections may be asymptomatic.

Most hermaphroditic fluke infections are asymptomatic or present with mild symptoms only and are rarely life-threatening; spontaneous recovery may even occur. Heavy worm loads produce symptoms related to the site of infection. Heavy intestinal infections may be marked by diarrhoea, nausea and vomiting, abdominal pain, haemorrhage and, in severe cases, ascites and obstruction. Symptoms of liver fluke disease may include abdominal discomfort, diarrhoea, nausea and vomiting, hepatomegaly, jaundice and, in severe cases, cholangitis. Lung fluke infection may result in a productive cough, haemoptysis, dyspnoea and chest discomfort.

Treatment

Treatment of trematode infections is by the administration of praziquantel (BNF 5.5.5).

Infections may be prevented by ensuring high standards of sanitation, changing particular eating habits, and treatment of all infected individuals in endemic areas. Skin contact with fresh water should be avoided as far as possible, and drinking water should be boiled in areas where schistosomiasis is prevalent.

5.7 Ectoparasitic infestations

Myiasis

Definition and aetiology

Myiasis is an infestation of living tissue of vertebrates by larvae (maggots) of several species of fly (e.g. greenbottle, bluebottle or house flies). It occurs most commonly in warm climates and Eastern Europe.

The condition is uncommon in humans and is usually the result of accidental inoculation of sleeping, debilitated or bedridden individuals. Poor living conditions and low standards of hygiene predispose to infestation. People working closely with animals (e.g. cattle or sheep) may also be at risk.

Symptoms

Symptoms vary according to the species of fly and site of body involved. The most common lesions are non-specific and may be asymptomatic if larvae are confined to superficial wounds. Dermal invasion may result in furuncular lesions, which are swollen and painful as a result of the larvae moving under the skin and feeding on tissue fluid.

Larvae may invade orifices and produce a variety of symptoms. Pain and discharge are symptoms of involvement of the ear, with two-thirds of such patients developing otitis media. Infestation of the eye (e.g. by sheep bot fly) may cause conjunctivitis, photophobia and swollen lids. Other sites of infestation include mouth, nose and anogenital orifices. Accidental ingestion of larvae in food may give rise to intestinal myiasis, although in some cases, the discomfort may only last until the larvae are passed in stools.

Creeping eruptions are caused by larvae migrating under the skin, usually in the search for an exit site to continue the next phase of the life-cycle. Warble fly larvae migrate through the body dorsally and may cause serious damage or even death.

Many flies carry pathogenic microorganisms, and secondary infections may complicate myiasis.

Treatment

The larvae may be removed by gentle compression and extraction with forceps, preferably using a local anaesthetic. Surgery or irrigation may be necessary to remove larvae from orifices. Application of an anti-infective skin preparation (BNF 13.10) may be needed to treat secondary infections.

Myiasis may be prevented by improving living conditions and standards of hygiene, including frequent dressing changes. People at risk should protect themselves against contact with flies (e.g. by using eye shields or sleeping nets).

Pediculosis

Definition and aetiology

Pediculosis is an infestation with lice, which are blood-sucking arthropods. Three different species affect different sites of the body.

Pediculosis capitis

Definition and aetiology

Pediculosis capitis is infestation of the scalp by *Pediculus humanus capitis*, which is transmitted by close personal contact or fomites (e.g. hats, pillows, combs or brushes). Contrary to popular belief, lice do not jump from one person to another.

The adult louse is between 2.5 and 3.5 mm in length, greyish in colour, and inhabits the scalp attached to the base of a hair. The average number per head is 10. Eggs (nits), which are yellowish-white in colour and approximately 0.8 mm long, are laid close to the hair base. They hatch in 3–14 days, the length of time increasing as environmental temperature decreases. The eggs cannot be dislodged, and remain on the hair as empty opalescent shells after hatching. With hair growth of about 1 cm per month, the distance of the nit from the scalp thus indicates the time of initial infestation. Lice survive for approximately three days away from the body and die quickly if damaged (e.g. by combing).

The condition is common in schoolchildren and is not particularly associated with social class, standards of cleanliness or length of hair.

Symptoms

Pediculosis capitis mainly affects the scalp, although other areas of facial hair (e.g. eyebrows, eyelashes or beard) may also be involved. The eggs are easier to see than the adult lice, and are found most frequently above the ears and close to the nape of the neck.

Symptoms of infestation include pruritus and cervical adenopathy. Severe excoriation may produce secondary bacterial infection (e.g. furunculosis or impetigo), although the lice themselves do not carry pathogenic microorganisms.

Treatment

Pediculosis capitis is treated by the topical administration of lotions of malathion, carbaryl or the pyrethroids (permethrin and phenothrin) (BNF 13.10.4). It is recommended that local policies should be adopted whereby only one of these insecticides is used for a given period, alternating with the other to prevent the emergence of resistant strains. Patients should be advised to follow instructions carefully to avoid the use of sublethal doses which encourage resistant strains; similarly, lotions or shampoos should not be used prophylactically.

Lice and eggs may be removed after treatment using a special nit comb with close-set teeth. All family and social contacts should be inspected and treated if infested. Fomites should also be disinfected. Vacuuming carpets may help to remove shed hairs with attached eggs.

The condition may be prevented by avoiding close head contact or sharing hats, towels or hairdressing implements with others. Thorough combing of hair every night may damage any lice present and prevent egg laying.

Pediculosis corporis

Definition and aetiology

Pediculosis corporis is infestation of the body by *Pediculus humanus corporis* (Figure 5.13a), which is associated with overcrowding and poor standards of hygiene.

The eggs and adults are similar in appearance to the head louse, although the adult body louse is slightly larger (3–4.5 mm long). The eggs hatch within 6–15 days. They inhabit clothing fibres more frequently than body hairs, particularly clothes in close contact with skin.

The body louse also acts as a vector for some microorganisms that cause disease (e.g. epidemic typhus fever).

Symptoms

Symptoms include pruritus and urticaria, particularly on the shoulders, abdomen and buttocks. Small red punctate marks may be seen at the bite site.

Treatment

The treatment of pediculosis corporis is as for pediculosis capitis (*see above*). Resistant strains of the body louse are less common, and benzyl benzoate or lindane may also be effective.

Contacts should similarly be inspected and treated if necessary, and all bedding and clothing laundered in hot water and ironed.

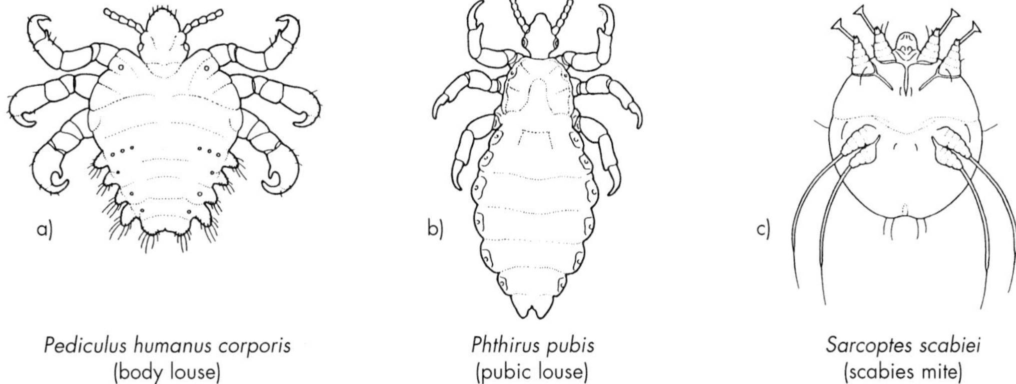

Figure 5.13 Examples of ectoparasites.

Pediculosis pubis

Definition and aetiology

Pediculosis pubis (crabs) is infestation of the hairs in the pubic and anogenital region by *Phthirus pubis* (Figure 5.13b). The eyelashes may also be affected.

It is generally transmitted by sexual contact, and only rarely by fomites, as the adult louse does not leave the body unless damaged.

The adult is approximately 1–2 mm in length and breadth and grey-white or yellow-brown in colour.

Symptoms

Pediculosis pubis is characterised by small, non-pruritic, greyish-blue macules, irregular in outline. However, the condition itself may be irritating, and excoriation may give rise to erythematous pustules.

Treatment

Treating and preventing further infestation is as for the other forms of pediculosis.

Scabies

Definition and aetiology

Scabies is a contagious skin infestation caused by a mite, *Sarcoptes scabiei* (Figure 5.13c). It is transmitted mainly by close personal contact as the mite does not survive for more than two to three days away from the host. The incidence of scabies is not significantly linked to poor living conditions.

The female mite, which is approximately 300 μm in breadth and 400 μm in length, burrows in the stratum corneum at a rate of 2 mm a day, and lays eggs. The larvae hatch in three to four days and mature about 10 days later.

Symptoms

Scabies is characterised by severe pruritus, particularly at night. Pruritus does not commence until at least two weeks after initial infestation, and is probably an allergic reaction to the presence of the mite. A variety of lesions may arise as a result of scratching, including urticarial papules, macules, vesicles, pustules or haemorrhagic crusts. Eczema may develop and be particularly severe in infants; secondary infection may also complicate scabies.

The actual burrow can easily be overlooked in the presence of other lesions. It is grey in colour, slightly raised, often curved, and between 3 and 15 mm long. Common sites include finger webs, hands, wrists, elbows, ankles, and feet. The nipples in women and male penis may be similarly affected. Palms and soles are less frequently affected in adults and the face and scalp only in infants.

Treatment

Treatment consists of the application of an appropriate parasiticidal preparation (BNF

13.10.4). Pruritus may persist for several weeks after eradication of the mite, but the patient should be advised not to reapply the parasiticide. Administration of oral antihistamines (BNF 3.4.1), the application of a topical antipruritic preparation (BNF 13.3), or both may be of value. Secondary infections may need treatment with appropriate antibacterial drugs (BNF 5.1).

All family and social contacts should be inspected and treated if necessary. Clothing and bedding should be laundered in the usual manner.

5.8 Sexually transmitted diseases

Chancroid

Definition and aetiology
Chancroid is a bacterial infection caused by *Haemophilus ducreyi*, a Gram-negative bacillus. It is endemic in parts of Africa and Asia and occurs sporadically throughout the rest of the world. Its incidence appears to be associated with poor living conditions and low standards of hygiene.

The infection is transmitted sexually, invading the host through small abrasions. The incidence is greatest in men, although the exact number of cases in women is difficult to assess as lesions are less obvious.

Symptoms
The incubation period is usually less than a week, but may be as long as two to three weeks.

A small painful papule develops at the inoculation site (usually in the perianal or genital area), and rapidly develops into a pustular vesicle which ulcerates. The ulcer is shallow, painful and tender with ragged margins and an erythematous border; there is a purulent necrotic base. Lesions may be multiple, arising as a result of auto-infection. In over 50% of cases, there may also be unilateral enlargement of the inguinal lymph nodes, which may fuse to form painful buboes. Large buboes may spontaneously suppurate through a sinus.

The lesions may persist for several months, causing tissue destruction which may be exacerbated by secondary infection. The condition is, however, often self-limiting and the ulcers heal with scar formation.

Treatment
Treatment consists of the administration of co-trimoxazole (BNF 5.1.8), erythromycin (BNF 5.1.5) or tetracycline (BNF 5.1.3). Buboes may require aspiration.

All sexual contacts should be screened and treated if necessary. Use of condoms during sexual intercourse, or thorough cleansing of genitalia subsequently may help to prevent chancroid developing.

Condylomata acuminata

Definition and aetiology
Condylomata acuminata (anogenital warts) are caused by the human papillomavirus, which is usually transmitted sexually. There may be an association between some subtypes of this virus and cervical cancer.

Symptoms
The average incubation period is two to three months, with a range of three weeks to nine months.

Condylomata acuminata may occur anywhere in the genital or perianal area of males and females. They are small, soft, pointed, pink, fissured lesions of varying shape. They grow rapidly, become pedunculated and, because several usually occur at the same site, can resemble a cauliflower; single lesions are infrequent. They may become more widespread during pregnancy, which favours even more rapid growth. Spontaneous resolution may occur.

Treatment
Treatment consists of the topical application of preparations containing podophyllin (BNF 13.7) for warts and calluses, cryosurgery or surgical removal.

All sexual contacts should be treated, although up to one-third of patients may relapse, but not necessarily as a result of re-infection.

Gonorrhoea

Definition and aetiology
Gonorrhoea is a bacterial infection caused by *Neisseria gonorrhoeae*, a Gram-negative aerobic

diplococcus. Humans are the natural host and the disease occurs worldwide.

In addition to sexual transmission, gonorrhoea may be acquired by an infant from an infected mother during birth. It is rarely transmitted via fomites, as the microorganism does not survive for long outside the body.

Symptoms

The incubation period is shorter in men (range 2–14 days) than in women (range 7–21 days).

Gonorrhoea is frequently asymptomatic, particularly in women who may remain carriers for weeks. Almost all infected males present with symptoms, the most common complaint being urethritis, characterised by dysuria, frequency and urgency. A yellowish, purulent, urethral discharge may also occur. Complications are rare if treatment is prompt, but may include epididymitis, prostatitis and urethral stricture. Post-gonococcal urethritis may develop after successful treatment.

The most common site of infection in females is the endocervix, and symptoms include vaginal discharge and occasionally abnormal menstrual bleeding. Symptoms of gonorrhoea in women may be masked by those of trichomoniasis, with which it is often associated. The most serious complication is salpingitis, which may lead to pelvic inflammatory disease and infertility. Other sites which may become infected in both sexes include the rectum and pharynx, and in females, the urethra.

Disseminated gonococcal infection is a serious complication affecting women more than men. Symptoms vary in severity from mild fever and arthralgia to destructive arthritis and prostration. Bacteraemia may lead to further complications (e.g. hepatitis, meningitis, endocarditis, myocarditis and pericarditis).

The eyes are most frequently affected in neonates (*see* Ophthalmia neonatorum, Section 5.2), although other sites may include the pharynx, larynx and rectum.

Treatment

The prognosis of gonorrhoea in the absence of serious complications is good. The infection may resolve spontaneously without treatment, although lasting immunity does not develop.

Treatment comprises the administration of appropriate antibacterial drugs (BNF 5.1, table 1 and BNF 5.1.1.1) or, if the microorganism has developed a resistance to penicillin, the administration of spectinomycin (BNF 5.1.7), ciprofloxacin or ofloxacin (BNF 5.1.12).

Complete control of gonorrhoea is difficult due to the large numbers of asymptomatic carriers. Diagnosis and treatment should be undertaken at specialist centres and sexual contacts traced and treated. Further spread may be prevented by abstaining from sexual intercourse until treatment is complete. Use of condoms during sexual intercourse may afford some protection against infection; counselling may also be of value.

Syphilis

Definition and aetiology

Syphilis is a chronic, contagious, bacterial infection caused by *Treponema pallidum*, a microaerophilic spirochaete. The disease occurs worldwide, although in western countries the number of cases in the late stages is declining. The number of patients presenting with early syphilis is, however, increasing.

The microorganism gains entry into a new host via mucous membranes and skin, and rapidly disseminates throughout the body. Transmission in blood transfusions is a possibility, although other mechanisms (e.g. fomites) are rare as the microorganism cannot survive for long outside the body. Congenital transmission across the placenta does occur, although the incidence is waning as a result of antenatal screening and treatment.

Symptoms

The incubation period is usually about three weeks, although it may be as long as three months depending on inoculum size.

The first stage of syphilis (primary syphilis) is characterised by a lesion (the chancre) appearing at the inoculation site. The site is usually the genitalia, although other areas (e.g. mouth, finger or anus) may be involved. Initially, it is a painless papule which becomes ulcerated with hardened edges, and heals spontaneously within two to six weeks. The chancre may be accompanied by enlarged lymph nodes.

The secondary stage follows several weeks later, or in some cases, after several months. Conversely, some individuals may show an overlap between these first two stages. There is a macular or papular, non-pruritic, symmetrical rash characteristically covering the palms and soles; it is also evident on the trunk and limbs. Accompanying symptoms include enlarged lymph nodes, malaise, nausea, fatigue, mild fever, headache, anorexia, arthralgia and myalgia. Condylomata lata are highly infectious, papular, pinkish-grey, discoid lesions arising in areas where two skin surfaces are in contact (e.g. axillae, perineum and under the breasts). Greyish-white infectious mucous patches, surrounded by a red margin, develop in the oropharynx and on the genitalia. Other organs which may also be affected during secondary syphilis are the eyes, liver, spleen, kidneys and meninges. The secondary stage resolves after a few months, although recurrences may occur in 20% of patients. Most patients enter a latent period after one year and are generally not infectious, although women who become pregnant may transmit the infection to the fetus.

After several years, some patients progress to a late non-infectious tertiary stage, whose manifestations are currently changing and becoming atypical. The classical benign lesion, which is now less commonly seen, is the gumma. This is a granulomatous lesion appearing on the face, legs, buttocks and upper trunk as single or multiple punched-out ulcers. Mucosal gummas in the oropharynx may destroy the hard palate and nasal septum. Periostitis may affect bones and cause pain, particularly at night.

Cardiovascular syphilis may arise 20–30 years after infection. The most common manifestations are aortic aneurysm and insufficiency of the aortic valve, resulting in congestive heart failure and death.

The earliest manifestation of neurosyphilis, appearing five years after infection, is meningovascular syphilis. Characteristic symptoms include headache, dizziness, neck stiffness, blurred vision, papilloedema, insomnia, poor concentration and confusion. Thrombosis and infarction may occur.

General paresis, occurring after 10–20 years, is now very rare. It is the result of meningoencephalitis and has an insidious onset. It starts with fatigue, headache, irritability, personality changes, confusion, delusions and convulsions. Patients gradually deteriorate physically and mentally until they are completely unable to look after themselves.

Tabes dorsalis is a degenerative condition commencing 20–30 years after infection. It is gradually progressive with an insidious onset. The first symptom is often severe repetitive lightning pains in the legs and feet, which cease as abruptly as they start. There may also be severe abdominal pain, loss of sensation in the feet, ataxia, optic atrophy, destruction of the large joints, faecal or urinary incontinence, and impotence.

The symptoms of congenital syphilis increase in severity the more recent the mother's infection. Symptoms appearing within 2–10 weeks of birth represent early congenital syphilis; after two years of age, the condition is referred to as late congenital syphilis. Symptoms at birth are rare, but if present, offer a poor prognosis. Early symptoms resemble the secondary stage of acquired syphilis in adults, although the lesions (which are infectious) are often bullous. In addition, there may be lymphadenopathy, hepatosplenomegaly, rhinitis, failure to thrive and osteochondritis causing immobility in the limbs.

Many children do not develop late symptoms but remain in the latent period for the rest of their lives. In late congenital syphilis, cardiovascular symptoms do not occur, but neurological symptoms are more common than in adults. These may include interstitial keratitis, deafness and optic atrophy. General paresis can occur between 8 and 15 years of age, although tabes dorsalis rarely occurs. Periostitis may cause misshaping of bone, resulting in bowed tibia, bossed frontal and parietal skull bones, and a saddle nose. The maxillae remain underdeveloped, and mucocutaneous gummas may cause destruction of the palate and nasal septum. Permanent teeth show a characteristic central notch and are widely spaced (Hutchinson's teeth).

Treatment

All stages of syphilis and congenital syphilis may be treated by the administration of penicillin (BNF 5.1, table 1). In late cases, treatment may prevent further damage but cannot reverse that already done. Follow-up examinations are required for up to a year in primary and secondary stages of syphilis, into adult life for congenital cases, and possibly for life in late cases.

Diagnosis and treatment should be undertaken at specialist centres and sexual contacts traced and treated. Further spread may be prevented by abstaining from sexual intercourse until treatment is complete. Use of condoms during sexual intercourse may afford some protection against infection; counselling may also be of value. Individuals at greatest risk (e.g. prostitutes and homosexuals) should be encouraged to attend for regular check-ups.

All pregnant women should be routinely screened and treated if necessary to minimise the effects on the fetus. Treatment before 16 weeks of pregnancy may totally prevent any damage.

6

Endocrine disorders

6.1 Pituitary and hypothalamic disorders

Acromegaly

Definition and aetiology

Acromegaly is a rare disorder in which there is hypersecretion of growth hormone, usually caused by a pituitary adenoma.

Symptoms

It is characterised by enlargement of the hands and feet, and coarsening of the facial features (e.g. large nose, full lips, large tongue, prominent brow and protrusion of the jaw). The onset is usually insidious and the presenting symptoms may be arthralgia, sweating, paraesthesia or pain and stiffness in the hands and feet. Headache and visual disturbances may be caused by the pituitary tumour. Other symptoms may include deepening of the voice, diabetes insipidus, hirsutism, hypertension, impaired glucose tolerance or occasionally diabetes mellitus, kyphosis, muscle weakness, progressive heart failure, skin thickening and seborrhoea, and thyroid disorders.

Treatment

Treatment consists of surgery (hypophysectomy), external irradiation, implantation of radioactive materials, or the administration of bromocriptine (BNF 6.7.1).

Diabetes insipidus

Definition and aetiology

Diabetes insipidus results from impaired water reabsorption by the kidney. This is caused by a deficiency of vasopressin (cranial diabetes insipidus) or, occasionally, by insensitivity of the renal tubules to vasopressin (nephrogenic diabetes insipidus).

Cranial diabetes insipidus may be idiopathic or caused by trauma, pituitary surgery, or cranial tumours or metastases. Rarely it may be caused by granulomas, infections (e.g. meningitis and encephalitis) or vascular lesions. Nephrogenic diabetes insipidus may be caused by hypercalcaemia, hypokalaemia, hydronephrosis, pyelonephritis, or may be drug-induced (e.g. by lithium or demeclocycline). Diabetes insipidus may be chronic or temporary.

Symptoms

It is characterised by polyuria with the loss of fluid ranging from 3 to 20 litres daily. This results in excessive thirst, and nocturia is also common. Dehydration occurs if patients are deprived of water.

Treatment

Treatment is directed towards removing the underlying cause. Cranial diabetes insipidus may be treated by replacement therapy with vasopressin and its analogues (BNF 6.5.2). Thiazide and related diuretics may be used in the treatment of cranial and nephrogenic diabetes insipidus (BNF 6.5.2). Chlorpropamide and carbamazepine have also been used for partial cranial diabetes insipidus.

Growth hormone deficiency

Definition and aetiology

A lack of growth hormone secreted by the anterior pituitary in childhood results in dwarfism. It is commonly caused by pituitary tumours, but is not often recognised until the child starts school and comparisons with other similarly aged children are made.

Symptoms

Size at birth is usually normal, but growth rate is slower during childhood. Hypoglycaemic episodes may accompany the short stature, and other outward signs include plump and immature features, and small hands, feet and genitalia. Normal muscular development is often retarded, with 'baby fat' being more persistent. If the condition remains untreated, puberty may be delayed. However, unlike other causes of dwarfism, intelligence is not impaired.

Treatment

Treatment comprises the administration of somatropin (synthetic human growth hormone) (BNF 6.5.1). Therapy must continue until an acceptable adult height is reached.

Hyperprolactinaemia

Definition and aetiology

Hyperprolactinaemia is excessive secretion of prolactin and increased plasma prolactin concentrations. It may be of non-pathological origin (e.g. pregnancy, breast feeding, sleep or emotional disturbances) or may be due to hypothalamic or pituitary tumours (e.g. prolactinomas) or granulomatous disease (e.g. sarcoidosis). It may also be iatrogenic (e.g. caused by phenothiazines, haloperidol, methyldopa, cimetidine, metoclopramide or oestrogens) or idiopathic (functional hyperprolactinaemia). Other causes include hyperthyroidism and chronic renal failure.

Symptoms

Hyperprolactinaemia is more common in women, and is characterised by amenorrhoea or oligomenorrhoea, galactorrhoea, infertility and hirsutism. In men, symptoms include impotence, galactorrhoea, oligospermia, infertility and feminine-type distribution of body fat.

Treatment

Treatment consists of surgery (hypophysectomy) to remove any underlying prolactinoma, and radiotherapy or medical treatment with bromocriptine (BNF 6.7.1) and other dopamine-receptor stimulants, or both.

Hypopituitarism

Definition and aetiology

Hypopituitarism is reduced or absent function of the pituitary gland. There may be a deficiency of only one or of all pituitary hormones (panhypopituitarism). Hypopituitarism in the adult usually occurs as a result of destruction of the pituitary gland by a pituitary or local tumour, or metastases. Associated pressure on the optic chiasma may result in visual impairment. Pituitary damage may also be caused by infections (e.g. tuberculosis and syphilis), granulomatous disease (e.g. sarcoidosis) or trauma. It may also follow pituitary surgery, radiotherapy or prolonged treatment with target-organ hormones (e.g. steroids and thyroxine), or occur secondary to hypothalamic disease. In women, pituitary infarction and necrosis may occur in association with postpartum haemorrhage, and results in lack of prolactin. When hypopituitarism occurs before puberty, it is usually partial rather than complete, and is dominated by growth hormone deficiency, which causes short stature. Additionally the onset of puberty is delayed or may not occur; the cause may be congenital.

Symptoms

Deficiency of a single pituitary hormone results in the deficient function of the target organ of that hormone. Panhypopituitarism results in a syndrome characterised by the total lack of pituitary hormones and of the hormones from the target glands. Lack of thyrotrophin results in fatigue and cold intolerance (*see* Hypothyroidism, Section 6.2). Lack of adrenocorticotrophin (ACTH) results in secondary adrenocortical insufficiency, hypotension, fluid retention, pallor and a tendency to develop coma through hypoglycaemia. Lack of gonadotrophins (i.e. follicle-stimulating hormone and luteinising hormone) results in loss of libido, impotence, infertility, atrophy of the genitalia and loss of body hair (*see* Hypogonadism, Section 6.5). Lack of vasopressin results in the passage of large volumes of dilute urine (*see* Diabetes insipidus). Lack of prolactin results in failure of lactation. Patients become weak and easily fatigued, and personality changes may occur.

Treatment

Hypopituitarism is treated by replacement therapy (BNF 6.3.1, 6.4.2, 6.5.1) of the missing hormone(s), allied to surgical removal of any underlying tumour or treatment of any causal infection.

6.2 Thyroid and parathyroid disorders

Hyperparathyroidism

Definition and aetiology

Hyperparathyroidism is the excessive secretion of parathyroid hormone by one or more parathyroid glands. Primary hyperparathryoidism is usually caused by an adenoma of a parathyroid gland, but may also be due to hyperplasia and rarely carcinoma of the glands. It usually occurs in patients over 50 years of age and is more common in women.

Secondary hyperparathyroidism arises as a result of an abnormal physiological state (e.g. deficiency of vitamin D, vitamin D-resistant osteomalacia or rickets, malabsorption of calcium, chronic renal disease or renal tubular acidosis) which leads to hypocalcaemia. The hypocalcaemia results in hyperplasia of the parathyroid glands. Occasionally (e.g. in renal transplant patients, or patients with chronic malabsorption or chronic renal failure), long-standing hypocalcaemia may give rise to autonomous parathyroid secretion and hypercalcaemia (tertiary hyperparathyroidism).

Symptoms

Primary hyperparathyroidism is characterised by hypercalcaemia and hypophosphataemia, although some patients may be normocalcaemic. A large proportion of patients are asymptomatic. General symptoms include depressive disorders, malaise and hypertension. Reabsorption of calcium from bones is increased and results in skeletal rarefaction, the formation of cysts, and weakness of the bones; bone pain and tenderness may occur but are more common in secondary hyperparathyroidism. Kidney involvement may be marked by renal calculi and polyuria.

Treatment

Hyperparathyroidism is treated by surgical removal of parathyroid tissue (parathyroidectomy) or treatment of any underlying condition.

Hyperthyroidism

Definition and aetiology

Hyperthyroidism (thyrotoxicosis) results from an excess of circulating thyroxine or liothyronine, or both. It is usually due to diffuse hyperplasia and hypertrophy of the thyroid gland (Graves' disease), which is associated with circulating thyroid-stimulating immunoglobulins. Less commonly, it is caused by a single toxic adenoma or by multiple toxic nodular goitres (Plummer's disease). Rarely, hyperthyroidism may be caused by a well-differentiated thyroid cancer, Hashimoto's thyroiditis, or subacute thyroiditis.

Symptoms

Hyperthyroidism is characterised by an increased metabolic rate, which causes weight loss, increased appetite, fatigue, emotional disturbances, heat intolerance and sweating, diarrhoea or increased frequency of defecation, muscle weakness, and tachycardia or atrial fibrillation. Ocular symptoms (e.g. retraction of the upper eyelid, exophthalmos and eyelid lag) are common, especially in Graves' disease. Hyperthyroidism is associated with a goitre (Figure 6.1) in most patients. Other symptoms include alopecia, angina pectoris, heart failure, nausea and vomiting, and tremor. Menstrual disorders

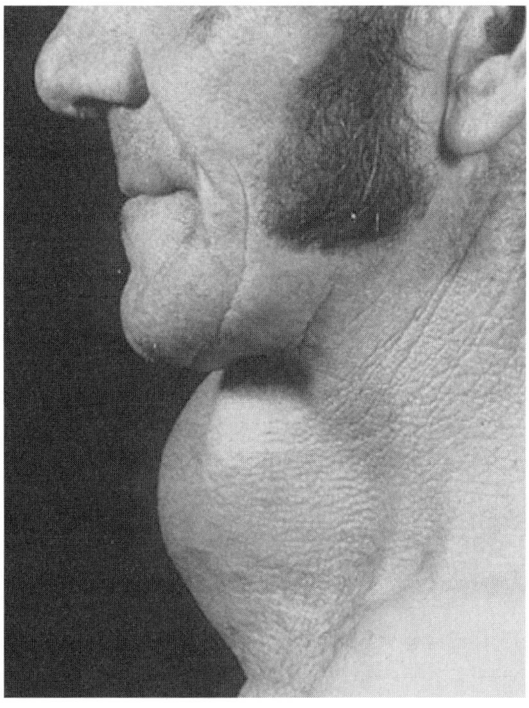

Figure 6.1 Goitre. (Reproduced with permission of Biophoto Associates/Science Photo Library.)

(e.g. oligomenorrhoea) or gynaecomastia may also occur. A 'thyroid storm' is an abrupt onset of highly visible symptoms of hyperthyroidism, and can be a clinical emergency.

Treatment

Hyperthyroidism is treated by the administration of antithyroid drugs (BNF 6.2.2), radioactive sodium iodide, or by surgery (thryoidectomy). Certain beta-adrenoceptor blocking drugs (BNF 2.4) are used pre-operatively and in the treatment of 'thyroid storm'.

Hypoparathyroidism

Definition and aetiology

Hypoparathyroidism is a reduced secretion of parathyroid hormone and is characterised by hypocalcaemia and hyperphosphataemia. It is usually the result of removal of parathyroid tissue during thyroidectomy, parathyroidectomy or laryngeal surgery, but may also be idiopathic (e.g. due to autoimmune disease of the parathyroid glands, congenital absence of parathyroid tissue, or may be familial). It may also be a consequence of severe and prolonged magnesium depletion. Neonatal hypoparathyroidism occurs as a result of maternal hypercalcaemia. Idiopathic hypoparathyroidism may also be associated with Addison's disease, candidiasis, malabsorption syndromes, osteomalacia and megaloblastic anaemia.

Symptoms

Hypoparathyroidism results in a decreased reabsorption of skeletal calcium and a reduced absorption of calcium from the intestine. The immediate effect of hypoparathyroidism is hypocalcaemia. Longer term consequences include mental disorders, epilepsy, cataracts, alopecia, brittle deformed nails and dry skin. Papilloedema and other signs of raised intracranial pressure indicate calcification of the basal ganglia. Mental retardation and dental abnormalities may occur in children.

Treatment

Severe hypocalcaemia due to hypoparathyroidism is treated initially by intravenous injection of calcium gluconate (BNF 9.5.1.1). Plasma calcium is maintained in the long term by the administration of vitamin D preparations (BNF 9.6.4).

Hypothyroidism

Definition and aetiology

Hypothyroidism is a deficiency of circulating thyroid hormones. It may occur congenitally (cretinism), occurring in about 1 in 4000 births, or may arise later in life. Adult hypothyroidism is often termed myxoedema. Cretinism may be caused by iodine deficiency, absence of the thyroid gland, a defect in hormone synthesis, or maternal ingestion of antithyroid drugs. Hypothyroidism in later life may be primary, due to disease of the thyroid gland (e.g. Hashimoto's thyroiditis or idiopathic atrophy), or to prolonged treatment with antithyroid drugs, sodium aminosalicylate, or lithium salts. It may also arise secondary to pituitary and hypothalamic disorders.

Hypothyroidism may also be caused by excessive thyroidectomy or irradiation of the thyroid. Myxoedemic coma may be precipitated by exposure to cold, infections and drugs (e.g. phenothiazines, opioid analgesics or anaesthetics).

Symptoms

Early symptoms of hypothyroidism in neonates are non-specific and vague, but include constipation, lethargy, feeding difficulties, jaundice and respiratory distress. Later symptoms include a bloated face, large tongue, umbilical hernia, and dry skin and hair. If untreated, cretinism leads to physical and mental retardation.

The onset of hypothyroidism in later life (usually between 35 and 50 years of age) is insidious and is characterised by a gradual increase in fatigue and cold intolerance, weight gain and constipation. There may also be swelling of the skin with mucinous infiltration (myxoedema), characterised by coarsening of the features and puffy eyes. Other symptoms may include alopecia, angina pectoris, anaemia, arthralgia, bradycardia, depressive disorders, coarsening of the voice, dry skin and hair, goitre, heart failure, menorrhagia and myalgia.

Treatment
Hypothyroidism is treated by replacement therapy with thyroid hormones (BNF 6.2.1). Myxoedemic coma is treated by intravenous injection of liothyronine (BNF 6.2.1), and appropriate adjunctive therapy.

Cretinism is prevented by routine screening of neonates for thyroid function.

Thyroiditis

Definition and aetiology
Thyroiditis is inflammation of the thyroid gland which may be acute (rare), subacute or chronic (e.g. Hashimoto's thyroiditis).

Subacute thyroiditis (de Quervain's thyroiditis) is a disease of unknown aetiology, although a viral origin has been proposed. Hashimoto's thyroiditis (lymphocytic thyroiditis) is a very common chronic autoimmune disease. It is often familial and women are affected more frequently than men.

Symptoms
Subacute thyroiditis is characterised by an acutely tender goitre, fever and sweating. It most commonly affects young women and may start insidiously with features of an upper respiratory-tract infection, occasionally with dysphagia. Hyperthyroidism may develop, and very rarely the disease may progress to permanent hypothyroidism as a result of destruction of the gland.

Hashimoto's thyroiditis is characterised by a firm, well-defined goitre or hypothyroidism, or both. Very rarely, Hashimoto's thyroiditis may be associated with clinical hyperthyroidism. Other autoimmune diseases may occur concurrently.

Treatment
Subacute thyroiditis is usually self-limiting and may be treated symptomatically with non-opioid analgesics (BNF 4.7.1). More severe disease may require treatment with corticosteroids. Treatment of Hashimoto's thyroiditis consists of replacement therapy with thyroid hormones (BNF 6.2.1).

6.3 Adrenal disorders

Addison's disease

Definition and aetiology
Addison's disease (primary adrenocortical insufficiency) is a rare chronic insufficiency of the adrenal cortex, with less than one case per 100 000 population. It results in the reduced secretion of glucocorticoids, mineralocorticoids and sex hormones. Adrenocortical insufficiency is usually caused by idiopathic atrophy often attributable to autoimmune processes, or to destruction of adrenal glands (e.g. by tuberculosis or metastases). Total adrenalectomy for the treatment of Cushing's syndrome may also result in Addison's disease. Secondary adrenocortical insufficiency is usually caused by corticosteroid therapy or hypopituitarism. It results in a deficiency of glucocorticoids and androgenic secretions, but not of aldosterone.

Symptoms
Addison's disease is characterised by progressive fatigue and weakness, weight loss, hypotension and gastrointestinal disturbances (e.g. abdominal pain, anorexia, nausea and vomiting, and diarrhoea). Skin pigmentation or vitiligo are classical symptoms, but are not always present. The symptoms of secondary adrenocortical insufficiency are similar to, though milder than, those of Addison's disease, and pigmentation of the skin does not occur.

Treatment
Addison's disease is treated by replacement therapy with hydrocortisone (BNF 6.3.2) and a mineralocorticoid (e.g. fludrocortisone, BNF 6.3.1). Mineralocorticoids are not required in secondary adrenocortical insufficiency.

Adrenal virilisation

Definition and aetiology
Adrenal virilisation is virilisation produced by an excess of adrenal androgens. It may be caused by adrenal hyperplasia (either congenital or

acquired, as in Cushing's syndrome) or by virilising adrenal adenomas or adenocarcinomas. Mild hirsutism and virilisation may also be produced by the polycystic ovary syndrome.

Symptoms

Symptoms depend on the sex and age of the patient at the onset of the disease. Virilisation is not usually noticeable in male adults. In adult females, symptoms include hirsutism, alopecia, acne, amenorrhoea, deepening of the voice, atrophy of the uterus, clitoral hypertrophy, decreased breast size and increased muscularity. In mild cases, hirsutism may be the only feature. Congenital adrenal hyperplasia may cause masculinisation of the female external genitalia or enlargement of the penis in boys. Affected children grow at an accelerated rate, and show advanced skeletal maturation and precocious puberty in boys. Females undergo slow and progressive virilisation.

Treatment

Treatment depends on the underlying cause. Surgery may be required for adrenal adenomas. Dexamethasone and betamethasone (BNF 6.3.2) are used in the treatment of congenital adrenal hyperplasia.

Adrenocortical insufficiency, acute

Definition and aetiology

Acute adrenocortical insufficiency is an acute deficiency of corticosteroid hormones caused by an exacerbation of Addison's disease by stress or infections, abrupt withdrawal of maintenance corticosteroid therapy, or attributed to adrenal haemorrhagic necrosis caused by an overwhelming infection (e.g. meningococcal septicaemia). It may also occur as a complication of anticoagulant therapy, or be precipitated by abrupt or too fast withdrawal of corticosteroids used in the treatment of other conditions.

Symptoms

The condition is rapid in onset and is characterised by extreme weakness, apathy, abdominal pain, hypotension, myalgia, nausea and vomiting, diarrhoea, and shock followed by oliguria. In the absence of treatment, death will follow.

Treatment

Immediate intravenous administration of corticosteroids (BNF 6.3.2) and intravenous fluid replacement (BNF 9.2.2) are required. Replacement therapy with corticosteroids (BNF 6.3.1) may subsequently be required. During surgery or infection and in times of stress, the physiological requirements for corticosteroids are increased, and maintenance dosage should therefore be raised accordingly.

Cushing's syndrome

Definition and aetiology

Cushing's syndrome is a chronic overproduction of hydrocortisone by the adrenal gland that occurs most commonly in women. Most cases are caused by bilateral adrenal hyperplasia, which arises through excessive secretion of adrenocorticotrophin by a pituitary tumour (Cushing's disease). Cushing's syndrome may also be caused by benign or malignant adrenocortical tumours or the production of adrenocorticotrophin by carcinomas. However, it most commonly arises through the administration of high doses of corticosteroids.

Symptoms

Cushing's syndrome is characterised by obesity of the trunk and neck, facial rounding (mooning) and reddening, muscle weakness and atrophy, skin atrophy, livid striae, spontaneous bruising and osteoporosis. Growth arrest and obesity are characteristic in children. Other common symptoms include acne, hypertension, impaired glucose tolerance or diabetes mellitus, hirsutism, oedema, oligomenorrhoea and psychiatric disturbances.

Treatment

Adrenal hyperplasia may be treated by irradiation of the pituitary by X-rays or heavy particles, by implantation of radioactive materials, by pituitary surgery, or by total adrenalectomy. Tumours of the adrenals may be removed, and iatrogenic Cushing's syndrome may be treated by reducing the dose of corticosteroid. Drugs that have been used in the treatment of Cushing's syndrome are metyrapone (BNF 6.7.3), aminoglutethimide (BNF 8.3.4.1), trilostane (BNF 6.7.3) and ketoconazole (BNF 5.2).

Primary aldosteronism

Definition and aetiology
Primary aldosteronism (Conn's syndrome) is characterised by excessive production of the adrenocortical hormone aldosterone. The condition may be classified as aldosterone-producing adenoma, idiopathic hyperaldosteronism (commonly due to adrenal hyperplasia) and glucocorticoid-remediable hyperaldosteronism. All three classifications produce a similar spectrum of symptoms, although their treatment is varied.

Symptoms
Primary aldosteronism may initially present with hypertension which may be severe and associated with renal damage, retinal damage and hypokalaemia. Normally, aldosterone causes the retention of sodium and the loss of potassium in the distal kidney tubules. Excess retention of sodium causes an expansion of the plasma volume which results in hypertension. Depletion of body potassium levels produces muscular weakness, which may manifest as tetany, cramp, paraesthesia and paralysis. An inability to concentrate urine results in polyuria and polydipsia. Personality disturbances, hyperglycaemia and glycosuria may also occur.

Treatment
Removal of the adenoma by surgery will reverse hypertension and hypokalaemia in 50–60% of cases. In idiopathic hyperaldosteronism, potassium-sparing diuretics (BNF 2.2.3) will correct electrolyte abnormalities and improve hypertension. Glucocorticoid-remediable hyperaldosteronism may be treated with dexamethasone (BNF 6.3.2), possibly in conjunction with potassium-sparing diuretics (BNF 2.2.3). Trilostane (BNF 6.7.3) may be of value.

6.4 Pancreatic disorders

Diabetes mellitus

Definition and aetiology
Diabetes mellitus is characterised by persistent hyperglycaemia, usually with glycosuria, caused by a deficiency, or diminished effectiveness, of insulin. The condition may be of multifactorial origin in which hereditary factors, age, sex, pregnancy, obesity, autoimmune factors, infections and emotional disturbances may be important. It may be precipitated by pancreatic disorders, hormonal disorders (e.g. acromegaly and Cushing's syndrome), or by administration of drugs (e.g. corticosteroids or diuretics, especially thiazides). Diabetes mellitus is classified as type I and type II, although the clinical distinction may be blurred.

Type I diabetes

Definition
Type I diabetes (insulin-dependent diabetes mellitus, IDDM) usually develops during the first 30 years of life, but can occur at any age. It is usually caused by the autoimmune destruction of the islets of Langerhans. There are about 30 cases per 100 000 population in the UK, and the disease affects predominantly the white Caucasian population.

Symptoms
The onset of symptoms is frequently abrupt, but may be insidious. Classical symptoms include polydipsia, polyuria and nocturia, dehydration, fatigue and weight loss. Blurred vision, paraesthesia in the hands and feet, nocturnal leg cramps and constipation may occur. Some patients develop a craving for sweet foods. Pruritus vulvae is common. The presence of ketonuria is an early indication of progression towards diabetic ketoacidosis and hyperglycaemic coma. Ketones, which arise as a result of abnormal breakdown of fats by the liver, accumulate in the blood. They are excreted in the urine and on the breath, which develops a sweet, sickly smell. Ketonuria may be associated with a dry furred tongue, cracked lips, rapid pulse and hypotension. Mental confusion and apathy may also be present.

Treatment
Type I diabetes is treated by long-term replacement therapy with insulin (BNF 6.1.1) and a controlled diet. Diabetic ketoacidosis and hyperglycaemic coma are treated by intravenous or intramuscular administration of insulin (BNF 6.1.3) and intravenous fluid replacement (BNF

9.2.2). Hypoglycaemia is treated by administration of glucose or glucagon (BNF 6.1.4). Diabetics should be counselled about diet control, insulin administration, urine testing and the symptoms of hypoglycaemia.

Type II diabetes

Definition and aetiology
Type II diabetes (non-insulin-dependent diabetes mellitus, NIDDM) develops most commonly in middle-aged or elderly patients, who are often obese. There is a marked familial tendency. The condition is much more common than type I diabetes mellitus, with between 8% and 12% of the UK population affected.

Symptoms
The onset is insidious and the disease is usually mild. Ketoacidosis and other classical symptoms are often absent, but there may be pruritus vulvae. The presence of chronic recurrent infections, neuropathy and retinopathy may be indicative of long-standing diabetes.

Treatment
Type II diabetes may be controlled by diet alone, but if this is unsuccessful it may be possible to obtain control by diet together with the administration of oral antidiabetic drugs (BNF 6.1.2) or insulin (BNF 6.1.1).

Self-help organisations
Diabetes Foundation
Diabetes UK
Medic-Alert Foundation

Hypoglycaemia

Definition and aetiology
Hypoglycaemia is an abnormally low plasma glucose concentration. It occurs commonly in diabetes mellitus as a complication of insulin therapy and occasionally of therapy with oral antidiabetic drugs, but is otherwise uncommon in adults. Spontaneous hypoglycaemia may be precipitated by fasting for several hours, following which symptoms commonly occur during the night or on waking. It may also occur in severe hepatic disease or as a consequence of insulinoma. Alcohol can induce hypoglycaemia in fasting alcoholics. Rarely, spontaneous hypoglycaemia can arise in patients with Addison's disease or hypopituitarism, or as a result of large extra-pancreatic sarcomas.

Reactive (postprandial) hypoglycaemia occurs 2–5 hours after eating. It may be idiopathic or occurs as an early symptom in patients with mild type II diabetes.

Symptoms
Hypoglycaemia produces adrenergic symptoms (e.g. pallor, sweating, tachycardia, tremor, weakness, hunger and nervousness) and neurological symptoms (e.g. confusion, lack of coordination, mental and visual disturbances, and transient stroke). The neurological symptoms may progress to loss of consciousness, convulsions, coma and, if untreated, death.

Treatment
Treatment of acute hypoglycaemia consists of oral or intravenous admininistration of glucose or glucagon injected by any route (BNF 6.1.4). Any underlying cause should also be treated. Diazoxide (BNF 6.1.4) may be useful in the management of chronic intractable hypoglycaemia (e.g. due to a non-operable insulinoma). All type I diabetics should carry a readily absorbed form of glucose.

6.5 Gonadal disorders

Hypogonadism

Definition and aetiology
Hypogonadism is the deficiency or absence of testicular function in men, or of ovarian function in women. It may be hereditary (e.g. caused by Turner's or Klinefelter's syndromes), caused by the destruction of the gonads by irradiation, caused by infections (e.g. tuberculosis, syphilis or mumps), or by surgical removal of the gonads. It may also be secondary to a hypothalamic disease or hypopituitarism, in which lack of gonadotrophins results in gonadal atrophy. A

reversible state of hypogonadism also occurs in patients with anorexia nervosa.

Symptoms
If hypogonadism occurs before puberty, the expected pubertal changes do not take place during adolescence. If it occurs in the adult, there is regression of some secondary sexual characteristics.

In the prepubertal female, hypogonadism results in primary amenorrhoea, the absence of mammary development or growth of body hair, and failure of the bony epiphyses to close resulting in excessive growth of the long bones. In the adult female, there is atrophy of the breasts and external genitalia, loss of libido, amenorrhoea, and infertility.

In the prepubertal male, hypogonadism results in non-development of the genitalia or muscles, the absence of erection or ejaculation, failure of the voice to break, absence of facial and body hair, and failure of the bony epiphyses to close. In the adult male, there is regression of muscle development, smoothing of the skin, loss of beard and body hair, atrophy of the external genitalia, loss of libido, infertility and the development of obesity and mental lethargy.

Treatment
Hypogonadism is treated by replacement therapy with androgens (BNF 6.4.2) or oestrogens (BNF 6.4.1) as appropriate. This will promote pubertal changes or the return of secondary sexual characteristics, but will not confer fertility. If hypogonadism is due to hypothalamic or pituitary disorders, fertility may be restored by treatment with gonadotrophins.

Precocious puberty

Definition and aetiology
Precocious puberty is the premature occurrence of puberty, which occurs much more frequently in girls than boys. It may be complete (true precocious puberty) or incomplete (e.g. pseudoprecocious puberty, in which testicular enlargement or ovulation does not occur). The onset of menstruation (menarche) in girls before eight years of age, or the development of secondary sexual characteristics in boys before nine years of age, is considered abnormal. Precocious puberty is commonly idiopathic (especially in girls), but may also be caused by lesions affecting the hypothalamus, intracranial tumours, hypothyroidism, adrenal virilisation, ovarian tumours or testicular cancer, or ingestion of oestrogens, androgens or anabolic steroids. Iatrogenic precocious puberty may also be precipitated in boys treated with large doses of chorionic gonadotrophin for cryptorchidism.

Symptoms
In boys, precocious puberty is characterised by the development of facial, axillary, pubic and body hair, penile growth, and deepening of the voice. In girls, it is characterised by growth of pubic and axillary hair, development of the breasts and external genitalia, and menarche. Initially, rapid linear growth may occur in both sexes, but premature closure of the bony epiphyses results in short adult stature.

Treatment
Treatment is dependent on the underlying cause. Idiopathic precocious puberty may be treated with gonadorelin (gonadotrophin-releasing hormone, BNF 6.5.1) analogues by depot injection. Cyproterone acetate (BNF 6.4.2) is the drug of choice for pseudoprecocious puberty.

6.6 Anatomy and physiology of the endocrine system

The endocrine system consists of a group of diverse tissues located throughout the body that exert their effects on metabolism through the secretion of hormones. The hormones interact with specific target structures, triggering reactions within that structure.

The integration of the activity of the endocrine glands is carried out by the hypothalamus, which forms part of the floor of the third ventricle. The hypothalamus secretes 'releasing factors', which are secreted into the hypophyseal portal veins and carried to the anterior pituitary (adenohypophysis). The output of the anterior pituitary gland is regulated by the action of hypothalamic releasing factors. The secretion of releasing factors from the hypothalamus is modulated by a negative feedback mechanism. When the levels of circulating hormone released from the target gland reach a certain concentration in the plasma, the hypothalamus responds by decreasing its output of the corresponding releasing factor.

The pituitary gland

The pituitary gland (hypophysis) is located on the underside of the brain immediately above the sphenoidal sinus (*see* Figure 12.3), and in close anatomical relationship with the hypothalamus. The posterior portion of the gland (neurohypophysis) secretes hormones produced by the hypothalamus (vasopressin and oxytocin). However, the posterior pituitary is normally considered part of the nervous system rather than of the endocrine system.

The anterior pituitary consists of three types of cells. The chromophobes are resting cells. The trophic hormones, which act on the target endocrine glands, are secreted by the basophils, while the acidophils produce prolactin and growth hormone. The trophic hormones released by the anterior pituitary are:

- Thyrotrophin (thyroid-stimulating hormone), which acts on the thyroid gland to increase the rate of secretion of thyroid hormones.
- Adrenocorticotrophin (ACTH), which stimulates the release of cortisol from the adrenal cortex.
- The gonadotrophins, luteinising hormone (LH) and follicle-stimulating hormone (FSH), which act on the ovaries and testes to stimulate the release of oestrogens, progesterone and testosterone. FSH also assists in the development of the ova and initiates spermatogenesis. In the female, LH induces the release of an ovum from the ovary and prepares the uterine structure to receive the fertilised ovum.

Two other hormones are secreted by the anterior pituitary, but are not classed as trophic hormones as they exert their effects directly on the target sites and not through intermediate glands. Prolactin acts on the mammary glands to produce enlargement and induce milk production during pregnancy and lactation. Growth hormone stimulates the growth activity of cells, particularly skeletal and soft tissues. This is achieved through influencing the rate of protein synthesis, the breakdown of fat, and the conversion of glycogen into glucose.

The thyroid gland

The two lobes of the thyroid gland are situated on both sides of the upper trachea (Figure 6.2). The lobes are joined by a central isthmus, which lies in front of the trachea, and they receive an abundant blood supply from the superior and inferior thyroid arteries. The gland is made up of follicles whose interior is lined by a unicellular wall which extracts iodine from the blood. The central cavity of each follicle is filled with thyroglobulin, which stores the thyroid hormones. The combination of iodine and the amino acid tyrosine within thyroglobulin produces liothyronine (tri-iodothyronine or T_3) and thyroxine (T_4). The complex of thyroglobulin and thyroid hormones are stored as the thyroid colloid. The release of liothyronine and thyroxine into the bloodstream is under the control of thyrotrophin secreted from the anterior pituitary. Excessive concentrations of circulating thyroid hormones decrease the amount of thyrotrophin produced by the pituitary.

Thyroxine is widely distributed within the body and acts to increase the rate of metabolism of all tissues. In the young, its presence is essential for the development and maturation of the nervous system and for normal growth. In adults, it is required for continued normal mental and physical activity.

The cells which fill the spaces between the follicles have been shown to release the hormone calcitonin, which acts to increase the uptake of calcium into bone, and consequently decrease plasma calcium concentrations.

The parathyroid glands

The four approximately spherical parathyroid glands are symmetrically located on the posterior surface of the thyroid gland (Figure 6.3). The glands secrete parathyroid hormone which has the overall effect of increasing the plasma calcium

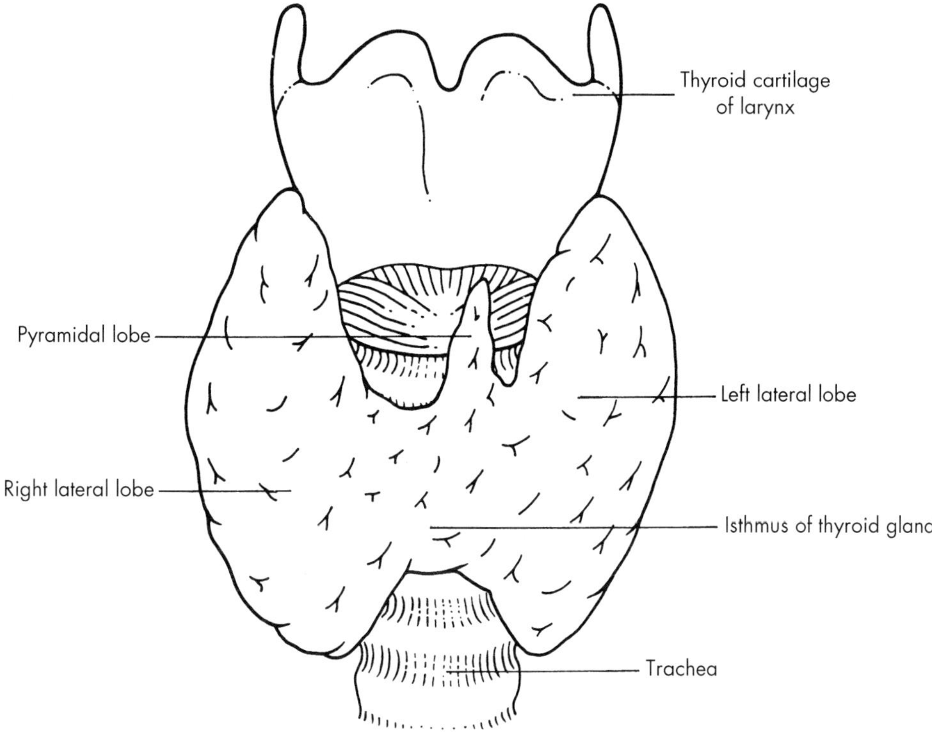

Figure 6.2 Anterior view of the thyroid gland.

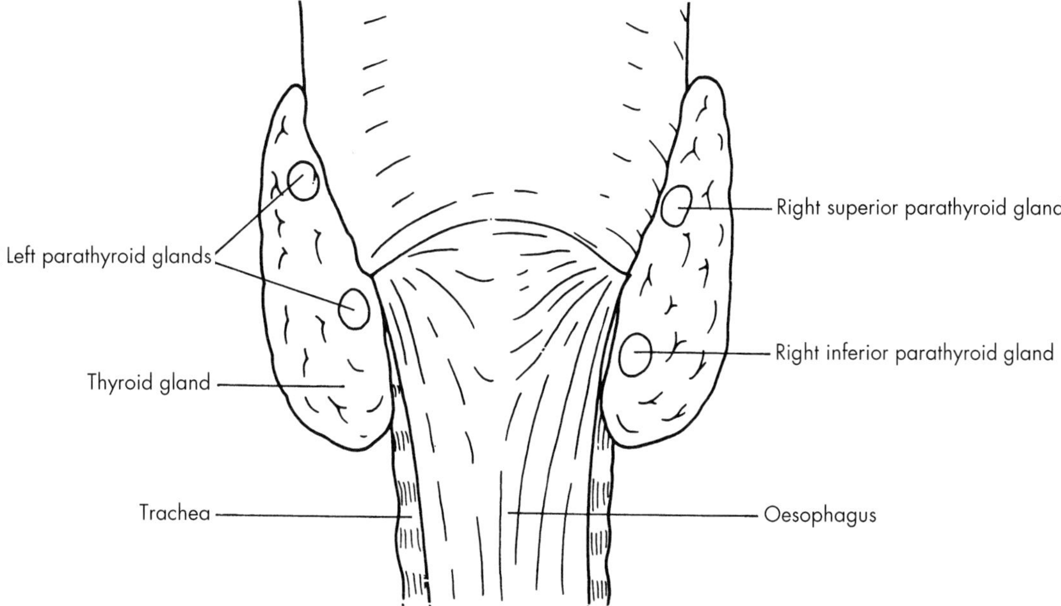

Figure 6.3 Posterior view of thyroid and parathyroid gland.

concentration. This is achieved by increasing the reabsorption of calcium from bone, decreasing the amount of calcium excreted by the kidneys, and stimulating an increased absorption of calcium from the gastrointestinal tract. The release of parathyroid hormone is regulated by the parathyroid glands themselves which monitor the concentrations of circulating calcium (there is no direct pituitary involvement in the maintenance of hormone secretion). Normal physiological plasma calcium concentrations are maintained by the balance between the secretion of parathyroid hormone and calcitonin.

The adrenal glands

The two adrenal (suprarenal) glands, which lie adjacent to the upper surface of the kidneys (Figure 6.4), are anatomically and functionally divided into two regions.

The outermost tissue, the adrenal cortex, is composed of three unequal layers. The external layer, the zona glomerulosa, consists of aggregates of small cells which secrete mineralocorticoids. The centrally sited zona fasciculata, which covers the largest area, is composed of columns of cells which produce glucocorticoids and small quantities of sex hormones. The internal layer, the zona reticularis, contains 'reserve' cells whose secretory activity may be called upon when the capacity of the other cells is overstretched.

The hormones secreted by the adrenal cortex are all derived from cholesterol. The mineralocorticoids, of which aldosterone is the most important, regulate the permeability of cell membranes to the passage of electrolytes, especially sodium and potassium ions. In the kidney, aldosterone increases the reabsorption of sodium ions and decreases the reabsorption of potassium ions into the bloodstream, and thereby regulates ionic and water homeostasis. This regulation is achieved by several mechanisms. Ionic exchange of plasma hydrogen ions for sodium ions maintains the electrostatic equilibrium, but decreases blood acidity. The movement of sodium ions generates a positively charged environment in the blood vessels in the kidney tubules. As a result, anions (e.g. chloride and bicarbonate ions) are drawn from the urine into the blood. The increase in plasma sodium concentration leads to the flow of water from urine into the blood by osmosis.

The control of the release of aldosterone is a complex process, involving the adrenal glands and the kidneys. When the blood pressure falls (e.g. as a result of haemorrhage, dehydration or hyponatraemia), the kidney secretes an enzyme, renin, into the bloodstream. Renin converts angiotensinogen, a plasma protein, into angiotensin I, which is further modified to angiotensin II by a pulmonary plasma enzyme. Circulating angiotensin II stimulates the release of aldosterone from the adrenal cortex, producing retention of sodium and water to restore blood volume. The complex control system is described as the renin–angiotensin system.

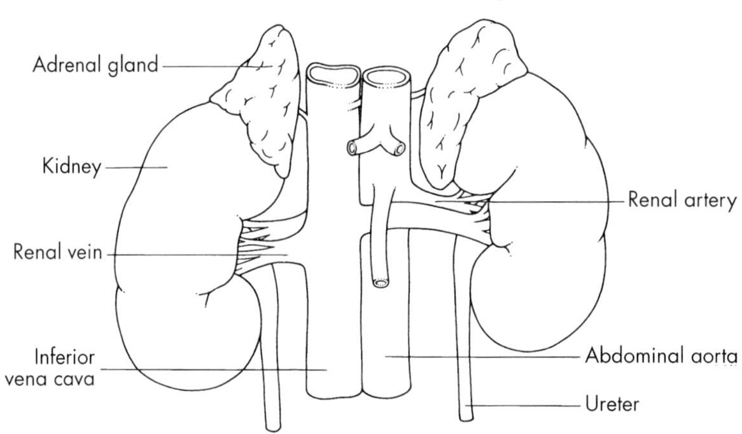

Figure 6.4 Position of adrenal glands.

The glucocorticoids are a triad of hormones, hydrocortisone (cortisol), corticosterone and cortisone, of which hydrocortisone is the dominant member. The hormones increase the rate of catabolism of protein, converting the resultant amino acids to energy if the stores of fat and glycogen are low (gluconeogenesis). Other fat stores are also mobilised to provide energy (e.g. fatty acids). The provision of an adequate energy source is critical for normal body metabolism, and may also assist the body to respond to stress (e.g. surgery, severe infection, extreme cold and fright). The vasoconstrictor effects of the glucocorticoids may be of benefit if the induced stress is as a result of haemorrhage.

The glucocorticoids suppress inflammatory and allergic responses through a range of mechanisms (e.g. stabilisation of lysosomal membranes and reduction in the secretion of histamine). However, excessive secretion of these hormones may retard wound healing and suppress immune responses.

The adrenal medulla is both an endocrine gland and an important part of the sympathetic nervous system. It secretes the catecholamines adrenaline (epinephrine) and noradrenaline (norepinephrine) into the bloodstream from chromaffin cells. Adrenaline stimulates the breakdown of muscular and hepatic glycogen, providing an important source of energy in an emergency. Noradrenaline and adrenaline increase the metabolic rate of certain organs of the body, and supplement the activity of the sympathetic nervous system.

The pancreas

The pancreas is both an endocrine and exocrine organ. It is divided into a head, tail and body, the head portion lying closest to the junction with the duodenum (*see* Figure 1.4). Exocrine secretions from the pancreas are transported to the duodenum through the pancreatic duct. The bulk (99%) of the pancreas is composed of exocrine cells, the acini, which secrete pancreatic juice (*see* Section 1.10). The endocrine secretions of the pancreas are produced by the islets of Langerhans which are subdivided as alpha, beta and delta cells according to their secretions.

The largest cells, the alpha cells, secrete glucagon, a polypeptide whose principal action is to increase the level of circulating glucose. This is achieved by stimulating the hepatic formation of glucose from glycogen (glycogenolysis), and amino acids, lactic acid and glycerol (gluconeogenesis). The release of glucagon is controlled by a negative feedback mechanism which monitors plasma glucose concentrations.

The beta cells secrete insulin. Insulin is a hypoglycaemic agent by virtue of its effects on the transport and utilisation of glucose. It increases the rate of uptake of glucose from the blood into tissues, and the conversion of glucose into glycogen. Insulin also prevents glycogenolysis and gluconeogenesis (*see above*). Fatty acid formation (lipogenesis) and protein synthesis are promoted in the presence of insulin. The secretion of insulin is regulated directly by plasma glucose concentrations, but indirect control may also be exerted by the action of other hormones. Growth hormone secretion and the release of glucocorticoids caused by the secretion of ACTH induce hyperglycaemia, which in turn increases the secretion of insulin.

The delta cells of the pancreas secrete growth hormone-inhibiting factor (somatostatin), but are not normally considered an integral part of the endocrine system.

The gonads

The gonadal endocrine glands in the female are the ovaries (*see* Figure 7.2 and Section 7.6), and in the male, the testes. The ovaries are the primary reproductive organs of the female, responsible for the secretion of oestrogens and progesterone and the production of ova. The oestrogens, of which estradiol is the most important, are responsible for the development and maintenance of the female secondary sexual characteristics (e.g. the shape of the pelvis, the pitch of the voice and the distribution of body fat). They exert control over the menstrual cycle (e.g. by stimulating the production of luteinising hormone from the anterior pituitary) and increase the likelihood of successful fertilisation (e.g. by decreasing the viscosity of cervical mucus at the time of ovulation). If conception is successful, the oestrogens assist in the maintenance of pregnancy and the preparation of the mammary glands for lactation.

The release of progesterone is responsible for the preparation of the endometrium on the assumption that fertilisation will occur. Its release and steady accumulation from day 14 of the menstrual cycle increases the vascularity and thickness of the lining of the uterus to receive the fertilised ovum. If fertilisation and implantation of the ovum does not occur, the continued secretion of progesterone inhibits the release of luteinising hormone. Consequently, the concentrations of oestrogens and progesterone decline through the destruction of their source and lead to shedding of the proliferative endometrium (menstruation).

The release of progesterone assumes greater importance in the event of fertilisation and implantation. It reduces the risk of premature labour by preventing uterine contractions, and, in combination with oestrogen, inhibits further ovulation during the pregnancy. Progesterone is also secreted from the developing placenta.

The male gonadal glands, the testes, are suspended in two scrotal sacs outside the abdominal wall. The sperm are produced within the tightly coiled seminiferous tubules. Interstitial Leydig cells are located within the spaces between the seminiferous tubules, and are responsible for the secretion of testosterone, the male sex hormone. Like oestrogen in the female, testosterone is necessary for the development of male secondary sexual characteristics (e.g. deepening of the voice, muscular and skeletal development, and the production and distribution of facial, body and pubic hair). The production of testosterone is controlled by the secretion of luteinising hormone from the anterior pituitary.

7

Obstetric, gynaecological, renal and urogenital disorders

7.1 Obstetric disorders

Abortion

Abortion is the termination of pregnancy before the fetus is considered viable legally (i.e. before the 28th week of pregnancy).

Spontaneous abortion occurs without external stimuli. During the first trimester of pregnancy, spontaneous abortion is usually due to fetal abnormalities, but in later weeks it is commonly due to maternal factors (e.g. abnormalities of the genital tract).

Habitual abortion is repeated spontaneous abortion. The usual criterion is the occurrence of three consecutive, unexplained abortions, usually in a woman who has never had a successful pregnancy. Causes of habitual abortion include endocrine and metabolic disease (e.g. hypothyroidism or hyperthyroidism, diabetes mellitus or chronic renal failure), anatomical uterine abnormalities and incompetence of the cervix. Defective function of the corpus luteum is a common cause. Progestogens have been used to maintain the endometrium, but their efficacy is doubtful. Suturing of the cervix may prevent abortion in cases of cervical incompetence.

Threatened abortion is uterine bleeding in the presence of an apparently intact pregnancy. The usual treatment is bed rest for several days or until the bleeding stops, and avoidance of coitus.

Inevitable abortion occurs when, in addition to vaginal bleeding in early pregnancy, there are uterine contractions accompanied by pain and passage of fetal or placental tissue. Abortion occurs soon after the onset of symptoms. If abortion is incomplete (i.e. products of conception remain in the uterus), it may be completed by curettage.

Missed abortion is the retention of the products of conception within the uterus for a prolonged period after the death of the fetus. There is cessation of growth or diminution in the size of the uterus. The pregnancy test becomes negative, but there is no expulsion of uterine contents. Complete abortion is achieved by stimulation of the uterus with prostaglandins and oxytocics, or by curettage.

Septic abortion occurs when the contents of the uterus become infected by bacteria before, during or usually after, an abortion. Chills, fever, septicaemia and peritonitis may occur and septic shock may develop. It is treated with antibacterial drugs.

Therapeutic abortion is the elective termination of pregnancy. Very early abortion can be carried out using a fine cannula passed into the uterine cavity, and sucking out the contents. After 14 weeks gestation, instillation of prostaglandins via the cervix or injection into the amniotic cavity results in evacuation, usually within 8–18 hours. Oxytocin infusion may also be required, and retained uterine contents must sometimes be removed under anaesthetic. Rarely pregnancy may be terminated by hysterotomy.

Self-help organisations
Birth Control Trust
British Pregnancy Advisory Service
Family Planning Association
Marie Stopes International
National Abortion Campaign
Pregnancy Advisory Service

Ectopic pregnancy

Definition and aetiology

An ectopic pregnancy is a pregnancy in which a fertilised ovum implants and begins to develop outside the endometrium. The majority occur within the Fallopian tubes, although other possible sites include the ovaries, cervix and peritoneal cavity. Tubal ectopic pregnancies occur more commonly in patients with partial tubal obstruction, usually as a consequence of salpingitis. The incidence of ectopic pregnancy is also increased in women who become pregnant in the presence of an intra-uterine device and in those who have had a previous ectopic pregnancy.

Symptoms

Symptoms may include slight vaginal bleeding ('spotting') and colicky lower abdominal pain. This is usually followed by abrupt severe lower abdominal pain, marked vaginal bleeding, and syncope caused by rupture of the Fallopian tube and intra-abdominal haemorrhage; hypotension and shock may develop.

Treatment

Treatment consists of surgical removal of the fetus, placenta, and part or all of the affected tube. Transfusion may be required.

Hydatidiform mole

Definition and aetiology

Hydatidiform mole is a benign tumour of the trophoblastic tissue. It occurs in abnormal pregnancies when a degenerating ovum fails to abort spontaneously. The trophoblastic tissue continues to proliferate, resulting in a fleshy tumour in which the villi are grossly distended with fluid (hydropic). Hydatidiform mole occurs most commonly in females at the two extremes of their reproductive life: in the very young (17 years of age) and in those over 40 years of age.

Symptoms

It is characterised by abnormally rapid uterine enlargement, severe nausea and vomiting, and vaginal bleeding, eventually followed by spontaneous abortion. Patients with hydatidiform mole may later develop choriocarcinoma. In other patients, the mole may be locally invasive and there may be distant spread. Metastases formed as a result may regress after removal of the mole. Other complications include intra-uterine infections, haemorrhage, septicaemia and pre-eclampsia.

Treatment

Abortion may be induced with prostaglandins (BNF 7.1.1) or by suction curettage. Patients require careful follow-up to detect choriocarcinoma. Antimetabolites (BNF 8.1.3) or cytotoxic antibiotics (BNF 8.1.2), or both, may be required in the treatment of invasive moles.

Postpartum haemorrhage

Definition and aetiology

Primary postpartum haemorrhage is characterised by significant blood loss (at least 500 mL) occurring after birth and within 24 hours. It may be caused by an atonic uterus, retained products of conception, lacerations or hypofibrinogenaemia. It usually occurs soon after parturition and before complete delivery of the placenta, but may occur as long as one month after delivery.

Secondary postpartum haemorrhage occurs after 24 hours and usually within several weeks. Its aetiology may be the same as the primary form, or it can be caused by uterine infection.

Treatment

Postpartum haemorrhage may be prevented or controlled by the routine administration of ergometrine and oxytocin (BNF 7.1.1). The placenta should be examined for completeness and any retained products of conception removed from the uterus. If haemorrhage does occur, the risk of serious blood loss may be reduced by intravenous injection of ergometrine, by intravenous oxytocin infusion when the patient does not respond to ergometrine, and repair of lacerations. Hypotension should be treated promptly to prevent pituitary necrosis. Antibacterial drugs (BNF 5.1) may be required for infection.

Pre-eclampsia and eclampsia

Definition and aetiology

Pre-eclampsia (toxaemia of pregnancy) is characterised by hypertension, proteinuria and oedema. Its presence results in increased fetal and, to a lesser extent, maternal morbidity and mortality. Pre-eclampsia usually occurs in the latter half of the pregnancy and resolves soon after delivery. It occurs more frequently in first pregnancies, older women, and in multiple pregnancies, although its aetiology is uncertain. Eclampsia refers to convulsions in late pregnancy, labour or the puerperium and can lead to coma. It is often preceded by pre-eclampsia. Fetal morbidity and mortality is very high.

It is a common occurrence, with estimates ranging from between 1 in 20 and 1 in 30 pregnancies in the UK. An arbitrary blood pressure reading of 140 mmHg/90 mmHg is taken as the threshold for hypertension associated with proteinuria to define pre-eclampsia.

Eclampsia affects about 1 in 2000 pregnancies in the UK, and has a high (2%) maternal death rate.

Symptoms

The only symptoms of pre-eclampsia are oedema and weight gain. In impending eclampsia, headache, visual disturbances and vomiting can occur. There may also be epigastric pain and reduced urinary volume.

Treatment

Pre-eclampsia responds to rest and careful observation. Hospitalisation is necessary for all cases considered more than mild, in an attempt to prevent eclampsia. Should it develop, early delivery may be required. Antihypertensive therapy (BNF 2.5), antiepileptics (BNF 4.8), and hypnotics and anxiolytics (BNF 4.1) may be necessary.

7.2 Gynaecological disorders

7.2.1 GENERAL DISORDERS

Endometriosis

Definition and aetiology

Endometriosis (Figure 7.1) is a condition in which functioning endometrial tissue is found in an abnormal location. It occurs most commonly between 30 and 40 years of age. Common sites for the ectopic endometrium include the ovary, Fallopian tubes, vagina, myometrium, uterine ligaments, uterorectal pouch, rectum and sigmoid colon (Figures 7.2 and 7.3). The endometrial tissue may form a small nodule often with surrounding fibrosis. In the ovaries, lesions are commonly cystic and respond to the cyclic changes in oestrogen and progesterone by repeated swelling (causing pain) and bleeding (causing fibrosis) at the time of menstruation. In ovarian cysts some of the fluid may be of a chocolate and tarry consistency, and the cyst may grow as large as an orange. Its rupture may result in multiple adhesions.

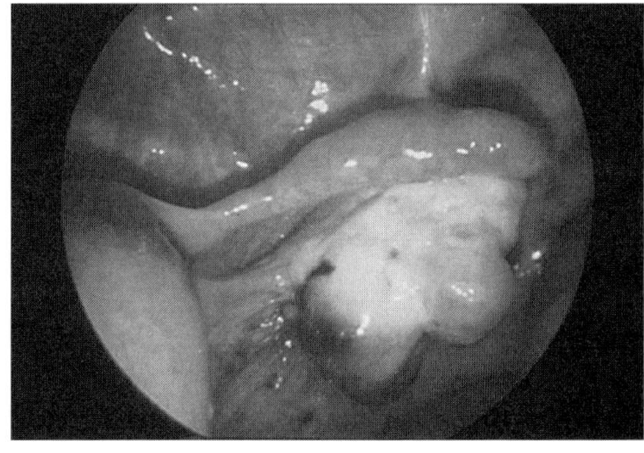

Figure 7.1 Endometriosis as seen at laparoscopy. (Reproduced with permission of Mike Wyndham/BV Lewis.)

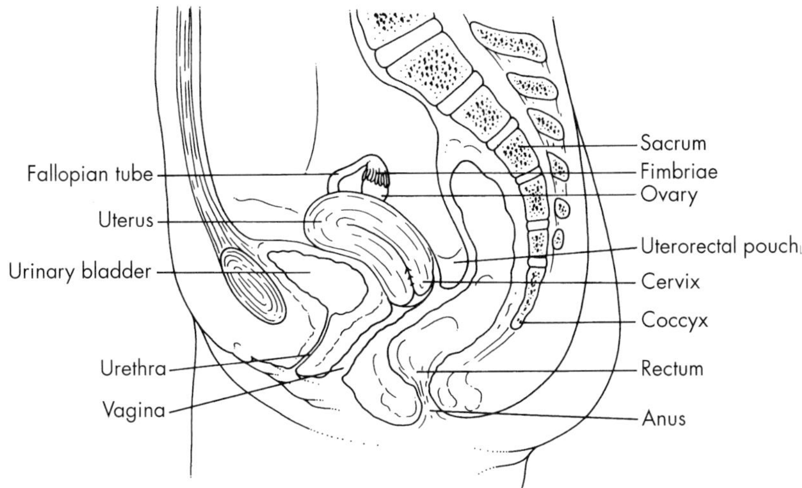

Figure 7.2 Female pelvic organs (sagittal section).

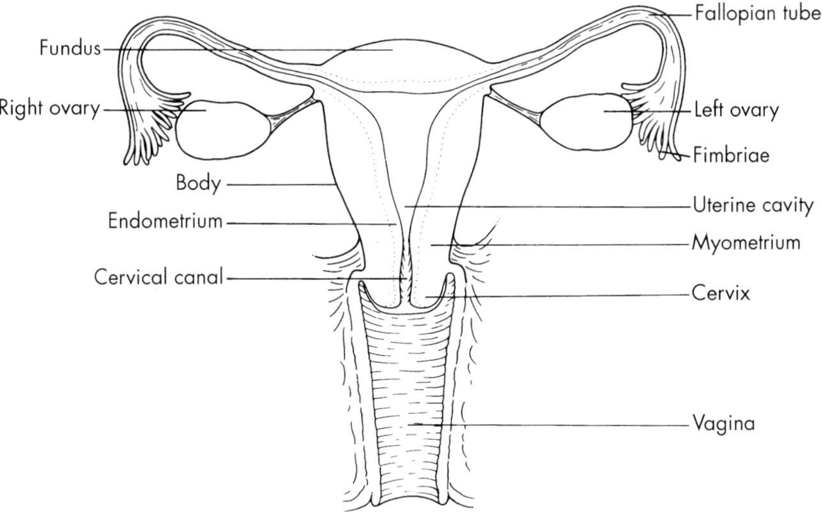

Figure 7.3 Female reproductive system.

Symptoms

The symptoms of endometriosis are varied, depending upon location, but usually include dysmenorrhoea, dyspareunia, menorrhagia, intermenstrual pelvic pain and back pain. Infertility occurs in about 30–40% of patients. If the rectum or sigmoid colon is involved, there may be cyclic rectal pains, pain on defaecation, and occasionally mild diarrhoea and tenesmus. Dysuria may occur if the bladder is involved.

Treatment

Treatment depends on the severity of symptoms and the age and parity of the patient. Endometriosis is suppressed by pregnancy and the menopause. Progestogens (BNF 6.4.1.2) may be given continuously for several months; alternatively cyclical or continuous treatment with combined oral contraceptives (BNF 7.3.1), gonadorelin analogues (BNF 6.5.2) or danazol (BNF 6.7.2) may be useful. Fertility may be enhanced on the withdrawal of such treatment. Surgery (usually hysterectomy) may be required in more severe cases.

Hirsutism

Definition and aetiology

Hirsutism is excessive facial and body hair growth, especially in women. It may be idiopathic or caused by increased testosterone production, usually as a result of polycystic ovary syndrome. Rarer causes include adrenal or ovarian tumours, Cushing's disease, acromegaly and juvenile hypothyroidism. Hirsutism may also be induced by drugs (e.g. anabolic steroids, androgens, corticosteroids, phenytoin, diazoxide and minoxidil).

Treatment

Treatment is dependent on the underlying cause. Idiopathic hirsutism may be treated by local removal of unwanted hair. Severe cases may be treated with cyproterone acetate (BNF 6.4.2) or combined oral contraceptives (BNF 7.3.1).

Infertility

Definition and aetiology

Infertility is the reduced or absent ability to conceive children. It affects 10–15% of couples and may be caused by abnormalities in either partner; it may also be psychogenic. Failure to conceive after 12 months is considered abnormal as 90% of fertile couples achieve conception within that time.

Age is an important factor in determining fertility. Conception rates after 35 years of age are half those below 25 years of age. The increasing maternal age of the first conception (with a mean of about 27 years of age) has increased the incidence of infertility.

In males, infertility may occur as a result of impaired spermatogenesis caused by endocrine disturbances (e.g. hyperprolactinaemia, hypogonadism, hypopituitarism, prolonged fever, testicular infection or injury, cryptorchidism, or varicocele). Spermatogenesis may also be affected by drug administration (e.g. testosterone) or environmental toxins (e.g. heavy metals). Infertility may also arise from obstruction of the seminal ducts due to congenital abnormalities, infection, stricture or surgery. In addition, sperm may not be deposited in the vagina as a result of certain disorders (e.g. impotence or premature ejaculation).

In females, infertility may arise through abnormal ovarian function as a result of endocrine disorders and polycystic ovary syndrome. Fallopian tube defects may be present as a consequence of congenital abnormalities or infection (e.g. salpingitis). Congenital uterine defects may also exist or conditions in the cervix may not be ideal for the transmission of sperm.

Treatment

Treatment is aimed at the underlying cause. Corrective surgery may be necessary in the case of anatomical abnormalities, and *in vitro* fertilisation may be considered in selected cases.

Self-help organisations

British Pregnancy Advisory Service
Child
Family Planning Association
ISSUE (National Fertility Association)
Marie Stopes International

Menopause

Definition and aetiology

The menopause (climacteric) is the cessation of menstruation. It usually occurs between 45 and 55 years of age (although it can occur any time after puberty), during which time the ovaries progressively secrete less oestrogen and progesterone. This results in increased plasma gonadotrophin concentrations and menstrual irregularities, culminating in the cessation of menstruation.

Symptoms

Clinical features of the menopause are primarily due to oestrogen deficiency. They include vasomotor symptoms (e.g. hot flushes, sweating and headache), insomnia, irritability, loss of libido, anxiety and depressive disorders. Long-term effects of endocrine changes, which may appear in postmenopausal women combined with the effects of ageing, include osteoporosis and atrophy of the breasts, endometrium, myometrium, vagina and vulva. Atrophy of pelvic muscles and ligaments may lead to uterine prolapse. The incidence of ischaemic heart disease is increased postmenopausally.

Treatment
Symptomatic treatment with clonidine (BNF 4.7.4.2) for hot flushes, and anxiolytics (BNF 4.1.2) and antidepressant drugs (BNF 4.3) may be necessary. Symptoms may also be treated by hormone replacement therapy, with oestrogens given cyclically with a progestogen (BNF 6.4.1.1 and 6.4.1.2) or combined preparations (BNF 6.4.1.3). Hormone implants may also be used. The majority of women, however, may be successfully treated by counselling and reassurance alone.

Polycystic ovary syndrome

Definition and aetiology
The polycystic ovary syndrome (Stein-Leventhal syndrome) is characterised by the presence of multiple bilateral ovarian cysts and stromal hyperplasia. It may be associated with the conditions of hypersecretion of androgens (e.g. congenital adrenal hyperplasia and Cushing's syndrome).

Symptoms
It usually occurs in young women and is characterised by menstrual irregularities (e.g. secondary amenorrhoea or oligomenorrhoea) and impaired fertility. Hirsutism and obesity commonly occur and occasionally other signs of virilisation may be present.

Treatment
Infertility arising from the polycystic ovary syndrome may be treated by administration of clomiphene or chorionic gonadotrophin (BNF 6.5.1), or both. Oral contraceptives (BNF 7.3.1) are the first line of treatment for hirsutism.

Turner's syndrome

Definition and aetiology
Turner's syndrome is a rare form of defective gonadal development in females associated with the complete or partial absence of the second X-chromosome.

Symptoms
It is characterised by primary amenorrhoea, short stature and numerous skeletal abnormalities (e.g. webbing of the neck, shield-like chest, metacarpal abnormalities and cubitus valgus). Other signs include poorly developed secondary sexual characteristics, hypertension, lymphoedema, a low posterior hairline and multiple naevi. Cardiovascular and renal abnormalities are common. Turner's syndrome is associated with an increased incidence of Hashimoto's thyroiditis, diabetes mellitus and infertility.

Treatment
Treatment consists of replacement therapy, initially with ethinylestradiol (BNF 6.4.1.1) for several months and subsequently with a combined oral contraceptive (BNF 7.3.1); infertility is irremediable. Antihypertensive therapy (BNF 2.5) may be required.

Vaginitis

Definition and aetiology
Vaginitis is inflammation of the vagina which may be infectious or atrophic.

Infective vaginitis

Definition and aetiology
Infective vaginitis may be caused by a variety of microorganisms (e.g. *Chlamydia trachomatis*, *Candida albicans*, *Trichomonas vaginalis* and *Neisseria gonorrhoeae*) or may be non-specific. Vaginal candidiasis may be precipitated by diabetes mellitus, pregnancy, or the administration of antibacterials, corticosteroids and possibly combined oral contraceptives. Non-specific vaginitis is thought to be due to infection with *Gardnerella vaginalis*, although other causes include foreign bodies (e.g. retained tampons) and local irritants (e.g. douches, deodorants or spermicides).

Symptoms
In vaginal candidiasis, the discharge is usually thick, white and caseous and is accompanied by vulvitis and marked pruritus. In vaginal trichomoniasis, the discharge is usually offensive, yellowish, and may be frothy and profuse with

soreness and pruritus. In non-specific vaginitis, the discharge is usually greyish, frothy and malodorous (fishy smell).

Treatment
Treatment is dependent on the underlying cause. Vaginal candidiasis is treated with anti-infective drugs (BNF 7.2.2). Vaginal trichomoniasis and *Gardnerella* infections are treated systemically with metronidazole or tinidazole (BNF 5.4.2).

Atrophic vaginitis

Definition and aetiology
Atrophic (senile) vaginitis occurs in postmenopausal women and is associated with oestrogen deficiency. Abnormal vaginal discharge may also be caused by malignancy, foreign bodies, cervical erosions or strictures, radiotherapy or sexually transmitted diseases.

Symptoms
Atrophic vaginitis may be asymptomatic in many, but a discharge, if present, is usually thin and watery. Many patients experience pruritus, and soreness may cause pain during sexual intercourse.

Treatment
Atrophic vaginitis may be treated with topical oestrogens (BNF 7.2.1) or, in severe unresponsive cases, by systemic hormone replacement therapy with oestrogens and progestogens (BNF 6.4.1).

Vulvitis

Definition and aetiology
Vulvitis is inflammation of the vulva. It may accompany atrophic or infective vaginitis or may be due to local allergic reactions, poor hygiene, bacterial, fungal, parasitic or viral infections, or malignant or sexually transmitted diseases.

Symptoms
It is characterised by local erythema and oedema, burning pain, and pruritus vulvae. Ulceration may be present and atrophy (kraurosis vulvae) may occur in postmenopausal women.

Treatment
Treatment is dependent on the underlying cause. Topical corticosteroids (BNF 13.4) may be required for local allergic reactions; local anaesthetic and antipruritic preparations (BNF 13.3) may provide symptomatic relief; topical hormones (BNF 7.2.1) may be indicated for kraurosis vulvae; anti-infective drugs (BNF 7.2.2) may be required for vulval infections.

7.2.2 BREAST DISORDERS

Benign mammary dysplasias

Definition and aetiology
Benign mammary dysplasias (cystic mastopathy or chronic cystic mastitis) are a group of benign breast changes which frequently occur in premenopausal women and are the commonest cause of breast lumps.

Symptoms
The changes occur mainly in the lobular and terminal ducts and include formation of cysts, epitheliosis (hyperplasia of the ductular epithelium), adenosis and fibrosis. Any one of these changes may predominate and they may occur in any combination. Cysts are usually multiple and bilateral, although solitary cysts may occur.

Treatment
Treatment is not usually required, although aspiration and biopsy may be necessary to differentiate the condition from breast cancer.

7.2.3 MENSTRUAL DISORDERS

(The menstrual cycle in the absence of fertilisation is illustrated in Figure 7.4.)

Amenorrhoea

Definition and aetiology
Amenorrhoea is the absence of menstruation. In primary amenorrhoea the menarche fails to occur

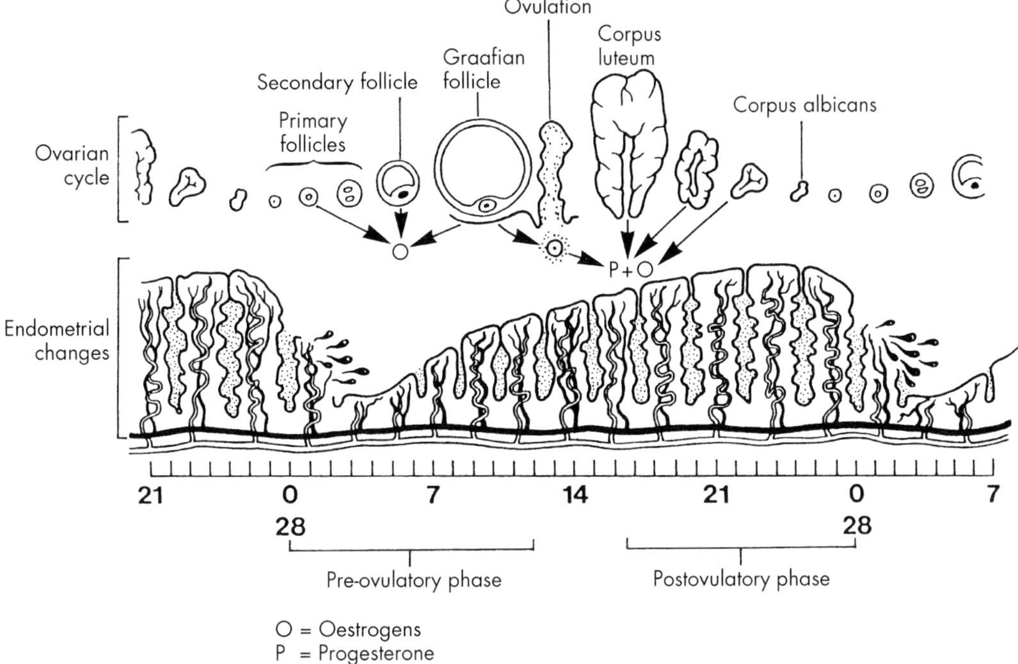

Figure 7.4 Menstrual cycle (in the absence of fertilisation).

by 16 years of age. Secondary amenorrhoea is the absence of menstruation for six months or longer in a female who has previously been menstruating. It may be physiological (e.g. due to pregnancy, lactation or the menopause) or pathological. Amenorrhoea is usually a symptom of an underlying disorder and can be caused by disturbances of the hormonal regulation of the menstrual cycle.

Amenorrhoea is commonly associated with endocrine disease. Primary causes include pituitary or hypothalamic disorders (e.g. hyperprolactinaemia and hypopituitarism). Secondary causes include other endocrine pathology, ranging from thyroid disorders (e.g. hyperthyroidism) and adrenal disorders (e.g. adrenal virilisation) to gonadal disorders (e.g. hypogonadism). Amenorrhoea may also be associated with anorexia nervosa and obesity. Emotional disturbances, excessive exercise and severe systemic illness (e.g. malignant disease) may also cause amenorrhoea. Amenorrhoea may also be drug-induced (e.g. due to antipsychotic drugs or corticosteroids) or may follow discontinuation of oral contraception. Rarely, primary amenorrhoea may be due to structural uterine or vaginal abnormalities.

Treatment

Treatment is dependent on the underlying cause. Oestrogens (BNF 6.4.1.1) may be used to induce artificial menstruation in primary amenorrhoea. They are usually given cyclically with a progestogen (BNF 6.4.1.4), or a combined oral contraceptive (BNF 7.3.1) may be used. Clomiphene or cyclofenil (BNF 6.5.1) may be used to induce ovulation in patients with idiopathic secondary amenorrhoea or amenorrhoea caused by the polycystic ovary syndrome.

Dysmenorrhoea

Definition

Dysmenorrhoea is painful menstruation which may be primary or secondary.

Primary dysmenorrhoea

Definition and aetiology

Primary (spasmodic) dysmenorrhoea is caused by uncoordinated uterine contractions which occur as the endometrium is shed and expelled. There is increasing evidence of a role for prostaglandins in its aetiology.

Symptoms
It is common in young nulliparous women, and is characterised by colicky lower abdominal, back and leg pain, which usually starts on the first day of menstruation and lasts for up to 48 hours. Occasionally, the pain may precede menstruation. Dysmenorrhoea may be associated with abdominal distension, nausea and vomiting, diarrhoea, headache, premenstrual syndrome and urinary frequency.

Treatment
It may be treated with anti-inflammatory non-opioid analgesics (BNF 4.7.1), myometrial relaxants (BNF 7.1.3), or in severe cases with progestogens (BNF 6.4.1.2) or combined oestrogen/progestogen preparations (BNF 7.3.1). Application of local heat, adequate rest and regular exercise may also be beneficial.

Secondary dysmenorrhoea

Definition and aetiology
Secondary (congestive) dysmenorrhoea is pain secondary to various disorders (e.g. endometriosis, fibroids, salpingitis or chronic pelvic inflammatory disease).

Symptoms
The pain usually occurs as a dull ache in the lower abdomen and back, commencing several days before menstruation and often relieved within 24 hours of its onset, although it may persist throughout menstruation. Abdominal distension and the premenstrual syndrome may also occur.

Treatment
Treatment should be directed at the underlying cause. Measures indicated in primary dysmenorrhoea may also be useful.

Premenstrual syndrome

Definition and aetiology
Premenstrual syndrome usually starts 7–10 days before menstruation and commonly disappears a few hours after the onset of menstruation.

Symptoms
It is characterised by emotional lability, irritability, nervousness, depressive disorders, weight gain, abdominal distension and breast tenderness. Headache, fatigue and oedema may also occur.

Treatment
A wide variety of treatment measures have been tried. Many women benefit from explanation and reassurance. A wide variety of drugs have been used, with varying degrees of success. These include pyridoxine (BNF 9.6.2), diuretics (BNF 2.2), progestogens (BNF 6.4.1.2), combined oral contraceptives (BNF 7.3.1) and gonadorelin analogues (BNF 6.7.2). Antidepressant drugs (BNF 4.3) have been used for emotional instability.

7.3 Male genital disorders

Benign prostatic hypertrophy

Definition and aetiology
Benign prostatic hypertrophy is a non-malignant condition in which the prostate gland becomes large and nodular. It is common (occurring in about one in five) in men over 50 years of age, and results in varying degrees of urethral obstruction. Its cause is unknown, but it is thought to be associated with the endocrine disturbances of ageing.

Symptoms
The symptoms are associated with obstruction of the urethra. Difficulty in urination is common, with a decrease in the volume and force of the urine flow, terminal dribbling and incomplete bladder emptying. Urinary frequency and nocturia usually follow. Urinary retention may become total and severe pain develops as a result of pressure build-up. Urinary-tract infection is a common complication. If urinary retention is prolonged, renal failure may develop.

Treatment
Patients should avoid anticholinergic and narcotic drugs, which can induce obstruction. Catheterisation may be performed in order to drain the bladder. Drug management can be

achieved with finasteride (BNF 6.4.2), which reduces prostate size and improves urinary flow rate. Surgical resection (prostatectomy) may be necessary either via the urethra (transurethral resection) or by an abdominal incision.

Cryptorchidism

Definition and aetiology

Cryptorchidism is a developmental defect in which one or both testes fail to descend into the scrotum, but remain in the abdominal cavity or inguinal canal (normal descent commonly occurs before birth or during the first two years of life). The cause is not known, but endocrine or anatomical abnormalities may be responsible. Infertility caused by impaired spermatogenesis is likely to develop, particularly if the defect persists after five years of age. There is also a greater likelihood of malignant disease in undescended testes.

Treatment

Chorionic gonadotrophin and gonadorelin (BNF 6.5.1) have been used in the treatment of cryptorchidism. The standard treatment is surgical relocation and fixation in the scrotum (orchidopexy). If the defect persists after puberty, orchidectomy may be carried out because of the risk of malignancy.

Klinefelter's syndrome

Definition and aetiology

Klinefelter's syndrome is a familial condition in males associated with the presence of one or more extra X-chromosomes in at least one cell line.

Symptoms

It is characterised by infertility due to azoospermia or oligospermia, small firm testes, and variable degrees of masculinisation; hypogonadism and gynaecomastia may occur. Patients are often tall with long limbs, and mental retardation is common; skeletal abnormalities may occur. There is an increased incidence of breast cancer compared with other males, and an increased frequency of impaired glucose tolerance and diabetes mellitus.

Treatment

Hypogonadism may be treated by replacement therapy with androgens (BNF 6.4.2), but infertility is irremediable.

Torsion of the testis

Definition and aetiology

Torsion of the testis occurs when a testis twists on the spermatic cord within the membranous covering (tunica vaginalis) of the testis. This may occur spontaneously and at any age, although it is more common during puberty. It may follow vigorous physical activity, particularly if there is a pre-existing anatomical defect. Torsion results in venous obstruction which may lead to local oedema, haemorrhage, arterial obstruction and infarction.

Symptoms

Symptoms include extreme pain and tenderness in the testis, and the patient may be unable to walk. The scrotum and testis become inflamed and swollen. Fever, nausea and vomiting, and very occasionally dysuria and frequency, may develop.

Treatment

Surgical investigation of any suspected torsion must be carried out urgently. Delay reduces the chances of the testis remaining viable. In severe cases, orchidectomy may be indicated.

Varicocele

Definition and aetiology

Varicocele is a varicose condition of the veins within the scrotum. It is usually left-sided.

Symptoms

It is characterised by scrotal swelling (often described as a 'bag of worms') which disappears on lying down. The swelling is often accompanied by a constant, dragging, dull pain. Blue discoloration may be visible through the scrotal skin. Varicocele is a common cause of infertility.

Treatment

A scrotal support (or similar garment) may be all that is required. Surgery, by ligation of the

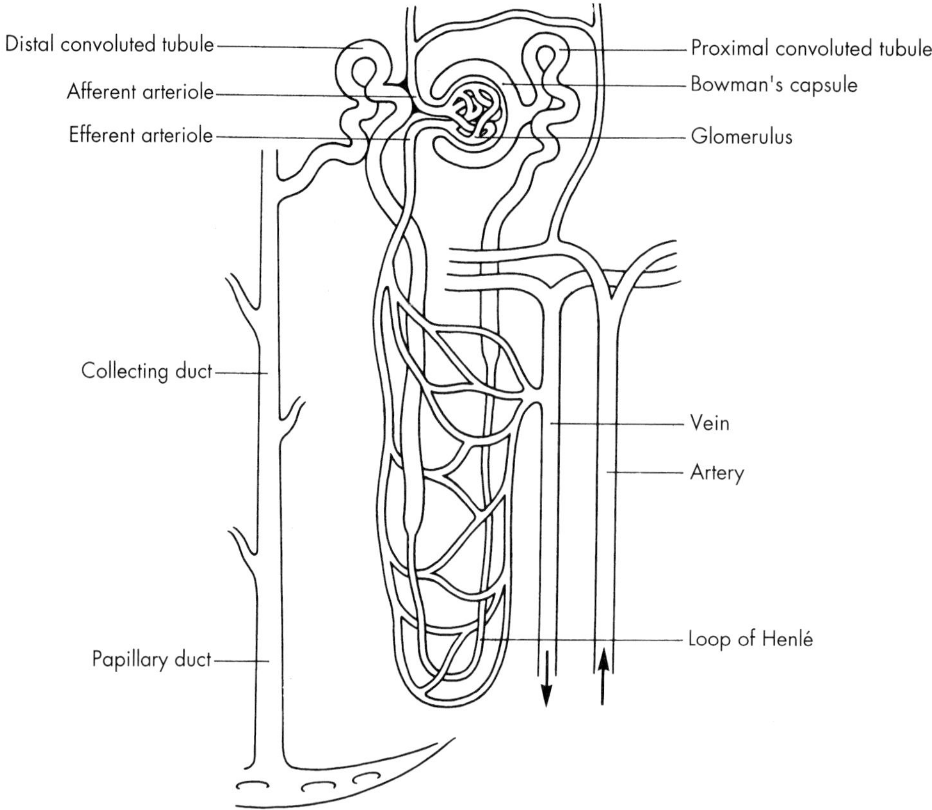

Figure 7.5 Nephron.

spermatic vein, may be necessary if infertility develops or the symptoms are unacceptable.

7.4 Renal disorders

Glomerulonephritis

Definition

Glomerulonephritis (Bright's disease) is characterised by inflammation of renal glomeruli which may be acute or chronic. (The structure of a healthy nephron is illustrated in Figure 7.5.)

Acute glomerulonephritis

Definition and aetiology

Acute (postinfectious) glomerulonephritis is usually preceded by a group A β-haemolytic streptococcal infection, often of the pharynx or skin. It is associated with the laying down of antigen–antibody complexes in the glomeruli.

Symptoms

It is most common in children and young adults. The onset is usually sudden in children, occurring two to three weeks after the infective episode, but slower in adults. Symptoms include fever, headache, malaise, nausea and vomiting, and oedema with hypertension and dyspnoea. Proteinuria and haematuria are almost always present, and abdominal and back pain may occur. The probability of recovery is favourable, especially in children, although progressive renal impairment may develop in some and culminate in renal failure.

Treatment

Treatment consists of bed rest and, in the presence of residual streptococcal infection, the administration of an appropriate antibacterial drug (BNF 5.1). Diuretics (BNF 2.2) and antihypertensive therapy (BNF 2.5) may be necessary. An adequate fluid intake should be maintained and dietary protein and sodium restricted.

Chronic glomerulonephritis

Definition and aetiology
Chronic glomerulonephritis is a syndrome which may follow any one of a number of inflammatory glomerular disorders. A history of acute glomerulonephritis is, however, uncommon.

Symptoms
The onset is insidious and usually occurs in adults. Persistent proteinuria and haematuria are usually present and common symptoms, associated with renal impairment, include dyspnoea, fatigue, nausea and vomiting, and pruritus. Oedema may occur and hypertension is common. Death may occur as a result of renal failure.

Treatment
Treatment is generally ineffective. Antihypertensive therapy (BNF 2.5) may be useful and dialysis may be necessary in severe renal failure. Dietary sodium and protein should be restricted, while maintaining an adequate fluid intake.

Self-help organisation
British Kidney Patient Association
National Kidney Federation
The National Kidney Research Fund and Kidney Foundation

Interstitial nephritis

Definition and aetiology
Interstitial nephritis is characterised by inflammation of the renal interstitial tissue, including the tubules. It may be acute or, more commonly, chronic. It has a wide variety of causes. These include toxicity due to drugs (e.g. analgesics and antibacterials) or heavy metals (e.g. lead), metabolic disorders (e.g. hypokalaemia and gout), immunological disorders (e.g. systemic lupus erythematosus), urinary-tract infection, obstruction and vascular abnormalities (e.g. renal artery obstruction). It may also be idiopathic.

Symptoms
The acute form of the disease, which is most often due to drug toxicity, may present with oliguria, fever and occasionally arthralgia. Renal failure may develop. In chronic interstitial nephritis, there are few symptoms before the onset of renal failure and uraemia. Subsequent symptoms include anaemia, anorexia, fatigue, nausea and vomiting, and weight loss. Hypertension may occur in severe cases. Renal failure is a common complication, which may prove fatal.

Treatment
Treatment in acute disease comprises the administration of corticosteroids (BNF 6.3.4). In the chronic form, treatment is aimed at the underlying cause. Antibacterial drugs (BNF 5.1) may be used in the presence of infection, and surgery may be indicated in the presence of urinary-tract obstruction. In both forms of the disease, dialysis or transplantation may be necessary if chronic renal failure develops.

Nephrotic syndrome

Definition and aetiology
The nephrotic syndrome is characterised by increased glomerular permeability to protein, resulting in more than 3–5 g in the urine each day. The most common cause is glomerulonephritis, but occasionally diabetes mellitus, malignant disease or systemic lupus erythematosus may be responsible. It may also arise as an adverse effect of drug administration (e.g. penicillamine and sodium aurothiomalate).

Nephrotic syndrome occurs at any age, but is more common in young children under four years of age.

Symptoms
The onset is usually insidious and symptoms include persistent severe proteinuria and hypoproteinaemia, leading to salt and water retention, and marked generalised oedema. An increased susceptibility to infection is common, and other complications include hypertension and renal failure.

Treatment

Treatment consists of bed rest and a high-protein, low-sodium diet. Specific treatment depends on the underlying disorder. Diuretics (BNF 2.2) may be administered; corticosteroids (BNF 6.3.2) may be helpful. Cyclophosphamide has also been used. Antibacterial drugs (BNF 5.1) and antihypertensive therapy (BNF 2.5) may be necessary.

Oedema

Definition and aetiology

Oedema is the presence of abnormally large amounts of fluid in the intercellular tissue spaces of the body. It is usually detected by the accumulation of fluid in the subcutaneous tissues and is accompanied by retention of sodium and chloride ions. It may be localised, caused by venous (*see* Embolism, Section 9.1.1) or lymphatic obstruction, or by increased vascular permeability. It may also be generalised, caused by systemic heart disease, hepatic disease or renal disease.

Symptoms

It is commonly characterised by an increase in weight, facial puffiness, and swelling of other parts of the body (e.g. ankles, hands, and wrists, Figure 7.6). Effusions into body cavities may occur (e.g. ascites).

Treatment

Treatment is directed at the underlying disease. The administration of diuretics (BNF 2.2) may be indicated.

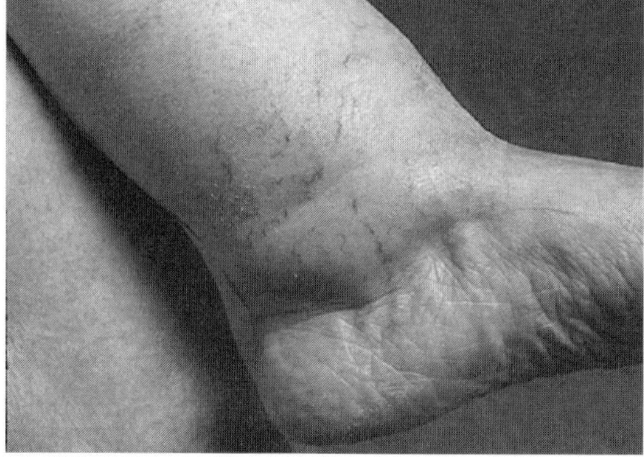

Figure 7.6 Ankle oedema. (Reproduced with permission of Alain Dex, Publiphoto diffusion/Science Photo Library.)

Polycystic kidney disease

Definition and aetiology

Polycystic kidney disease is an autosomally dominant inherited disease in which normal kidney tissue is replaced by cysts. Its cause is unknown. It has an incidence of about 1 in 1000, and almost all patients over 80 years of age have some sign of the disease. It also occurs in 5–10% of patients with end-stage renal disease.

Symptoms

The onset of the disease usually occurs between 30 and 40 years of age. Common symptoms include abdominal and back pain, haematuria, hypertension and urinary-tract infections. Polycystic kidney disease is a common cause of chronic renal failure. Hepatic cysts may accompany the renal cysts.

Treatment

No specific treatment exists, although drug treatment is indicated in the presence of hypertension and urinary-tract infection. Patients with chronic disease may eventually require dialysis or transplantation.

Renal calculi and colic

Definition and aetiology

Renal calculi (kidney or urinary stones) are abnormal hard concretions, composed mainly of mineral salts. The calculi are formed in the kidney and may be found in any part of the urinary tract (i.e. kidney, ureter, bladder and urethra). Calcium calculi are most common and may be associated with dehydration, hypercalcaemia or hypercalciuria. A low urinary pH or gout may result in the formation of uric acid calculi. Calculi of mixed composition (e.g. calcium phosphate and magnesium ammonium phosphate) may arise due to high urinary pH or after urinary-tract infection.

Symptoms

The presence of large calculi retained in the kidney may be asymptomatic. Most very small calculi are spontaneously voided in the urine. Calculi in the kidney may, however, cause loin pain, and a ureteric calculus may produce severe colicky pain (ureteric or renal colic) radiating from loin to groin. Bladder calculi may produce strangury, and urine flow may be interrupted by urethral calculi. Other symptoms include dysuria and frequency, haematuria and proteinuria, and recurrent urinary-tract infections. The pain of renal colic is very severe and often accompanied by retching and vomiting.

Treatment

Calculi associated with urinary-tract obstruction and infection should be surgically removed (lithotomy). Extraction via the urethra may be possible, and ultrasonic destruction (lithotripsy) may be used. In other cases, treatment is conservative. Any identifiable cause should be treated and patients should be maintained on a high fluid intake. Drugs which alter urinary pH may be of value (BNF 7.4.3). An opioid analgesic (BNF 4.7.2) may be required for renal colic and an injectable non-steroidal anti-inflammatory drug (BNF 10.1.1) has been shown to be of benefit.

Renal failure

Definition

Renal failure is the failure of the kidney to excrete metabolic waste products or to maintain plasma electrolytes at normal concentrations in the presence of normal dietary intake. It may be acute or chronic. In either case it is characterised by the development of uraemia. Drugs that are excreted by the kidney (e.g. many antimicrobials) will remain in the body for longer than is normal, and when used in renal failure their dosage will require adjustment.

Uraemia

Definition

Uraemia is a clinical state associated with advanced renal impairment and retention of nitrogenous waste products in the blood.

Symptoms

Initially it is characterised by fatigue, insomnia, lethargy and general malaise. This is followed by gastrointestinal symptoms (e.g. anorexia, diarrhoea, gastrointestinal bleeding, hiccup, and nausea and vomiting). If water intake is reduced, dehydration may occur because urine of a fixed osmolality is produced. Conversely, water retention may arise if fluid intake is increased. Hypertension together with sodium and water retention are common, and may lead to heart failure and resultant peripheral and pulmonary oedema. There may be pericarditis, and anaemia is a common sign.

Neurological symptoms include confusion with loss of concentration, muscle twitching and peripheral neuropathy. Convulsions and coma may develop. Infection, particularly of the urinary tract, is a common complication and may lead to septicaemia. Metabolic acidosis can occur and hyperphosphataemia may lead to hypocalcaemia. Hyperkalaemia may develop and result in sudden death.

Treatment

Haemodialysis or peritoneal dialysis will remove nitrogenous waste products from the blood and delay the onset of uraemia.

Acute renal failure

Definition and aetiology

Acute renal failure is a rapid, severe deterioration in renal function, resulting in acute uraemia. Acute failure may be caused by hypovolaemic shock, acute tubular necrosis, interstitial nephritis, acute glomerulonephritis, renal vascular abnormalities or urinary-tract obstruction. It may also arise as a result of drug administration (e.g. analgesics and antibacterials), septicaemia or heavy metal poisoning (e.g. lead). Other causes include burns, crushing injuries, malignant hypertension or heart failure. It may also occur after surgery.

Symptoms

By definition, the onset of acute renal failure is sudden. The only initial symptoms may be oliguria, back pain and tenderness, but these are followed by anuria and uraemic symptoms.

Treatment

Acute renal failure is a medical emergency. The underlying cause should be treated if possible. Hyperkalaemia must be treated immediately and a calcium salt (BNF 9.5.1.1) or glucose (BNF 9.2.2), or both, with or without insulin, may be given intravenously. In addition, an ion-exchange resin (BNF 9.2.1.1) may be used. A loop diuretic (BNF 2.2.2) may be administered, although fluid replacement may be necessary if the patient becomes dehydrated. Metabolic acidosis should be treated with an infusion of sodium bicarbonate with isotonic sodium chloride (BNF 9.2.2). Antiepileptics (BNF 4.8) and antihypertensive therapy (BNF 2.5) may be necessary. The patient should be maintained on a low-protein diet (BNF appendix 7) with fluid and electrolyte intake regulated. Dialysis may be indicated.

Chronic renal failure

Definition and aetiology
Chronic renal failure is a chronic reduction in renal function which is characterised by the progressive development of uraemia. It commonly arises as a result of glomerulonephritis, interstitial nephritis or pyelonephritis. Other causes include urinary-tract obstruction, hereditary abnormalities (e.g. polycystic kidney disease), or systemic disorders (e.g. diabetes mellitus, gout or systemic lupus erythematosus). It may also be due to nephrotoxic drugs (e.g. analgesics and antibacterials) or heavy metals (e.g. lead).

Symptoms
Initially, compensation for the loss of renal function may occur and the only symptoms of failure may be an impaired power of urine concentration and clearance, resulting in polyuria, nocturia and thirst. Pruritus and increased skin pigmentation may occur. Only when excretion fails to keep pace with production does uraemia develop.

Treatment
Treatment is as for acute renal failure (*see above*). Phosphate-binding agents (BNF 9.5.2.2) may be required to treat hyperphosphataemia, and a vitamin D analogue (BNF 9.6.4) to prevent renal osteodystrophy. Long-term dialysis or renal transplantation may prevent the fatal outcome of chronic renal failure.

Self-help organisations
British Kidney Patient Association
National Kidney Federation
The National Kidney Research Fund and Kidney Foundation

Renal osteodystrophy

Definition and aetiology
Renal osteodystrophy (renal rickets) is a collective term for a group of skeletal disorders which occur as a result of chronic renal failure. These disorders include osteitis fibrosa, osteomalacia and osteoporosis. They may occur singly or in combination, and are due to the development of hyperphosphataemia and hypocalcaemia together with hyperparathyroidism, and disturbed vitamin D metabolism. All of these can occur as a result of chronic renal failure. Renal osteodystrophy may be exacerbated by corticosteroid administration, and by aluminium retention resulting from dialysis.

Symptoms
Symptoms include bone pain and tenderness, fractures, joint disease, skeletal deformity and soft-tissue calcification. Growth retardation (renal dwarfism) may occur in children.

Treatment
Treatment consists of the administration of a phosphate-binding agent (BNF 9.5.2.2) and a vitamin D preparation (BNF 9.6.4). Calcium (BNF 9.5.1.1) and vitamin supplements without vitamin A (BNF 9.6) may be required. A reduction in dialysis fluid aluminium concentration may be helpful. If drug treatment is ineffective, parathyroidectomy may be considered.

7.5 Urinary-tract disorders

Urinary incontinence

Definition and aetiology
Urinary incontinence is characterised by constant or frequent involuntary urination.

Urge incontinence is involuntary urination which occurs as soon as the desire to urinate becomes apparent. It may be a consequence of dementia, stroke or urinary-tract infection, or caused by an instability of bladder smooth muscle (unstable detrusor muscle).

Stress incontinence occurs more commonly in women and is characterised by the leakage of urine as a result of stress (e.g. coughing, laughing or lifting). It is usually due to weakness of the pelvic floor muscles and may occur as a result of childbirth, the menopause, pregnancy or uterine prolapse. It may occur in men subsequent to prostatectomy.

Urinary incontinence may also occur as a result of drug administration (e.g. diuretics and hypnotics), neurological disorders (e.g. multiple sclerosis), or spinal cord injury (e.g. neurogenic bladder).

Treatment

Treatment comprises bladder training, the use of incontinence aids, and physiotherapy to strengthen the pelvic floor muscles. Catheterisation may be indicated in severe cases. Anticholinergic drugs or certain tricyclic antidepressants (BNF 7.4.2) may be helpful in urge incontinence, and surgery may be required in severe cases of stress incontinence.

Nocturnal enuresis

Definition and aetiology

Nocturnal enuresis is persistent involuntary urination during sleep. It occurs normally in young children, but is abnormal if it continues after the age at which control is usually achieved. It is most common in boys and a family history often exists. It is often associated with deep sleep and may be due to some underlying physical cause (e.g. phimosis, spina bifida or urethral stricture). Urinary-tract infection (e.g. cystitis and urethritis) may be responsible and it may be psychogenic.

Treatment

Appropriate antibacterial therapy (BNF 5.1) is indicated in the presence of urinary-tract infection. Enuretic alarms may be used, psychotherapy is beneficial in some patients, and surgical correction is required in others. In refractory cases, drug treatment comprises the administration of certain anticholinergic, sympathomimetic or tricyclic antidepressant drugs (BNF 7.4.2) . Bladder training, however, may be all that is required.

7.6 Anatomy and physiology of the genital, renal and urinary-tract systems

The male and female genital systems

The female reproductive organs

The female reproductive system (Figure 7.3) consists of the ovaries, the Fallopian tubes (oviducts), the uterus (womb), the vagina, and the external organs. The breasts are also considered to be part of the system.

The two ovaries, located one on each side of the uterus in the pelvic cavity, are the primary organs of the female system and are responsible for the maturation of the ova and the secretion of the reproductive hormones, the oestrogens and progesterone. Approximately 18 000 primary oocytes (the precursor cells from which the ova develop) are formed by the third month of fetal development and stored within the ovaries. The ovaries are suspended by ligaments immediately outside the open ends of the Fallopian tubes. The two Fallopian tubes provide the channels along which the ovum is transported from the ovary to the uterus. The movement of the ovum is assisted by peristaltic contractions of the muscular layer and surface cilia of the Fallopian tubes.

The uterus is the central feature of the female reproductive system. It is the site of origin of the elements in menstrual flow, the site of implantation and nurture of a fertilised ovum, and the tissue which expels the developed fetus from the mother's body. It is anatomically divided into the innermost fundus, the central tube-shaped body, and the outermost narrow neck of the uterus (the cervix). The outer surface of the uterine wall forms part of the peritoneum. The uterovesical and uterorectal pouches denote the front and rear projections of the peritoneum over the bladder and rectum respectively (*see* Figure 7.2). The muscular central portion of the uterus wall is the myometrium. The inner surface of the uterus (the endometrium) is highly vascularised and undergoes cyclical changes to its structure and thickness (*see below*).

The uterine orifice at the cervix is held tightly closed except during childbirth, although the opening is sufficient to allow the passage of sperm. The channel from the cervix to the exterior is formed of a muscular passageway (the vagina) which can dilate to accommodate the penis during sexual intercourse and to allow the passage of the fetus at birth.

The outermost organ of the female reproductive system is the vulva, which comprises the clitoris, the labia majora and minora, and the prepuce.

The menstrual and ovarian cycles

The ovum is produced within the ovary from the primary oocyte by meiosis (oogenesis). At puberty and cyclically until the menopause, an ovum develops each month during the first two weeks of the menstrual cycle (*see* Figure 7.4). The ovum is formed within a fluid-filled Graafian follicle and at ovulation it is released from the follicle into the pelvic cavity. The ovum is guided into the funnel-shaped infundibulum of the Fallopian tube by finger-like ciliary projections (the fimbriae). The remnants of the Graafian follicle in the ovary multiply rapidly and form the yellow, highly vascularised corpus luteum. The corpus luteum secretes oestrogens and progesterone, which act on the endometrium to increase its blood supply and thickness in preparation for the receipt of a fertilised ovum. If the ovum is not fertilised, the corpus luteum degenerates. The resultant decline in progesterone and oestrogen levels leads to menstruation through the breakdown and shedding of the endometrium (*see also* Section 6.6).

The mammary glands

The development of the mammary glands at puberty is stimulated by increased secretion of oestrogens and the presence of progesterone. Each gland (Figure 7.7) consists of 15–20 lobes separated by adipose tissue, the quantity of which determines the size of the breast. The lobes are subdivided into lobules consisting of connective tissue in which clusters of milk-secreting cells (the alveoli) are embedded. Milk is transported from the alveoli through the mammary ducts to storage compartments, the ampullae, and is then released to the nipple through lactiferous ducts.

The male reproductive organs

In the male, the organs analogous to the female ovaries are the testes. They are formed on the fetal posterior abdominal wall and descend before birth into a sac (the scrotum) located outside the body cavity (Figure 7.8). The position of the testes in an environment maintained 3 or 4°C below body temperature is important for the production and survival of sperm.

The testes are internally divided into 200–300 lobules, which each contain one to three highly convoluted seminiferous tubules of up to 60 cm in length. The spaces between the tubules are occupied by the interstitial cells of Leydig which secrete testosterone. The process of sperm production (spermatogenesis) starts at puberty and continues throughout life. It begins in the basement membrane of the seminiferous tubules with the formation of the spermatogonia, which become primary spermatocytes on detachment from the membrane. Meiotic division results in the formation of spermatids which develop into spermatozoa. The spermatozoa are transported from the seminiferous tubule to the epididymis where they undergo final maturation. Approximately 300 million spermatozoa reach full maturity each day.

The epididymis, which lies on the rear surface of the testis (Figure 7.9), consists of a tightly coiled tube which may extend to up to 6 metres in length. Spermatozoa may reside within the tube for up to four weeks but if they are not ejected within this period they are reabsorbed. Sperm are transported from the epididymis along the vas deferens (ductus deferens) into the ejaculatory duct located at the back of the bladder. The vas deferens is supported and protected by the spermatic cord (comprising arteries, veins, nerves, lymphatic vessels and muscle). From the ejaculatory duct, sperm enter the urethra which passes through the prostate gland and into the penis.

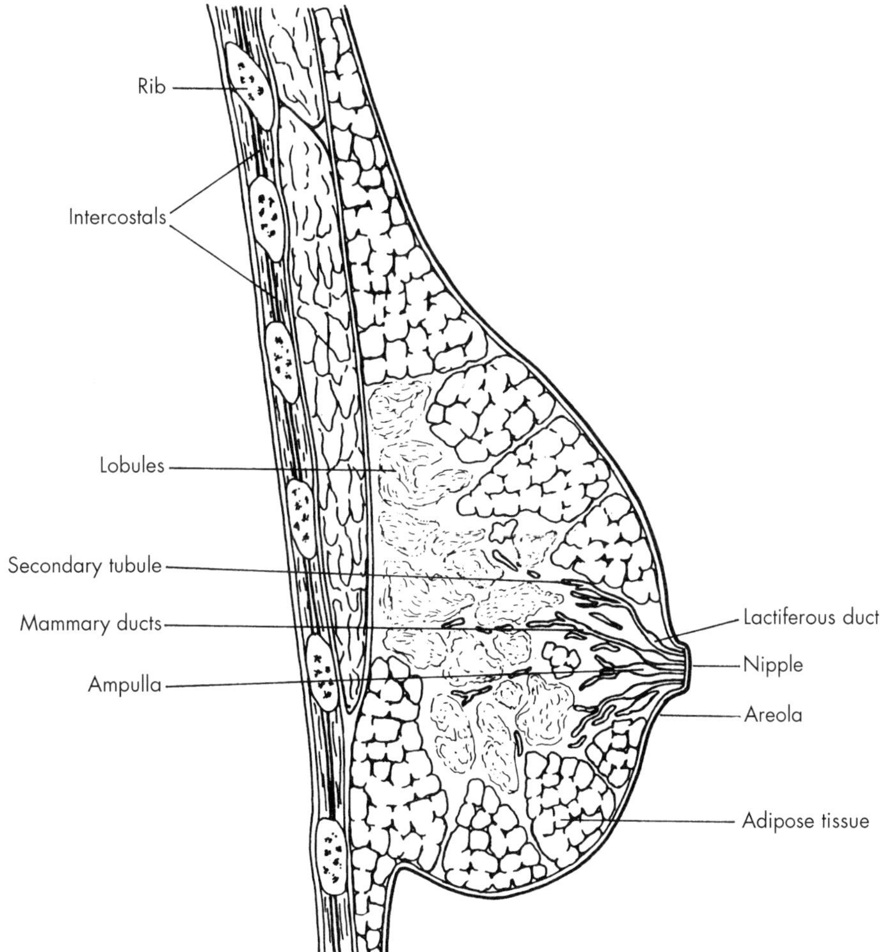

Figure 7.7 Breast (sagittal section).

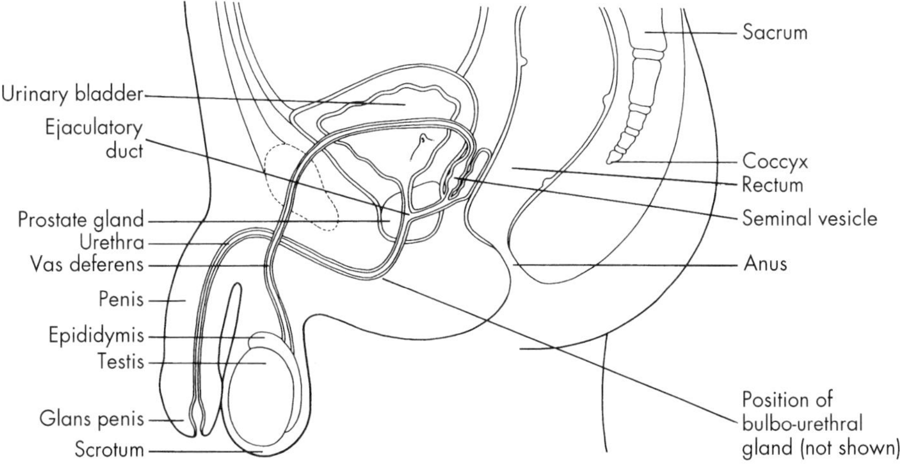

Figure 7.8 Male pelvic organs.

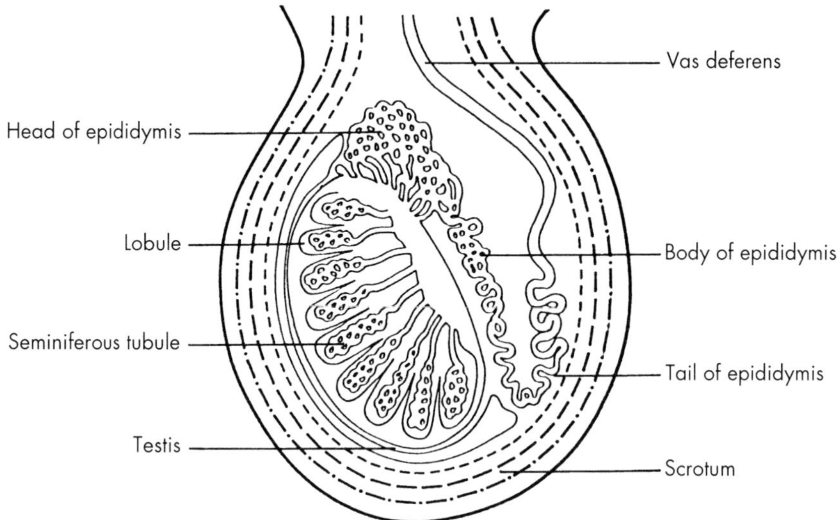

Figure 7.9 Cross-section of a testis.

The sperm are maintained within a fluid which is secreted by the prostate gland, the seminal vesicles, and the bulbo-urethral (Cowper's) glands. The prostate gland encircles the neck of the bladder and its alkaline secretions, which impart a milky appearance to seminal fluid, are added to the spermatozoa through numerous ducts into the prostatic portion of the urethra.

The seminal vesicles are a pair of sac-like structures lying on each side of the lower surface of the bladder. Their secretions, which include fructose in an alkaline medium, are added to the sperm in the vas deferens immediately before they enter the ejaculatory duct.

The bulbo-urethral glands are located underneath the prostate gland and secrete an alkaline fluid into the urethra.

The renal and urinary-tract systems

The kidneys are located within the rear of the abdominal cavity on either side of the vertebral column and are partially protected by the lowest pairs of ribs (Figure 7.10). They lie outside the peritoneal cavity (i.e. retroperitoneally) and are surrounded by a protective mass of fat, the adipose capsule.

Internally, the kidney consists of the renal parenchyma which is divided into an outer cortex and an inner medulla. The medulla contains from 5 to 14 pyramidal structures. The base of each pyramid forms the boundary between the cortex and medulla and the apex points towards the renal pelvis. The pyramids appear striated due to the presence of linear blood vessels and tubules. The renal pelvis is the collecting chamber for urine, which subsequently drains into the ureters, bladder and urethra.

Each kidney contains approximately one million nephrons which are the basic functional units. The head of the nephron is formed of a cup-shaped tubule (the Bowman's capsule) which embraces a capillary network (the glomerulus). Nephrons may be classed as cortical if the glomerulus lies in the outer cortex, or as juxtamedullary if the glomerulus lies within the cortex but close to the cortico-medulla border.

Beyond the Bowman's capsule the nephron consists sequentially of the proximal convoluted tubule, the loop of Henlé, the distal convoluted tubule and the collecting duct (*see* Figure 7.5).

The kidney receives approximately 25% of the blood output of the heart and is abundantly supplied with blood vessels. Blood enters the kidneys via the renal artery which subdivides into individual afferent arterioles for the glomerulus of

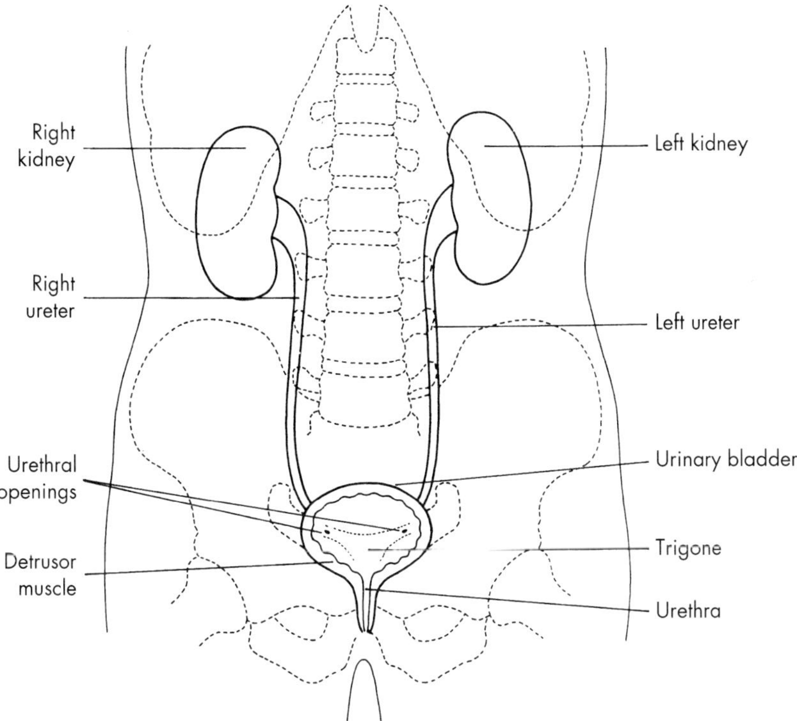

Figure 7.10 Position of kidneys and bladder.

each nephron. The network of capillaries which comprise the glomerulus rejoin to form the efferent arteriole (not an efferent venule). Capillaries branch off from the efferent arteriole to produce a meshwork of blood vessels around the convoluted tubules and loop of Henlé. These peritubular capillaries eventually reunite to pass blood to the renal vein which leaves the kidney near the renal pelvis.

The kidney carries out its roles of controlling blood volume and solute concentration, regulation of blood pH, and removal of toxic waste materials by the processes of glomerular filtration, tubular reabsorption and tubular secretion. Approximately 10% of the 1300 mL of blood which enters the glomerulus each minute is forced through the glomerular–Bowman's capsule interface. The pressure for filtration derives primarily from the hydrostatic pressure within the blood vessel but is opposed by osmotic pressure generated by the presence of plasma protein and the pressure of fluid already within the kidney tubule. Under normal circumstances, the filtrate consists of all blood components with the exception of blood cells and the larger proportion of plasma protein. In a healthy adult, the glomerular filtration rate is approximately 125 mL per minute, but of this only 1% is excreted as urine.

As the fluid passes along the nephron, essential materials are conserved through their transfer into the peritubular capillaries by the processes of diffusion, active reabsorption and electrostatic attraction. Under normal circumstances, all the glucose, amino acids and potassium ions present in the filtrate are actively reabsorbed in the proximal convoluted tubule.

Sodium ions are actively transported by the 'sodium pump' from the nephron, mainly in the proximal convoluted tubule and the loop of Henlé, but also in the distal convoluted tubule. The passage of sodium ions into the blood creates a temporary electropositive environment which is balanced by the reabsorption of chloride ions from the nephron.

The return of sodium ions into the plasma leads to the reabsorption of an iso-osmotic equivalent of water, and accounts for the reabsorption of approximately 80% of all water retained. The remainder is reabsorbed in the distal and collecting tubules under the influence of vasopressin, and it is this component which significantly affects the blood volume.

The homeostatic regulation of blood pH is achieved by the secretion of potassium and hydrogen ions in the distal convoluted tubule. Hydrogen ions, commonly in combination with ammonia produced by the deamination of amino acids, are secreted in exchange for the reabsorption of sodium ions, causing the pH of blood to rise. (Urea, another deamination waste product, is also excreted by the nephron.)

Hydrogen ions are also removed from the blood through the formation of carbonic acid. Carbon dioxide from the plasma diffuses into the cells lining the distal and collecting duct tubules. In these cells, it combines with water to form carbonic acid which can then dissociate to produce hydrogen ions and bicarbonate ions. If the pH of the blood is low (i.e. there is a high hydrogen ion concentration), a diffusion concentration gradient is established between the capillaries and the tubule, and hydrogen ions enter the urine. The electrostatic balance in the tubule cells is maintained by the reabsorption of a cation, usually sodium, from the urine. Sodium ions then combine with bicarbonate ions in the tubule cell and the product is absorbed into the blood. As a result, the pH of the blood is raised and the presence of sodium bicarbonate acts as a buffer to prevent a further fall in blood pH.

The end-product of the processes of filtration, reabsorption and secretion which occur in the kidney is urine. The volume of urine excreted each day varies from 1 to 2 litres and is influenced by many factors (e.g. blood pressure, temperature and fluid intake). Urine passes from the collecting ducts of each nephron into the renal pelvis. From the pelvis, a funnel-like neck narrows to form the ureter, a long muscular tube, which leads to the urinary bladder.

Urine flows down the ureter partially by gravity, but its passage is considerably assisted by peristaltic contractions of the muscular wall of the ureter. The waves of contraction cause the urine to enter the bladder in spurts occurring every 10–60 seconds.

The bladder is a muscular reservoir, which in the male lies directly in front of the rectum, and in the female is situated in front of the vagina and below the uterus. The ureters have to pass beneath the bladder to reach the openings, which arise on its floor in a triangular non-elastic muscular region, the trigone. This anatomical arrangement means that, despite the absence of reflux valves, the backflow of urine towards the kidneys is prevented by the pressure of the expanding bladder on the underlying ureters. The ureteral openings are situated at the two rear apices of the trigone, and the urethral orifice lies at the front apex.

As the bladder fills with urine, the muscular layer within its wall, the detrusor muscle, relaxes. When the volume within the bladder exceeds approximately 200–400 mL, stretch receptors in the detrusor muscle are stimulated, leading to the desire to void urine (micturition). The bladder initiates emptying by contraction of the detrusor muscles and relaxation of the internal bladder sphincter. Urine is voided by the conscious relaxation of the external sphincter which lies in the urogenital diaphragm (pelvic floor) and is composed of skeletal muscle.

The urethra is the vessel that carries urine from the base of the bladder to the outside. In males it is approximately 20 cm in length, but in females it is much shorter (approximately 4 cm).

8

Malignant disease

8.1 Malignant neoplasms of the gastrointestinal tract

Cancer of the gall bladder and bile ducts

Definition and aetiology
Cancer of the gall bladder is uncommon, but occurs more frequently in the elderly, particularly women. There may be an association with obesity and the presence of gallstones.

Bile-duct cancers are most commonly adenocarcinomas, slow-growing, and occur predominantly in the middle-aged and the elderly. An increased incidence may be associated with chronic ulcerative colitis.

Symptoms
In gall-bladder cancer, periodic pain and dyspepsia may be present for several years prior to diagnosis. Later symptoms, which indicate an advanced stage of the disease, may include

weight loss, severe pain particularly located in the right upper abdominal quadrant, and jaundice. A firm tender mass may also be felt at the site of the pain. Confirmation of diagnosis may be achieved with ultrasound or computerised tomography (CT).

Cancer of the bile ducts may produce symptoms of progressive obstruction. Jaundice, pruritus and weight loss may occur, together with dark urine and pale stools. Vomiting, and diarrhoea or constipation may also develop.

Treatment

The prognosis is poor in cancer of the gall bladder, but can be variable in cancer of the bile ducts. Surgical removal of the gall bladder and liver resection may be attempted in cancer of the gall bladder, often with very limited success. It is not usually possible to excise the slower growing bile-duct tumour, although drainage of bile can be facilitated by the insertion of prostheses.

Cancer of the liver

Definition and aetiology

Cancer of the liver is a disease with a grim outlook. It commonly occurs secondary to cancer in another organ and only infrequently as a primary malignancy (hepatocellular carcinoma).

Metastatic carcinoma of the liver

Definition and aetiology

The passage of blood through the liver may act as a source of metastases, particularly from the gastrointestinal tract and respiratory system. The breast may also be a primary source of the cancer. Initial diagnosis of the primary cancer, particularly in the elderly, may be shown through the presence of liver metastases.

Symptoms

Non-specific symptoms include weight loss, anorexia and fever. The degree of hepatomegaly may correspond to the stage of advancement of the disease. Splenomegaly and ascites may also occur and, in later stages, jaundice may develop. Liver function tests may initially remain normal, although alkaline phosphatase levels may rise steadily as the disease progresses.

Treatment

Treatment is commonly ineffective.

Hepatocellular carcinoma

Definition and aetiology

Hepatocellular carcinoma is a primary malignant disease that is less common than metastatic carcinoma of the liver. The condition is comparatively rare in the western world, but has a higher incidence in Africa and South East Asia. It is most commonly associated with pre-existing cirrhosis, although chronic hepatitis B virus infections have also been implicated.

Symptoms

The onset may be insidious. Presenting symptoms include right upper abdominal pain, fever and weight loss. Abdominal swelling may be caused by hepatomegaly, in the presence or absence of ascites. The tumour may rupture, causing intraperitoneal bleeding.

Treatment

The mean survival time is limited to several months. Improvement in survival time may only be achieved by transplantation or complete resection, although surgical resection is frequently hampered by the presence of cirrhosis. Chemotherapy may be beneficial, with a positive response sometimes obtained following intravenous administration of doxorubicin (BNF 8.1.2).

Cancer of the stomach

Definition and aetiology

Stomach cancer is commonly an adenocarcinoma. It has a varied geographical distribution, and has been tentatively linked to genetic factors because of a higher incidence in people of blood group A. Environmental and dietary factors are more important, and proposed factors include ingestion of pickled foods and alcohol, and inhalation of smoke and dust particles. Interest has been expressed in the levels of nitrates in water or food, as they are converted to potentially carcinogenic nitrosamines by bacteria in the intestine.

Stomach cancer is predominantly a condition of old age, with the highest incidence in those of 60–70 years of age. It is the third most common fatal cancer in the UK, with an incidence of about 8 per 100 000. Its incidence appears to be declining, although the reason for this is unknown.

Symptoms

Early disease may be asymptomatic, and many patients do not present until the condition is advanced. Dyspepsia, epigastric pain, and a feeling of fullness after eating may be early signs which are difficult to distinguish from peptic ulceration. Later signs may include anorexia, nausea and vomiting, and weight loss, resulting in weakness. Anaemia may also occur as a result of occult blood loss. Metastases may cause abdominal swelling due to ascites, or jaundice due to liver involvement. Metastases may also arise in bone, brain and lungs.

Treatment

Early surgical removal of the tumour (partial gastrectomy) provides the best prognosis, giving a five-year survival rate of 90%. However, few tumours are diagnosed sufficiently early. The survival rate in advanced disease is considerably reduced. Total parenteral nutrition (BNF 9.3) may be required. Chemotherapy has been used with limited success.

Carcinoid syndrome

Definition and aetiology

The carcinoid syndrome (argentaffinoma syndrome) comprises a varied and complex group of symptoms occurring in patients with malignant carcinoid tumours (argentaffinoma). The primary tumour may originate in the argentaffin cells of the gastrointestinal tract (most commonly in the terminal ileum, appendix and rectum), lung tissue, ovaries and testes. Most patients with carcinoid tumours do not, however, get the syndrome. Whereas symptoms of the syndrome may be produced by primary lung and gonadal tumours, they do not develop from primary gastrointestinal tumours unless hepatic metastases have arisen. This is because the biologically active agents (e.g. serotonin and prostaglandins) released from these tumours are metabolised in the hepatic-portal system before they can reach the general circulation.

Symptoms

The syndrome is characterised classically by flushing. This may be accompanied by a sensation of intense heat, hypotension and tachycardia. The flush, which ranges from redness to cyanosis, typically affects the head and neck, but in severe cases may spread to the trunk and limbs. The duration of the flush ranges from minutes to almost continuous. Flushing may be precipitated by alcohol, caffeine, food, emotional disturbances and other forms of stress. Other symptoms include bronchospasm, diarrhoea (which is often severe and may be associated with abdominal pain), nausea and vomiting, weight loss and wheezing. Complications include obstruction of the small intestine, pellagra, and pulmonary and tricuspid stenosis, causing dyspnoea and oedema as a result of right ventricular failure.

Treatment

Treatment is directed towards alleviating the symptoms. Surgical removal of the primary tumour is indicated only if it is situated in the lungs, ovaries or testes. Surgery to remove liver metastases or selective embolisation via the hepatic artery may help relieve symptoms. Flushing may be controlled by avoidance of precipitating factors, and by the administration of alpha-adrenoceptor blocking drugs (BNF 2.5.4), or phenothiazines (BNF 4.2.1). Antihistamines (BNF 3.4.1) and H_2-receptor blocking drugs (BNF 1.3) may also be used. The use of corticosteroids (BNF 6.3.2) is reserved for severe and protracted attacks.

Diarrhoea may be treated with antidiarrhoeal drugs which reduce motility (BNF 1.4.2); colestyramine (BNF 1.5) may reduce bile acid-induced diarrhoea in patients with a resected ileum. Specific serotonin antagonists such as cyproheptadine (BNF 3.4.1) or methysergide (BNF 4.7.4.2) may be effective in controlling intractable diarrhoea and flushing, but methysergide should be used with caution in view of the risk of retroperitoneal fibrosis. Nicotinamide (BNF 9.6.2) and adequate protein intake are required to prevent and treat pellagra.

Colorectal cancer

Definition and aetiology

Cancers in the large intestine may be classified as adenomas found as polyps, which are frequently precancerous, and adenocarcinomas found in colorectal cancer.

A significant proportion of cancers of the large intestine occur in the rectum and sigmoid colon. Colonic cancer is more common in women, whereas rectal cancer is twice as common in men. Most cancers are adenocarcinomas, slow-growing and form discrete anatomical entities that can be easily removed. Metastases may develop in the liver and bladder.

The incidence has been related to the intake of fat, meat, processed foods and alcohol, with diets high in fibre producing a low incidence. Ulcerative colitis may also be a predisposing factor. With the exception of those cases associated with genetic factors (e.g. familial adenomatous polyposis, *see* Polyps, Section 1.1), most cases of colorectal cancer arise in the middle-aged and the elderly.

Colorectal cancer is the second most common cause of new cases of cancer in the western world, after lung cancer. The disease usually appears after 40 years of age, reaching a peak between 60 and 75 years of age.

Symptoms

Symptoms in the early stages may include occult blood in the stools, fatigue and weakness. Patients may also report a change in bowel habits. Late symptoms may occur (e.g. pain and weight loss) and a detectable mass may be caused by the tumour or blockage of faeces.

Treatment

Surgery is the primary form of treatment. Colorectal carcinomas may be surgically excised and the large intestine resected. If the anal sphincter is involved, the formation of a colostomy is required. Radiotherapy may be beneficial, particularly for patients who are experiencing significant pain. Some patients may respond to chemotherapy with fluorouracil (BNF 8.1.3).

Screening for the prevention and early detection of the disease is possible and should be carried out in any cases of undiagnosed bowel habit changes.

Oesophageal cancer

Definition and aetiology

Malignant tumours in the oesophagus arise predominantly in the middle and lower portions. They are commonly squamous cell carcinomas, although a small proportion may be adenocarcinomas. Oesophageal tumours have been associated with heavy alcohol and tobacco consumption. Poisoning with corrosive agents may also increase the likelihood of cancer due to oesophageal damage. Achalasia has also been linked with oesophageal cancer.

Symptoms

The commonest symptom is dysphagia, initially only present on ingestion of solids, but subsequently also associated with fluid intake. The presence of persistent chest pain warns of infiltration, with metastases commonly arising in the liver, gastric glands, lungs and aorta. Weight loss and anorexia may develop, possibly associated with difficulty in swallowing. In advanced stages of the disease, anaemia may also occur.

Treatment

Symptomatic relief may be obtained by oesophageal dilatation. Surgery may be useful, particularly in adenocarcinoma, but is often associated with a high incidence of mortality. Chemotherapy is of little value, but radiotherapy and laser photocoagulation may provide temporary relief. The prognosis is poor following diagnosis, with an expected five-year survival rate of less than 5%.

Pancreatic (exocrine) cancer

Definition and aetiology

Pancreatic (exocrine) cancer is an invariably fatal disease and is usually an adenocarcinoma. Most malignancies arise in the head of the gland although, because early diagnosis is difficult, dissemination to many sites may occur prior to initial identification. Metastases to the lung and liver are common.

Pancreatic cancer occurs most commonly in patients of 50 years of age and over and is more common in men and in smokers than non-smokers. A high incidence has also been correlated with a high dietary fat content, alcohol intake, and with diabetes mellitus.

Symptoms
The predominant symptom is usually pain, commonly arising in the upper abdomen. The pain may be aggravated by food and relieved by changes in posture. Obstructive jaundice may develop due to blockage of the bile duct or gall bladder. Other non-specific symptoms may include a progressive loss of weight, anorexia and lassitude. If the tumour is initially localised to the body or tail of the gland, gastric and oesophageal varices may occur in association with splenomegaly and gastrointestinal haemorrhage.

Treatment
Most measures which may be taken after diagnosis are palliative only. Surgery (e.g. total pancreatectomy) may be carried out but must be followed by pancreatin supplements (BNF 1.9.4) and insulin therapy (BNF 6.1.1). Chemotherapy has not proved effective, although fluorouracil (BNF 8.1.3) in combination with radiotherapy has shown a slight improvement in life expectancy. However, most patients do not survive beyond nine months.

8.2 Malignant neoplasms of the respiratory system

Cancer of the pleura and peritoneum

Definition and aetiology
Cancer of the pleura and peritoneum may arise as a primary malignancy or as a metastasis. Primary cancer, which usually takes the form of a mesothelioma, commonly arises through exposure to asbestos. Unlike lung cancer, it is not related to smoking. The mesothelioma usually arises in the pleura, but it may also originate in the peritoneum.

Metastatic pleural cancer can occur as a consequence of cancer of the lung, breast and ovaries, and may develop unilaterally or bilaterally.

Symptoms
Symptoms of primary malignancy may be ill-defined and include dyspnoea, dull chest pain and weakness. Cough, pyrexia and weight loss are less common symptoms. Radiography may reveal massive pleural effusions.

Treatment
Surgery is not feasible, whereas radiotherapy and chemotherapy may be beneficial in a minority of early cases. The accumulation of pleural fluid may be retarded by intrapleural injection of tetracycline (BNF 5.1.3), bleomycin (BNF 8.1.2) or thiotepa (BNF 8.1.1). These irritant substances produce adhesion between the inner surfaces of the pleural membranes and are injected following drainage of the pleural fluid. The prognosis is grim, with an average survival of 8–10 months.

Lung cancer

Definition and aetiology
Lung cancer (bronchial carcinoma) may arise primarily in the bronchi, or as a secondary growth from other parts of the body (e.g. pancreas, breast, colon and bone). It occurs most frequently between 50 and 70 years of age. It is the most common cause of death from cancer in males in the UK; the incidence is relatively constant in women. It accounts for 35 000 deaths each year in England and Wales.

Well-documented statistical studies have linked the development of lung cancer to various factors, the most common being smoking (cigarette, cigar and pipe). The incidence may be related to the amount smoked each day, the depth of inhalation, number of puffs and the type of tobacco smoked. All tobacco smoking can cause lung cancer, but the incidence is greatest in cigarette smoking. There is also a correlation between the degree of risk and how young the individual is when smoking is started. Individuals subjected to continual smoke-filled atmospheres also have a higher risk of developing lung cancer through passive smoking.

Other causes of lung cancer include ionising radiations, asbestos, and possibly air pollution. Occupations associated with a high risk of lung cancer include workers exposed to tar in steel and aluminium industries, and environments where a high level of polycyclic hydrocarbons may be introduced into the atmosphere.

The classification of lung cancers has been devised by the World Health Organization (WHO). Epidermoid (squamous) cell cancers give rise to bulky tumours and are commonly attributable to smoking. They occur predominantly in the larger bronchi and are spread through the lymphatic system. Small (oat) cell cancers are undifferentiated cells which may arise anywhere within the proximal large bronchi. The cells are rapid-growing, are commonly induced by ionising radiations, and are highly invasive. Adenocarcinomas, which appear in the periphery of the lung and are spread through the bloodstream, are less directly the consequence of smoking. The remainder of the cell types which appear in lung cancer are grouped under the classification of large cell carcinomas. They are commonly caused by smoking and, like adenocarcinomas, are spread through the bloodstream.

Symptoms

The symptoms of lung cancer are varied and depend on various factors. These include the type of cancer cell; the direct spread of the tumour to adjacent tissues and indirect metastasis via the blood and lymphatic system; and the secretion of hormones and other agents from the tumour which may give rise to metabolic, endocrine and neurological symptoms.

Cough is commonly the primary symptom. A smoker may cough as a result of chronic bronchitis, and a change in the nature and severity of the cough may be an important indication of the development of cancer. Excess sputum in the bronchial tree (produced as a direct consequence of the tumour, from infection due to blockage, or the presence of the tumour itself) may cause the entrapment of air in the alveoli, leading to wheezing and atelectasis. Haemoptysis, commonly seen as streaking in the sputum, may occur in up to 50% of patients. Less clearly defined symptoms, but whose presence may indicate a deterioration in general health, include chest pain or ache, dyspnoea, weight loss, lack of energy and a loss of interest.

Complications may develop from the pressure of the growth on adjacent structures or from the presence of metastases. The superior vena cava may become compressed, resulting in distension of the veins of the neck, thorax and upper arms. Associated symptoms may include oedema of the face and neck, headache, and pleural effusions. Speech impairment may be a consequence of compression of the laryngeal nerve, and dysphagia can occur as a result of oesophageal constriction. Metastases are common in the skeleton (e.g. the humerus, ribs and vertebrae), liver and brain.

Endocrine complications occur due to the production of polypeptides which mimic the action of endogenous hormones (e.g. vasopressin, adrenocorticotrophin, parathormone and gonadotrophin).

Treatment

With the exception of the majority of small cell lung cancers, surgery is the most effective means of treatment. Surgical excision (thoracotomy) of a well-formed mass may give a better prognosis, although surgery may be contraindicated in patients with cardiac or respiratory impairment, and in those with distant metastases.

Radiotherapy is used primarily for the relief of symptoms, although it has been employed as an adjunct before and after surgery. It is effective in reducing the pain of bone and brain metastases.

Chemotherapy is used predominantly for the treatment of small cell lung cancers. Drugs are most effective when used in combinations of up to four agents (BNF 8.1) comprising members from each of the classes of cytotoxic drugs. Survival times for patients with localised small cell cancer may be up to 18 months and for patients with extensive disease up to 12 months. Other drugs may be required to treat the complications of lung cancer. Antibacterial drugs (BNF 5.1) may be used for respiratory infections and dexamethasone (BNF 6.3.4) for the control of cerebral oedema from brain metastases.

8.3 Malignant neoplasms of the central nervous system

Intracranial tumours

Definition and aetiology

Intracranial tumours constitute a wide variety of cell types which produce a broad spectrum of disease. The classification of malignant and benign is less important in the brain than in other tissues of the body, as the ability of the brain to accommodate any growth is extremely limited.

Tumours may arise from the meninges, the skull, or any component of the central nervous tissue. Primary tumours predominate, although approximately 25% of all intracranial tumours may arise as metastases from the lungs, kidneys, breast, thyroid and melanomas. Central nervous tissue is the second most common site for primary tumours in childhood. No causative agents have been linked to the incidence, but certain primary tumours (e.g. meningioma and optic glioma) have been associated with von Recklinghausen's neurofibromatosis.

The commonest form of intracranial tumours develops from neural tubes and is classed as gliomas. These are further subdivided as astrocytomas, oligodendrogliomas and medulloblastomas. Astrocytomas may be benign or malignant and occur at any age. They may be well circumscribed and slow-growing, producing few early clinical symptoms, or rapidly proliferating and invasive and causing significant cerebral oedema. Oligodendrogliomas are extremely slow-growing and only appear in adulthood. Medulloblastomas usually develop in the roof of the fourth ventricle, are extremely malignant, and appear in childhood. Unlike the majority of other intracranial tumours, they form metastases in bone and bone marrow.

The second largest group of tumours is classed as meningiomas. They occur predominantly in adults of 40–60 years of age, are commonly benign, and usually develop from arachnoid cells to appear on the dorsal surface of the brain and the base of the skull. If there is a rich vascular supply to the tumour, it may be described as angioblastic, and on enlargement may cause erosion of the skull.

Schwannomas (neurilemmomas or neurinomas) are derived from Schwann cells (which supply the myelin sheath) and are benign. The presence of a Schwannoma on the acoustic nerve may affect hearing as a result of pressure on the nerve.

Pituitary tumours may develop from the remnants of the pituitary stalk (craniopharyngiomas) and cause compression of the optic nerve and chiasma, hypopituitarism and hydrocephalus. Pituitary adenomas are more common and usually benign. They may be secreting, producing a range of pituitary hormones (e.g. adrenocorticotrophin, growth hormone and prolactin), or non-secreting, causing compression of normal pituitary tissue and resulting in hypopituitarism.

Haemangioblastomas are benign tumours of uncertain origin but are normally classed as vascular tumours. They are commonly found in the cerebellum of adolescents and young adults, and usually arise singly and are cystic.

Other less common forms of intracranial tumours include colloid cysts and choroid plexus papillomas.

Symptoms

The symptoms of an intracranial tumour vary according to its size, location, morphological characteristics and rate of growth. Symptoms may be attributed to raised intracranial pressure, epilepsy and localised neurological changes.

Raised intracranial pressure produces headache, vomiting, drowsiness and visual disturbances. Headache commonly occurs early in the morning or may wake the patient from sleep. It may be aggravated by factors that further increase intracranial pressure (e.g. coughing). In the presence of a tumour in the fourth ventricle, vomiting may occur on its own or as a precursor to headache. Drowsiness, increased lethargy and tiredness indicate depression of the central nervous system and are signs of severe worsening of the patient's condition. Deterioration in vision, commonly due to enlargement of the blind spot as a result of papilloedema, also requires urgent investigation.

The development of epilepsy or changes in the nature of epileptic attacks, particularly when accompanied by changes in behaviour, are positive warnings of intracranial tumours. Seizures may be generalised or focal, and the type of seizure may provide an indication of the site of the lesion.

Localised neurological changes may be subtle and identified only by those who have irregular contact with the patient. The most common changes include reduced memory, increased irritability, reduction in coordination, dizziness, fatigue and lethargy. Personality changes may be apparent and, in the later stages of the condition, stupor, confusion and dementia may develop.

Other symptoms may reflect the changes in pituitary function (e.g. acromegaly, amenorrhoea and hyperprolactinaemia) and hypothalamic function (e.g. diabetes insipidus and disturbed temperature regulation).

Treatment

Suspected intracranial tumours may be investigated by computerised tomography (CT) scanning, radioisotopic brain scanning and nuclear magnetic resonance (NMR) scanning. Treatment may involve relieving severe symptoms or specific measures to remove as great a proportion of the tumour tissue while preserving brain function intact.

Non-specific emergency measures may include the use of intravenous antiepileptics (BNF 4.8) and the administration of dexamethasone (BNF 6.3.4) to counteract cerebral oedema. Headache may be treated with non-opioid (BNF 4.7.1), or non-depressant opioid (BNF 4.7.2), analgesics.

Surgery may be used to completely remove the tumour or to relieve intracranial pressure. Complete excision may be impracticable due to the diffuse boundary between tumour and healthy tissue, and the need to limit the damage to surrounding structures. Hydrocephalus produced as a result of raised pressure within the cerebral ventricles may be relieved by insertion of a ventriculo-atrial or ventriculo-peritoneal shunt.

External irradiation may be carried out over a period for the treatment of malignant primary and secondary tumours, although meningiomas are insensitive to radiotherapy. Improved results may be obtained with less malignant growths and in patients who have previously had intracranial pressure reduced surgically.

Chemotherapy is ineffective for the treatment of primary intracranial tumours, but may be used in secondary deposits.

Spinal cord tumours

Definition and aetiology

Tumours within the spinal cord may be classified as extramedullary, occurring outside the spinal cord but within the surrounding membranes, or intramedullary. All tumours of the spinal cord are rarer than intracranial tumours and tend to develop in middle life. The majority are extramedullary, malignant and spread rapidly. Primary tumours include neurofibromas (which develop from the Schwann cells of the spinal roots), meningiomas and astrocytomas. Metastatic tumours are also common and may develop from almost any site (e.g. breast, lung or from lymphomas).

Symptoms

Most symptoms of spinal cord tumours arise as a result of compression of the spinal cord and spinal nerve roots. Initial symptoms, which include pain and paraesthesia, may develop insidiously and commonly occur in areas below the site of the lesion. Pain may be localised, mild or severe, and located to one or both sides of the spine. Sensory loss, muscle weakness and muscle wasting along the distribution of the affected nerves may ensue. Progressive growth of the tumour may lead to spasticity, and loss of control of bladder and bowel function. Intramedullary tumours may produce symptoms which mimic syringomyelia. Some secondary tumours can produce paraplegia within hours or days.

Treatment

Surgical excision may be possible for extramedullary primary tumours, although only partial excision may be practicable to retain function. Radiotherapy may be necessary postoperatively. Intramedullary and non-operable extramedullary tumours may benefit from radiotherapy in isolation or following surgical decompression. Corticosteroids (BNF 6.3.2) may be used to reduce spinal cord oedema.

8.4 Endocrine malignant neoplasms

Pancreatic endocrine tumours

Definition
Pancreatic endocrine tumours must be differentiated from pancreatic cancer, which involves the exocrine functions of the pancreas (*see above*). Endocrine tumours may secrete a particular hormone in isolation (*see below*) or in combination (multiple endocrine adenomatosis), giving rise to varied clinical syndromes. The tumours commonly occur in association with other forms of neoplasm (e.g. pituitary adenomas).

Insulinoma

Definition and aetiology
Insulinomas are rare adenomas of the beta-cells of the pancreas and are responsible for the continued secretion of insulin even in the presence of fasting. The tumour is usually small and slow-growing and may develop in any part of the pancreas. The condition can develop at any age, but there is a peak incidence between 40 and 60 years of age. Only approximately 10% of cases are malignant.

Symptoms
Symptoms are related to the development of hypoglycaemia and may be especially prominent several hours after a meal or on exercise. Central nervous system symptoms include headache, drowsiness on waking, confusion and lightheadedness. Palpitations, sweating and hunger may also develop. In severe forms, unconsciousness, convulsions and coma may develop. Some patients may become obese as frequent meals prevent symptoms, although most patients do not experience a change in weight.

Malignant insulinomas may produce metastases (e.g. in the liver), and uncontrollable hypoglycaemia may be fatal.

Treatment
Surgical excision is the treatment of choice. Deep-set adenomas may require distal subtotal pancreatectomy. If symptoms persist, total pancreatectomy may be necessary. Diazoxide (BNF 6.1.4) is used to treat hypoglycaemia. Streptozocin, fluorouracil or doxorubicin, alone or in combination, may be used for treatment of metastases.

Glucagonoma

Definition and aetiology
Glucagonoma is a very rare alpha-cell tumour of the pancreas, which occurs in adulthood with a mean onset at 50 years of age. The majority of tumours occur in women and are malignant.

Symptoms
Patients commonly present with insulin-dependent diabetes mellitus and a distinctive rash. A chronic necrolytic migratory rash may occur on the extremities and the perineum, and is accompanied by bullae which break down, heal and subsequently recur at a different position. The lesions are reddish-brown and exfoliating. Other symptoms include a vermilion tongue, cheilitis, weight loss, diarrhoea and crumbling nails.

Treatment
Reversal of the rash and diabetic symptoms may be obtained by surgical excision of the tumour. If metastases have been produced or the tumour is not resectable, streptozocin and doxorubicin may be useful. The rash may also respond to administration of oral corticosteroids (BNF 6.3.2) and oral tetracycline (BNF 5.1.3).

Zollinger–Ellison syndrome

Definition and aetiology
The Zollinger–Ellison syndrome is a condition in which there is an increased plasma gastrin concentration and hypersecretion of gastric acid. Peptic ulceration or diarrhoea, or both, may also occur. The increased plasma gastrin is usually due to a gastrin-secreting tumour of the pancreas (gastrinoma) which may be malignant.

Symptoms
The syndrome is characterised by diarrhoea, and abdominal pain due to peptic ulceration; steatorrhoea may sometimes occur. Multiple ulcers are

frequently present, but occasionally diarrhoea may occur in the absence of ulceration. Haemorrhage or perforation occurring soon after gastric surgery is characteristic of the syndrome.

Treatment

Treatment involves the administration of omeprazole (BNF 1.3.5), together with an antimuscarinic (BNF 1.2) if necessary. Resection of the tumour and selective vagotomy may be carried out, and total gastrectomy may be required if medical treatment is ineffective.

Phaeochromocytoma

Definition and aetiology

A phaeochromocytoma is a catecholamine-producing tumour arising from chromaffin tissue usually in the adrenal medulla but sometimes in other sites; the tumours are usually benign. Phaeochromocytomas are often familial and may be associated with other disorders (e.g. von Recklinghausen's neurofibromatosis).

Symptoms

Phaeochromocytoma is characterised by hypertension, which may be paroxysmal or sustained, with exacerbations occurring during paroxysmal attacks. In a minority of patients, hypotension may develop, often following a paroxysmal hypertensive attack. Severe headache, tachycardia, pain in the chest and abdomen, sweating, apprehension, nausea and vomiting, orthostatic hypotension, weight loss, hyperglycaemia, and glycosuria may occur. Paroxysmal attacks may occur several times a day or sometimes less frequently. They usually last between 15 and 60 minutes and are followed by exhaustion, weakness and aching muscles. Pallor commonly occurs but may be followed by cyanosis. Paroxysmal attacks may be precipitated by changes in posture, emotional stress, exercise, straining during defecation, abdominal pressure and administration of anaesthetics.

Treatment

Phaeochromocytoma is treated by the surgical removal of the tumour. Alpha-adrenoceptor blocking drugs (BNF 2.5.4) are used in conjunction with beta-adrenoceptor blocking drugs (BNF 2.4) for short-term management of paroxysmal attacks. Metirosine (BNF 2.5.7) may be used alone or in combination with an alpha-adrenoceptor blocking drug in pre-operative treatment and in patients with inoperable tumours.

Thyroid cancer

Definition and aetiology

Thyroid cancer is a comparatively rare form of cancer of uncertain aetiology (although it is the most common endocrine gland cancer). Its incidence has been related to the former practice of irradiation of the head, neck and upper thorax for the treatment of minor illnesses of childhood (e.g. thymic enlargement, tonsillitis and acne), although the time lag between irradiation and the development of thyroid cancer may be up to 30 years.

The majority of primary thyroid malignancies are papillary carcinomas. These are slow-growing, and may infiltrate the local lymph nodes, neck muscles, lungs, bone and the trachea. They occur primarily between 20 and 40 years of age. Follicular carcinomas occur later in life, predominantly in women, and have a greater malignant potential than papillary carcinomas. They may spread to the lungs and bone through the blood. Other rarer forms of thyroid cancer are medullary and anaplastic carcinomas.

Symptoms

The presence of thyroid cancer may be asymptomatic apart from the presence of a palpable mass in the neck region. The distinction between a thyroid nodule and the presence of thyroid cancer may be difficult.

Treatment

Small discrete papillary carcinomas may be surgically excised, although the amount of tissue removed from larger tumours may be determined by the degree of spread of the carcinoma. Unilateral lobectomy is preferred but greater tissue involvement may require total or subtotal thyroidectomy. Follicular carcinoma invariably requires total thyroidectomy.

Thyroxine (BNF 6.2.1) may be administered to suppress regrowth and to reduce the secretion of thyroid-stimulating hormone. Radioactive iodine (^{131}I) may be used to ablate remaining thyroid tissue, in which case subsequent thyroxine administration is essential. The prognosis for papillary and follicular carcinomas is good, although the outlook for rarer forms is less good.

8.5 Malignant neoplasms of the gynaecological and genito-urinary systems

8.5.1 GYNAECOLOGICAL MALIGNANT NEOPLASMS

Breast cancer

Definition and aetiology
Breast cancer is the most common fatal cancer in women, accounting in the developed world for approximately 20% of all female deaths from cancer. It is rare in women under 30 years of age, but its incidence increases with age, particularly after the menopause. Breast cancer is commonly an adenocarcinoma.

The incidence of breast cancer has been linked to hormonal and genetic factors. The combination of an early menarche and late menopause, and the greater the age at the time of the first pregnancy, have been associated with increased rates. Breast-feeding does not protect against the development of breast cancer, although the age at which lactation is initiated may be important. The risk is approximately trebled if there is a family history of breast cancer, suggesting an aetiological role for genetic factors.

Breast cancer may also occur rarely in men (e.g. in Klinefelter's syndrome and other male genital disorders).

Clinically, breast cancer may be classified as stage I (early stages of the disease with negligible lymph node involvement) through to stage IV (the presence of tumours of greater than 5 cm diameter and metastases). Tumours may also be categorised as oestrogen-receptor protein positive or negative, depending on their ability to bind radiolabelled estradiol, and this may be important for drug therapy (*see below*).

Metastases are common (e.g. in the liver, pleura and bone) and may arise by direct invasion of localised tissue or via the lymphatics and bloodstream.

Symptoms
The detection of a slow-growing, single, painless lump in the breast, especially in women in high-risk groups, is often presumed to indicate breast cancer until proved otherwise. There may be vague discomfort, but more serious signs include a retracted nipple, bleeding from the nipple, distorted breast contour, oedema of the skin of the breast, skin dimpling and ulceration above the site of the lesion, and enlargement of localised lymph nodes. The breast mass may become attached to the surrounding chest wall. Diagnosis may be aided by mammography.

Treatment
Radical mastectomy (in which pectoral muscles are removed as well as mammary tissue and axillary lymph nodes) is now less widely used. It has been superseded by the cosmetically more acceptable modified radical mastectomy in which the pectoral muscles are retained. The 10-year survival rates for both procedures are less than 50%.

Conservative surgery (partial mastectomy) may be possible for primary stage I and II tumours, followed by radiotherapy. This gives excellent cosmetic results, and is replacing both forms of radical mastectomy. Radiotherapy may also be used following surgery if metastases of the lymphatic system are found.

Hormonal therapy may be used to relieve the symptoms and retard the development of the disease. It may be combined with radiotherapy in recurrent cases following surgery, or in advanced disease. Oestrogens (BNF 8.3.1) may be used in post-menopausal women and are particularly effective in those who are oestrogen-receptor protein positive. Progestogens (BNF 8.3.2) may be reserved for refractory cases. The most successful form of hormonal treatment in pre- and post-menopausal women is the use of tamoxifen (BNF 8.3.4.1), although the majority of successful cases are oestrogen-receptor protein positive. Goserelin

(BNF 8.3.4.2) is used for premenopausal and trilostane (BNF 8.3.4.1) for postmenopausal breast cancer. Anastrozole, letrozole, formestane and exemestane (BNF 8.3.4.1) are all used in the treatment of advanced postmenopausal breast cancer.

Cervical cancer

Definition and aetiology

Cervical cancer is the second most common cancer of the female reproductive tract and the incidence appears to be increasing, particularly in young women. There is a higher incidence in women from a poor social background and a number of other risk factors have been identified. There may be a higher risk in women who have had a large number of sexual partners, and a greater risk exists the earlier the age at which sexual intercourse first took place. The disease has been shown to be linked to the presence of sexually transmitted disease, commonly a human papillomavirus. There may be an association between the development of the disease and the use of oral contraceptives and with heavy smoking.

Cervical carcinoma is commonly a squamous cell carcinoma, with a minority appearing as adenocarcinomas. Early pathological changes may be detected by the proliferation of cells in the lower third of the cervical epithelium (minimal cervical dysplasia) and these may be detected by cervical smear testing. Many of these abnormalities may spontaneously regress, but some may progress to carcinoma *in situ*. The further spread of these cells may occur to adjacent organs.

A positive diagnosis is staged as a means of indicating the spread of the cancer.

Stage	*Spread of cancer*
0	Pre-invasive
I	Confined to the cervix
II	Spread beyond cervix, but not onto pelvic wall
III	Spread onto pelvic wall
IV	Widespread dissemination

About 1% of women in the UK are diagnosed with invasive cervical cancer during their lifetime, and about 0.4% die from it.

Symptoms

Early disease may be asymptomatic, and the disease is usually well advanced before symptoms arise. These may include malodorous vaginal discharge, bleeding that can often occur after intercourse, abdominal pain, dyspareunia and low back pain. Following widespread dissemination, urinary and rectal symptoms may develop.

Treatment

The treatment depends on the stage of the disease and the age of the patient. Early stages may be managed by cryotherapy, laser treatment and diathermy. Hysterectomy at this stage may be reserved for older women who have completed a family, or those who are likely to be unreliable in attending follow-up examinations. Radiotherapy, surgery, or both, may be used for more extensive forms, particularly when there is lymph node involvement, although proctitis and cystitis are major complications. Chemotherapy is of limited value, and drug administration may be reserved for the treatment of pain.

Prophylaxis by cervical screening (Pap test) of all sexually active women has reduced the development of the disease by increased early detection. Screening is carried out every three years, although high-risk groups may need more frequent checks.

Choriocarcinoma

Definition and aetiology

Choriocarcinoma is a rare malignant tumour of the trophoblastic (placental) tissue which characteristically secretes chorionic gonadotrophin. The term choriocarcinoma is also applied to certain types of testicular teratomas and ovarian cancers that secrete chorionic gonadotrophin. Most cases occur in females as a result of malignant degeneration of a hydatidiform mole, but the tumour may also develop after spontaneous abortion or after a period of months or years as a sequel to normal pregnancy.

Symptoms

Choriocarcinoma may present with abnormal uterine bleeding, rapid uterine enlargement or symptoms of disseminated disease. The tumour produces metastases at an early stage via the circulation to the lungs, liver, brain or vaginal wall. Pulmonary embolism or pulmonary hypertension may occur. In males, choriocarcinoma may present with testicular pain, accidental discovery of a hard testicular mass or signs of disseminated disease.

Treatment

Choriocarcinoma is treated with the administration of antimetabolites (BNF 8.1.3). Surgery, radiotherapy and chemotherapy may be indicated for testicular or ovarian tumours.

Endometrial cancer

Definition and aetiology

Endometrial cancer is the third most common malignancy affecting women (after breast and colorectal cancers). It is commonly an adenocarcinoma and is more prevalent in developed societies. Unlike cervical cancer, women who have not had children are at greatest risk, but it is unrelated to the number of sexual partners. There is a peak incidence postmenopausally between 50 and 60 years of age. A higher incidence has been linked to an early menarche and late menopause (as in breast cancer).

The condition has been linked to the secretion of oestrogen predominantly in the absence of progestogen secretion. Hypersecretion of oestrogen may occur in oestrogen-secreting tumours and polycystic ovary syndrome. Predisposition to endometrial cancer may occur in other conditions in which oestrogen secretion can be unopposed (e.g. diabetes mellitus, hypertension and obesity). Obesity can increase the risk of cancer from 3 to 10 times.

Symptoms

The presence of unexpected uterine bleeding between menstrual periods (in premenopausal women) and in others postmenopausally is a potent indicator of endometrial abnormalities. Bleeding may be preceded by a watery discharge. Diagnosis may be confirmed by fractional dilatation and curettage. Unlike in cervical cancer, a Pap test does not detect endometrial cancer. Staging of the progress of the disease is carried out, as in cervical cancer.

Treatment

Surgery may be possible in many cases and involves hysterectomy and removal of the Fallopian tubes and ovaries. Progestogens (BNF 8.3.2) may be used indefinitely for advanced disease or relapses and may prove effective in retarding the development of metastases. Combined cytotoxic (doxorubicin and cisplatin) (BNF 8.1) and progestogen therapy may also be beneficial in the treatment of metastases and in prevention of recurrence. The five-year survival rate is approximately 60%, although age and staging of the disease may significantly affect the prognosis.

Ovarian tumours

Definition and aetiology

Cancer of the ovaries accounts for 2.3% of all cancers and 2.7% of all cancer deaths. It is the most severe of the gynaecological cancers.

Ovarian cancer (Figure 8.1) comprises a range of histological entities, the most common of which are adenocarcinomas. Approximately 75% are benign, although the proportion which are

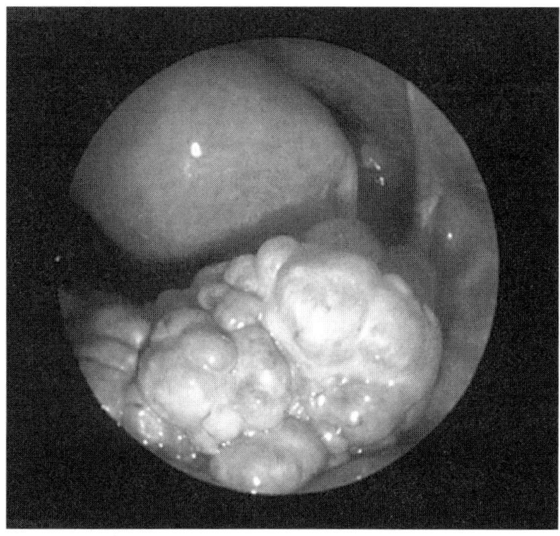

Figure 8.1 Ovarian cancer, laparoscopic view. (Reproduced with permission of Mike Wyndham/BV Lewis.)

malignant increases with age. The incidence of the cancer increases with high standards of living and with an early menarche linked to a late menopause. A decreased incidence has been associated with increased parity and oral contraceptive use.

There may be a familial history of the cancer in up to 40% of patients. It is more common in the same family if there is also a history of breast, endometrial and colonic cancer.

Symptoms

The tumour may be asymptomatic until it has spread to other structures within the pelvis. The presence of a palpable mass may indicate the presence of a tumour, but cysts must also be considered. Early signs may be non-specific and include vague abdominal discomfort and gastro-intestinal disturbances. Ascites, anaemia and pelvic pain may be associated with late stages of the disease. Rarely, tumours may secrete one or more hormones. The secretion of oestrogens may lead to precocious puberty in girls and endometrial proliferation in postmenopausal women. Other hormones secreted may include serotonin, thyroxine and chorionic gonadotrophin.

Treatment

Treatment depends upon the stage of the disease. Localised tumours may be surgically excised conservatively, preserving reproductive function. In advanced disease, hysterectomy and salpingo-oophorectomy with omentectomy, may be necessary. Three or more cytotoxic drugs may be used in combination (e.g. cisplatin, ifosfamide and doxorubicin), and the addition of a progestogen (BNF 8.3.2) may improve the outcome. The five-year survival rate may range from 15% to 45%.

8.5.2 GENITO-URINARY SYSTEM MALIGNANT NEOPLASMS

Bladder cancer

Definition and aetiology

Bladder cancer is usually a transitional cell carcinoma, which may be localised or highly invasive. Squamous cell carcinoma, which has a poor prognosis due to its high invasiveness, occurs less frequently and may be associated with parasitic infection.

The cancer accounts for 4.6% of all cancers and 3.4% of cancer deaths. It occurs in more than three times as many men as women. Aetiological factors which have been identified include smoking, occupational exposure to aromatic amines used in the dyeing, cable and rubber industries, and administration of cyclophosphamide. Parasitic infection (e.g. with *Schistosoma haematobium*) may produce cancer as a result of chronic irritation.

Symptoms

Haematuria without pain is the initial presenting symptom, and is accompanied by dysuria, urinary frequency and pyuria. Pain in the lower abdomen may develop in the later stages of the disease.

Treatment

Superficial lesions of the bladder wall may be surgically excised by endoscopic resection, although the procedure may need repeating. Partial or total cystectomy may be necessary for tumours which have infiltrated the bladder wall. Urostomy formation is required in total cystectomy. Local cystodiathermy is also widely used.

Radiotherapy may be beneficial post-operatively and can be curative on its own. Chemotherapy is of limited use, although direct instillation of alkylating drugs (BNF 8.1.1) and cytotoxic antibiotics (BNF 8.1.2) into the bladder has been attempted.

Prostatic cancer

Definition and aetiology

Cancer of the prostate gland is invariably an adenocarcinoma and most cases occur in men over 50 years of age. It is the most common cancer in men over 50. Metastases may frequently be present on diagnosis, commonly occurring in the lymph nodes, bone, lung and liver.

The identification of androgen receptors in approximately 75% of patients may be a useful marker to predict the effectiveness of hormonal therapy.

The incidence is increasing due to the increasing number of elderly people. No definite causative factors have been identified, but an increased incidence has been associated with sexually transmitted diseases, sedentary occupations and sexual activity. A hormonal link has been suggested on the basis that castrated males do not develop the disease.

Symptoms

Early stages of the disease may be asymptomatic. Later symptoms may only develop once the disease is well advanced and include urinary outflow obstruction and, less commonly, haematuria and pyuria. In some patients, the presenting symptom may be bone pain caused by metastases. Rectal examination may identify the presence of a firm nodule.

Treatment

Localised disease may be managed symptomatically, especially as the mean age of presentation is 70 years and other pathology is invariably present. In more diffuse disease, and in the absence of lymph node involvement, treatment by prostatectomy or radiotherapy may be attempted. However, elderly patients may suffer more from the complications of treatment (e.g. urinary incontinence and diarrhoea) than from the tumour itself.

A significant proportion of patients have metastases at presentation and they may benefit from hormonal therapy and orchidectomy. Oestrogens suppress plasma levels of testosterone. Medical orchidectomy may also be carried out by the administration of gonadorelin analogues (BNF 8.3.4).

Renal cancer

Definition

Renal cancer is very common, comprising 1–2% of adult cancers. The classification is based upon the cell types. Renal tubule epithelium cells may give rise to renal cell carcinomas (hypernephromas). A tumour arising from the embryonic renal tissue is described as a Wilms' tumour (nephroblastoma). Urothelial tumours arise from transitional cells, and rarely from squamous cells.

Renal cell carcinomas

Definition and aetiology

Renal cell carcinoma occurs predominantly in adults, with a higher incidence in males. Its occurrence has been tentatively linked to smoking. The tumour may occur singly or as multiples in one or both kidneys. It is encapsulated, but metastases may occur via the bloodstream to the lungs, liver, and bone and by direct invasion into adjacent tissues.

Symptoms

Initial non-specific symptoms may include weakness, anorexia and weight loss. The classical symptoms are pain, haematuria and the presence of a palpable mass. Pain may be experienced as a dull ache in the loin. Other symptoms may be due to substances released by the tumour or by invasion of other structures. Fever may be produced by the secretion of pyrogens; the secretion of renin can lead to hypertension. Endocrine effects may occur (e.g. hypercalcaemia caused by the secretion of parathormone, and polycythaemia due to the secretion of an erythropoietin-like substance). Varicocele may develop as a result of dissemination of the tumour into the renal vein and the resultant occlusion of the testicular vein.

Treatment

Nephrectomy may be carried out if only one kidney is affected. If both are involved, partial nephrectomy may be attempted. The use of radiotherapy, chemotherapy and immunotherapy has not proved beneficial. The five-year survival rate may be as high as 60% in localised disease.

Wilms' tumour

Definition and aetiology

Wilms' tumour is a solid tumour of childhood, with the majority identified before three years of age. The tumour consists of connective tissue, epithelial cells and muscle cells and is rapid-growing, often reaching enormous proportions.

Tumours usually arise unilaterally, but may also occur bilaterally. Metastases (e.g. to the lungs, liver and bone) may be formed at an early stage via the bloodstream, and by direct local invasion.

Symptoms
A palpable mass may be found in the abdomen and is associated with abdominal pain, nausea and vomiting, anorexia, fever, haematuria and weight loss.

Treatment
The tumour, which is commonly encapsulated, may be surgically removed or nephrectomy carried out. Radiotherapy may be used pre-operatively to promote shrinkage of the tumour or post-operatively to treat any leakage of cells. Vinca alkaloids (BNF 8.1.4) and cytotoxic antibiotics (BNF 8.1.2) may be administered following nephrectomy. Five-year survival rates are approximately 65%.

Urothelial tumours

Definition and aetiology
Urothelial tumours may occur not only in the renal pelvis, but also in the epithelium of the ureter, urethra and urinary bladder (*see also* Bladder cancer). Those of the renal pelvis and ureter are usually only of low-grade malignancy and they may be papillary or solid. They have been linked to occupational exposure (e.g. to aromatic amines used as dyes), the ingestion of phenacetin, to schistosomiasis, and to chronic inflammation (e.g. caused by indwelling catheters).

Symptoms
The most prominent symptom is haematuria. Obstruction to the outflow of urine may produce renal colic, but the tumour only rarely becomes large enough to be palpable. If the tumour develops in the ureter, the presence of only a small mass may cause urinary obstruction.

Treatment
Complete removal of the kidney and ureter may be necessary, although local dissection of the tumour may be effective in some cases. Radiotherapy may be used post-operatively. Tumours may give a five-year survival rate of 50% overall, ranging from 90% for localised tumours to virtually zero for those that have spread to tissues around the ureter.

Testicular cancer

Definition and aetiology
Although testicular cancer is rare, it is the most common cancer in young men, and consists of two cell types. Teratomas, which are of uncertain origin, have a peak incidence at approximately 20 years of age. Seminomas, which arise from the germinal cells, occur most commonly at approximately 30 years of age. Tumours may rarely occur in older men and are usually lymphomas.

The disease has been associated with a high standard of living. Predisposing factors include undescended testes and testicular feminisation syndrome.

Symptoms
The presence of an enlarging firm mass in the scrotum may cause discomfort. If bleeding into the tumour develops, the mass may be tender with extreme local pain. Metastases to the lymph nodes, lungs and liver may occur.

Treatment
Identification of the cell type provides the basis for treatment. Seminomas may respond to radiotherapy and have a five-year survival rate of at least 80%. Teratomas and other cell types may require lymph node dissection and combination chemotherapy with cytotoxic drugs (BNF 8.1), and have a poorer prognosis than seminomas.

8.6 Haematological malignant neoplasms

Leukaemias

Definition and aetiology
Leukaemias are characterised by the uncontrolled proliferation of blood-forming elements arising from progenitor bone-marrow cells. The

normal bone marrow is replaced and the production of normal cellular components is reduced, leading to anaemia, thrombocytopenia and neutropenia.

Leukaemias are classified as acute or chronic, depending on the maturity of the cell populations. In acute forms, immature leucocytes proliferate and fail to reach maturity. In chronic forms, mature leucocytes are not removed from the circulation but accumulate. Leukaemia is also classified by the identity and origins of the dominant cell as lymphoid (lymphocytic, lymphatic or lymphogenous) or non-lymphoid (myeloid, granulocytic, myelocytic or myelogenous). Recent advances in immunological science has greatly assisted the understanding of the classification and aetiology of the leukaemias, such that the immunophenotype of the disease is also used for classification purposes.

The aetiology of the leukaemias is unknown in the majority of cases, although a higher incidence has been linked to a number of factors. Exposure to environmental or occupational radiation may predispose to leukaemia. Occupational contact with benzene, administration of some cytotoxic drugs (e.g. alkylating drugs), and exposure to viruses may also contribute to the development of leukaemia. Genetic defects (e.g. Down's syndrome) may produce a higher incidence.

The acute forms are considered jointly, but the more clinically variable chronic forms are discussed separately.

Acute leukaemias

Definition and aetiology

Acute leukaemias may be classified as acute lymphatic leukaemia (ALL) (acute lymphoblastic leukaemia) and acute non-lymphoid leukaemia, which includes acute myeloid leukaemia (AML).

About two-thirds of cases of ALL occur in children, with a peak between two and five years of age. It is the most common form of cancer in childhood. A smaller peak of incidence, which is equivalent in males and females, starts at about 60 years of age.

The incidence of AML increases with age, with 80% of all patients over 60 years of age.

Symptoms

Non-specific early symptoms may include the progressive development of pallor, weakness and lethargy, like a prolonged and unfinished bout of influenza. The predominant features relate to the replacement of normal bone marrow with malignant cells.

Infection, haemorrhage and anaemia are common. Infection may arise in any tissue but occurs most commonly in the lungs, mucous membranes and skin. Skin lesions may be extremely slow to heal and, if infected, may be characterised by the absence of pus. Septicaemia may suddenly develop and prove rapidly fatal. The presence of herpes and candidal infections may complicate the development of fulminant oral aphthae. Haemorrhagic lesions are common. Petechiae, bruising and purpura may develop spontaneously and persistent epistaxis can occur.

Bone pain may be a prominent feature, caused by the presence of a tumour mass or infarction in the bone marrow. Later symptoms may be due to infiltration of the central nervous system and include irritability, headache and vomiting.

Treatment

Prior to treatment, laboratory assessment of blood is essential to differentiate between ALL and AML. The aim of treatment is to remove the leukaemic cells from the blood and bone marrow and to allow its repopulation by normal cells. Chemotherapy is the mainstay of treatment, and is sometimes used in conjunction with radiotherapy, but all schedules are complex and undergoing continual revision. Bone-marrow transplantation is considered for those patients who are suitable.

Remission is induced in ALL by oral prednisolone (BNF 6.3.4), intravenous vincristine (BNF 8.1.4), and intramuscular L-asparaginase (BNF 8.1.5) over a three- to four-week period. This has been shown to be effective in more than 95% of children and 80% of adults. Improved 'clear-up' is assisted by the administration of cytosine arabinoside and daunorubicin. The role of bone-marrow transplantation in ALL is controversial.

In AML, remission is induced by a combination of cytosine arabinoside and an anthracycline (e.g. aclarubicin or idarubicin) for 7–10 days' treatment. The vinca alkaloids (BNF 8.1.4) have also proven successful in inducing remission. Once an improved blood profile has been achieved methotrexate (BNF 8.1.3), and possibly radiotherapy, may be used in the prophylaxis of CNS complications. Varying periods of maintenance therapy using antimetabolites (BNF 8.1.3) may be administered to minimise the occurrence of relapses. Relapses may occur in the bone marrow, CNS and testes, of which the most serious is the bone marrow. The five-year survival rate is 50%, although the prognosis is worse in boys because of the risk of testicular relapses, and is dependent on the leucocyte cell count on diagnosis.

Chronic lymphoid leukaemia

Definition and aetiology

The presence of small immature lymphocytes in the bone marrow and blood is indicative of chronic lymphoid leukaemia (CLL) (chronic lymphatic leukaemia). Its incidence increases with age and it affects about twice as many men as women. CLL accounts for about 25% of all cases of leukaemia. Staging of the disease to indicate probable prognosis has assisted the effective management of the condition.

Other closely related, but much rarer, forms of leukaemia are hairy cell leukaemia and prolymphocytic leukaemia.

Symptoms

Approximately 25% of cases may be asymptomatic. In patients with symptoms, there may be an insidious development. Non-specific symptoms can include anaemia, weight loss, anorexia, fever, dyspnoea on exertion, and a sense of abdominal fullness. Lymphadenopathy and splenomegaly may be present. Macules and plaques can develop during the course, and these may ulcerate. Later symptoms include petechiae, bruising and bleeding.

Complications can arise from the increased susceptibility to infection. Herpes zoster infection and recurrent chest infections are a major cause of morbidity and mortality. Haemolytic anaemia may occur as a result of an autoimmune reaction.

Treatment

Patients diagnosed with CLL who are asymptomatic do not require treatment, although some may be given chlorambucil, with or without prednisolone, as a pre-emptive action. Treatment may be indicated in the presence of bone-marrow failure, lymphadenopathy, systemic symptoms or the appearance of complicating symptoms.

Radiotherapy may be used for treatment and the relief of symptoms (e.g. lymphadenopathy and splenomegaly). Combinations of drugs may be given: cyclophosphamide, oncovin and prednisolone (COP) or CHOP (COP plus doxorubicin). Nucleoside analogues (fludarabine and 2-deoxycoformycin) have also been shown to be of benefit. It should be recognised, however, that treatment programmes are continually being updated and improved.

Chronic myeloid leukaemia

Definition and aetiology

Chronic myeloid leukaemia (chronic myelocytic leukaemia, chronic granulocytic leukaemia or chronic myelogenous leukaemia) is a rare form of leukaemia which predominantly affects those over 40 years of age. It may be associated with exposure to ionising radiations or to chemicals (e.g. benzene). The condition has been linked to a chromosomal abnormality (the Philadelphia chromosome) and to the presence of a chimaeric gene, *BCR-ABL*.

Symptoms

The progression of chronic myeloid leukaemia may be considered to consist of two stages. The chronic phase is of widely variable duration (typically two to six years) and the symptoms may be controlled by treatment. The accelerated phase represents a considerable worsening of the condition which may be associated with dissemination of the tumour to other sites (e.g. skin and bone), although the transition in symptoms between the two phases may be ill-defined.

The condition may be characterised by the insidious onset of non-specific symptoms. These may include anaemia, a sense of abdominal fullness, anorexia, weight loss and night sweats.

Abdominal pain may occur due to infarction of the spleen, and splenomegaly may be severe and accompanied by hepatomegaly. Later symptoms may include the development of large haematomas.

Treatment

The condition can only be cured by bone marrow transplantation. Treatment is intended to arrest its development. This may be possible during the chronic phase with the administration of interferon-α or hydroxyurea (BNF 8.1.5). Radiotherapy of the spleen may be used as an adjunct to chemotherapy, but resistance to irradiation may develop. There is no effective treatment of the accelerated phase of the condition.

Lymphomas

Definition

Lymphomas are neoplasms of the lymphoid tissue which are progressive, destructive and invasive, and which cause swelling of the lymph nodes and spleen. They are differentiated from infections, which may also cause swelling of lymphoid tissue. Lymphomas give rise to approximately 5% of all cancers.

Hodgkin's disease

Definition and aetiology

Hodgkin's disease rarely occurs before 10 years of age and has peak incidences in early adulthood (25–35 years of age) and in middle to old age. Its aetiology is uncertain, although certain infections have been implicated. The disease may be caused by chromosomal abnormalities, but no specific characteristics have been universally noted.

The disease is clinically staged through localised involvement (stage I) to widely disseminated disease (stage IV), and subclassified according to the presence of systemic symptoms.

Symptoms

Early disease may be characterised by enlarged lymph nodes (e.g. in the neck and axillae) which are usually painless. As the disease spreads through the reticulo-endothelial system, systemic symptoms may appear. Severe pruritus may be an early symptom that may lead to extensive excoriation. More widespread disease may be indicated by drenching night sweats, fever and weight loss, which may be caused by involvement of internal lymph nodes (e.g. in the retroperitoneum), bone marrow or liver. Bone pain may be a consequence of bone infiltration.

The presence of an enlarged lymphoid mass may cause obstruction of other tissues and organs. Oedema of the face and neck may result from superior vena cava obstruction, and bile-duct obstruction may cause jaundice. Advanced disease may be characterised by hepatomegaly.

The progressive deterioration in cell-mediated immunity may predispose patients with advanced disease to opportunistic infectious diseases (e.g. herpes zoster and *Pneumocystis carinii* pneumonia).

Treatment

Radiotherapy may be used to treat patients with localised disease. Adjacent uninvolved lymph nodes may also be irradiated. Chemotherapy is used in other cases of localised disease and in all disseminated states. Combination therapy with cytotoxic drugs is used (as many as eight different drugs may be used), with 28- or 42-day cycles of treatment repeated up to six times to ensure remission. Chemotherapy may also be used in the event of relapse following initial radiotherapy or chemotherapy.

Complications of successful chemotherapy and radiotherapy may occur with the development of secondary malignancies (e.g. acute non-lymphoid leukaemia). The five-year survival rate for Hodgkin's disease without treatment was approximately 10%. With the introduction of chemotherapy, this has increased to approximately 75%, and most patients do not suffer relapses.

Non-Hodgkin's lymphoma

Definition and aetiology

Non-Hodgkin's lymphoma comprises a diverse range of lymphomas. The incidence is greater than Hodgkin's lymphoma and it is predominantly a disease of the elderly. It is of unknown aetiology, although viral associations have been suggested. The conditions are staged similarly to Hodgkin's lymphoma (i.e. stage I to stage IV) and the classification of the disease ranges from low-grade with reasonable prognosis to high-grade with potentially poor prognosis. Approximately 80% of non-Hodgkin's lymphomas are of B-cell origin; the remainder are of T-cell origin.

The disease is uncommon in patients under 40 years of age, and peaks in those between 60 and 70 years of age.

Symptoms

Lymphadenopathy (Figure 8.2) characterised by the presence of large rubbery nodes may be the only presenting symptom. The distribution of nodal involvement may be similar to that in Hodgkin's disease, although popliteal nodes and pharyngeal lymphoid tissue may also be affected. Extranodal tissue is also commonly involved (e.g. the skin, bone marrow and gastrointestinal tract) and may produce varied symptoms (e.g. malabsorption syndrome). Anaemia, neutropenia and thrombocytopenia may occur. Night sweats, weight loss and fever may indicate disseminated disease.

Central nervous system disease may develop due to spinal cord compression, especially in high-grade lymphomas. Depressed immunoglobulin production may predispose to infection.

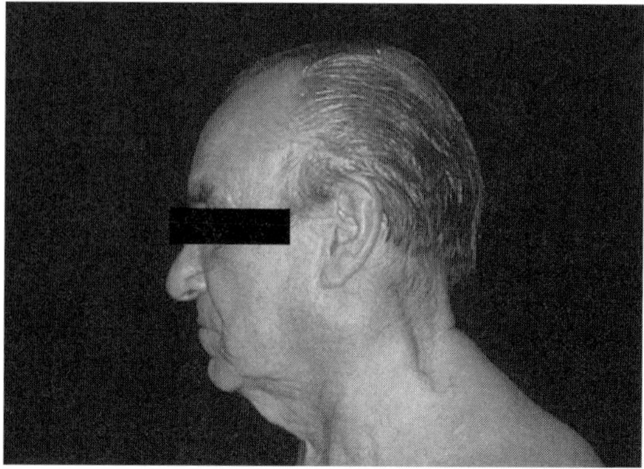

Figure 8.2 Lymphoma, elderly man. Lymphadenopathy, neck. (Reproduced with permission of Mike Wyndham.)

Treatment

Most patients will have high-grade disease at presentation and, despite appropriate treatment, the prognosis is poor. Treatment is directed towards relief of symptoms and prolongation of life. Localised low-grade disease may be treated by radiotherapy, although relapse to other sites is common. Disseminated low-grade disease may be treated with a single agent or combination therapy with cytotoxic drugs (BNF 8.1). Advanced disease may respond to treatment with interferons (BNF 8.2.4), although high-dose multiple drug regimens may also be used.

The prognosis of non-Hodgkin's lymphoma is poorer than Hodgkin's lymphoma. The prognosis for high-grade lymphomas has improved with the introduction of aggressive chemotherapy, and cure may be possible.

Myeloma

Definition and aetiology

Myeloma is a paraproteinaemia in which the plasma concentration of a single immunoglobulin is increased due to the monoclonal proliferation of B-cells. It is characterised by the presence of plasma-cell tumours in the bone marrow. It affects predominantly those over 40 years of age, with an average age at diagnosis of 62. The disease has a slow course.

Symptoms

Patients may be asymptomatic apart from a general malaise. The most common early symptom is bone pain, which may affect predominantly the back and the ribs and may be aggravated by movement. Diffuse osteoporosis or erosion of the skeleton may be caused by the tumour or a tumour secretion (osteoclast-activating factor), and may lead to vertebral collapse or pathological fracture. Hypercalcaemia may be associated with bone erosion, leading to depression, vomiting and anorexia. Gradual renal impairment may be due to the deposition of immune complexes within the renal tubules. Spontaneous bleeding may be caused by impairment of renal and platelet function. Hyperviscosity of the circulation due to the excess presence of immunoglobulins may cause neurological disturbances (e.g. visual disturbances, headache and peripheral neuropathy). The patient may be predisposed to the development of infections caused by depressed immunoglobulin function.

Treatment
Treatment is symptomatic. Localised myeloma may be treated by radiotherapy, but most cases are disseminated and require chemotherapy. Alkylating drugs (BNF 8.1.1) are given singly, although the addition of corticosteroids (BNF 8.2.2) may improve the response. Bone-marrow transplantation may be successful in a minority of cases. Interferons (BNF 8.2.4) may achieve limited remission when used as a first-line treatment.

General measures include the use of radiotherapy in the relief of bone pain, and the patient should be encouraged to remain ambulant. Improvement in renal function may be noted if the fluid intake is greatly increased, particularly in the presence of hypercalcaemia. Opportunistic infections should be immediately treated with antibacterial drugs.

8.7 Malignant neoplasms of the skin

Basal cell carcinoma

Definition and aetiology
A basal cell carcinoma (rodent ulcer) is the most common malignant disease of the skin, arising from the basal layer of the epidermis. It rarely forms metastases but is capable of invading and destroying local tissues. It may occur in areas damaged by ionising radiation or ultraviolet light, or in scar tissue (e.g. from burns and vaccinations). It is more common in males and usually occurs after middle-age, although it is also common in young immunocompromised patients. It is also more common in fair-skinned people, and is very rare in people with black skin.

Symptoms
The most common sites for basal cell carcinoma are the face, head and neck. The appearance may take several forms, but they are most commonly seen in early stages as small, firm, pearly, raised nodules that are covered by a thin epidermis. The thin epidermis may rupture, resulting in ulceration, and later stages are characterised by a pearly border with superficial telangiectasia surrounding the ulcer. Death may result in rare cases due to an untreated basal cell carcinoma destroying underlying structures (e.g. cartilage or bone).

Treatment
Treatment comprises removal by chemosurgery, cryosurgery, radiotherapy or surgery. It is essential that the excision is complete to prevent recurrence.

Kaposi's sarcoma

Definition and aetiology
Kaposi's sarcoma is a form of vascular tumour which arises in the dermis and may spread to the epidermis. It is caused by herpesvirus type 8, and may arise in three forms: indolent, lymphadenopathic and AIDS-related. In the latter form, it becomes widely disseminated to the gastrointestinal tract, lymph nodes and brain.

Symptoms
The indolent form may be characterised by the formation of a nodule, often appearing on the leg or foot, or by the presence of a brown, plaque-like lesion which may penetrate soft tissue and enter bone. Kaposi's sarcoma in AIDS may produce red or pink plaques or papules, initially occurring on the upper torso, but rapidly spreading to other parts. Mucous membranes may also be involved.

Treatment
Radiotherapy may be used to treat indolent forms of the disease, depending on the depth of the lesions. Chemotherapy using vinblastine or combinations of up to six cytotoxic drugs may be used in aggressive forms of the disease. The tumour may respond to treatment with interferons (BNF 8.2.4).

Melanoma

Definition and aetiology
Melanoma (malignant melanoma) (Figure 8.3) is a malignant disease of the skin arising from melanocytes in the epidermis. Approximately

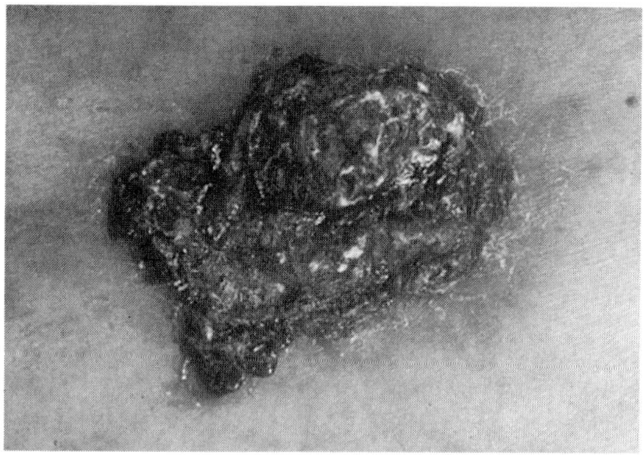

Figure 8.3 Melanoma. (Reproduced with permission of James Stevenson/Science Photo Library.)

50% of all melanomas arise from an existing lentigo, mole or naevus, while the rest occur in previously unblemished skin. Ultraviolet light (e.g. through chronic sun exposure) appears to be the most likely significant causative agent. Melanomas are more common in females and prognosis is related to the stage of the disease, thickness of the tumour and its site.

Symptoms

Melanomas occur in various forms and all have the ability to invade and form metastases. The only common symptom is mild pruritus and a tingling sensation. They may be classified according to their appearance and behaviour.

Nodular melanoma, which usually occurs in middle-age, may be dark brown, greyish-black, or virtually colourless. The initial nodule is raised and rapidly invades the dermis with little lateral growth. The lesion is usually asymptomatic until ulceration occurs.

Superficial spreading melanoma develops most frequently on female legs and on the male torso, occurring commonly at middle-age. The lesion is slightly raised with a well-defined but irregular margin, brown or black with red, white, or blue spots, and spreads horizontally. Peripheral inflammation may also be present. Vertical dermal invasion may eventually occur and result in bleeding and crusting.

Lentigo maligna melanoma arises from flat uniformly brown lesions (lentigo maligna) and occurs on the face in elderly patients. As malignancy develops, the margins become irregular and the colour changes to brownish-black and blue. Dermal invasion may occur after years of lateral growth and results in a raised nodule.

Treatment

Successful treatment relies upon early diagnosis and consists of wide surgical excision with, in some cases, skin grafts. Lymphadenectomy may be necessary when deep invasion and metastasis has occurred. Chemotherapy with cytotoxic drugs (BNF 8.1) may also be of value, especially in the presence of metastases.

8.8 Miscellaneous neoplasms

Cancer of the bone

Definition and aetiology

Cancer of the bone may arise as a primary tumour or as a metastasis. Primary bone tumours are rare and occur predominantly in children and young adults; metastatic bone tumours are more common in adults. Immunodeficiency may be a causative factor and the degree of immunocompromise may have a bearing on the course of the disease.

The most common forms of primary malignant bone tumour are osteosarcoma (osteogenic sarcoma), Ewing's sarcoma (Ewing's tumour) and chondrosarcoma. Osteosarcomas may occur at any age, but have the greatest incidence at 10–20 years of age. Metastases to the lung are common. Ewing's sarcoma has a similar age profile and has a higher incidence in males. Chondrosarcoma is a cartilaginous sarcoma and occurs in an older age group, with peak incidence occurring in patients of 40–60 years of age.

Symptoms

Osteosarcoma occurs predominantly around the knee and is characterised by the presence of pain and swelling. The mass may be firm and tender and its presence may restrict joint movement. Similar symptoms may be present in Ewing's sarcoma, which occurs commonly in the femur and the pelvis. Accompanying symptoms may include fever and weight loss. Chondrosarcomas are slow-growing and commonly arise in the pelvis and less frequently in the femur, humerus, ribs and scapula. Early disease may be asymptomatic, although pain and swelling may arise as the disease progresses.

Treatment

In osteosarcoma, amputation of the limb may be required, although more conservative measures may be attempted initially (e.g. removal of the tumour and reconstruction of the limb). Cytotoxic antibiotics (BNF 8.1.2) and cisplatin (BNF 8.1.5) may be used pre- and post-operatively and may be effective at preventing metastases. Ewing's sarcoma may be treated by a combination of surgery, radiotherapy, and intensive chemotherapy and may give five-year survival rates of 30–60%. Chondrosarcomas appear to be resistant to radiotherapy and chemotherapy and therefore must be treated by surgical removal or amputation.

Cancer of the head and neck

Definition and aetiology

Cancer of the head and neck constitutes a diverse group of cancers of the upper respiratory and gastrointestinal tracts. Many individual conditions are uncommon, but as a group they form approximately 4% of all cancers. The most common aetiological factor is tobacco and alcohol consumption. Poor dental and oral hygiene may also be contributory factors. The majority are squamous cell carcinomas; the remainder are melanomas, lymphomas and sarcomas.

Cancer of the larynx

Definition and aetiology

Cancer of the larynx forms the largest single group of head and neck cancers. A strong causative link with smoking and alcohol intake has been established. It is commonly caused by a squamous cell carcinoma and the site of origin is predominantly the glottis.

Symptoms

A common early symptom is hoarseness. Other and subsequent symptoms are linked to the presence of the tumour above or below the glottis. If the tumour arises above the glottis, dysphagia may occur. Subglottal carcinoma may be accompanied by dyspnoea and stridor.

Treatment

Treatment of localised glottal cancer consists of a combination of radiotherapy and, where necessary, surgery. For advanced disease, laryngectomy may be required, although voice preservation or substitution is often attempted. Speech therapy is also necessary for many patients.

Cancer of the mouth

Definition and aetiology

Cancer of the mouth encompasses all tumours which arise on the lip, tongue, gingiva, floor and inner lining of the mouth, and hard and soft palate. The incidence of disease increases with age and is twice as common in males. The incidence has been linked to smoking (with pipes and cigars more strongly implicated than cigarettes), poor oral hygiene and regular alcohol consumption. Infective agents may also be important in the development of the disease, and leucoplakia may be a predisposing factor. Local infiltration of lymph nodes may occur to produce metastases.

Symptoms

An early warning of cancerous changes in the mouth may be the development of a dry mouth, although some patients, especially those with large tumours, may salivate excessively. Cancer of the lip, gingiva and tongue may be characterised by an ulcerated lesion with an indurated base, which can be extremely reluctant to heal. Cancer of the tongue may cause pain and earache. Alternatively, an oral tumour may present as a single or multiple firm mass which gradually increases in size and interferes with eating and speech.

Treatment

Good results may be obtained by surgical removal of the lesion and surrounding tissues. Radiotherapy may be used as a primary treatment for cancer of the lip or as an adjunct to surgery or in refractory cases. Chemotherapy may also be successful in management of the condition. The patient should be advised to stop smoking, and improved oral hygiene should be recommended. The prognosis is variable depending on the site. The five-year survival rate for cancer of the lip is 80%, while the prognosis of other forms may range from 20% to 50%.

Cancer of the pharynx

Definition and aetiology

Cancer of the nasopharynx is largely localised to Chinese populations, including those who have settled in the west. The unusual distribution may be attributed to dietary factors or localised infective agents. It occurs equally in children and adults, but has a higher incidence in males.

Oropharyngeal cancer occurs predominantly in patients over 50 years of age and has a significant male preponderance. Smoking or chewing tobacco have been identified as causative factors. Hypopharyngeal carcinomas have a similar aetiology.

Many pharyngeal neoplasms are non-Hodgkin's lymphomas, and these may spread to other tissues (e.g. paranasal sinuses and the stomach).

Symptoms

Cervical lymph node involvement is often the presenting symptom in cancer of the nasopharynx. Unilateral nasal obstruction may also occur, and sero-mucinous otitis media may lead to deafness as a result of Eustachian tube obstruction. Pain may be produced by involvement of the cranial nerves which pass through the sinuses.

Oropharyngeal cancer may produce tonsillar enlargement which causes dysphagia, and occasionally dysarthria may arise if the posterior tongue is affected. Pain may be referred to the ear, and ulceration may produce blood-stained saliva.

Cancer of the hypopharynx may cause dysphagia and referred earache. Spread of the tumour may lead to hoarseness, dyspnoea, stridor or anorexia.

Treatment

The mainstay of treatment and the relief of symptoms is intensive radiotherapy. Surgery is reserved for advanced stages of disease and in patients who are refractory to radiotherapy. The overall prognosis is poor, with five-year survival rates of approximately 30%.

Cancer of the salivary glands

Definition and aetiology

Cancer of the salivary glands is of unknown aetiology and occurs largely in the parotid glands, although the minor salivary glands (e.g. in the cheeks, lips and palate) may also be affected. They may be benign (mainly pleomorphic adenomas) or malignant (e.g. muco-epidermoid carcinomas). The disease occurs primarily in patients over 50 years of age.

Symptoms

The gradual development of a painless encapsulated mass may lead to facial distortion. The presence of facial palsy may indicate infiltration of the facial nerve by a malignant growth, and acute swelling of the parotid gland may cause discomfort.

Treatment

The tumour is removed by surgery. For malignant tumours, surgery may be followed by radiotherapy if complete excision is not possible or a recurrent tumour is undergoing removal. Radiotherapy may also be used as a primary therapy for malignant tumours if surgery is contraindicated (e.g. in the elderly).

Blood, nutritional and metabolic disorders

9.1 Blood and lymph disorders

9.1.1 GENERAL DISORDERS

Agranulocytosis

Definition and aetiology
Agranulocytosis is characterised by a marked decrease in the number of granulocytes, which results in an increased susceptibility to infection. It may be acute or chronic, and is due to decreased production of granulocytes in the bone marrow, or to increased destruction or utilisation. Impaired production invariably results from the toxic effects of certain drugs (e.g. phenylbutazone, antithyroid drugs, cytotoxic drugs, phenothiazines or sulphonamides) on the bone marrow. In addition, production may be impaired by irradiation or malignant bone-marrow disease. Agranulocytosis may also be inherited.

Symptoms
Symptoms are a direct consequence of an increased susceptibility to bacterial and fungal infection. The mouth and throat appear to be particularly at risk, and ulceration and dysphagia are common. Initial symptoms may include fever, rigors and prostration. Localised infections of the gastrointestinal and respiratory systems and the skin may also occur and, if untreated, may progress to septic shock and death.

Treatment
The offending agent should be withdrawn immediately and any serious infection treated by the administration of an appropriate antimicrobial drug (BNF 5.1 and 5.2). Antimicrobials may also be given as prophylaxis. Corticosteroids (BNF 6.3.2) may be given to treat shock, and lithium carbonate has been used in attempts to stimulate granulocyte production. Mouth ulcers may require local treatment.

Amyloidosis

Definition and aetiology
Amyloidosis is an uncommon disorder characterised by the deposition of a glycoprotein, amyloid, in a wide variety of body tissues. Amyloid is synthesised by reticulo-endothelial cells and is not normally found in the body in significant amounts. In amyloidosis, amyloid invades and displaces parenchymal cells, thus impairing the function of the affected organ. Amyloidosis may be idiopathic, but is often associated with chronic infections and inflammatory or malignant diseases (e.g. Hodgkin's disease, myeloma, rheumatoid arthritis, ankylosing spondylitis and tuberculosis). It may be inherited.

Symptoms
Symptoms are related to the site of amyloid deposition. They include arrhythmias, heart failure, nephrotic syndrome, renal failure, macroglossia, hepatomegaly, splenomegaly, diarrhoea and haemorrhage in the gastrointestinal tract. Amyloid may also accumulate in skin.

Treatment
The underlying disease should be treated. There is no specific treatment for amyloidosis, although

colchicine, corticosteroids, cytotoxic drugs and dimethyl sulfoxide have been used.

Embolism and venous thrombosis

Embolism

Definition and aetiology
An embolism is an obstruction of a blood vessel by a mass of undissolved material or gas (an embolus) which has been transported from another part of the circulation.

An embolus may consist of a thrombus (thromboembolus) or may be composed of gas, fat or tumour cells. Thromboemboli usually arise in the leg veins (*see* Deep vein thrombosis *below*) or in the heart. Air emboli may be introduced into the circulation during surgical procedures. Gas embolism may also be caused by bubbles of nitrogen appearing in the circulation of subjects who undergo rapid decompression (e.g. divers). Fat embolism may occur as a result of bone marrow entering the circulation following the fracture of a long bone. Malignant cells from a tumour may enter the circulation to form an embolism. Common sites of embolism are the arteries of the brain (*see* Stroke, Section 4.2), the lungs (*see* Pulmonary embolism *below*), and the legs.

Symptoms
Embolism in a major artery of the leg may result in acute limb ischaemia. Symptoms include pain and pallor of the affected limb. Claudication (limping) may be present. Chronic limb ischaemia is characterised by intermittent claudication (pain on exercise of the leg muscle which is relieved by rest). Pain on rest, however, may occur, and ulceration and gangrene of the limb may develop.

Treatment
Emergency surgery may be required for embolism in a major artery to restore the circulation. In chronic ischaemia, patients should be advised to exercise, reduce weight and avoid smoking. In order to avoid infection, great care must be taken when trimming nails, and attention to cleanliness of the affected limb is important. If symptoms are severe and persistent, treatment is by surgery (embolectomy). Amputation may occasionally be necessary.

Deep vein thrombosis

Definition and aetiology
Venous thrombosis is the formation of a blood clot (thrombus) within a vein and is usually accompanied by inflammation of the vein (thrombophlebitis). It is usually caused by venous stasis (e.g. during chronic illness or after surgery), venous damage (e.g. in infection), or as a result of disruption of clotting mechanisms (e.g. in malignant disease or oral contraceptive administration). Venous thrombosis most commonly affects the veins of the legs.

Symptoms
In deep vein thrombosis, no local symptoms may be produced. However, warmth, aching and swelling of the calf or thigh may develop, together with erythema. Severe pain may occur. The thrombus may become detached and be transported to the lung, resulting in pulmonary embolism (*see below*). This may be the presenting symptom.

Treatment
Treatment consists of the administration of heparin (BNF 2.8.1) and oral anticoagulants (BNF 2.8.2), analgesics (BNF 4.7) and bed rest. Fibrinolytic drugs (BNF 2.10) may also be used in severe cases. Surgery may be required. Prophylactic measures include limb compression (e.g. with graduated compression hosiery) and elevation, and the use of anticoagulants.

Superficial thrombophlebitis

Definition and aetiology
Superficial thrombophlebitis (phlebitis) is thrombosis of a superficial vein which occurs as a result of inflammation.

Symptoms
Superficial thrombophlebitis is characterised by local pain and tenderness, erythema, oedema and

local warmth. The thrombosed vein may be felt as a hard 'cord'. It rarely results in embolism.

Treatment

Treatment consists of rest, limb elevation and the administration of analgesics (BNF 4.7). The condition is usually self-limiting.

Pulmonary embolism and infarction

Definition and aetiology

Pulmonary embolism is the blockage of the pulmonary artery or one of its branches by an embolus, which leads to a reduction in pulmonary blood flow. It may be associated with necrosis of lung tissue (pulmonary infarction). It is almost always due to thrombi, which pass into the pulmonary circulation from a deep vein thrombosis (*see above*). Rarely, the embolus consists of air, fat or tumour cells.

Symptoms

The symptoms of pulmonary embolism depend on the extent and duration of the embolus. In minor disease, patients may be asymptomatic, although sudden acute chest pain and haemoptysis are common and are associated with pulmonary infarction. In more severe cases, these symptoms are less likely, although right heart failure may develop and be associated with anginal pain. Other symptoms include acute dyspnoea, tachypnoea and cyanosis. Syncope may occur as a result of a reduction in cardiac output, and may be fatal. Pulmonary hypertension and a rise in venous pressure may occur in subacute and chronic cases.

Treatment

Treatment is symptomatic in mild disease, although in severe cases emergency resuscitation may be necessary. In such cases, treatment may include oxygen therapy (BNF 3.6) and the administration of opioid analgesics for chest pain (BNF 4.7.2), parenteral (BNF 2.8.1) and oral anticoagulants (BNF 2.8.2), and fibrinolytic drugs (BNF 2.10). Surgical embolectomy may be necessary if symptoms are life-threatening. Anticoagulant prophylaxis using low-dose heparin or warfarin may be necessary for patients at risk.

Polycythaemia

Definition and aetiology

Polycythaemia is a myeloproliferative disorder characterised by an increased mass of erythrocytes in the circulatory system. It may be of unknown aetiology (e.g. polycythaemia vera, *see below*), or be caused by a decreased total blood volume produced by severe dehydration or burns, diuretic therapy or endocrine disorders (relative, pseudo-, or stress polycythaemia). Erythrocytosis (secondary polycythaemia) occurs as a physiological response to tissue hypoxia encountered in heart, pulmonary or renal diseases. It may also occur in healthy individuals who live at high altitude.

Polycythaemia vera

Definition and aetiology

Polycythaemia vera is a chronic myeloproliferative disorder characterised by proliferation of the bone marrow, resulting in an increased erythrocyte count and often accompanied by an increase in leucocytes, platelets and total blood volume. It occurs most commonly between 50 and 60 years of age, but its exact cause is unknown.

Symptoms

The onset of polycythaemia vera may be insidious. Its presence may be initially diagnosed during an investigation of gout. Patients may have a ruddy complexion and initially suffer non-specific symptoms (e.g. fatigue, headache, tinnitus, vertigo and visual disturbances). Severe pruritus, especially after bathing, is common. Cardiovascular symptoms, due to increased blood viscosity, may develop and include angina pectoris and thromboses. Abnormal platelet function may result in haemorrhage, and abdominal pain may arise from peptic ulceration and splenomegaly. Death may follow haemorrhage or thrombosis, or the disease may progress to acute leukaemia.

Treatment

Treatment is controversial, but may include venesection and removal of 300–500 mL blood every other day, and the administration of radioactive phosphorus-32 or certain cytotoxic drugs (BNF 8.1).

Splenomegaly and hypersplenism

Definition and aetiology

Splenomegaly is enlargement of the spleen which may be accompanied by hypersplenism (*see below*). Splenomegaly usually occurs as a result of some other primary disorder. Common causes include infections (e.g. malaria and typhoid), inflammatory diseases (e.g. rheumatoid arthritis, sarcoidosis and amyloidosis), chronic haemolytic anaemias (e.g. hereditary spherocytosis and thalassaemias), portal hypertension, malignant disease or physical trauma.

Symptoms

In addition to palpable splenic enlargement, splenomegaly is often accompanied by abdominal pain, oesophageal varices, a feeling of satiety (due to pressure on the stomach) and purpura. Hypersplenism may occur and is characterised by a reduction in the number of circulating blood cells and a compensatory proliferation of bone marrow.

Treatment

Treatment is by the correction of the underlying primary disorder. Because of the inherent dangers (i.e. thrombosis and infection), splenectomy should only be performed in restricted circumstances (e.g. chronic haemolytic disorders and severe physical trauma).

9.1.2 ANAEMIAS

Anaemias

Definition and aetiology

Anaemia is a reduction in the concentration of erythrocytes or haemoglobin, or both, in the blood. In addition, the size and shape of erythrocytes may be altered. Anaemias may occur as a result of any condition in which there is defective production (e.g. iron, folic acid or vitamin B_{12} deficiency), or increased destruction (e.g. by drugs) or loss (e.g. haemorrhage) of erythrocytes.

Symptoms

The symptoms of anaemias are related to a reduction in the oxygen-carrying capacity of the blood and arise from tissue hypoxia. Mild anaemias may be asymptomatic, although fatigue, general weakness and pallor may be evident. In more severe disease, a wide variety of additional symptoms are likely and may include angina pectoris, dyspnoea, heart failure with peripheral oedema, and tachycardia. Drowsiness, headache, irritability, tinnitus and vertigo may also occur. Gastrointestinal symptoms include anorexia, constipation, diarrhoea and nausea. Menstrual disturbances and loss of libido may develop.

Treatment

For treatment of the anaemias, see under individual conditions.

Aplastic anaemia

Definition and aetiology

Aplastic anaemia arises as a result of bone-marrow degeneration and is characterised by a failure to produce adequate numbers of erythrocytes, leucocytes and platelets. Those erythrocytes which are produced are, however, normal in size and haemoglobin content. It occurs most commonly in adolescents and young adults. Aplastic anaemia may occur as a result of exposure to chemicals (e.g. benzene), drugs (e.g. chloramphenicol, chlorpromazine, cytotoxic drugs, phenylbutazone or phenytoin), or to radiation. It may also follow a viral infection or very rarely be inherited (e.g. Fanconi's anaemia).

Symptoms

Symptoms include those stated under anaemias (*see* Anaemias *above*). In addition, the likelihood of infections is increased as a result of leucopenia, haemorrhage may occur due to thrombocytopenia, and these often prove fatal.

Treatment

Treatment comprises the avoidance of causative agents, reducing sources of infection, and the prompt administration of antimicrobial drugs (BNF 5.1) for any existing infection. The treatment of choice for older patients or those without a compatible donor is equine antithymocyte globulin (ATG). Ciclosporin (BNF 8.2.2) has also been shown to be effective, either on its own or in combination with ATG. Blood transfusion may be necessary, and anabolic steroids and corticosteroids (BNF 9.1.3) have been used. It may be necessary to administer a chelating compound and ascorbic acid (BNF 9.1.3) to treat iron overload arising from repeated transfusion. Bone-marrow transplantation is indicated in intractable disease.

Haemolytic anaemias

Definition and aetiology

Haemolytic anaemias are characterised by an increased destruction of erythrocytes, although those that remain are of normal size and haemoglobin content. They may be caused by defective erythrocyte formation, they may be inherited (e.g. sickle-cell anaemia and beta thalassaemia), or may be due to the action of some other factor (e.g. blood transfusion, drug administration, infection or other systemic disease, or autoimmune mechanisms).

Symptoms

Symptoms are as stated under anaemias (*see* Anaemias *above*), but haemolytic anaemias may also be accompanied by hepatomegaly and splenomegaly, hyperbilirubinaemia or jaundice. Haemoglobinuria and oliguria may occur.

Treatment

Treatment comprises the identification and withdrawal of the underlying cause. Anabolic steroids, corticosteroids and pyridoxine (BNF 9.1.3) have been used.

Beta thalassaemia

Definition and aetiology

Beta thalassaemia is an inherited, chronic, haemolytic anaemia occurring most commonly in Mediterranean and some Eastern races. There is a reduction in (beta thalassaemia minor) or complete absence of (beta thalassaemia major) production of beta chains, which are one type of polypeptide chain contributing to the structure of normal adult haemoglobin (haemoglobin A). The eventual result is ineffective erythropoiesis and failure of the red cells to mature.

Symptoms

Symptoms of beta thalassaemia major often occur in the first year of life. They include failure to thrive, short stature, bossed skull with prominent jaw and a muddy complexion. There may be marked hepatomegaly with abdominal distension in addition to the symptoms stated under anaemias (*see* Anaemias *above*). Infection is a common complication. Iron overload is common as a result of repeated transfusion and heart failure may occur. Beta thalassaemia major is often fatal. The minor variant is usually asymptomatic, although intermediate forms of the disease do exist.

Treatment

Prevention in future generations may be achieved by genetic counselling or antenatal screening. Treatment is by repeated transfusion or more recently by bone-marrow transplantation. The maintenance of an adequate diet and the prophylactic administration of folic acid (BNF 9.1.2) may be beneficial. The administration of a chelating compound and ascorbic acid (BNF 9.1.3) may be required to treat iron overload.

Sickle-cell anaemia

Definition and aetiology

Sickle-cell anaemia is a severe inherited haemolytic anaemia characterised by the presence of sickle-shaped erythrocytes. 'Sickling' occurs as a result of the formation of abnormal haemoglobin. The disease occurs most commonly in black people, in whom it affects as many as 0.5%; between 8% and 13% are carriers of the disease.

Symptoms

Mild forms of the disease may be asymptomatic and only discovered during hypoxic episodes (e.g. during anaesthesia). Symptoms may be mild or severe. All the symptoms stated under anaemias (*see* Anaemias *above*) may be present, but severe infection (e.g. bronchitis) and painful swelling of the hands and feet (hand and foot syndrome) may also occur, particularly during the first year of life. Thromboses may develop as a result of the abnormally shaped erythrocytes, and crises are likely, particularly in the presence of infection. Initial symptoms may include severe bone pain in the limbs and back. Dyspnoea with chest pain may occur. There may be marked splenomegaly and hepatomegaly together with acute abdominal pain (which may occasionally be the major symptom). Complications include convulsions, jaundice, meningitis and osteomyelitis. Sickle-cell anaemia is often fatal, commonly due to renal impairment.

Treatment

There is no effective cure for the disease. Prevention may be achieved by genetic counselling or antenatal screening. In the presence of the disease, prompt antibacterial therapy (BNF 5.1) is indicated for the treatment of concurrent infection. Patients should be hospitalised at the time of a crisis, and oxygen therapy (BNF 3.6) and opioid analgesics (BNF 4.7.2) may be required. Transfusion may be indicated. Folic acid (BNF 9.1.2) may be administered prophylactically.

Haemolytic disease of the newborn

Definition and aetiology

Haemolytic disease of the newborn is caused by the passage of IgG antibodies from the mother across the placenta to the fetus. The antibodies can be derived from almost any source, but are most commonly caused by incompatability of rhesus factors in the maternal and fetal circulation. Haemolytic disease of the newborn caused by rhesus incompatability usually occurs in the second or subsequent pregnancies.

A second common, but less severe, cause of haemolytic disease is incompatibility between maternal and fetal ABO blood groups. This occurs predominantly when a fetus of blood group A or B is born to a mother of blood group O. Unlike in rhesus incompatability, ABO incompatibility can commonly produce symptoms in the first-born child.

Symptoms

In rhesus haemolytic disease, symptoms range from severe to mild. In severe cases, the fetus is usually prematurely delivered, has pronounced anaemia, and is usually born with hydrops fetalis. This syndrome consists of generalised oedema of the scalp, the lungs (pleurisy) and peritoneal cavity (ascites). The skin is extremely pale, the heart, liver and spleen are grossly dilated, and heart failure may occur. Death often occurs rapidly. In less severe cases, many of these symptoms are still present, although physiological jaundice may develop from the continued breakdown of erythrocytes. Excess levels of bilirubin can lead to kernicterus. In mild cases, anaemia may be only mild and jaundice may be absent.

The symptoms of ABO haemolytic disease are considerably less severe than the rhesus form. Raised bilirubin levels and haemolysis infrequently occur, and it is thought that hydrops fetalis never arises from ABO incompatability.

Treatment

In cases of severe anaemia or where there is a risk of kernicterus, freshly donated rhesus-negative blood must be given to the neonate by exchange transfusion. Phototherapy may also be beneficial. In hydrops fetalis, diuretics (BNF 2.2), positive inotropic drugs (BNF 2.1), and fluid and electrolytes (BNF 9.2) are also vital.

Prevention in the mother by administration of anti-D (Rh_0) immunoglobulin in rhesus-negative women who have previously carried a rhesus-positive baby or had an abortion has significantly reduced the incidence.

Iron-deficiency anaemias

Definition and aetiology

Iron-deficiency anaemias are due to inadequate iron intake (e.g. in dietary deficiency, malabsorption syndromes or pregnancy) or to iron loss by haemorrhage (e.g. gastrointestinal tumour, haemorrhoids, menorrhagia or peptic ulceration). The erythrocytes are small (microcytic) and deficient in haemoglobin (hypochromic).

Symptoms

The symptoms of iron-deficiency anaemias are as described under anaemias (*see* Anaemias *above*).

Treatment

Treatment is by the administration of iron salts (BNF 9.1) and correction of any underlying pathology.

Megaloblastic anaemias

Definition and aetiology

Megaloblastic anaemias are most commonly due to a deficiency of vitamin B_{12} or folic acid, or both, and are characterised by the failure of erythrocytes to mature. Despite a normal haemoglobin content (normochromic), the erythrocytes are fewer in number and larger (macrocytic) than usual. Vitamin B_{12} deficiency may occur in some vegetarians and vegans. If the intrinsic factor secreted by the gastric mucosa is absent, vitamin B_{12} is not absorbed. This is characteristic of pernicious anaemia and also occurs after total gastrectomy. Folic acid deficiency may occur in alcoholics, the elderly, during pregnancy, or in malabsorption syndromes. It may also arise as a side-effect of drug administration (e.g. methotrexate and phenytoin).

Symptoms

The symptoms of megaloblastic anaemias are as described under anaemias (*see* Anaemias *above*), but in addition they are associated with glossitis, leucopenia and thrombocytopenia. Vitamin B_{12} deficiency may also result in subacute combined degeneration of the spinal cord.

Treatment

Treatment comprises the identification of the specific deficiency and the administration of vitamin B_{12} or folic acid preparations (BNF 9.1.2), or both, as appropriate.

9.1.3 HAEMORRHAGIC DISORDERS

Haemophilia

Definition and aetiology

Haemophilia (classical haemophilia or haemophilia A) is an inherited haemorrhagic disorder occurring almost exclusively in males. It is characterised by a tendency to excessive haemorrhage in response to trivial injury. It arises as a result of a deficiency of the antihaemophilic factor, factor VIII, in blood. Women may carry the disease, but do not normally suffer from it. Men inherit it from their carrier mothers (i.e. it is an X-chromosome-linked disease).

Symptoms

The extent of this inherited deficiency varies between families. Some symptoms of haemophilia may occur in an individual in whom the haemostatic capacity of factor VIII is reduced to about 25–50% of normal. In infancy, bleeding is characterised by the appearance of cutaneous ecchymoses or haematomata in the soft tissues. In severely affected children whose factor VIII level is 1% or less, joint haemorrhages (haemarthroses) are likely to occur as soon as crawling or walking begins. If untreated, these haemorrhages result in severe pain, limitation of movement, destruction of joints and skeletal deformity. The knees, elbows and ankles are most commonly affected. Bleeding into muscle and gastrointestinal haemorrhage also occur. Excessive bleeding is also common after dental and surgical procedures, and major surgery or trauma may cause fatal haemorrhage.

Treatment

Prevention in future generations may be achieved by genetic counselling or antenatal screening. Haemorrhages may be treated by the intravenous administration of factor VIII, which may also be given as prophylaxis prior to dental or surgical procedures. Desmopressin may be used as an adjunct. Drugs which may precipitate haemorrhage (e.g. aspirin and indomethacin) must be avoided.

Christmas disease

Definition and aetiology

Christmas disease (haemophilia B), named after the patient first described with the condition, is an inherited haemorrhagic disorder characterised by a deficiency of factor IX. It is less common than haemophilia, and its inheritance and clinical presentation are identical to haemophilia A.

Symptoms and treatment
Symptoms and treatment are similar to that of haemophilia (*see above*), with the exception that factor IX is administered.

Purpuras

Definition and aetiology
Purpuras are a group of disorders. They are characterised by purple/red skin discoloration, which occurs, sometimes in the absence of physical trauma, as a result of leakage of blood from capillaries into the tissues.

Anaphylactoid purpura

Definition and aetiology
Anaphylactoid purpura (Henoch–Schönlein purpura) is thought to occur as a result of an anaphylactic response to an infective allergen. It is predominantly caused by an upper respiratory-tract infection, although no specific allergen has been identified. It commonly occurs in children between two and seven years of age, with a higher incidence in boys. It can, however, occur at any age.

Symptoms
The onset is usually sudden, with the appearance of characteristic symmetrical purpuras particularly on the lower limbs and buttocks. Somatic symptoms include abdominal pain with gastrointestinal haemorrhage, arthralgia, fever and malaise, and myalgia. Renal complications (e.g. glomerulonephritis) may produce oedema, haematuria and proteinuria. The disorder is usually self-limiting after about four weeks, although relapses are common. Death may infrequently occur as a result of gastrointestinal haemorrhage or renal failure.

Treatment
Treatment is not normally required, although corticosteroids (BNF 6.3.2) have been given in the presence of severe symptoms.

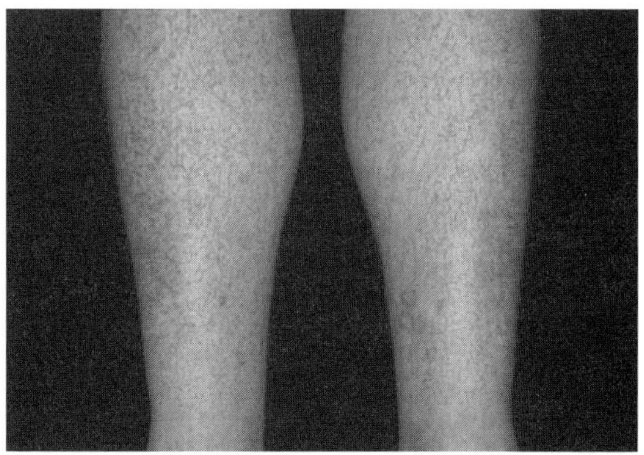

Figure 9.1 NSAID-induced vasculitis on the leg. (Reproduced with permission of Mike Wyndham.)

Vascular purpura due to drugs or infection

Definition and aetiology
Vasculitis (in the absence of thrombocytopenia) caused by blood-vessel wall damage may produce purpura during acute infections (e.g. meningitis). It may also follow drug therapy (e.g. with penicillin, chlorothiazides, non-steroidal anti-inflammatories or sulphonamides) (Figure 9.1).

Treatment
Exposure to known precipitating factors should be avoided.

Thrombotic thrombocytopenic purpura

Definition and aetiology
Thrombotic thrombocytopenic purpura is of unknown aetiology. It is characterised by histological and anatomical changes in small blood vessels and a decreased concentration of platelets, particularly in peripheral blood. It may be precipitated by an acute infection. The disorder may occur at any age and is more common in adult women.

Symptoms
The onset is sudden. Common symptoms include anaemia, convulsions, fever, haemorrhage (particularly of the gastrointestinal tract), psychiatric disturbances and purpura. Symptoms may last for days or weeks, and acute relapses are

common. Death may occur as a result of severe haemorrhage, renal failure or stroke.

Treatment
Treatment is non-specific and symptomatic. Transfusion may be required for anaemia, and dialysis for renal failure. Other methods of treatment have included the administration of anticoagulant and antiplatelet drugs, splenectomy and exchange transfusion.

Thrombocytopenia

Definition and aetiology
Thrombocytopenia is a deficiency of blood platelets (below the normal range of 140 000–400 000/μL) which results in spontaneous haemorrhage. It may be caused by a decrease in the production of platelets or an increase in their rate of destruction. Thrombocytopenia caused by failure of platelet production may occur in aplastic anaemia, megaloblastic leukaemia or malignant bone disease. Excessive platelet destruction may occur as a result of an autoimmune mechanism (idiopathic thrombocytopenic purpura) and may be acute or chronic. In addition, thrombocytopenia may be secondary to some other condition (e.g. hypersplenism or systemic lupus erythematosus). It may also follow transfusion or an acute infection, or arise as a side-effect of drug administration (e.g. quinidine). A transient thrombocytopenia may occur in infants born to mothers suffering from idiopathic thrombocytopenic purpura.

Symptoms
The acute idiopathic disease occurs most commonly in children, is usually of rapid onset and short duration, and is characterised by petechiae. Chronic disease is marked by bruising, scattered petechiae and mucous membrane bleeding. Epistaxis, gastrointestinal haemorrhage and menorrhagia may occur. Relapses may be frequent and death is common.

Treatment
Idiopathic disease is treated by the administration of corticosteroids (BNF 9.1.4); splenectomy may be indicated in the chronic form. Other drugs, including azathioprine, danazol and vinca alkaloids (BNF 9.1.4), have been used. In drug-induced disease, the offending agent should be withdrawn. Any primary blood or other systemic disorder should be treated.

9.1.4 LYMPHATIC DISORDERS

Lymphangiectasia

Definition and aetiology
Lymphangiectasia is the dilatation of lymphatic vessels in the small intestine. It may be congenital or acquired, occurring secondary to malignant disease, pericarditis or pancreatitis.

Symptoms
It is characterised by mild diarrhoea or steatorrhoea, or both, hypoproteinaemia and oedema.

Treatment
Treatment consists of adoption of a low-fat diet. Surgical resection may be possible for localised disease.

9.2 Nutritional disorders

9.2.1 GENERAL DISORDERS

Anorexia nervosa

Definition and aetiology
Anorexia nervosa is characterised by a distorted perception of body image associated with marked anxiety regarding weight gain and physical appearance. It is a condition of unknown aetiology which predominantly affects females between 10 and 30 years of age, and may be chronic. The disease has been reported as affecting between 0.25 and 14 per 100 000 female population, and the incidence has increased in recent years.

Symptoms
Anorexia results in weight loss of at least 25% of original body-weight caused by insufficient food

intake, and may be accentuated by self-induced vomiting, purgation or excessive exercise. There may also be evidence of emotional disturbance (e.g. bereavement or examinations) and family tensions. The patient may be withdrawn, depressed and may suffer from insomnia and have difficulty in concentrating. There is usually denial of any illness.

Physical signs include wasting of subcutaneous fat, resulting in hollow cheeks, stick-like limbs, shrunken breasts, flat abdomen, and wasted thighs and buttocks. The hands and feet are usually cold, and the skin is dry and covered with an excess of downy hair (lanugo) over the neck, cheeks, forearms and legs. Bradycardia and hypotension are usually present and amenorrhoea, loss of libido and impotence usually appear at an early stage due to endocrine disturbances.

Treatment

Severe cases should be treated in hospital, with psychological support aimed at gaining the patient's confidence, restoring body-weight, and reducing the duration of the condition. Intravenous (BNF 9.3) or enteral nutrition (BNF Appendix 7) may also be necessary. Long-term treatment with supportive psychotherapy is directed at preventing relapses.

Bulimia nervosa

Definition and aetiology

Bulimia nervosa is associated with anorexia nervosa and is characterised by episodes of gross overeating, followed by a pathological fear of getting fat. This causes the patient to self-inflict vomiting or purgation, or both, often using fingers or a toothbrush to induce the gag reflex. The condition commonly arises in women who are slightly older than those presenting with anorexia nervosa alone.

It has an incidence of between 1% and 2% amongst young women, and has become the most common eating disorder.

Symptoms

Overeating and vomiting occur at least once daily, rising to an incidence of up to 40 times in severe forms. Persistent vomiting causes depletion of body fluids and electrolytes, resulting in hypokalaemia, hyponatraemia and alkalosis. Consequently, muscle weakness, tetany and convulsions may occur, with urinary-tract infections, and renal failure resulting from loss of potassium. There may be depressive symptoms of gloom, irritability and occasionally suicidal contemplations. Body-weight may be normal, and menstruation and fertility are not impaired.

Treatment

Severe cases are treated in hospital, but most cases respond to counselling or group therapy. Treatment is directed towards the restoration of normal eating habits, and convincing the patient to accept a higher body-weight. Antidepressant drugs (BNF 4.3) may have a beneficial effect.

Obesity

Definition and aetiology

Obesity is characterised by an increase in body-weight in excess of physical requirements, and results from excessive accumulation of body fat. It is most commonly caused by a dietary intake which exceeds that required for physical activity, tissue repair and vital functions. However, obesity may very occasionally arise from genetic disorders, often in association with hypogonadism. Endocrine causes of obesity are rare, but may include Cushing's syndrome or hypothyroidism. Obesity may also be drug induced (e.g. by corticosteroids, oral contraceptives or phenothiazines). A family history of obesity is common in overweight individuals, and the condition is often considered to have an emotional or behavioural component.

Complications

Obesity is often responsible for a deterioration in health and, in severe cases, can lead to premature death. Obesity may be associated with an increased likelihood of cardiovascular disease (e.g. angina pectoris, heart failure, hypertension and stroke), diabetes mellitus and gastrointestinal disease (particularly of the colon or gall bladder), some of which may be life-threatening. Obese women may suffer from menstrual disorders. All overweight individuals are more susceptible to back pain, osteoarthritis, respiratory disorders and varicose veins. Severely obese patients are also at greater risk during surgery involving general anaesthesia.

Treatment
Treatment is primarily by dietary management which is usually necessary on a permanent basis. A group approach (e.g. weight-watchers) is often beneficial. Behaviour modification may be tried in some patients and psychological support is often valuable. Appetite suppressants (BNF 4.5) are available and may be of some short-term value in selected patients. Surgical techniques (e.g. gastrointestinal bypasses and jaw wiring) have been used in severe cases.

9.2.2 INTOLERANCE CONDITIONS

Lactose intolerance

Definition and aetiology
Lactose intolerance is an inability to metabolise and absorb lactose. It arises as a result of a deficiency of the enzyme, lactase, which is responsible for converting lactose to galactose and glucose in the small intestine. As a result, lactose accumulates and is subject to fermentation. Lactase is synthesised by the intestinal mucosa and deficiency may arise from an intestinal disorder (e.g. coeliac disease, Crohn's disease, gastroenteritis and short-bowel syndrome).

Lactase deficiency occurs normally in about 75% of adults, except for adults from north-western Europe in whom the incidence is less than 20%.

Symptoms
The characteristic symptom is explosive, frothy diarrhoea associated with abdominal cramps and distension, and nausea and vomiting. Affected children fail to gain weight.

Treatment
Treatment is by the introduction of a lactose-free diet (BNF Appendix 7), with supplements of calcium (BNF 9.5.1).

9.2.3 DEFICIENCY DISORDERS

Beri-beri

Definition and aetiology
Beri-beri is caused by dietary thiamine (vitamin B_1) deficiency. It occurs as a result of starvation (or high carbohydrate intake following starvation), and may occasionally occur in chronic alcoholism. Beri-beri may also arise due to increased requirements for vitamin B_1, in hyperthyroidism, pregnancy, lactation and fever.

Symptoms
Early symptoms (e.g. general weakness) are vague. Subsequently, cardiovascular symptoms may predominate (wet beri-beri), and these include congestive heart failure with marked oedema and dyspnoea. Polyneuropathy may occur (dry beri-beri) and paraesthesia and cramps of the legs are common. Ataxia, confusion, nystagmus and speech disorders may develop. In untreated cases, encephalopathy, coma and death may result.

Treatment
Treatment is by the oral or parenteral administration of thiamine hydrochloride (BNF 9.6.2).

Pellagra

Definition and aetiology
Pellagra is caused by a deficiency of nicotinic acid, although other vitamin deficiencies are often present. It commonly occurs as a result of poor diet (e.g. in areas where maize forms a major part of the diet), but may also arise as a result of malabsorption disorders, diarrhoea or alcoholism.

Symptoms
It is characterised by a symmetrical erythematous rash (pellagra dermatitis) followed by hypertrophy and subsequently atrophy of the skin. Diarrhoea and dementia are common, but encephalopathy only rarely develops.

Treatment
Treatment is by the administration of nicotinamide (BNF 9.6.2). Accompanying nutritional deficiencies may also require treatment.

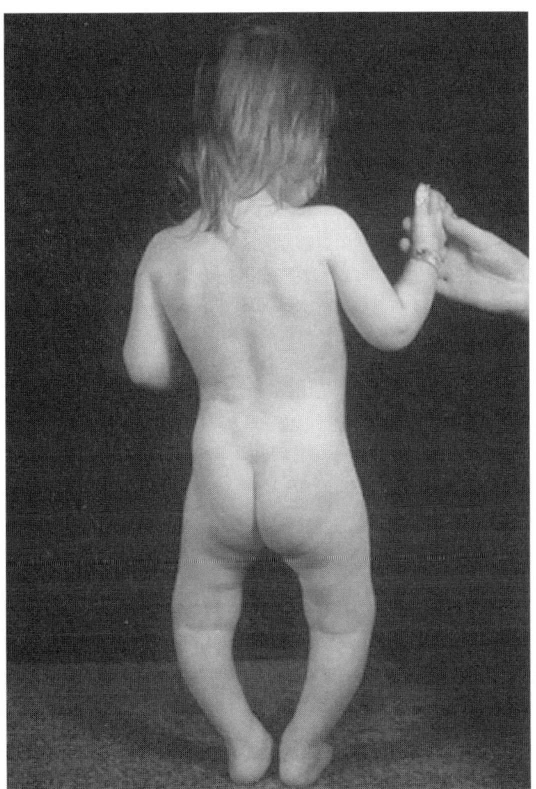

Figure 9.2 Rickets. (Reproduced with permission of Biophoto Associates/Science Photo Library.)

Rickets and osteomalacia

Definition and aetiology

Vitamin D deficiency is characterised in growing infants and children by rickets (Figure 9.2), and in adults by osteomalacia. The deficiency is often of dietary origin, but it may also be caused by inadequate exposure to sunlight, particularly in the elderly and in Asians, or by the administration of antiepileptics. Occasionally a malabsorption disorder may be responsible. Rarely it may be caused by an inherited renal tubular disorder (i.e. hypophosphataemic vitamin D-resistant rickets). Vitamin D deficiency results in decreased gastrointestinal absorption of calcium and phosphate, which leads to the defective mineralisation of bone. Osteomalacia is more common in women as a result of the additional nutritional demands exerted by pregnancy.

Symptoms

Rickets is characterised by a reduced growth-rate and skeletal deformities (e.g. bowing of the long bones, enlargement of epiphyses and bossing of the skull). Chest and spinal deformities may also be evident, and muscle weakness may occur.

In osteomalacia, bone pain and tenderness are common, and fractures (e.g. of the neck of the femur) may occur. Muscle weakness may reduce the patient's mobility, causing a waddling gait, difficulty in climbing and descending stairs and in standing from low chairs.

Treatment

Treatment is similar for both rickets and osteomalacia. Vitamin D preparations (BNF 9.6.4) may be given in combination with calcium, and also as prophylaxis. A phosphate supplement (BNF 9.5.2.1) may be required in hypophosphataemic rickets. An appropriate diet should be maintained, and adequate exposure to sunlight is beneficial. Any underlying primary disorder should be treated.

Scurvy

Definition and aetiology

Scurvy is caused by a dietary deficiency of ascorbic acid (vitamin C) and is characterised by impaired collagen synthesis. It is most common in elderly or alcoholic patients, but may occur in artificially fed infants.

Symptoms

In adults, the onset is usually insidious and is marked by anorexia, fatigue and general malaise. Other common symptoms include haemorrhage in, and inflammation of, the gums, gingival infection and loose dentition. Haemorrhages may also occur in the gastrointestinal or urinary tracts, the muscles, nose and skin, and wound healing may be impaired. In infants, subperiosteal haemorrhage with pain and tenderness of the legs may occur, but gingival symptoms are less common.

Treatment

Treatment consists of the administration of ascorbic acid (BNF 9.6.3), which may also be given as prophylaxis.

Vitamin A deficiency

Aetiology

Vitamin A deficiency is usually due to an inadequate diet and is often accompanied by protein deficiency. It may also result from a malabsorption syndrome or hepatic impairment.

Symptoms

Visual symptoms are characteristic of vitamin A deficiency. Dark adaptation is impaired and night blindness often follows. The cornea may become soft (i.e. keratomalacia) and dry. Blindness may occur if the deficiency is untreated. Other non-specific symptoms are anaemia, growth retardation and increased susceptibility to infection.

Treatment

Treatment is by the administration of vitamin A (BNF 9.6.1), which may also be given as prophylaxis. An adequate diet should be introduced and any underlying disorder treated.

Vitamin B deficiencies

(*See also* Beri-beri *and* Pellagra *above*.)

Riboflavine deficiency

Aetiology

Riboflavine (vitamin B_2) deficiency is due to an inadequate diet.

Symptoms

Symptoms are usually mild, and include fissuring and scaling of the lips (cheilosis) and of the angles of the mouth (angular stomatitis). Glossitis and seborrhoeic dermatitis may also occur.

Treatment

Treatment is by the administration of riboflavine (BNF 9.6.2). An adequate diet should be introduced.

Pyridoxine deficiency

Aetiology

Pyridoxine (vitamin B_6) deficiency may occasionally arise from an inadequate diet, but may also result from a malabsorption syndrome or may be drug-induced (e.g. by isoniazid).

Symptoms

Symptoms include anaemias, cheilosis, seborrhoeic dermatitis, glossitis and peripheral neuropathy. Convulsions may occur in infants.

Treatment

Treatment is by the administration of pyridoxine hydrochloride (BNF 9.6.2), which may also be given as prophylaxis to prevent drug-induced deficiency. Any underlying cause should be treated.

Vitamin K deficiency

Aetiology

Vitamin K deficiency may occur in underweight neonates through inadequate synthesis. Breast-fed infants may also suffer deficiency as breast milk is a poor source of vitamin K. Other causes include decreased absorption due to obstructive jaundice or malabsorption syndromes. Drugs may antagonise vitamin K (e.g. coumarin anticoagulants) or inhibit its synthesis (e.g. sulphonamides).

Symptoms

The most common symptom, which results from low prothrombin concentrations, is haemorrhage. Likely sites of bleeding include the gastrointestinal tract, gums, nose, and wounds. Intracranial haemorrhage may occur at birth.

Treatment

Treatment is by the administration of vitamin K preparations (BNF 9.6.6), which may also be given routinely to all neonates or to mothers prior to delivery.

Zinc deficiency

Aetiology

Zinc deficiency may occur as a result of inadequate dietary intake (e.g. in young children fed on milk products which are low in zinc). Zinc may be chelated by dietary fibre or phytate, and this may also lead to deficiency. Patients suffering from malabsorption syndromes, physical trauma, burns, and those fed intravenously are also susceptible to zinc deficiency. Acrodermatitis enteropathica, a previously fatal inherited disorder, is now known to be caused by zinc malabsorption.

Symptoms
Anorexia, growth retardation, hypogeusia and hypogonadism may occur in children. Impaired dark adaptation and night blindness may also develop and wound healing may be impaired. Acrodermatitis enteropathica is characterised by alopecia, eczema, diarrhoea, growth retardation and paronychia.

Treatment
Treatment is by the administration of zinc salts (BNF 9.5.4) and dietary management.

9.3 Metabolic disorders

9.3.1 GENERAL DISORDERS

Gout

Definition and aetiology
Gout (Figure 9.3) is a disorder of purine metabolism characterised by hyperuricaemia, followed by deposition of urate crystals in joints and other tissues. Hyperuricaemia is caused by an increase in production, or decrease in renal excretion, or both, of uric acid. It may be idiopathic, inherited, secondary to some other disorder (e.g. polycythaemia vera or renal failure), or may be due to the administration of drugs (e.g. loop or thiazide diuretics). A diet high in purines (e.g. brain, game, kidney, liver, meat extracts and sea foods) and alcohol consumption may be contributory factors.

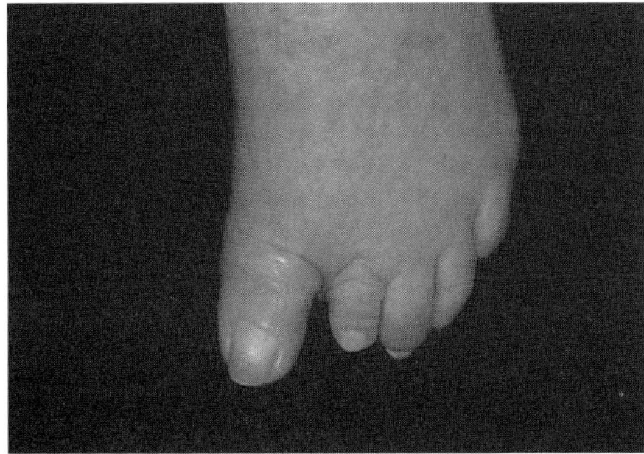

Figure 9.3 Gout. (Reproduced with permission of Mike Wyndham.)

Symptoms
Symptoms usually occur only after prolonged hyperuricaemia. The onset, however, is sudden and is characterised by severe pain and inflammation of a single joint, often the metatarsophalangeal joint of the great toe. This may be accompanied by fever and rigors. These initial symptoms commonly disappear within a few days or weeks. Recurrent attacks are likely, however, with the joints of all limbs eventually becoming chronically affected. Urate deposits (tophi) may develop in other tissues (e.g. bursae, cartilage of the pinna and tendon sheaths) and may also occur in the kidney, leading to renal impairment and even renal failure. Renal calculi are common.

Treatment
Acute gout attacks may be treated by the administration of non-steroidal anti-inflammatory drugs (BNF 10.1.1), although salicylates must not be used. Colchicine (BNF 10.1.4) may also be useful and corticotrophin may be used in unresponsive cases.

Long-term management and prophylaxis comprises the administration of a xanthine-oxidase inhibitor or a uricosuric drug (BNF 10.1.4). These must not be given during, or just after, an acute attack. Patients should be encouraged to avoid excessive consumption of foods high in purines, and of alcohol.

Hyperlipidaemias

Definition and aetiology
Hyperlipidaemias are a group of disorders characterised by increased plasma lipid concentrations (i.e. cholesterol, triglycerides, or both). Disorders which may be inherited (primary hyperlipidaemias) include common hypercholesterolaemia, familial combined hyperlipidaemia, and familial hypercholesterolaemia. They may also be acquired (secondary hyperlipidaemias),

commonly through excess alcohol consumption or hypothyroidism. Other causes include cholestasis, chronic renal failure, diabetes mellitus and gout. The administration of drugs (e.g. oral contraceptives, thiazide diuretics or chlorthalidone) may also precipitate hyperlipidaemia.

Symptoms

The most important implication of hyperlipidaemias is the consequent development of atherosclerosis with attendant ischaemic heart disease and stroke. The accumulation of yellowish lipid deposits under the skin (i.e. xanthomas) may occur in some types of hyperlipidaemia, and common sites include the eyelids (xanthelasma), elbows and knees.

Treatment

The detection and treatment of hyperlipidaemia are important factors in the prevention of atherosclerosis and heart disease. Dietary intake of saturated fats should be restricted and body-weight controlled. The administration of lipid-lowering drugs (BNF 2.12) may be indicated.

9.3.2 CARBOHYDRATE METABOLIC DISORDERS

Galactosaemia

Definition and aetiology

Galactosaemia (galactose intolerance) is an autosomal inborn error of metabolism which may occur in two forms. It is most commonly due to a deficiency of the enzyme galactose 1-phosphate uridyl transferase and a consequent inability to metabolise galactose. As a result, galactose 1-phosphate and galactose accumulate in the tissues. It may also be due to galactokinase deficiency, in which galactose accumulates in the blood and tissues.

Symptoms

In galactose 1-phosphate uridyl transferase deficiency, symptoms develop in the first few days of life. Diarrhoea is followed by dehydration and hypoglycaemia. Other symptoms include a failure to thrive, cataract formation, hepatomegaly, jaundice and vomiting. Mental retardation may occur. The disorder may be fatal in the absence of treatment, and some degree of handicap may persist even in treated patients. Antenatal brain damage may occur.

Cataract formation is the only symptom of galactokinase deficiency.

Treatment

Early treatment is essential and comprises the adoption of a galactose-free lactose-free diet. Special foods and milk substitutes are available (BNF 9.4.1 and Appendix 7). Prevention may be possible by prenatal diagnosis of the carrier state.

Glycogen storage diseases

Definition and aetiology

Glycogen storage diseases are a group of inherited metabolic disorders. Several types have been identified, and each type is characterised by deficiency of a different enzyme (e.g. glucose 6-phosphatase and glycogen synthetase) involved in glycogen metabolism. Almost all these deficiencies result in the accumulation of glycogen in body tissues.

Symptoms

Symptoms, which vary according to enzyme deficiency and body system affected, include heart failure, hepatomegaly, hypoglycaemia, physical and mental retardation, and muscle cramps and weakness.

Treatment

Some types of glycogen storage disease respond to frequent carbohydrate feeds, and special foods are available (BNF 9.4.1 and Appendix 7). Others, however, do not respond to any treatment and result in early death.

Hereditary fructose intolerance

Definition and aetiology

Hereditary frucose intolerance is an autosomal inborn error of metabolism caused by decreased activity of the enzyme fructose 1-phosphate aldolase, and a consequent inability to metabolise fructose.

Symptoms
Symptoms occur in infants soon after introducing fructose into the diet. Vomiting, anorexia and a failure to thrive are common, and are accompanied by fructosaemia, fructosuria and hypoglycaemia. Other symptoms include hepatomegaly, jaundice, proteinuria and renal impairment. Untreated cases may be fatal.

Treatment
Treatment consists of the adoption of a diet completely free of fructose, sorbitol and sucrose.

9.3.3 ELECTROLYTE DISORDERS

Acidosis

Definition
Acidosis is a disturbance of acid–base balance characterised by an accumulation of acid or depletion of alkaline content of extracellular fluid. There is an increase in the hydrogen ion concentration (i.e. a fall in pH). Acidosis may be metabolic or respiratory (*see below*), although their aetiology and mechanisms of compensation may be closely interrelated.

Metabolic acidosis

Definition and aetiology
Metabolic acidosis is caused by a metabolic disturbance in which acid accumulates in, or bicarbonate is lost from, the extracellular fluid. It may be due to shock or cardiac arrest, in which tissue hypoxia causes anaerobic metabolism and the production of lactic acid (i.e. lactic acidosis). Severe diarrhoea may also result in a metabolic acidosis through increased excretion of hydroxyl ions in the faeces. Uncontrolled diabetes mellitus and starvation may cause metabolic acidosis through increased production of organic acids (i.e. diabetic ketoacidosis). In chronic renal disease, the distal tubules may fail to excrete hydrogen ions and a metabolic acidosis develops (i.e. renal tubular acidosis). Other causes of metabolic acidosis include ingestion of acid and ethanol poisoning.

Symptoms
Mild metabolic acidosis may be asymptomatic, but it can be accompanied by fatigue, and nausea and vomiting. Rapid deep respiration (hyperpnoea) is characteristic, however, and severe acidosis may lead to the development of shock and be fatal.

Treatment
Any underlying disorder must be treated. Severe acidosis is treated by the administration of sodium bicarbonate (BNF 9.2.2) preceded by isotonic sodium chloride intravenous infusion.

Respiratory acidosis

Definition and aetiology
Respiratory acidosis is an acidosis arising from the accumulation of carbon dioxide caused by hypoventilation. There is a rise in the partial pressure of carbon dioxide (i.e. an increase in PCO_2). It may be due to respiratory depression (e.g. by drugs), chronic obstructive airways disease (e.g. chronic bronchitis or emphysema), or obstruction of the larynx or trachea.

Symptoms
Respiratory acidosis produces vasodilatation, leading to encephalopathy with headache and drowsiness. Stupor and coma may develop.

Treatment
Treatment is as for metabolic acidosis (*see above*). Assisted ventilation and oxygen therapy (BNF 3.6) may be required.

Alkalosis

Definition
Alkalosis is a disturbance of acid–base balance characterised by the accumulation of base or the

depletion of acid in the extracellular fluid. There is a decrease in the hydrogen ion concentration (i.e. a rise in pH). Alkalosis may be metabolic or respiratory (*see below*), although their aetiology and mechanisms of compensation may be closely interrelated.

Metabolic alkalosis

Definition and aetiology
Metabolic alkalosis is due to a metabolic disturbance in which bicarbonate accumulates in, or acid is lost from, the extracellular fluid. It may arise through persistent vomiting (e.g. in pyloric stenosis) resulting in the loss of gastric acid, renal retention of bicarbonate, excessive ingestion of alkali, potassium depletion or volume depletion (e.g. in burns or diuretic therapy).

Symptoms
Common symptoms include irritability and neuromuscular excitability. Tetany may develop.

Treatment
The underlying disorder should be corrected. In mild alkalosis, treatment may be unnecessary. In more severe cases, fluid replacement (BNF 9.2.2) may be undertaken and potassium and sodium depletion may require correction (BNF 9.2.2).

Respiratory alkalosis

Definition and aetiology
Respiratory alkalosis is an alkalosis arising from excessive elimination of carbon dioxide in expired air. It occurs as a result of hyperventilation and is characterised by a fall in the partial pressure of carbon dioxide (i.e. a decrease in PCO_2). Hyperventilation may result from a central nervous system disorder (e.g. stroke or meningitis), anxiety, exertion at high temperature or altitude, or from excessive assisted ventilation (e.g. during anaesthesia). It may also be due to drug administration (e.g. salicylates).

Symptoms
Respiratory alkalosis is marked by tetany with spasm of the hand muscles and acroparaesthesia. Convulsions may occur and respiratory arrest may develop. Peripheral vasoconstriction is likely, resulting in pallor.

Treatment
Treatment may consist of rebreathing expired carbon dioxide. Any underlying disorder should be treated and anxiolytics (BNF 4.1.2) may be beneficial. Excessive assisted ventilation should be corrected by appropriate adjustment of the equipment.

Hypercalcaemia

Definition and aetiology
Hypercalcaemia is an increase in the plasma-calcium concentration above normal (i.e. >2.6 mmol/L). It usually occurs as a result of calcium reabsorption from bone into the bloodstream or a decrease in the renal excretion of calcium. The most common cause is primary hyperparathyroidism, although malignant diseases with bony metastases, vitamin D administration or excessive calcium ingestion (e.g. milk-alkali syndrome) may be responsible. Other causes include Addison's disease, diuretic therapy and sarcoidosis.

Symptoms
Mild hypercalcaemia may be asymptomatic, but if symptoms develop, they may include abdominal pain, anorexia, constipation, fatigue, nausea and vomiting, and polyuria with nocturia and thirst. Severe cases are characterised by confusion, delirium and psychosis. Stupor and coma may also develop. Marked muscle weakness may occur, or renal impairment may develop as a result of calculi formation. This may progress to renal failure which may be fatal.

Treatment
The underlying cause should be identified and treated. Intravenous fluid replacement (BNF 9.2.2) and the restriction of dietary calcium may, however, be the only treatment required. The administration of binding or chelating agents (BNF 9.5.1.2) may be beneficial. In severe hypercalcaemia, a calcitonin preparation (BNF 6.6.1) or a corticosteroid (BNF 6.3.4) may be given to inhibit calcium reabsorption from bone.

Hyperkalaemia

Definition and aetiology

Hyperkalaemia is an increase in the plasma potassium concentration above normal (i.e. >5 mmol/L). It usually occurs as a result of defective excretion arising from renal failure, although excessive potassium administration or potassium-sparing diuretic therapy may also be responsible.

Symptoms

Hyperkalaemia may be initially asymptomatic, although a flaccid paralysis occasionally occurs. Characteristic ECG changes may occur, and the development of asystole is often associated with sudden death.

Treatment

In mild cases, a reduction in potassium intake or the discontinuation of potassium-sparing diuretics may be sufficient, although an ion-exchange resin (BNF 9.2.2.1) may be beneficial. Marked hyperkalaemia (i.e. >6.5 mmol/L) constitutes a medical emergency and urgent treatment (*see* Acute renal failure, Section 7.4) is essential.

Hypernatraemia

Definition and aetiology

Hypernatraemia is an increase in the plasma-sodium concentration above normal (i.e. >148 mmol/L). It usually occurs as a result of fluid loss in excess of sodium loss. This may arise as a result of diarrhoea or vomiting, excessive sweating, diabetes insipidus or osmotic diuresis. In addition, hypernatraemia may be caused by inadequate fluid intake (particularly in infants, elderly or unconscious patients) or to excessive intake of sodium (e.g. in inappropriate intravenous fluid therapy or dialysis).

Symptoms

Thirst is less marked than might be anticipated. Symptoms may include confusion, drowsiness and lethargy, dry skin, hypotension, muscle twitching and peripheral vasoconstriction. Coma may develop. Hypernatraemia is especially dangerous when it occurs suddenly, and thromboses may occur in infants. Brain cells may become dehydrated, resulting in cerebral, subarachnoid or subdural haemorrhage.

Treatment

Treatment is by the gradual correction of fluid balance and may comprise the intravenous (BNF 9.2.2) or oral (BNF 9.2.1) administration of fluid.

Hypocalcaemia

Definition and aetiology

Hypocalcaemia is a reduction in the plasma calcium concentration below normal (i.e. <2.1 mmol/L). It is an infrequent occurrence, but may develop as a result of hypoparathyroidism, vitamin D deficiency, renal disease, magnesium depletion, acute pancreatitis or hypoproteinaemia.

Symptoms

Hypocalcaemia is often asymptomatic. However, symptoms may develop depending on the severity, and include paraesthesia of the face, fingers and toes, tetany, or prolonged tonic spasms of muscles due to neuromuscular instability. This may result in laryngeal spasm and stridor. Convulsions and psychosis may also occur.

Treatment

Treatment depends upon the underlying disorder. Intravenous infusion of calcium salts (BNF 9.5.1.1) or oral calcium, sometimes in combination with vitamin D, may be used in hypoparathyroidism. Dietary phosphorus restriction or phosphate-binding agents (BNF 9.5.2.2) may be beneficial in renal failure.

Hypokalaemia

Definition and aetiology

Hypokalaemia is a reduction in the plasma potassium concentration below normal (i.e. <3.5 mmol/L). It may occur as a result of potassium loss in the urine, renal disease or in diuretic therapy (e.g. with thiazide or loop diuretics). Excess potassium may also be lost in the faeces and may occur as a result of diarrhoea or laxative abuse. Other causes include Cushing's syndrome, corticosteroid therapy, diabetes mellitus, hyperaldosteronism (*see* Primary aldosteronism, Section 6.3), or vomiting. Dietary deficiency may occur in elderly patients.

Symptoms
Hypokalaemia may be characterised by neuromuscular disturbances, cramps, muscle weakness and tetany. In severe cases, muscle weakness may progress to paralysis and respiratory failure. Arrhythmias may also develop, particularly in patients receiving cardiac glycosides.

Treatment
Any underlying cause should be corrected. If diuretics are being given, a potassium-sparing drug (BNF 2.2.3 and 2.2.4) should be used, especially in those patients also receiving cardiac glycosides. The administration of oral potassium supplements (BNF 9.2.1.1) may be indicated, and intravenous therapy (BNF 9.2.2) may be necessary in severe hypokalaemia.

Hyponatraemia

Definition and aetiology
Hyponatraemia is a reduction in the plasma sodium concentration below normal (i.e. <135 mmol/L), although it is more commonly associated with an excess of water in the absence of reduced plasma sodium concentrations. Sodium depletion may be caused by loss via the gastrointestinal tract (e.g. diarrhoea or vomiting) or the kidney (e.g. in polycystic kidney disease or pyelonephritis), or as a result of excessive sweating. It may also arise from the administration of loop or thiazide diuretics. Water excess (i.e. water intoxication) may be caused by increased fluid ingestion, inappropriate post-operative intravenous fluid therapy or acute renal failure.

Symptoms
Symptoms include orthostatic hypotension and reduced skin turgor. Confusion may occur, and convulsions may develop in severe cases. Water intoxication, however, is marked by anorexia, heart failure, hypertension, muscle weakness and oedema.

Treatment
Hyponatraemia may be corrected by an increased dietary salt intake. Oral sodium supplements (BNF 9.2.1.2) may be indicated in some patients, although the administration of sodium chloride intravenous infusion (BNF 9.2.2) may be necessary.

Pseudohypoparathyroidism

Definition
Pseudohypoparathyroidism is a rare hereditary condition in which there is failure of the target tissues to respond to parathyroid hormone.

Symptoms
Clinically it resembles hypoparathyroidism, with symptoms produced through hypocalcaemia. However, pseudohypoparathyroidism is also associated with certain developmental abnormalities (e.g. round face, short stature and shortening of the metacarpals and metatarsals). Other associated disorders include amenorrhoea, diabetes mellitus, hypothyroidism and Turner's syndrome.

Treatment
Treatment consists of correction of hypocalcaemia by administration of vitamin D preparations (BNF 9.6.4), initially with calcium supplements (BNF 9.5.1.1) if necessary.

9.3.4 INBORN ERRORS OF METABOLISM

Hepatolenticular degeneration

Definition and aetiology
Hepatolenticular degeneration (Wilson's disease) is a rare, autosomal, inborn error of metabolism characterised by the accumulation of copper in the brain, kidneys, liver and certain other tissues. It is a progressive disorder which is usually fatal in the absence of treatment.

Symptoms
The onset, which is insidious, usually occurs in childhood or adolescence, but it may not develop until the fifth decade. It is characterised by the

development of neurological and hepatic symptoms. Common neurological symptoms include akinesia and rigidity, chorea, convulsions, drooling, dysphagia, speech disorders, muscle wasting and weakness, and tremor. The presence of a golden-brown ring around the outer edge of the cornea (Kayser-Fleischer ring) is a positive diagnostic feature. Behaviour and personality disorders are common and may be extreme, and untreated patients become immobile, demented and mentally impaired. Cirrhosis, hepatitis and jaundice are common hepatic symptoms, and ascites and hepatic coma may develop.

Treatment

Treatment, which comprises the long-term administration of a copper-chelating agent (BNF 9.8), must begin as soon as the disorder is diagnosed. Prompt treatment produces successful control and a correspondingly favourable prognosis. Patients should be advised to avoid foods rich in copper (e.g. shellfish and liver).

Maple-syrup urine disease

Definition and aetiology

Maple-syrup urine disease is a rare inborn error of amino acid metabolism. It occurs as a result of a reduction in the activity of the enzyme keto-acid decarboxylase, which is responsible for the metabolism of the keto acids formed from certain amino acids (e.g. isoleucine, leucine and valine).

Symptoms

Symptoms vary according to the severity of the disorder. In the most severe (classical) form, symptoms develop soon after birth and include convulsions, feeding problems, lethargy and metabolic acidosis. Patients have a characteristic maple-syrup odour caused by excretion of keto acids in sweat and urine. This form of the disorder is often fatal and those who survive may suffer severe brain damage. Other patients suffer from an intermittent form of the disorder and only experience episodic symptoms, which are usually precipitated by an acute infection. Such patients remain well between episodes, although they may suffer some psychomotor impairment. Milder forms of the disorder, with continuous but less marked symptoms, also exist.

Treatment

Treatment is by the dietary restriction of the relevant amino acids and, if begun immediately after birth, is usually successful. Special foods are available (BNF Appendix 7). One of the mild forms of the disorder responds to treatment with thiamine. Dialysis or exchange blood transfusion may be required during acute attacks and any infection should be treated immediately.

Phenylketonuria

Definition and aetiology

Phenylketonuria is an autosomal, recessive, inborn error of metabolism. It is characterised by deficiency of the enzyme phenylalanine hydroxylase and a consequent inability to convert phenylalanine to tyrosine. This results in the accumulation of phenylalanine in the blood and tissues.

Symptoms

Affected neonates may appear normal at birth, but phenylalanine accumulation gives rise to brain damage with mental retardation. The degree of retardation may vary, but is marked if the condition is not treated. Other symptoms include convulsions, eczema, hyperkinesia, microcephaly, light pigmentation and a 'mousy' body odour.

Treatment

Early diagnosis is essential and is usually achieved soon after birth by routine screening using the Guthrie test. Genetic counselling may be beneficial as a means of prevention in future generations.

Treatment comprises the prompt introduction of a diet low in phenylalanine but adequate in other nutrients, and special foods are available (BNF Appendix 7).

Porphyrias

Definition and aetiology

The porphyrias are a group of rare inherited disorders resulting from disturbed porphyrin metabolism, which under normal conditions contributes to the formation of the iron-containing complex, haem. Attacks may be spontaneous and sporadic, but may be precipitated by drug administration (e.g. barbiturates, oestrogens and some antiepileptic drugs) or by alcohol consumption. Infection, menstruation and pregnancy have also been implicated as contributory factors.

Symptoms

The passage of dark urine is the most usual common factor in the different forms of porphyria. Acute intermittent porphyria is the most serious of the acute forms and may be fatal. Common symptoms include acute abdominal pain with vomiting and constipation or diarrhoea, peripheral neuritis with limb pain and paralysis, psychiatric disturbances (e.g. anxiety and psychosis), and convulsions. Hypertension and tachycardia are common cardiovascular symptoms. Variegate porphyria and hereditary coproporphyria are other acute forms, and are characterised by skin photosensitivity in addition to the above symptoms. Porphyria cutanea tarda and erythropoietic porphyria are non-acute forms of the disorder, and are also characterised by photosensitivity.

Treatment

Precipitating factors must be identified and removed. A high-carbohydrate diet should be maintained during attacks to reduce excessive production of porphyrins. Treatment of acute attacks is symptomatic and the administration of analgesics (BNF 4.7), anti-emetics (BNF 4.6), antiepileptics (BNF 4.8), antipsychotic drugs (BNF 4.2) and beta-adrenoceptor blocking drugs (BNF 2.4) may be indicated. Care must be taken to avoid drugs contraindicated in porphyrias. In addition, fluid and electrolytes (BNF 9.2) may be necessary and physiotherapy may be beneficial for paralysis. No specific treatment exists for skin symptoms, although beta-carotene has been used in erythropoietic porphyria.

9.4 Anatomy and physiology relevant to blood and lymph disorders

Introduction

Each cell within the body is a discrete unit, carrying out the functions for which it is genetically programmed. However, despite their apparent independence, cells are kept in continual contact with one another and with other parts of the body by the inward transmission of fluids containing nutrients, hormones, enzymes, and the outward flow of toxic and waste materials through the cell wall. The medium for the delivery and the removal of cellular components is the compartmentalised body fluid.

The largest compartment is the intracellular fluid in which the activities of the cell are carried out. The cell's intimate contact with the environment outside its walls is maintained by the presence of fluid around the cell wall, the interstitial (tissue) fluid. The third compartment of fluid is the blood plasma and lymph, which transports materials to and from the interstitial fluid. The interstitial fluid and the plasma are together referred to as the extracellular fluid.

It is vital that the plasma, lymph and the interstitial fluid are maintained free of the potentially harmful elements introduced into the body (e.g. by absorption from the gastrointestinal tract). The main circulatory defence mechanism within the body is the lymphatic system which collects material from the interstitial fluid.

Blood

Blood is a complex fluid, consisting of cellular components (approximately 45% of the total volume) suspended in a fluid environment, the plasma. An average adult male has about 5–6 litres of blood, whilst the blood volume in an average adult female is 4–5 litres.

Erythrocytes

The majority of blood cells are erythrocytes (Figure 9.4), which number approximately 5 million per mm^3 (5×10^{12}/L). The process of formation of erythrocytes (erythropoiesis) is carried out in the red bone marrow (myeloid tissue) of the sternum, vertebrae, ribs, femur, humerus and pelvis. Development within the bone marrow proceeds via erythroblasts (in which haemoglobin is synthesised) and reticulocytes. The reticulocytes become denucleated before they leave the bone marrow, and develop into erythrocytes within one to two days of entering the general

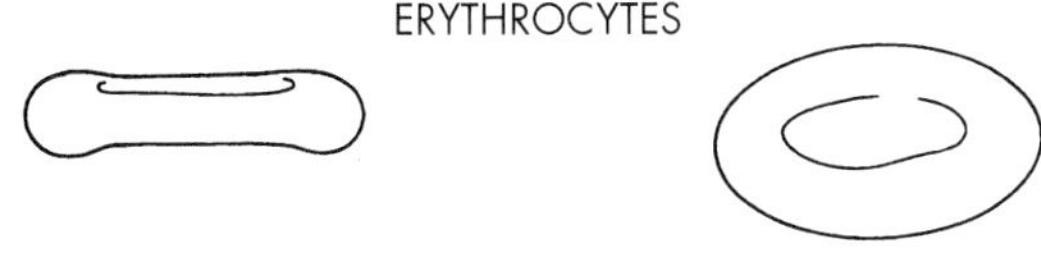

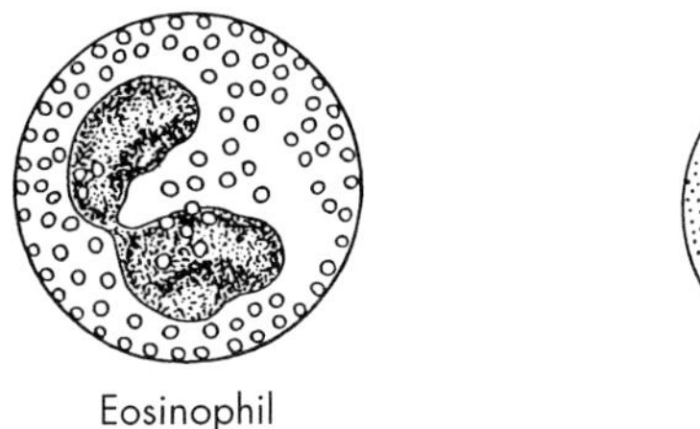

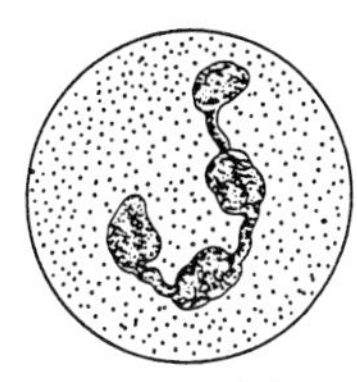

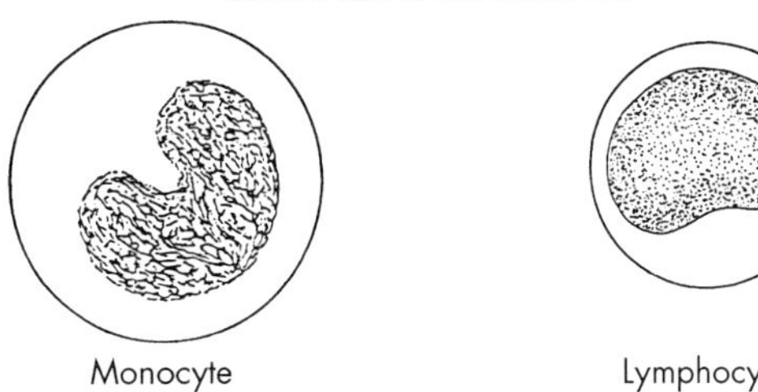

Figure 9.4 Erythrocytes and leucocytes.

circulation. Erythrocytes have a lifespan of approximately 120 days, at the end of which time they are destroyed by macrophage engulfment in the liver, spleen and bone marrow.

Each erythrocyte is a biconcave disc about 8 μm in diameter, consisting of a lipoprotein membrane surrounding cytoplasm and a red pigment, haemoglobin. The role of haemoglobin is crucial. Each haemoglobin molecule contains four haem molecules which are structurally derived from the porphyrin ring. Each ring contains an iron atom and can bind reversibly to oxygen. Haem combines with inhaled oxygen in the ratio of one haem molecule to one oxygen molecule to form oxyhaemoglobin. Once haemoglobin has divested itself of oxygen, the proteinacious globin portion combines with waste carbon dioxide to form carbaminohaemoglobin, which is transported to the lungs for dissociation and exhalation.

At the end of the life of the erythrocyte, haemoglobin is broken down into haemosiderin (which may be stored and reused to make new haemoglobin), bilirubin (secreted by the liver in the bile), and globin.

Leucocytes

There are between 5000 and 7000 leucocytes per mm^3 of blood ($5–7 \times 10^9$/L). They are classified into two main groups, the granular leucocytes (granulocytes) and the agranular leucocytes. Granular leucocytes are subdivided into neutrophils (polymorphs), eosinophils, and basophils. Agranular leucocytes are subdivided into lymphocytes and monocytes.

The myeloid tissue of the red bone marrow is the origin of agranular and granular leucocytes. Agranular leucocoytes are also produced in lymphoid tissue. The three different types of granular leucocytes are produced from a common myeloblast, whereas monocytes and lymphocytes develop from monoblasts and lymphoblasts respectively. The proportion of each type of leucocyte is an important gauge of the state of health of the body. In health, the bulk of the elements are formed of neutrophils (60–70%) and lymphocytes (20–25%), but changes in the ratios may indicate allergic reactions, infection or antigen–antibody reactions.

The principal function of the leucocytes is to counteract potentially pathogenic invasion of the body, and each leucocytic element is modified to provide a particular aspect of the defence mechanism.

Neutrophils (polymorphonuclear leucocytes) consist of a nucleus which is divided into three to five lobes linked by thin strands. They ingest bacteria by phagocytosis and secrete the bactericidal enzyme lysozyme. They are also attracted by chemicals released at the site of tissue damage (chemotaxis).

Eosinophils are structurally similar to neutrophils, although the nucleus generally consists of only two linked lobes. Their functions, however, are different and may involve a role in the immune response. They may modulate the severity of the antigen–antibody reaction and counteract the release of histamine from mast cells in allergic reactions. They may also enhance the body's resistance to re-infection with helminths.

The granules in basophils contain a range of components (e.g. heparin, serotonin and histamine) which play a role in the mediation of allergic reactions. Basophils may also be the precursors of the mast cells from which the basophilic granules are released.

Lymphocytes play a fundamental role in the immune response. They are functionally divided into T-cells (thymus-dependent cells) and B-cells.

The T-cells derive their immune competence within the thymus gland during fetal development. They are distributed throughout the body by the bloodstream and the lymphatic system. They are activated in response to a specific foreign agent (an antigen) to which they become attached and which they ultimately destroy. The response of T-cells is referred to as cell-mediated immunity as the antigen (e.g. a virus, cancer cell or a transplanted tissue) is attacked within the cell. Several subdivisions of T-cells have been identified (e.g. killer, helper and suppressor T-cells). The presence of T-helper cells is essential to enable B-cells (*see below*) to divide and produce plasma cells. Conversely, T-suppressor cells prevent the production of antibodies possibly through an effect on the corresponding helper cells for that antibody. T-cytotoxic cells kill specific cells (e.g. those infected with a virus). Null cells are non-specific cytotoxic T-cells, which comprise natural killer cells, lymphokine-activated killers and killer cells.

The B-cells (so-called because in birds they develop in the bursa of Fabricius) are thought to mature in the bone marrow, liver and spleen and are transported to the lymphoid tissue for storage. These cells are the precursors of plasma cells which produce antibodies and provide humoral (circulating) immunity. The antibodies are produced from the plasma cell within the storage tissue and are specific for a particular antigen. Memory cells are also produced from the B-cells, and these may generate a more rapid and much greater antibody response should the antigen be identified on a subsequent occasion.

Monocytes, like neutrophils, are attracted to the site of infection by chemotaxis, and ingest bacteria and dead material by phagocytosis. As monocytes, these cells are short-lived but they enlarge to form highly efficient and long-lived phagocytic cells, the macrophages. The macrophages circulate widely throughout the body, but are also concentrated in certain tissues (e.g. bone marrow, liver, lungs and spleen). These fixed macrophages are described as the cellular components of the reticulo-endothelial system, which plays an important role in clearing the blood of bacteria and particulate matter.

Platelets

The sequence of platelet (thrombocyte) formation starts in the red bone marrow from megakaryoblasts, which mature into megakaryocytes. Multiple fragmentation of the cytoplasm of the megakaryocyte leads to the production of tiny packets which become enclosed within a cell membrane. Platelets of 2–4 μm diameter are formed in this way from each 40 μm megakaryocyte. There are between 150 000 and 400 000 platelets per mm^3 of blood ($150–400 \times 10^9$/L). The lifespan of platelets is approximately 5–9 days, and they play an essential role in the processes of blood clotting. In trauma, they reduce the loss of erythrocytes from blood vessels by increasing in size and adhesiveness, resulting in the formation of plugs within arterioles, which also prevents fluid and cell loss. They also promote coagulation of blood through interaction with clotting proteins.

Blood groups

Except under emergency circumstances, it is not possible to transfuse blood from one patient to another without a knowledge of the blood group of the patient. An individual's blood group is determined by the presence or absence of specific antigens (agglutinogens) on the surface of the erythrocyte and of corresponding antibodies (agglutinins) in the plasma. In the ABO system of blood groups, the erythrocyte antigens are polysaccharides; the antigenic character of the rhesus system is unknown. The antibodies to both sets of blood groups are primarily IgG or IgM, or both.

The ABO system

In the ABO system, the presence of two surface antigens, A and B, determines the presence of antibodies anti-A and anti-B, and these are summarised in Table 9.1. Subgroups to group A and group AB exist and are described as A_2 and A_2B. It

Table 9.1 The ABO system of blood groups

Group	Antigens	Antibodies	Frequency (%) in UK population
A_1	A_1	anti-B	34
A_2	A_2	anti-B and anti-A in 10%	8
B	B	anti-A	9
A_1B	A_1 and B	neither anti-A nor anti-B	2.7
A_2B	A_2 and B	neither anti-A nor anti-B or, in 25%, anti-A_1	0.3
O	neither A nor B	anti-A and anti-B	46

is recommended that the terms 'universal donor' and 'universal recipient' are no longer used, partly because of the formerly unidentified presence of subgroups, and because other antigens, notably the rhesus factor, must also be considered in any proposed transfusion.

The rhesus system

Rhesus factors (so called after their initial identification in rhesus monkeys) are present on the membranes of erythrocytes of about 85% of the population in the UK, who are described as rhesus-positive. The most common rhesus factor is the D antigen, but unlike the ABO system in which antibodies to absent factors are always present in the blood, anti-D antibodies are only produced when a rhesus-negative person comes into contact with rhesus-positive blood. This most commonly occurs when a rhesus-negative mother carries a rhesus-positive fetus. Anti-D rhesus antibodies can be produced in the maternal circulation, particularly at parturition, when the mother's blood may mix with that of the neonate. If a subsequent fetus has rhesus-positive blood, the transplacental transfer of anti-D antibodies can cause the potentially fatal haemolytic disease of the newborn.

Lymphatic system

The lymphatic system is a specialised form of circulatory system that consists of lymph vessels and the lymphatic organs (the bone marrow, thymus, spleen, and lymph nodes). Lymph nodes (which are 1–25 mm in size and limited within a capsule) are located along the lymph vessels, usually in groups. The connective tissue present in some mucous membranes (e.g. in the tonsils, the Peyer's patches of the ileum, the appendix, the respiratory system, and the reproductive system) also contains unencapsulated non-nodular lymphatic tissue.

Lymph capillaries originate in the spaces between cells and consist of walls which allow the one-way inward transfer of material from the blood capillaries. The movement of fluid is dependent upon contractions within the smooth muscle of the vessels and skeletal muscle, as there is no pump comparable to the heart. The lymphatic vessels eventually merge to form two major channels, the thoracic (left lymphatic) duct and the right lymphatic duct.

The lymphatic system serves several purposes. Excess fluid and the small amount of protein which leaks from blood capillaries into the interstitial fluid cannot return directly to the capillaries, but passes to the lymph capillaries as lymph fluid. The fluid is then passed through the lymphatic system and is returned to the blood at the right and left internal jugular and subclavian veins.

The lymphatic system assists in the absorption of fat from the small intestine. Complexes of bile salt and fat diffuse into intestinal epithelial cells and combine with lipids and proteins to form small particles (chylomicrons). These are too large to be absorbed directly into the circulation and so they pass into the lymph vessels for indirect transfer to the blood.

Lymph nodes participate in the defence mechanisms of the body. As lymph passes into the nodes, unwanted materials are filtered and destroyed by the action of macrophages, T-cells and B-cells. Lymphocytes are also produced within the nodes and some are distributed to other parts of the body through the lymphatic and blood circulatory systems.

Spleen

The spleen is situated in the upper abdominal cavity and is the largest organ of the lymphatic system. It consists of red pulp, which occupies the venous sinuses and is filled with blood and splenic (Billroth's) cords, and white pulp which surrounds arteries and comprises white lymphatic tissue, consisting mainly of lymphocytes. Malpighian bodies, which are thickened lymphocytic nodules, are closely associated with the white pulp. Blood flows through the spleen in open and closed systems. The rate of blood flow through the closed system is fast and direct and this is the major route during health. Blood flows much more slowly through the open system as it has to negotiate a network of splenic cord spaces.

The spleen is responsible for the development of a small proportion of erythrocytes and lymphocytes in the fetus and newborn baby. This capacity is lost in early life but may be held in reserve in the event of haematological stress.

Splenic activity is responsible for reconditioning erythrocytes and destroying old erythrocytes and foreign material. As blood flows through the spleen, platelets and reticulocytes are temporarily removed for storage and maturation respectively. Blood is also stored in the spleen in the blood pool and this may be drawn on in the event of reduced blood volume (e.g. following haemorrhage).

The presence of the body's largest concentration of lymphocytes and stimulation of these cells by antigens results in antibody formation in the spleen.

The control of blood clot formation

Blood clotting (haemostasis), vasospasm and platelet plug formation are the mechanisms by which blood loss is minimised in the event of breakage of a blood vessel. These mechanisms are delicately balanced so that they are rapidly effective in the event of haemorrhage, but not so effective under normal circumstances that clot formation occurs spontaneously.

The message that trauma has occurred is amplified through a complex cascade of enzyme systems, which comprise the mechanisms of blood clotting. The key to the formation of fibrin is the production of prothrombin activator by one of two pathways (known as the intrinsic and extrinsic pathways) and the release of various coagulation factors (which are commonly designated by Roman numerals). The extrinsic pathway, which is the more rapid of the two, may produce prothrombin activator within a few seconds in the event of severe trauma. It is initiated by tissue factor III, a factor present in cell walls, which leads to the release of a group of substances referred to as tissue thromboplastin. In the presence of calcium ions and factor VIII (the antihaemophilic factor), thromboplastin activates factor X to form prothrombin activator.

The intrinsic pathway, which is more complex than the extrinsic pathway, may take up to several minutes to produce prothrombin activator, and is initiated within the blood by interaction between the collagen fibres of damaged blood vessels and the blood. This activates factor XII and causes the release of phospholipids from platelets. Factor XII activates factor XI, which in turn activates factor IX. The presence of calcium ions, factor VIII, activated factor IX and platelet phospholipids result in the activation of factor X. Prothrombin activator is finally formed in the presence of factor X, factor V, calcium ions and platelet phospholipids.

The complete clotting process may be considered to comprise three stages. The initial stage is the formation of prothrombin activator (*see above*), which then converts prothrombin in the plasma to thrombin. Thirdly, thrombin converts fibrinogen into fibrin, which forms intermolecular links to produce the network of threads which comprise the clot.

The prevention of unwanted thrombosis is due to the action of an endogenous fibrinolytic compound, plasmin, which is formed from its precursor, plasminogen.

The conversion of plasminogen to plasmin is catalysed by specific activators, plasminogen activators, which may be derived from the circulation, from local tissues, or by the action of drugs (e.g. streptokinase and urokinase).

10

Musculoskeletal and connective tissue disorders

10.1 General disorders

Back pain

Definition and aetiology

Back pain becomes more common with advancing age, and occurs most frequently in the lumbar (i.e. lumbago) or sacro-iliac regions. The cause is often uncertain, but the upright nature of the human posture results in shear strains which give rise to degenerative spinal joint disturbances. Back pain may also arise from inflammatory disease (e.g. ankylosing spondylitis), prolapsed (slipped) intervertebral discs, spinal nerve root compression (e.g. sciatica), osteoporosis, bony metastases, congenital spinal defects (e.g. spina bifida), fractures, infection, mechanical injury, and pelvic or retroperitoneal malignant disease. It may also be caused by strain arising from inappropriate lifting technique, obesity, poor posture or pregnancy. Back pain may also be psychogenic.

Symptoms

Pain may be local or diffuse and may radiate or be referred. It is, however, usually characterised by limitation of movement. If pain is exacerbated by movement and improved by rest, the cause is usually mechanical strain or injury; conversely, pain caused by inflammatory disease is usually worse after rest. Pain arising from nerve root compression may be exacerbated by coughing or sneezing. The onset of pain caused by disc, muscle or ligament injury is usually sudden. Pain caused by inflammatory disease often has a gradual onset.

Treatment

Treatment depends on the cause. Common treatment includes the administration of non-steroidal anti-inflammatory drugs (BNF 10.1.1), bed rest and physiotherapy. Patients should avoid lifting heavy weights, and be instructed in proper lifting techniques and maintaining an appropriate posture. Manipulation and traction may be beneficial in some patients and, very occasionally, laminectomy may be indicated.

Muscular dystrophy

Definition and aetiology

The commonest degenerative myopathy is Duchenne muscular dystrophy, which affects only boys, although cases in girls with Turner's syndrome have been reported. Duchenne muscular dystrophy is primarily a genetically inherited disorder, although cases do occur in the absence of known familial history. It is thought to be caused by the absence of a muscular protein, dystrophin. The absence of this protein permits the influx of calcium into the muscle cell, resulting in the activation of proteases which digest muscle fibres. The gene for dystrophin is located on the X-chromosome and is transmitted recessively to male offspring. Occasionally, gene mutation may give rise to the condition in the absence of familial history.

Symptoms

Early symptoms may be recognised with the late onset of walking at about 18 months of age, although other earlier developmental milestones (e.g. crawling) may also be delayed. Further disturbances of motor function (e.g. difficulty in climbing stairs, unsteadiness in walking and failure to run) can develop after three years of age. The majority of boys are diagnosed between four and six years of age. Compensatory hypertrophy of unaffected muscles (e.g. of the calf) may occur early in the disease, but disappears later. Obesity is common and mental retardation or impaired intellectual development can also occur. Contractures and scoliosis are common late symptoms. Continued development of muscular weakness is relentless, resulting in confinement to a wheelchair between 10 and 12 years of age, and death from respiratory failure, respiratory-tract infection or heart failure, often in the late teens or early 20s.

Treatment

There is no treatment for Duchenne muscular dystrophy. Palliative measures can be adopted to minimise the discomfort caused by contractures and scoliosis. Obesity should be treated with dietary control and physiotherapy may be helpful in the early stages. Carrier detection can be carried out in families with a history of the disease, followed by appropriate genetic counselling for affected females. Amniocentesis can detect affected males *in utero*.

Self-help organisation

Muscular Dystrophy Group

Sciatica

Definition and aetiology

Sciatica is a severe pain experienced along the course and distribution of the sciatic nerve in the buttocks, back of thigh and calf, and outer side of the calf and foot. It is usually caused by a prolapsed (slipped) lower lumbar intervertebral disc.

The prolapsed disc causes irritation and compression of one or more nerve roots of the cauda equina which usually lasts several weeks. There is often a history of low back injury and pain from lifting weights or sudden movement. Sciatic pain may also be referred from other structures within the nerve distribution of the spinal segments from which the sciatic nerve arises (e.g. the hip or sacro-iliac joints).

Symptoms
The pain usually begins in the lumbar region (lumbago) and extends along the course of the sciatic nerve. It may be aggravated by stooping, coughing or turning in bed.

Treatment
Treatment consists of bed rest and the administration of analgesics (BNF 4.7). To prevent relapse, the patient should be advised to avoid lifting objects with the back flexed. Chronic or recurrent sciatica may be treated surgically. Treatment of referred sciatic pain is directed towards the underlying cause.

Torticollis

Definition and aetiology
Torticollis (wry neck) is any condition in which rotating and tilting of the head to one side occurs. It may be spasmodic or permanent and although the cause is ill-defined, the most common form is due to spasm of the cervical muscles of the neck. It has been suggested that emotional disturbances may contribute. A history of an extrapyramidal disorder may be identified.

It has an incidence of about 3 per 10 000 persons.

Symptoms
The onset commonly occurs between 30 and 60 years of age, is usually gradual, but may occasionally be acute. It is characterised by painful spasms of the muscles on one side of the neck and the adoption of an unnatural head posture. The condition may be intermittent and mild, but may become chronic and produce immobility and deformity.

Treatment
Drug treatment and surgery are usually ineffective. The application of slight pressure to the jaw with the hand may give short-term relief in spasmodic torticollis. If emotional disturbance is a factor, psychiatric treatment may be beneficial.

10.2 Arthritis and related conditions

Ankylosing spondylitis

Definition and aetiology
Ankylosing spondylitis is a progressive chronic arthritis of the spine which most often occurs in men between 20 and 40 years of age. The disease usually has a milder course in women. It is characterised by inflammation of the sacro-iliac and intervertebral joints. Calcification and ossification may result in immobility and fusion (i.e. ankylosis) of these spinal joints. The cause of the disease is unknown, although a family history is often present.

Symptoms
Early symptoms include low back pain and morning stiffness which gradually progress up the back, sometimes reaching the neck. Pain around the ribs may develop and be exacerbated by deep breathing and coughing. Marked rigidity and kyphosis of the spine may occur. Some patients experience severe heel pain, and hip and shoulder joints may also be affected. Systemic complications include amyloidosis, cardiovascular disease (e.g. arrhythmias and aortic valve disease), iritis (*see* Uveitis, Section 11.1), and respiratory disease (e.g. cough, dyspnoea and infection). The disease may interfere significantly with the quality of life, although only a minority of patients suffer total spinal immobility.

Treatment
Treatment comprises vigorous physiotherapy and the administration of non-steroidal anti-inflammatory drugs (BNF 10.1.1). Pulse doses of corticosteroids (BNF 10.1.2.1) may be beneficial in unresponsive disease. Surgical straightening of the spine may be necessary in severe cases.

Radiotherapy has been successfully used, but there is a high risk of leukaemia following treatment.

Cervical spondylosis

Definition and aetiology

Cervical spondylosis is a common disorder characterised by degeneration of the intervertebral joints of the neck (cervical vertebrae) and the associated cartilage (intervertebral discs). Bony projections (osteophytes) may form, resulting in compression of spinal nerve roots or even of the cord itself. The cause of cervical spondylosis is unknown, although it is associated with advancing age.

Symptoms

Pain, stiffness and immobility of the neck are common. The pain may be mild or severe. Neurological symptoms, arising from spinal nerve root compression, may include severe pain in the arms and hands and sensory loss and weakness. In severe cases, the legs may become affected, paralysis can develop, and bladder function may be impaired.

Treatment

Treatment consists of providing a supportive collar and analgesics (BNF 4.7), muscle relaxants (BNF 10.2.2), and anti-inflammatory drugs (BNF 10.1.1) when necessary. Surgery is indicated only in severe intractable cases.

Chondrocalcinosis

Definition and aetiology

Chondrocalcinosis (pyrophosphate arthropathy) is characterised by the deposition of calcium salts (e.g. calcium pyrophosphate dihydrate) in articular cartilage and by their appearance in synovial fluid.

The cause of the disease is unknown, although a family history may be present, and it can occur in association with diabetes mellitus, gout, haemochromatosis and hyperparathyroidism.

Symptoms

Chondrocalcinosis may be asymptomatic, but the commonest symptom is osteoarthritis which may affect several joints simultaneously. Acute attacks of gout-like symptoms (pseudogout) may occur. Large joints, particularly the hip and knee, are most often affected. The periods between attacks are usually free of symptoms.

Treatment

Acute attacks may be treated by aspiration of the affected joint(s) and the administration of a non-steroidal anti-inflammatory drug (BNF 10.1.1). The intra-articular administration of a corticosteroid (BNF 10.1.2) may be beneficial.

Juvenile chronic arthritis

Definition and aetiology

Juvenile chronic arthritis (Still's disease) is a term used to describe a variety of conditions characterised by the development of inflammatory joint disease before 16 years of age. The cause of these diseases is unknown, but autoimmune mechanisms may be responsible. Juvenile rheumatoid arthritis is the childhood equivalent of rheumatoid arthritis. It has a poor prognosis. Juvenile ankylosing spondylitis is the childhood equivalent of ankylosing spondylitis. It is characterised by a peripheral arthritis, affecting predominantly the joints of the lower limbs.

Symptoms

Systemic juvenile chronic arthritis is characterised by a mild polyarthritis, irregular fever, lymphadenopathy, a rash and respiratory symptoms.

Polyarticular juvenile chronic arthritis is more common in girls. It may affect any joint and mild systemic symptoms usually develop. Rheumatoid factor (*see* Rheumatoid arthritis) is not detectable.

Pauci-articular juvenile chronic arthritis is characterised by the development of arthritis in a small number of joints, although only one joint may be affected. With the exception of iridocyclitis (*see* Uveitis, Section 11.1), systemic symptoms are rare.

Juvenile ankylosing spondylitis is characterised by a peripheral arthritis, affecting predominantly the joints of the lower limbs.

Treatment

Treatment comprises the measures described under rheumatoid arthritis.

Osteoarthritis

Definition and aetiology

Osteoarthritis (osteoarthrosis) is a non-inflammatory joint disease characterised by the degeneration of articular cartilage, the hardening (i.e. sclerosis) and refashioning of underlying bone, and the formation of bony projections (osteophytes) at the edges of the affected joint (Figure 10.1). Usually only one or two of the large weight-bearing joints are involved, most commonly those of the hip, knee, and spine. The smaller joints of the hands and feet may, however, also be involved. Osteoarthritis is very common, affecting more than 1 in 10 of the population, and is considered to be a normal sign of ageing (over half of those affected are over 60 years of age, although men tend to be affected at an earlier age than women). Predisposing factors include joint disease or injury, a family history, occupation, obesity and postural defects.

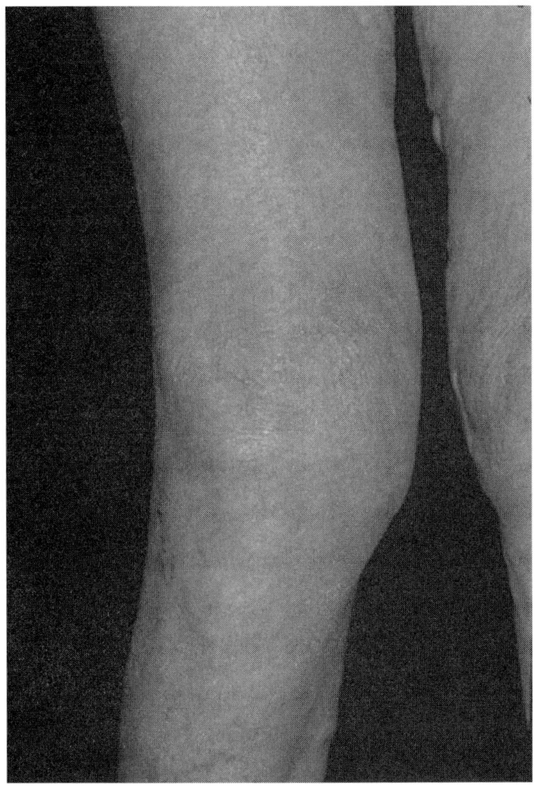

Figure 10.1 Osteoarthritis. (Reproduced with permission of Dr P Marazzi/Science Photo Library.)

Symptoms

The onset of symptoms, which usually occurs at about 50 years of age, is characterised by joint pain, stiffness and immobility. Transient stiffness after rest is common, although pain is exacerbated by movement and becomes more pronounced through the day. Affected joints may 'creak' on movement, and bony projections (Heberden's nodes) may be visible on the finger joints (Figure 10.2). Effusions can occur, and debilitating deformity may eventually develop.

Treatment

Treatment comprises the administration of non-opioid analgesics (BNF 4.7.1) or non-steroidal anti-inflammatory drugs (BNF 10.1.1) and gentle exercise, hydrotherapy, occupational therapy, physiotherapy and weight reduction. Affected joints should be kept warm and local heat treatment may be used. Domestic aids (e.g. handrails and specially designed furniture) and walking

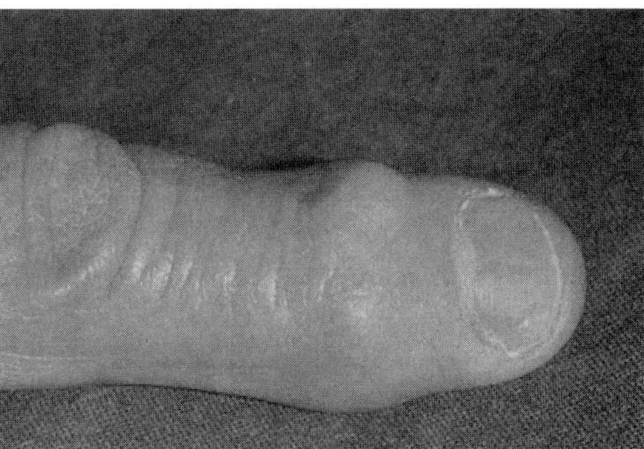

Figure 10.2 Heberden's node. (Reproduced with permission of Dr P Marazzi/Science Photo Library.)

frames or sticks are often beneficial. In severe cases, surgery may be required and osteotomy or total joint replacement may be indicated. The value of the intra-articular administration of corticosteroids (BNF 10.1.2) is controversial.

Psoriatic arthritis

Definition and aetiology

Psoriatic arthritis is arthritis which develops in the presence of psoriasis of the skin or nails. Very occasionally, arthritic symptoms precede the skin disorder. The cause is unknown, but psoriatic arthritis may be inherited and predisposing factors can include infection or trauma.

Symptoms

The interphalangeal joints are most commonly affected, and pitting and ridging of the nails often occur. Larger joints may also become involved and, in a minority of patients, ankylosis and marked deformity may develop. Ankylosing spondylitis may occur in association with psoriatic arthritis. Extra-articular symptoms are uncommon, although ocular complications (e.g. iritis and scleritis) may arise. Subcutaneous nodules do not develop. Although the erythrocyte sedimentation rate may be raised, rheumatoid factor is absent.

Treatment

The treatment for psoriatic arthritis is similar to that for rheumatoid arthritis, although antimalarials should not be given and penicillamine is ineffective. Immunosuppressants (BNF 10.1.3) may be given in unresponsive cases.

Rheumatoid arthritis

Definition and aetiology

Rheumatoid arthritis is a chronic systemic disorder. It is characterised by inflammatory changes in the peripheral joints and associated connective tissues, by the atrophy and rarefaction of bone, and by a variety of extra-articular symptoms. The cause of the disease is unknown, but an autoimmune mechanism may be responsible and viral infection may be a predisposing factor.

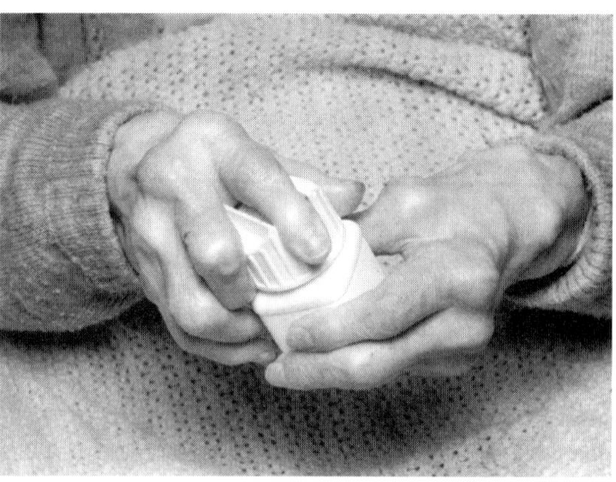

Figure 10.3 Rheumatoid arthritis. (Reproduced with permission from *Pharmaceutical Journal*.)

The condition affects about 1% of all populations, with women affected two to three times more commonly than men. Onset occurs at any age between 25 and 50 years of age.

Symptoms

The onset of rheumatoid arthritis may be acute or insidious. The small synovial joints of the feet and ankles, hands and wrists, knees, and cervical spine are most commonly affected, although any synovial joint may become involved. Affected joints become acutely painful, swollen and tender due to inflammation of the synovial membrane and the deposition of inflamed connective tissue (i.e. pannus) which destroys the articular cartilage. Ankylosis may occur and stiffness, particularly in the morning, is a common feature. As the disease progresses, partial joint dislocation may occur and marked deformity and disability may develop (Figure 10.3). Subcutaneous nodules may occur, particularly over pressure points.

General extra-articular symptoms include anaemia, fever, malaise, and weight loss. Vasculitis may occur and respiratory symptoms (e.g. pulmonary effusion and fibrosis) may develop. Pericarditis is common. Ocular manifestations include keratoconjunctivitis sicca (*see* Dry eye, Section 11.1), which in conjunction with rheumatoid arthritis or a connective tissue disorder (e.g. systemic lupus erythematosus) is referred to as Sjögren's syndrome. Scleritis, lymphadenopathy, peripheral neuropathy and renal impairment may develop. The erythrocyte sedimentation rate in patients suffering from rheumatoid arthritis is raised and this, together with the presence in the blood of an immunoglobulin known as rheumatoid factor, is diagnostic of the disease. Amyloidosis is a potentially fatal complication.

Prognosis is variable. The disease is subject to remission and relapse with exacerbation, and a minority of patients suffer severe disability.

Treatment

Treatment is long term and comprises adequate rest and gentle exercise, although joint immobilisation (i.e. splinting) may be necessary to relieve pain. Physiotherapy and treatment with heat, ice packs and ultrasound is beneficial. Occupational therapy and social support are often crucial, together with the provision of domestic and walking aids. Drug therapy is usually essential and includes the administration of non-steroidal anti-inflammatory drugs (BNF 10.1.1) and drugs which may affect the rheumatic disease process (e.g. gold compounds, sulfasalazine and penicillamine) (BNF 10.1.3). Intra-articular injections of corticosteroids (BNF 10.1.2.2) are used, but oral administration is usually avoided. Surgery may be indicated in severe cases, and procedures include joint fixation (arthrodesis), joint replacement (arthroplasty) and synovial membrane removal (synovectomy).

Self-help organisations

Arthritis Care
Leonard Cheshire Foundation
National Ankylosing Spondylitis Society

10.3 Bone disorders

Osteitis deformans

Definition and aetiology

Osteitis deformans (Paget's disease of bone) is a chronic bone disease characterised by alternate periods of increased bone reabsorption and excessive and disorganised bone repair. This increased bone turnover leads to destruction of normal bone structure and consequent bone weakness and enlargement. The cause of osteitis deformans is unknown, although viral infection may be a factor. There is a marked geographical variation in the incidence of the disease.

Symptoms

The onset of the disease usually occurs after 40 years of age and its incidence generally increases with age. Characteristic symptoms include bone deformity, fracture and pain. Common sites are the pelvis and spine and kyphosis is often seen. Bowing of the long bones (e.g. femur and tibia) may occur, and enlargement of the skull may be associated with nerve-compression deafness. Affected bones may become highly vascular and heart failure may result. Plasma calcium and plasma phosphate concentrations are usually normal, but there is marked elevation of plasma alkaline phosphatase concentrations. Cancer of the bone (e.g. sarcoma) may develop in some patients.

Treatment

Often no treatment is necessary. Non-opioid analgesics (BNF 4.7.1) may, however, be required for pain. Calcitonin (BNF 6.6.1) or disodium etidronate (BNF 6.6.2) may be given in severe unresponsive cases. Plicamycin has also been used. Surgery may be required.

Osteopetrosis

Definition and aetiology

Osteopetrosis (Albers-Schönberg disease or marble bone disease) is a rare inherited disease characterised by increased bone formation and density. The bones become abnormally hard and easily fractured. Osteopetrosis may be mild (benign) or severe, and it is thought to be caused by disturbed bone reabsorption.

Symptoms

In both forms, fractures are common and may result in osteomyelitis. Severe osteopetrosis develops in childhood and produces anaemia by invasion of the bone marrow, and sensorineural deafness or blindness by cranial-nerve compression. Growth and mental retardation may occur, and early death is common, due to repeated fractures with haemorrhage and infection. The mild form of osteopetrosis does not develop until adolescence or adulthood and may be asymptomatic.

Treatment

Treatment comprises dietary calcium restriction with bone-marrow transplantation. Corticosteroids have been given and blood transfusion or antimicrobial therapy may be indicated.

Osteoporosis

Definition and aetiology

Osteoporosis is characterised by a reduced bone mass in the presence of normal bone composition. It is caused by changes in bone metabolism which may arise from alcoholism, endocrine disorders (e.g. Cushing's syndrome and primary hyperparathyroidism), nutritional deficiency or malabsorption, prolonged corticosteroid administration, or immobility. It is most commonly associated, however, with advancing age, particularly in postmenopausal women, although it may very occasionally occur during childhood, pregnancy or in young adults.

Symptoms

Osteoporosis is characterised by brittle bones. Fractures, especially of the femoral neck, vertebrae and wrist, are common and result in pain and deformity. Multiple crush fractures of the vertebrae result in vertebral collapse, which causes chronic back pain and kyphosis, with a consequent decrease in height.

Treatment

Treatment is aimed at preventing further reduction in bone mass and comprises the administration of calcium supplements (BNF 9.5.1.1). Vitamin D preparations (BNF 9.6.4) may also be given. The treatment of postmenopausal osteoporosis includes the administration of oestrogens (BNF 6.4.1), and anabolic steroids (BNF 6.4.3) have also been given. A variety of drug therapies have been tried including calcitonin, parathormone hormone and sodium fluoride. Calcium may be administered as prophylaxis.

Analgesics (BNF 4.7.1) are often necessary, particularly for back pain, and a spinal support may be beneficial. Orthopaedic treatment is required for fractures. Physical activity should, however, be maintained.

10.4 Connective tissue disorders

Bursitis

Definition and aetiology

Bursitis, which may be acute or chronic, is inflammation of a bursa. The cause is frequently uncertain, but physical injury, infection or arthritic disease may be responsible.

Symptoms

Bursitis is characterised by local pain and tenderness, immobility, swelling and erythema. It commonly affects the shoulder (subacromial bursitis), although the elbow (olecranon bursitis or miner's elbow) or the knee (prepatellar bursitis, Figure 10.4; or housemaid's knee) may be affected. Bursitis may develop in association with deformity of the metatarsophalangeal joint of the great toe (i.e. a bunion). Popliteal bursitis (Baker's cyst) occurs when synovial fluid escapes from the knee-joint capsule and accumulates in the bursa in the popliteal space behind the knee joint.

Treatment

Treatment consists of the administration of non-steroidal anti-inflammatory drugs (BNF 10.1.1) or local corticosteroid injections (BNF 10.1.2.2). Aspiration of accumulated fluid or surgical removal of the affected bursa may be necessary in chronic cases.

Fibrositis

Definition and aetiology

Fibrositis (fibromyalgia) is a non-specific disorder of connective tissue characterised by generalised musculoskeletal pain, stiffness and tenderness in fibrous tissues, muscles, tendons and ligaments. It is often caused by physical injury, or exposure to cold or damp conditions.

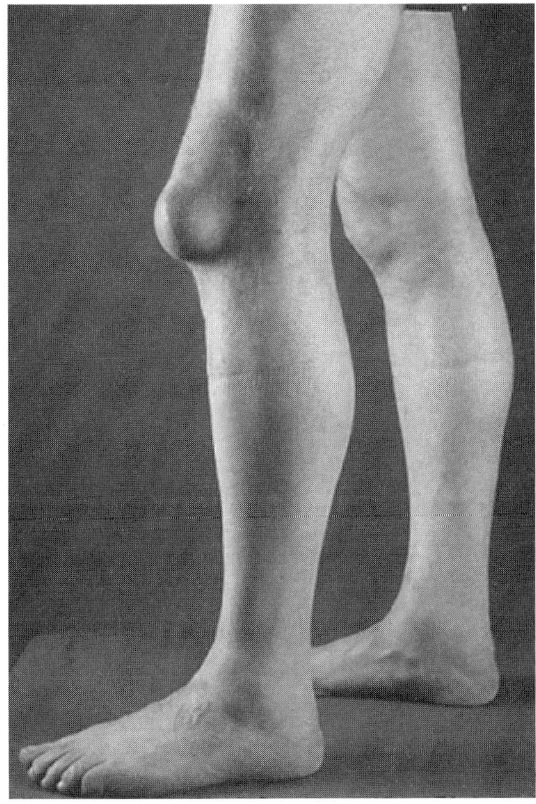

Figure 10.4 Bursitis. (Reproduced with permission of Princess Margaret Rose Orthopaedic Hospital/Science Photo Library.)

Other contributory factors include emotional disturbance and infection.

Symptoms
Symptoms may arise in almost any soft connective tissue, producing a variety of conditions (e.g. lumbago, torticollis and frozen shoulder). Onset may be sudden, and is marked by muscle pain with stiffness and tenderness. Symptoms are commonly aggravated by movement, but are often self-limiting and disappear within a few days or weeks. Tension headache and irritable bowel syndrome may accompany fibrositis.

Treatment
Treatment includes rest and the application of heat and gentle massage. Non-steroidal anti-inflammatory drugs (BNF 10.1.1) may be indicated, and the application of a rubefacient (BNF 10.3.2) may be beneficial. Antidepressants (BNF 4.3) and psychotherapy may be used for underlying psychological disturbances.

Frozen shoulder

Definition and aetiology
Frozen shoulder (adhesive bursitis, adhesive capsulitis or scapular arthritis) is characterised by an adhesive inflammation of the shoulder-joint capsule and associated cartilage. It is almost always due to overuse or physical injury.

Symptoms
The onset is usually gradual and is marked by increasing pain in the shoulder, stiffness and limitation of movement. Pain may be localised, but may also radiate into the neck (with muscle spasm) or the arm. Although the pain may be severe, it often resolves spontaneously. Joint mobility may, however, be permanently impaired.

Treatment
Treatment comprises adequate rest, physiotherapy, and the local application of heat or cold. Non-steroidal anti-inflammatory drugs (BNF 10.1.1) are often administered, and local corticosteroid injections (BNF 10.1.2.2) may be indicated. Attempts should be made to recommence use of the shoulder once the initial pain, muscle spasm and inflammation have been overcome. In severe cases, manipulation under anaesthesic may be necessary.

Giant cell arteritis

Definition and aetiology
Giant cell arteritis (cranial arteritis or temporal arteritis) is an inflammatory condition which may affect any of the larger arteries, especially the temporal and occipital arteries. The artery wall is damaged by granulomatous inflammation and, characteristically, giant cells are present which can cause thickening of the artery wall lining. Polymyalgia rheumatica frequently accompanies giant cell arteritis. It can affect 1 in 1000 patients over 50 years of age.

Symptoms

Giant cell arteritis rarely occurs under 50 years of age and may be preceded by a polymyalgic illness. Headache often occurs at a later stage and may be abrupt in onset with pain of great intensity and tenderness of the scalp, usually in the temporal region. The thickened temporal arteries may be tender and non-pulsatile, with erythema and oedema of the overlying skin. Up to 50% of patients have ocular disturbances which may result in irreversible blindness. Other symptoms are anaemia, fever, jaw pain (particularly on chewing) and weight loss.

Treatment

Early treatment with high-dose corticosteroids (BNF 10.1.2.1) is imperative to control inflammation and prevent blindness. Treatment should be continued for a minimum of two to three years at a reduced dose.

Polyarteritis nodosa

Definition and aetiology

Polyarteritis nodosa may affect any organ and is characterised by marked inflammation and necrosis of small and medium arteries. These result in weakening of the artery walls with consequent aneurysm formation, thrombosis and infarction. The cause is unknown, although it may be due to the formation of immune complexes, and hypersensitivity reactions (e.g. caused by penicillins or sulphonamides) have been implicated. The disorder is three times more common in men than women. It occurs generally between 40 and 50 years of age.

Symptoms

The onset of the disorder is characterised by non-specific symptoms (e.g. arthralgia, fever, malaise, myalgia and weight loss). Thereafter, any body system may be affected. Skin symptoms include nodule formation (due to aneurysms), ulceration and a wide variety of rashes. Renal complications characterised by hypertension are very common and are often fatal. Cardiac involvement frequently occurs and myocardial infarction, pericarditis and tachycardia may lead to death. Confusion, peripheral neuropathy and psychosis are symptoms of central nervous system involvement. Abdominal pain may arise as a result of gastrointestinal haemorrhage or infarction. Respiratory symptoms do not usually occur, although asthma can develop.

Treatment

Although no specific treatment exists, the combination of corticosteroids (BNF 6.3.4 and 10.1.2.1) and immunosuppressants (BNF 10.1.3) may retard the disease process and produce remission. Plasmapheresis has also been used.

Polymyalgia rheumatica

Definition and aetiology

Polymyalgia rheumatica is characterised by muscle pain and stiffness. It usually develops after 50 years of age and may occur in association with giant cell arteritis. The cause of the disorder is unknown, although a family history may exist.

Symptoms

The onset may be acute or insidious and is often marked by non-specific symptoms (e.g. malaise, apathy, weight loss and mild fever). Characteristic symptoms, however, include severe pain and early morning stiffness in the proximal muscles, particularly of the neck and shoulders. The disorder usually resolves spontaneously within 6–24 months, although it may persist for several years in a minority of patients.

Treatment

Treatment comprises the administration of corticosteroids (BNF 10.1.2.1), and non-steroidal anti-inflammatory drugs (BNF 10.1.1) may provide symptomatic relief.

Polymyositis and dermatomyositis

Definition and aetiology

Polymyositis is characterised by inflammatory and degenerative changes in muscle tissue. When the non-suppurative inflammation also involves subcutaneous tissue and the skin, the condition is called dermatomyositis. The cause is unknown, but immunological mechanisms may be responsible. Viral infection or a family history have also been implicated.

Symptoms

Onset, which may be acute or insidious, usually occurs between 30 and 60 years of age and is twice as common in women as it is in men. The most usual initial symptom is progressive proximal muscle weakness, often affecting the thigh muscles, and resulting in difficulty in climbing stairs and arising. Muscle atrophy and contractures may eventually develop, and dysphagia may be caused by disturbances of pharyngeal muscles. Respiratory muscles may also be affected, causing respiratory failure.

In dermatomyositis, a characteristic scaly erythematous rash covers the face and exposed areas, often in association with oedema. This rash often fades but is replaced by brown pigmentation. Although most patients recover, symptoms may be persistent and death may occur.

Treatment

Treatment involves bed rest and the administration of corticosteroids (BNF 10.1.2.1) or immunosuppressants (BNF 10.1.3), or both. Physiotherapy may be beneficial.

Sarcoidosis

Definition and aetiology

Sarcoidosis is a non-caseating granulomatous disorder characterised by the formation of epithelioid cell tubercles (i.e. sarcoid) in almost any organ or tissue. Secondary fibrosis and necrosis may develop. The cause of sarcoidosis is unknown.

Symptoms

The onset of the disorder may be acute or insidious, and usually occurs between 20 and 35 years of age. The organs most commonly affected include the eyes, liver, lungs, lymph nodes and skin, but small bones, the central nervous system, heart, joints, muscle or the spleen may also be involved. Common presenting symptoms are arthralgia, fever and weight loss, but symptoms generally depend on the organ affected. Erythema nodosum and lymphadenopathy are frequent symptoms, and pulmonary involvement may be marked by cough, dyspnoea and, eventually, pulmonary fibrosis and cor pulmonale. If the heart is affected, angina pectoris and heart failure may result. Spontaneous improvement and recovery is common, but sarcoidosis may become chronically progressive although death is uncommon.

Treatment

No specific treatment exists, although corticosteroids (BNF 6.3.4) may be useful in alleviating symptoms. Other drugs used include chlorambucil, chloroquine and methotrexate.

Systemic lupus erythematosus

Definition and aetiology

Systemic lupus erythematosus (SLE) is a generalised connective tissue disorder of unknown aetiology. It is associated with a series of autoimmune mechanisms which result in auto-antibody formation. Antinuclear antibodies specific to DNA are formed, together with a variety of organ-specific auto-antibodies. These lead to necrosis and fibrosis of small blood vessels, collagen and other connective tissues. The disorder occurs most commonly in black populations and in young women, and may be precipitated by drug administration (e.g. hydralazine), exposure to sunlight or viral infection. A family history may be present.

Symptoms

The onset of symptoms, which can be mild or severe, may be acute or insidious. Non-specific symptoms (e.g. fever and malaise, alopecia, aphthous stomatitis, and an erythematous rash on exposed areas) are common. A butterfly rash covering the cheeks and nose is characteristic. Musculoskeletal symptoms are very common and include arthralgia and myalgia. Central nervous system involvement is often prominent and may be characterised by convulsions, depressive disorders or psychosis. Renal impairment may occur and cause hypertension, oedema and proteinuria, and can lead to renal failure and death. Other symptoms include anaemia, keratoconjunctivitis sicca (*see* Dry eye, Section 11.1), hepatosplenomegaly, lymphadenopathy, pericarditis and pleurisy. The erythrocyte sedimentation rate is characteristically raised. The course of the disorder is often chronic with remissions and relapses, although the prognosis, even in the presence of renal involvement, is usually good.

Treatment

Exposure to precipitating factors should be avoided by susceptible patients. Sunscreening preparations may be useful (BNF 13.8.1). Drug treatment includes the administration of corticosteroids (BNF 6.3.2 and 10.1.2.1) and antimalarials or immunosuppressants (BNF 10.1.3). Non-steroidal anti-inflammatory drugs (BNF 10.1.1) are beneficial in treating musculoskeletal symptoms.

Self-help organisations

Arthritis Care
Leonard Cheshire Foundation
National Ankylosing Spondylitis Society

Systemic sclerosis

Definition and aetiology

Systemic sclerosis is a chronic disorder caused by increased collagen deposition and the obliteration of small blood vessels. The condition produces widespread fibrosis of internal organs (e.g. gastrointestinal tract, heart, kidneys and lungs). Involvement of skin is called scleroderma. The cause is unknown, although environmental factors (e.g. exposure to vinyl chloride) or a family history may be significant. The condition may arise at any age and is four times more common in women.

Symptoms

The initial symptom is often Raynaud's phenomenon (*see* Raynaud's syndrome, Section 2.5). Oedema of the hands and fingers is common and is followed by thickening and hardening (i.e. sclerosis) of the skin, which becomes hyperpigmented, shiny and tight. Cutaneous symptoms may spread to affect other areas (e.g. back, chest and legs) and facial telangiectasia is common. Cutaneous calcification, particularly of the fingertips, may occur.

Symptoms may be restricted to the skin for several years, but progression to the visceral organs may develop and is associated with a poor prognosis. Dysphagia may occur as a result of disordered oesophageal motility. Pulmonary fibrosis may lead to dyspnoea and pulmonary hypertension, and fibrosis of cardiac muscle may give rise to arrhythmias and heart failure. Renal involvement may lead to progressive renal impairment and is a significant cause of death. Arthralgia and myalgia are common.

Treatment

Treatment is chiefly symptomatic. Cutaneous symptoms may be alleviated by providing protective clothing and local heat. Physiotherapy may promote mobility. Antihypertensive drugs (BNF 2.5) may be indicated and non-steroidal anti-inflammatory drugs (BNF 10.1.1) may relieve musculoskeletal symptoms. Dialysis or transplantation may be necessary in the event of severe renal disorder. A variety of systemic drug therapies have been tried (e.g. chlorambucil, colchicine, corticosteroids and penicillamine) with variable success.

Tendinitis and tenosynovitis

Definition and aetiology

Tendinitis is inflammation of a tendon and tenosynovitis is inflammation of the tendon sheath enclosing it. The cause of these conditions, which often occur together, is unknown although they may be due to a primary systemic disease (e.g. gout and rheumatoid arthritis) or to physical trauma or unaccustomed exercise. It is a condition that increases in frequency with increasing age.

Symptoms

Tendinitis and tenosynovitis are characterised by local inflammation, swelling and tenderness. Pain, which may be severe, is usually exacerbated by movement. Common sites include the fingers and toes, hips, legs (e.g. hamstring or Achilles tendon) and shoulders.

Treatment

Treatment commonly includes immobilisation, the application of heat or cold, gentle exercise and physiotherapy. Non-steroidal anti-inflammatory drugs (BNF 10.1.1) may be indicated and local corticosteroid injections (BNF 10.1.2.2) may be beneficial.

10.5 Anatomy and physiology relevant to musculoskeletal and connective tissue disorders

Joints

A joint (articulation) is a junction between two bones or a bone and cartilage, and is classified according to its structure. If there is a space between the apposing surfaces and the structures are held together by a fibrous capsule, the joint is described as synovial. A joint with no space between the apposing surfaces may be held together by fibrous tissue (a fibrous joint) or by cartilage (a cartilaginous joint).

The most common type is the synovial joint (e.g. the knee, sacro-iliac and elbow). These are characterised by a space, the synovial cavity, between the bones and a lining of hyaline cartilage on the apposing bone surfaces. The two bones are held together by a capsule formed of an outer layer of connective tissue (the fibrous capsule) lined internally by a secretory membrane, the synovial membrane. The fibrous capsule may be modified in some joints to form bundles of parallel fibres (the ligaments), which enhance the strength of the fibrous capsule. Synovial fluid, which lubricates the joint and nourishes the cartilage, is secreted by the inner synovial membrane. This alkaline fluid also contains macrophages, which remove debris produced during normal working of the joint.

A further layer of cartilage, the articular discs, may be present in synovial joints. The cartilage divides the synovial cavity and allows opposite bones of different shapes to form effective joints.

The potential for friction between moving bones and the overlying skin, tendons, ligaments and muscles is reduced by the cushioning effect of sac-like fluid-filled cavities (the bursae).

Fibrous joints are characterised by irregular surfaces and are held together by a layer of fibrous connective tissue. The fibrous layer may be thin (e.g. the sutures between the bones of the skull) ensuring the complete absence of movement, or comparatively thick (e.g. the lower joint between the tibia and fibula) permitting small amounts of movement.

Cartilaginous joints are linked by a layer of hyaline cartilage or by fibrous tissue and cartilage. One example of a joint that is linked by hyaline cartilage is the one between the first rib and the sternum. This is immovable and cartilage is gradually replaced by bone during adult life. The joints between the bodies of vertebrae are formed of discs of fibrocartilage and allow a minute degree of movement.

Bone and skeleton

The skeletal system is the framework on which the organs and tissues of the body are supported. It provides protection for body systems, and acts as a lever for the action of muscles in the production of movement. It is also involved in homeostatic mechanisms in the body in its role as a storage compartment for minerals and the production of blood cells.

Bone is a connective tissue in which bone cells (osteocytes) are separated by hardened intercellular collagenous material, rich in calcium salts. The strength and protection inherent in bones may be largely attributed to compact bone in which layers of osteocytes are arranged in concentric cylinders (Haversian canals) around a central channel which contains blood cells. Spongy bone contains a far less organised structure consisting of a network of thin plates of bone (trabeculae) interspersed in some bones by the marrow. In the mature skeleton, compact bone can be formed by the transformation of spongy bone (remodelling).

Although bone appears to be a permanent structure, it is continually being replaced throughout adult life, allowing damaged bone to be replaced and bones to be refashioned. This is carried out by the deposition and reabsorption of calcium ions from the bone and the bloodstream. A balance exists in the formation of bone cells through the action of osteoblasts (ossification) and the reabsorption of calcium by osteoclasts. The homeostatic balance is also controlled by the availability of vitamin D (which assists in the absorption of calcium from the gastrointestinal tract and prevents the loss of calcium through the kidneys), an adequate dietary intake of calcium and phosphorus, and the presence of growth hormone, calcitonin, parathormone hormone and the sex hormones in balanced quantities.

The skeleton is a complex structure consisting of 206 bones, the majority of which may be classed as long (e.g. the thigh bone and the bones of the fingers), short (e.g. ankle and wrist bones), flat (e.g. scapula and cranium), or irregular (e.g. facial bones and the vertebrae).

The skeletal system may be divided into the axial and appendicular divisions. The axial skeleton consists predominantly of the bones of the trunk and head and includes the skull, sternum, ribs and vertebral column. The appendicular skeleton is formed of the bones of the limbs and those that attach them to the axial skeleton.

The vertebral column (Figure 10.5) is the central pivot on which the axial skeleton (and the musculature of the back) is supported. It also supports the head and protects the spinal cord. The column is made up of 33 vertebrae although the lower nine vertebrae are fused into two chains. There are seven cervical vertebrae in the neck region, 12 thoracic vertebrae at the rear of the thorax, five lumbar vertebrae in the lower back region, 5 sacral vertebrae which are fused to form the sacrum, and four fused coccygeal vertebrae which form the coccyx.

The junction between the top of the vertebral column and the head is formed at the atlas (C1) vertebra, whose shape permits backward and forward movements, and the axis (C2) vertebra

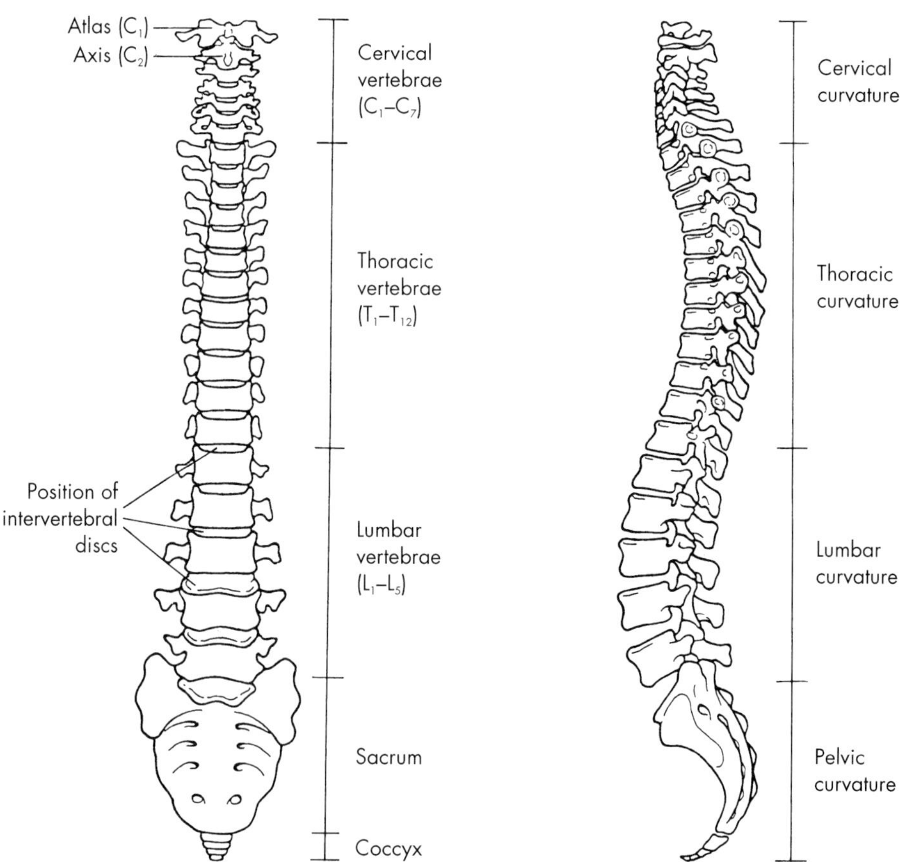

Figure 10.5 Vertebral column (lateral view).

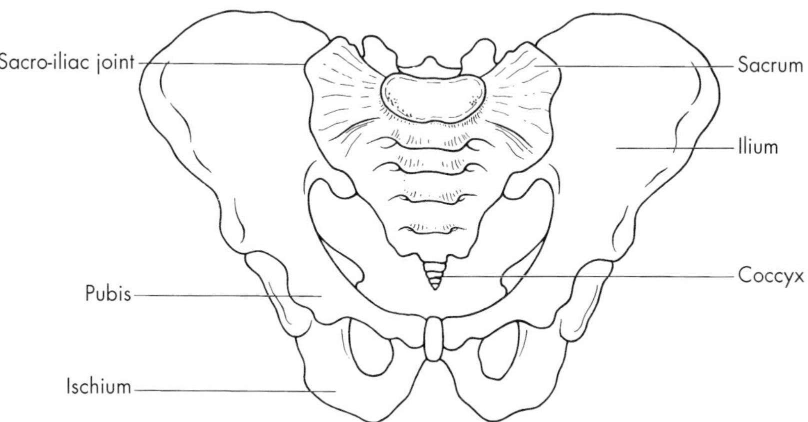

Figure 10.6 Pelvic girdle, male (anterior view).

which allows rotation. Individual vertebrae are linked through the intervertebral discs of fibrocartilage, which are formed of a hard exterior surrounding an inner elastic structure. The discs strengthen the vertebral column whilst at the same time being capable of distension and absorbing pressure changes created from above and below.

The sacral and coccygeal portions of the vertebral column and the pelvic girdle form the pelvis. The pelvic girdle (Figure 10.6) is formed of two hipbones and supports the abdominal contents. Although the hipbone is fused in the adult, in the neonate it is present as three separate bones, the ilium (which is the largest), the pubis and the ischium. The sacrum is attached to the ilium at the sacro-iliac joint.

Muscle

There are three types of muscle tissue in the body of which the greatest proportion is skeletal (striated) muscle. Skeletal muscle is responsible for the movement of bones and may be attached directly to the bone. However, where the presence of muscle tracts would interfere with the free movement of the bone, attachments are made through tendons. Tendons may also link muscles, and may be enclosed in a sheath of fibrous connective tissue. The sheath is similar in structure to bursae (*see above*) and permits the smooth movement of the tendon when the attached muscle contracts.

The fibres of skeletal muscle are formed of parallel, elongated, multinucleated cells enveloped within a plasma membrane, the sarcolemma. The muscle fibres are themselves built up of thousands of myofibrils which are subdivided by areas of dense tissue into compartments, the sarcomeres. The myofibrils consist of thin myofilaments composed predominantly of actin, and thick myofilaments formed of myosin. Cross bridges link the actin and myosin proteins on the two filaments.

Skeletal muscle contractions are voluntary, are initiated within the central nervous system, and pass to the muscle via the anterior spinal nerve roots and motor nerves. A muscle contraction is generated by the arrival of an action potential from the axon of a motor neuron at the sarcolemma of the muscle (the neuromuscular junction, Figure 10.7). The action potential within the nerve fibre causes the release of a neurotransmitter, acetylcholine, from the enlarged terminus of the axon, the synaptic bulb. This changes the permeability of the sarcolemma, causing a wave of excitation to pass through it which initiates muscle contraction.

Cardiac muscle is located exclusively in the heart wall and is structurally similar to skeletal muscle with the presence of actin and myosin, but only containing a single nucleus. The muscle fibres in cardiac muscle branch and are interconnected, permitting the rapid transmission of conduction from one filament to the next. The muscle also possesses an inherent ability to contract, and as a result requires a rich blood supply.

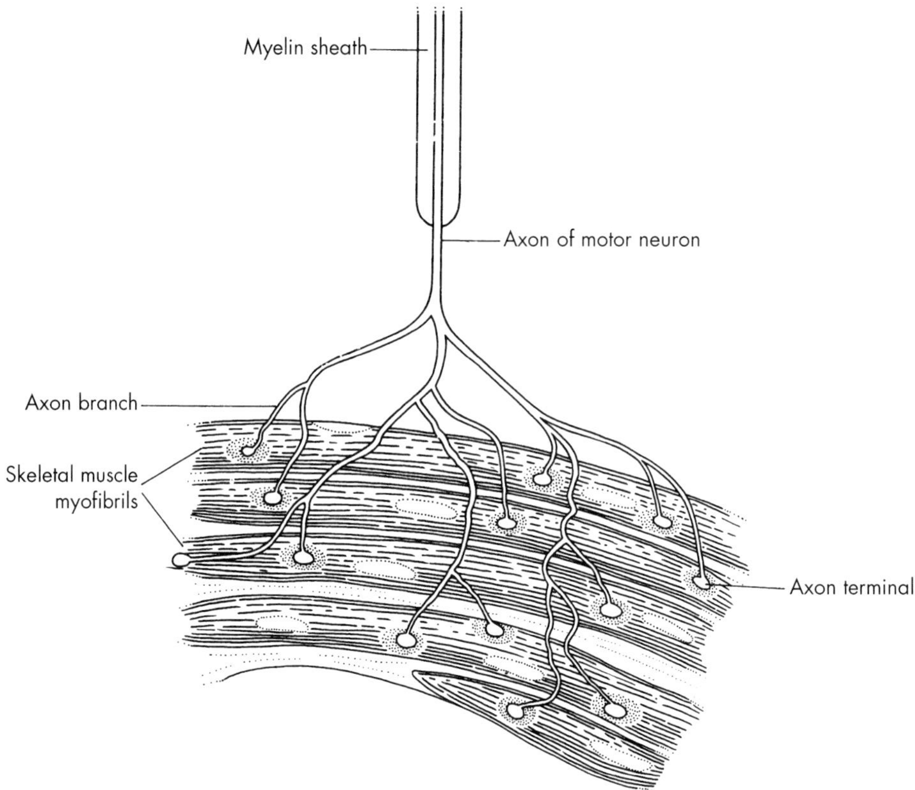

Figure 10.7 Diagrammatic representation of a neuromuscular junction.

The inherent rate of contraction may be modified by nervous stimulation.

Smooth (non-striated) muscle consists of sheets of spindle-shaped fibres each possessing a central oval nucleus. Smooth muscle found in the walls of small blood vessels and hollow organs (e.g. stomach, bladder and uterus) is termed visceral (single-unit) muscle tissue. Contraction of one cell is quickly passed to adjacent cells, because the fibres are closely interwoven into a continuous network. Contraction is usually initiated by the autonomic nervous system (i.e. it is under involuntary control) and the cells can contract even when they have been considerably distended (e.g. in the bladder).

Other smooth muscle (e.g. the walls of the bronchi, the walls of the large arteries and the intrinsic muscles of the eye) is formed of multi-unit tissues. These differ from single-unit fibres in that contraction of only one fibre can occur without spread to adjacent fibres.

Connective tissue

Connective tissue 'connects' organs and supports the body's structures. It may be classified as loose (areolar) connective tissue, adipose tissue, dense (collagenous) connective tissue, elastic connective tissue, and reticular connective tissue. Cartilage is also classified as connective tissue. Loose connective tissue consists of three types of fibres embedded within cells in a viscous intercellular substance called hyaluronic acid.

Bundles of collagenous fibres, which impart strength and flexibility in the tissue, are formed from the protein collagen. Elastic fibres, made of the protein elastin, provide strength and elasticity. Support within the fibril network is also provided by reticular fibres formed of collagen and glycoprotein. Cellular components of connective tissue include fibroblasts, macrophages, mast cells and plasma cells (*see* Section 9.4).

Adipose connective tissue contains cells modified for fat storage called adipocytes, and is located wherever there is loose connective tissue. It is primarily distributed in subcutaneous tissue of the skin, over the surface of the heart, and as padding around joints. The cells help prevent heat loss, act as an energy store and provide support.

Dense connective tissue fibres may be arranged irregularly or regularly. Irregularly orientated fibres contribute significantly to the fasciae and also occur in the protective fibrous capsules around organs. Fibres of dense connective tissue arranged in one direction impart strength but permit flexibility. These bundles form tendons and ligaments used to link muscles to bone, and bone to bone.

Elastic connective tissue has similar properties to regularly arranged dense tissuc, but the frequent branching of the fibres makes them better at imparting strength and elasticity to organ and vessel walls. The tissue is found in laryngeal cartilage, arterial walls and throughout the respiratory tree. It also links successive vertebrae and forms the vocal cords.

The liver, lymph nodes and spleen are supported by a fine network of reticular connective tissue. The tissue also binds cells of other smooth muscle tissue.

Cartilage (consisting of hyaline cartilage, fibrocartilage and elastic cartilage) is a resilient form of connective tissue characterised by the absence of blood vessels and nerve fibres. The cellular components are chondrocytes, which are embedded within spaces (lacunae) and are surrounded by dense tissue, the perichondrium.

11

Eye disorders

11.1 Disorders of the eye

Blepharitis

Definition and aetiology

Blepharitis (Figure 11.1) is inflammation of the margins of the eyelids. The cause is often unknown, although it may be allergic or occur in association with seborrhoea of the face and scalp (i.e. squamous blepharitis). Bacterial infection may, however, be responsible (i.e. ulcerative blepharitis).

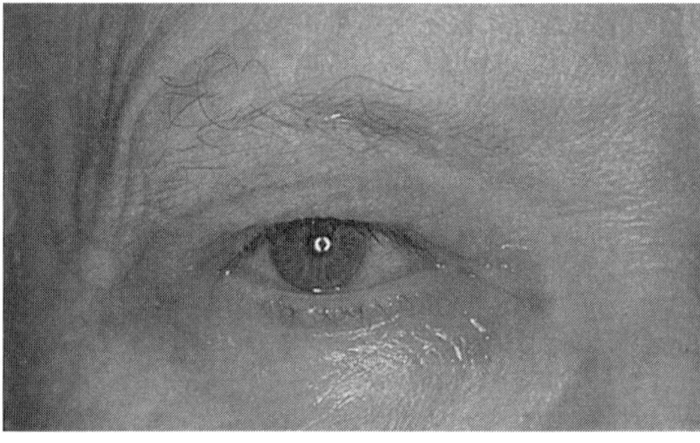

Figure 11.1 Blepharitis with punctate erosions. (Reproduced with permission of Mike Wyndham.)

Symptoms

Squamous blepharitis is characterised by local inflammation, scaling, pruritus and oedema. It is similar to seborrhoeic dermatitis of the scalp. In ulcerative blepharitis, yellow crusts form on the eyelashes, which may become stuck together. The eyelashes may be lost, lachrymation and photophobia may occur, and small ulcers can develop on the eyelid margins.

Both forms are subject to recurrence and may become chronic. Ulcerative blepharitis may be associated with the development of chronic conjunctivitis or corneal ulceration.

Treatment
The eyes should be cleansed with simple eye ointment or a suitably warmed eye lotion (BNF 11.8.1). In the presence of infection, an appropriate topical anti-infective preparation (BNF 11.3.1) should be used. Routine eye cleansing should be maintained and good hygiene encouraged. Rubbing or fingering the eyes must be avoided.

Cataract

Definition and aetiology
Cataract is any opacity of the lens of the eye or of its capsule. It may be inherited or may occur at, or soon after, birth (developmental cataract). It most commonly arises, however, as a result of degenerative changes associated with ageing (degenerative cataract). Other possible causes include diabetes mellitus, drug administration (e.g. corticosteroids), galactosaemia, ionising radiation, iritis (*see* Uveitis), and trauma.

Symptoms
Cataract is characterised by progressive visual impairment which varies according to the location and size of the opacity. Vision may eventually be significantly reduced with the lens becoming visibly opaque. Cataract is usually painless, but pain may occur if the cataract swells and secondary glaucoma develops. Cataract formation is usually bilateral.

Treatment
No effective medical treatment exists. The provision of appropriate spectacles may be sufficient initially. If vision is markedly impaired, treatment is by the surgical removal of the affected lenses or their contents, and the insertion of a prosthetic lens. Corrective spectacles or contact lenses may also be worn.

Chalazion

Definition and aetiology
A chalazion (Meibomian cyst or tarsal cyst) is an inflammatory granulomatous swelling on the eyelid or its margin. It occurs as a result of the blockage of one of the Meibomian glands which lubricate the eyelid. It is more common in adults than in children.

Symptoms
It is characterised by a painless slow-growing swelling which may be accompanied by conjunctival discoloration. Multiple swellings may appear but can disappear spontaneously. A chalazion may become so large, however, as to cause disfigurement, and secondary infection may occasionally develop.

Treatment
Treatment is often by surgical removal under local anaesthetic (BNF 11.7). An appropriate topical anti-infective preparation (BNF 11.3.1) may be necessary if infection occurs.

Conjunctivitis

Definition and aetiology
Conjunctivitis is an inflammation of the membrane that lines the eyelids (i.e. the conjunctiva). It may be acute or chronic and is most commonly due to allergy or viral infection. Other causes include bacterial infection, which may accompany upper respiratory-tract infection, and irritation caused by dust, smoke, wind or hand-to-eye contact (e.g. by contact-lens wearers).

Symptoms
Acute conjunctivitis is characterised by the production of a discharge which may be purulent, and by erythema and swelling of the eyelids. Local pruritus is a prominent feature if allergy is responsible. Chronic conjunctivitis is subject to remissions and relapses over a period of months or years. The symptoms are similar to those of the acute form, but less severe.

Treatment
The eyes should be kept clean and good hygiene should be encouraged. An appropriate topical anti-infective preparation (BNF 11.3) should be used if infection is responsible. In allergic conjunctivitis, a topical anti-inflammatory preparation may be administered.

Corneal ulceration

Definition and aetiology

Corneal ulceration may be described as the development of an area of necrosis in the tissue of the cornea. It is commonly caused by bacterial infection which occurs as a consequence of physical injury to the cornea. Viral infection may also be responsible, and dendritic ulcers are due to herpes simplex virus infection. Other possible causes include injury to, or defective closure of, the eyelids, or glaucoma.

Symptoms

Corneal ulceration is usually characterised by blinking, keratitis, lachrymation, pain and photophobia. Ulceration may spread across the surface of the cornea and visual impairment may occur. In severe cases, corneal scarring or perforation may develop and destruction of the eye may eventually occur.

Treatment

Prompt treatment under specialist supervision is essential and usually comprises the topical or systemic administration of an appropriate anti-infective preparation (BNF 11.3). In severe cases, surgical repair or corneal transplantation may be necessary.

Dacryocystitis

Definition and aetiology

Dacryocystitis (dacrycystitis) is inflammation of the lachrymal sac usually caused by obstruction of the nasolachrymal duct. This obstruction may arise as a result of nasal polyps, nasal septum deviation, rhinitis or trauma. In infants, it may be caused by congenital obstruction of the duct. Dacryocystitis is common and is often chronic.

Symptoms

The primary symptom is abnormal overflow of tears (i.e. epiphora), particularly on exposure to windy conditions. Local swelling and pain may occur. Chronic dacryocystitis is commonly progressive and may lead to the development of a lachrymal abscess.

Treatment

The condition usually resolves spontaneously in children. The application of hot compresses may be beneficial, and in the presence of an abscess, drainage and the administration of an appropriate anti-infective preparation (BNF 11.3) may be necessary. Dilatation of the nasolachrymal duct with a probe may be required in chronic cases. In unresponsive cases, surgical correction (i.e. dacryocystorhinostomy) is the only effective treatment.

Dry eye

Definition and aetiology

Dry eye (keratoconjunctivitis sicca) is a chronic condition characterised by dryness of the conjunctiva, cornea and sclera. It may be caused by a deficiency of conjunctival mucus (e.g. in Stevens–Johnson syndrome), corneal damage, eyelid disorders, or to tear deficiency arising from a systemic disease such as rheumatoid arthritis (i.e. Sjögren's syndrome).

Symptoms

Ocular irritation is the principal symptom, but photophobia and spasm of the eyelids (blepharospasm) may develop. Keratinisation of the cornea may eventually occur with ulceration, scarring and visual impairment.

Treatment

Treatment is by the frequent administration of a preparation for tear deficiency (BNF 11.8.1).

Ectropion and entropion

Definition and aetiology

Ectropion is the turning outward (i.e. eversion) and entropion is the turning inward (i.e. inversion) of the eyelid margins. Both conditions are usually associated with ageing, although they may arise as a result of scar formation on, or close to, the eyelid.

Symptoms

Ectropion is characterised by poor drainage of tears which consequently overflow (i.e.

epiphora). The eye becomes irritated and the exposed cornea may become ulcerated.

Entropion is marked by irritation of the eye due to the inverted eyelashes. This may lead to conjunctivitis and corneal ulceration, and scarring.

Treatment

Surgery is the only effective treatment.

Exophthalmos

Definition and aetiology

Exophthalmos (proptosis) is the abnormal protrusion of one or both eyeballs. It arises as a result of swelling of the orbital tissues and is most commonly caused by hyperthyroidism. Other causes include orbital inflammation (e.g. orbital cellulitis), oedema and malignant disease.

Symptoms

The surface of the eyeball becomes abnormally exposed. As a result, drying of the cornea may produce local infection or ulceration. Eye movement may be restricted and visual impairment may develop.

Treatment

The underlying cause should be treated. In some cases, exophthalmos may improve with the systemic administration of a corticosteroid, and surgery may be necessary.

Glaucoma

Definition and aetiology

Glaucoma is a group of ophthalmic disorders characterised by an increased intra-ocular pressure which results in damage to the optic disc and visual disturbances. Intra-ocular pressure increases through an imbalance between the production and drainage of aqueous humour. The cause of glaucoma is unknown, but a family history and hyperopia may be predisposing factors. Glaucoma may also arise secondary to an existing disease (e.g. uveitis and cataracts). It is the second most common cause of blindness.

Closed-angle glaucoma

Definition and aetiology

Closed-angle glaucoma (acute congestive, narrow-angle or obstructive glaucoma) is marked by a shallow anterior chamber and a narrow filtration angle which may be physically blocked by the iris. It may be acute or chronic. It is less common than open-angle glaucoma.

Symptoms

The acute form of the disorder is characterised by a sudden rise in intra-ocular pressure, accompanied by severe eye pain, headache, nausea and vomiting, and prostration. Symptoms may be preceded by short periods of visual disturbance (e.g. haloes around lights) which are a consequence of corneal oedema and pupil dilatation. Usually only one eye is affected but, in the absence of treatment, blindness may follow. The chronic form is characterised by similar, but less severe, recurrent attacks.

Treatment

Early treatment of glaucoma (BNF 11.6) is essential and includes the topical administration of a miotic. A carbonic anhydrase inhibitor may also be given for its systemic effect and the osmotic effect of glycerol or mannitol may be useful. Surgery (e.g. iridectomy) may be necessary in severe or intractable cases.

Open-angle glaucoma

Definition and aetiology

Open-angle glaucoma (simple, chronic simple or wide-angle glaucoma) occurs in the absence of any abnormality in the structure of the anterior chamber or filtration angle. The drainage of aqueous humour gradually becomes impeded over a period of years, leading to a slow increase in the intra-ocular pressure. The cause is unknown.

Symptoms

Open-angle glaucoma may be asymptomatic in the early stages, but is marked by a progressive loss of peripheral vision. Headache may occur, and central vision may deteriorate, eventually leading to blindness. Usually both eyes are affected.

Treatment
Drug treatment (BNF 11.6) comprises the topical administration of miotics, adrenaline or beta-adrenoceptor blocking drugs. A carbonic anhydrase inhibitor may also be given systemically. In severe cases, surgery may be required to facilitate drainage.

Macular degeneration

Definition and aetiology
Macular degeneration is an important cause of visual impairment in the elderly. It is associated with ageing and arises as a result of interference with the blood supply to the macula lutea, a modified area of the retina responsible for detailed central vision. Both eyes are usually affected and a family history is often present.

Symptoms
The onset is often gradual and is painless. It is characterised by the progressive impairment of central vision. Although peripheral vision is unaffected, the entire central field may eventually be lost.

Treatment
No effective treatment exists.

Optic neuropathies

Definition and aetiology
Optic neuropathy (optic neuritis) is inflammation of the optic nerve within the eyeball (i.e. papillitis) or behind it (i.e. retrobulbar neuritis). The cause is often unknown, but malignant disease, meningitis, multiple sclerosis, giant cell arteritis, chemical toxicity (e.g. caused by ethanol or lead) or viral infection may be responsible.

Symptoms
It is usually unilateral. Visual impairment may be slight or marked, and temporary blindness may develop and persist for many weeks. Movement of the eyeball may be painful. Although the condition usually remits spontaneously, relapses may occur, especially if multiple sclerosis is the cause.

Treatment
Any underlying cause should be treated. Systemic or retrobulbar and subconjunctival corticosteroid therapy may be beneficial.

Papilloedema

Definition and aetiology
Papilloedema (choked disc) is characterised by oedema of the optic disc. It is usually due to increased intracranial pressure (of which it is an important diagnostic sign) which may arise from intracranial tumours, cerebral haemorrhage, head injury, malignant hypertension or meningitis.

Symptoms
Vision may not be impaired initially, although the 'blind spot' becomes enlarged. In the absence of treatment, however, atrophy of the optic nerve may occur, with the eventual development of blindness.

Treatment
Treatment is by the reduction of intracranial pressure, according to the underlying cause.

Ptosis

Definition and aetiology
Ptosis is drooping of the upper eyelid. It may be partial or complete and may affect one or both eyes. It is most commonly congenital and results from defective muscular development. It may, however, also be acquired (e.g. through malignant disease, myasthenia gravis or physical injury).

Symptoms
Congenital ptosis is usually bilateral and acquired ptosis is usually unilateral. Visual impairment may occur, depending on the extent to which the pupil is obscured by the eyelid. As a result of trying to open the eyes, the head may be thrown back, the eyebrows raised, and the skin on the forehead may become wrinkled.

Treatment
Any underlying cause should be treated. Surgical correction may otherwise be necessary.

Retinal detachment

Definition and aetiology

Retinal detachment is a rare disorder. It usually occurs as a result of the leakage of vitreous humour through a hole or tear in the retina, causing the retina to become separated from its underlying pigmented epithelium. The detachment is localised initially but may extend in the absence of treatment. The most common cause is retinal degeneration, which occurs in association with ageing. Other causes include the production of exudate, haemorrhage, injury and malignant disease.

Symptoms

Retinal detachment is painless. Early symptoms include flashes of light and the appearance of 'floaters' in the field of vision. Central vision usually remains intact, but peripheral vision may become cloudy. As detachment progresses, the entire field of vision is lost and permanent blindness may follow through irreversible loss of retinal function. Retinal detachment usually affects only one eye at a time, but there is an increased likelihood of subsequent detachment in the other eye.

Treatment

Early diagnosis and location of offending retinal lesions is essential. Treatment is by surgery, and procedures used to repair retinal damage include cryosurgery, diathermy and photocoagulation. Retinal re-attachment usually follows, but regular screening of both eyes is desirable.

Scleritis and episcleritis

Definition and aetiology

Scleritis is deep-seated inflammation of the sclera. If the inflammation is superficial, the condition is known as episcleritis. These disorders are thought to develop as an allergic reaction in association with systemic diseases (e.g. rheumatoid arthritis).

Symptoms

Scleritis is marked by an intense purple discoloration of the sclera and discomfort or pain in the affected eye. Some visual impairment may develop and in severe cases perforation of the sclera may occur. The symptoms of episcleritis are similar, but milder.

Treatment

Treatment is by the administration of a topical corticosteroid or anti-inflammatory preparation (BNF 11.4), although a systemic preparation may be necessary in scleritis. Immunosuppressants have also been used in severe cases.

Strabismus

Definition and aetiology

Strabismus (cast, heterotropia or squint) is a lack of coordination of the eyes so that the visual axes assume an abnormal position relative to each other. It may be caused by paralysis of an eye muscle (i.e. paralytic strabismus), in which the degree of deviation varies according to the position of the eyes. It may also arise through defective insertion of the eye muscles (i.e. concomitant strabismus), in which case the degree of deviation is constant. Strabismus may be present at birth, but also often develops in early infancy. Irregular strabismus is a normal occurrence in the visual development of most babies and will normally resolve by three months of age. It is less common in adults in whom it is usually caused by a primary disease (e.g. brain injury, giant cell arteritis and hypertension).

Symptoms

Strabismus may be convergent, in which the eyes turn inwards towards each other, or divergent, in which the eyes turn outwards. A common symptom is diplopia, although children often do not develop diplopia as the images from the divergent eye are 'ignored' by the brain. Accordingly, this eye becomes 'lazy' and its vision impaired (i.e. amblyopia).

Treatment

Early investigation, diagnosis and treatment are essential. Eye exercises with occlusion (i.e. patching) of the normal eye may be helpful. Corrective spectacles, with or without patching, may be appropriate. In severe cases, surgical correction is often necessary. If untreated, strabismus may result in complete visual loss in the affected eye.

Uveitis

Definition and aetiology

Uveitis is inflammation of the uvea (uveal tract) and may be anterior or posterior. Anterior uveitis is characterised by inflammation of the iris (iritis), the ciliary body (cyclitis) or, more commonly, of both (iridocyclitis). Posterior uveitis is characterised by inflammation of the choroid (choroiditis) or, more commonly, of the choroid and retina (chorioretinitis). Uveitis is often idiopathic, but it may occur secondary to systemic infections (e.g. syphilis, toxoplasmosis and tuberculosis) or inflammatory disease (e.g. ankylosing spondylitis, rheumatoid arthritis and sarcoidosis). A primary infection, or allergic or hypersensitivity reactions may also be responsible.

Symptoms

Anterior uveitis is characterised by inflammation, lachrymation, pain and photophobia. The pupil becomes small, irregular and unreactive. Visual impairment may develop and, if the disease becomes chronic, iris–lens adhesions (i.e. synechiae) may occur. Possible complications include cataract formation and glaucoma. In posterior uveitis, pain and lachrymation are less common, but visual shapes and sizes become distorted and 'floaters' may be seen. Retinal detachment is a possible complication.

Treatment

Local hot applications may be soothing, but treatment usually comprises the administration of a cycloplegic and mydriatic (BNF 11.5) to prevent adhesions, and of a topical or systemic corticosteroid, or both.

11.2 Anatomy and physiology of the eye

Introduction

The eye (Figure 11.2) is a specialised visual structure into which light passes and within which it is focused onto a sensory surface. The image formed on the sensory surface is transmitted via the optic nerve to the visual cortex in the brain where the information received is interpreted by the surrounding occipital lobe of the cortex.

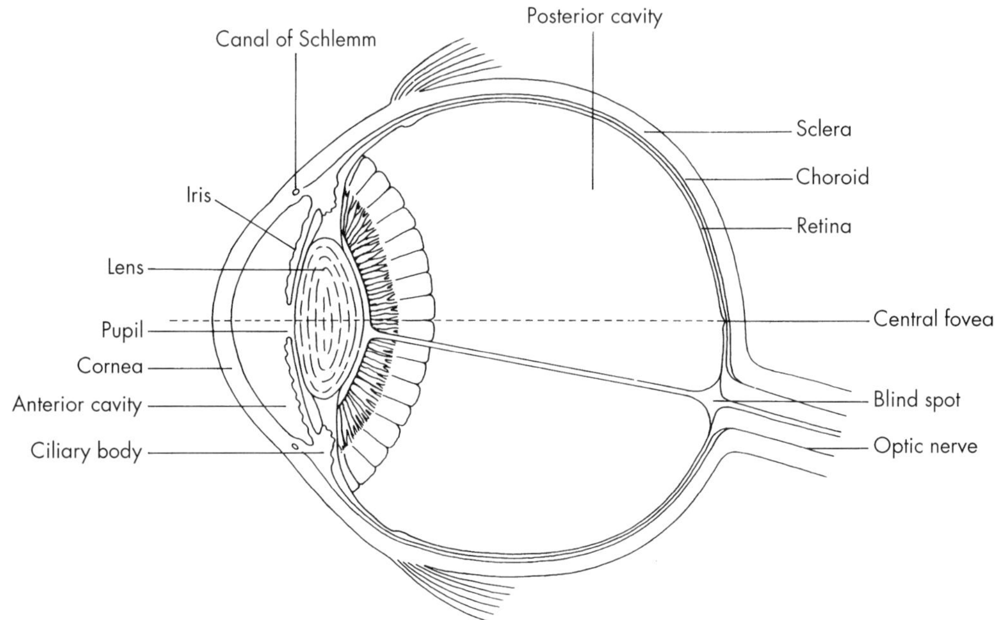

Figure 11.2 Structure of the eye (horizontal section).

Internal structure of the eye

The eye, which is a fluid-filled sphere, measures about 2.5 cm in diameter. The bulk of the orb is contained within a bony orbit, with only approximately one-sixth visible externally. The orb is protected by pads of fat and by the muscles which control and initiate its movement. The wall of the eyeball is composed of three coats of which the fibrous tunic is the outermost. The white fibrous layer at the rear of the eyeball, the sclera, is continuous with the transparent window, the cornea, at the front through which light enters the eye. The junction of the sclera and cornea is marked by the canal of Schlemm, which lies deep within the sclera.

The central layer of the wall of the eyeball, the vascular tunic, is composed of choroid, the ciliary bodies, and the iris which are collectively known as the uvea. The choroid is a dark, non-reflecting membrane, which is highly vascularised. The choroid becomes modified immediately behind the scleral–corneal junction to form the ciliary bodies and the iris. The ciliary bodies are formed of the ciliary processes, which secrete aqueous humour, and the ciliary muscle, which on relaxation or contraction alters the shape of the lens for accommodation. The iris consists of pigmented radial and circular muscle, at the centre of which is a hole, the pupil. The muscle of the iris relaxes and contracts to alter the amount of light entering the eye.

The inner surface of the eye is formed of the nervous tunic, the retina. Unlike the outer two coats, the retina is only present in the rear portion of the eye. It is a highly complex multilayered membrane, which may be broadly classified as nervous tissue with an outer pigmented layer. Blood vessels forming a random pattern over its surface may be readily seen in the retinal layer.

The nervous layer contains the morphologically descriptive rods and cones, which are the visual receptors. The rods, which number 70–140 million, operate in dim light and perceive different degrees of darkness and light. By comparison, there are only approximately 7 million cones, which are adapted for detecting colour and for the provision of visual acuity. The greatest concentration of cones occurs at a small depression, the central fovea, located in the middle of the yellow spot, the macula lutea. The central fovea is located at the visual axis of the eye and is the point of sharpest vision. The site at which the optic nerve leaves and at which the retinal blood vessels enter the eye is marked by the blind spot, optic disc. This lies close to the macula lutea and is marked by the absence of rods and cones.

The lens is a transparent proteinaceous body encapsulated in clear connective tissue. Its position forms the boundary between the anterior and posterior cavities of the eye. It is held in position and in a slightly stretched state by suspensory ligaments which arise in the ciliary bodies. The shape of the lens may be altered by the action of the ciliary muscles to allow light entering the eye to be sharply focused on the retina.

The shape of the anterior cavity, to the front of the lens, is maintained by the presence of a watery fluid, aqueous humour. Aqueous humour is continuously secreted by the ciliary body behind the iris and transported between the iris and lens through the pupil, and into the space between the lens and cornea. Normal pressure within the anterior cavity (about 16 mmHg) is maintained by the gradual drainage of aqueous humour through the canal of Schlemm into the blood.

The posterior cavity, behind the lens, is filled with a viscous fluid, the vitreous humour, which is formed *in utero* and, unlike the aqueous humour, is not recycled. It maintains the shape of the eyeball and helps to prevent distortion of the retinal membrane.

External structure of the eye

The eye is an extremely sensitive organ and requires protection from the external environment. The external surface of the eye and the inner lining of the eyelid are protected by a thin vascularised membrane, the conjunctiva, which in the space between the eyelid and the eyeball forms the conjunctival sac. Tears are secreted by the lachrymal glands (*see below*) into the upper conjunctival sac. The eyelids are formed of folds of muscle and skin above and below the eyeball.

The movement of the eyelids assists in the lubrication of the surface of the eyeball by tears, although the lower eyelid is more firmly fixed than the upper.

The eyelids are strengthened by the presence of a tarsal plate in which are embedded the sebaceous Meibomian (tarsal) glands. The glandular secretions reduce the loss of tears by evaporation and prevent the upper and lower eyelids from sticking to each other. The border of each eyelid is lined with short hairs, the eyelashes, at the base of which are sebaceous glands, the glands of Zeis.

The controlled secretion and drainage of tears (lachrymation) is essential for lubrication and the maintenance of a healthy eye. Tears are produced by the lachrymal glands located in the upper outer (i.e. furthest from the nose) portion of each eye orbit and contain an antibacterial enzyme, lysozyme. From the lachrymal gland, the tears are secreted through 6–12 lachrymal ducts onto the surface of the upper conjunctival membrane. Tears drain from the surface of the conjunctiva via the inner corner of each eye into the lachrymal sac, which is located along the side of the nose. The fluid drains into the nasolachrymal duct from the lachrymal sac and subsequently into the nasal cavity. Hence, eye-drops instilled into the conjunctival sac may end up in the nasal cavity to eventually be swallowed and absorbed.

12

Disorders of the ear, nose and oropharynx

12.1 Disorders of the ear

Deafness

Definition and aetiology

Conductive deafness is hearing loss which arises as a result of disturbance of the sound conduction mechanisms in the external auditory canal or the middle ear. Causes include physical obstruction (e.g. by ear wax), disease of the external or middle ear, perforation of the eardrum, or otosclerosis.

Sensorineural deafness is hearing loss characterised by disturbance of the inner ear or of the acoustic (eighth) nerve. It may be caused by neural or brain damage, loud noise (e.g. occupational deafness), or to the administration of drugs (e.g. aminoglycosides). Maternal rubella may produce congenital sensorineural deafness in neonates.

Treatment
Any underlying disorder must be identified and treated. Provision of a hearing aid may be beneficial.

Self-help organisations
Breakthrough
British Tinnitus Association
Council for the Advancement of Communication with Deaf People
Hearing Dogs for Deaf People
National Deaf Children's Society
National Deaf-Blind League
Royal National Institute for the Deaf
Scottish Association for the Deaf
SENSE
Wales Council for the Deaf

Labyrinthitis

Definition and aetiology
Labyrinthitis (otitis interna) is an uncommon disorder characterised by inflammation of the labyrinth which disturbs its function. It usually occurs as a complication of otitis media, in which the infection spreads from the middle ear. Viral labyrinthitis may occur as an epidemic.

Symptoms
The chief symptom is vertigo, which may be accompanied by severe nausea and vomiting. Nystagmus may occur and deafness may develop.

Treatment
Treatment comprises the administration of an anti-emetic (BNF 4.6). In severe cases, surgery (i.e. labyrinthectomy) may be necessary and antibacterial drugs (BNF 5.1) may be indicated in the presence of bacterial infection.

Mastoiditis

Definition and aetiology
Mastoiditis is inflammation of the bony mastoid process which lies behind the ear. It occurs as a serious complication of otitis media, with bacterial infection spreading to the mastoid air cells from the middle ear. It has become less common because of effective antibiotic therapy of otitis media.

Symptoms
Common symptoms include inflammation, pain and swelling over the mastoid process, and fever and malaise. The production of a profuse purulent discharge is also common and increasing conductive deafness may develop. Abscess formation may occur in severe cases.

Treatment
Treatment is by the oral or parenteral administration of an appropriate antibacterial drug (BNF 5.1). In severe cases, surgery (i.e. mastoidectomy) may be indicated in order to remove infected bone, and this may be followed by local topical treatment (BNF 12.1.2).

Ménière's disease

Definition and aetiology
Ménière's disease is a labyrinthine disorder associated with vertigo. It usually develops in middle or old age and may be mild or severe. It is due to damage to the receptor cells of the cochlea and vestibular system.

Symptoms
It is characterised by progressive deafness and tinnitus, eventually followed by recurrent attacks of vertigo. Deafness may become total. The vertigo is exacerbated by movement and may be accompanied by nausea and vomiting, and nystagmus. Attacks may last from several minutes to several hours.

Treatment
Treatment comprises the administration of drugs such as prochlorperazine, betahistine and cinnarizine (BNF 4.6), or ultrasonic irradiation. In extreme cases, it may be necessary to destroy the labyrinth by surgery or by chemicals, but deafness will result.

Otitis externa

Definition and aetiology
Otitis externa is characterised by inflammation of the external auditory canal. The acute form is

usually caused by bacterial infection, although fungal infection may be responsible. The entire canal may be involved or infection may be localised in the form of a furuncle. The chronic form of otitis externa is most often eczematous and is commonly associated with eczema occurring at other body sites. Contributory factors include mechanical trauma, chemical irritants (e.g. hair products) and dampness (e.g. after swimming).

Symptoms

Eczematous otitis externa is marked by itching of the auditory canal, which is often dry and scaly. Severe pain is characteristic of acute otitis externa and is often exacerbated by manipulation of the pinna. An offensive purulent discharge may be evident and the canal may become blocked as a result of local swelling and accumulated purulent debris. Accordingly, hearing may be impaired.

Treatment

The affected ear should be gently but thoroughly cleaned. The local application of warmth may be helpful and contributory factors should be avoided. A topical astringent or corticosteroid (BNF 12.1.1) may be administered in the presence of an eczematous reaction. If infection is responsible, however, an appropriate topical anti-infective preparation (BNF 12.1.1) should be used and an analgesic (BNF 4.7) may be required if pain is severe. In the presence of localised or unresponsive infections, a systemic anti-infective preparation may be indicated.

Otitis media

Definition

Otitis media (tympanitis) is inflammation of the middle ear. It may be classified as acute, chronic or sero-mucinous otitis media.

Acute otitis media

Definition and aetiology

Acute otitis media is usually due to bacterial infection (e.g. *Haemophilus influenza*, *Staphylococcus aureus* or *Streptococcus pyogenes*), although viral infection may be responsible. It is most common in young children and is often preceded by an upper respiratory-tract infection. Physical injury to the eardrum, however, may be a precipitating factor.

Symptoms

Acute otitis media is characterised by severe pain and a degree of conductive deafness. Fever, and nausea and vomiting are also common. A purulent exudate is produced and may accumulate in the middle ear. This may cause bulging, or even perforation, of the eardrum.

Treatment

The treatment of acute disease may include the administration of a non-opioid analgesic (BNF 4.7.1) and, in the presence of bacterial infection, an appropriate antibacterial drug (BNF 5.1, table 1). Antibacterial prophylaxis (BNF 12.1.2) may be considered. Surgical incision of the eardrum (i.e. myringotomy) may be necessary to drain accumulated exudate.

Chronic otitis media

Definition and aetiology

Chronic disease may follow an acute attack although its development may be insidious. It may also be associated with obstruction of the Eustachian tube or physical injury to the eardrum.

Symptoms

Chronic otitis media is marked by permanent painless inflammation of the middle ear and the production of a purulent discharge and perforation of the eardrum. Hearing impairment may be the presenting symptom.

Treatment

In the presence of chronic disease, the affected ear must be thoroughly cleaned. Topical treatment similar to that for otitis externa may be beneficial. A systemic antibacterial (BNF 12.1.2) may be indicated in severe cases. Surgical repair may be necessary.

Sero-mucinous otitis media

Definition and aetiology

Sero-mucinous otitis media ('glue ear' or secretory otitis media) is characterised by the accumulation of a viscous mucinous fluid in the middle ear. It is most common in children and often follows repeated attacks of acute otitis media arising from upper respiratory-tract infections. It may also be associated with obstruction of the Eustachian tube, allergic reactions, or inflammation of the adenoids or sinuses.

Symptoms
Sero-mucinous otitis media is characterised by varying degrees of conductive deafness. Deafness may become permanent in the absence of treatment and can cause learning difficulties and speech disorders in children. Pain and discharge are often absent, although discharge will become evident if perforation of the eardrum (myringotomy) is carried out.

Treatment
Expert supervision is essential. If an infection is thought to be responsible, an appropriate antibacterial drug (BNF 5.1) may be administered. A systemic nasal decongestant (BNF 3.10) or an antihistamine (BNF 3.4.1) may be beneficial in relieving Eustachian tube obstruction or allergy. Surgical incision of the eardrum may be necessary to drain off accumulated fluid, and a small drainage tube (i.e. a grommet or stopple) may be inserted in the eardrum. Any primary disorder of the nasopharynx should be corrected. Mucolytics have been used with varying success.

Otosclerosis

Definition and aetiology
Otosclerosis is characterised by the immobilisation of the stapes in the middle ear and is caused by abnormal formation of new bone around the stapes and the oval window. Its aetiology is unknown, although a family history is often present. It is a common cause of deafness, occurs more frequently in women, and is exacerbated by pregnancy.

Symptoms
Otosclerosis is marked by the progressive development of conductive deafness and may be accompanied by tinnitus and vertigo. Both ears are usually affected and total deafness may occur in the absence of treatment.

Treatment
Treatment consists of the surgical removal of the stapes (i.e. stapedectomy) followed by replacement with a prosthesis. The provision of a hearing aid may be helpful.

12.2 Disorders of the nose

Rhinitis

Definition and aetiology
Rhinitis is inflammation of the nasal mucosa which may be of allergic, infective (*see* Common cold, Section 5.3) or vasomotor origin.

Allergic rhinitis

Definition and aetiology
Allergic rhinitis may be seasonal (i.e. hay fever) and occur at specific times of year as a result of allergy to plant pollens (e.g. trees or grasses). Alternatively, it may be perennial (i.e. non-seasonal) and arise from exposure to other allergens (e.g. animal danders, feathers, fungal spores or house-dust mite).

Symptoms
Hay fever is characterised by the sudden onset of symptoms. These include lachrymation, rhinorrhoea and sneezing with itching of the eyes, ears, nose and palate. Coughing, wheezing and nasal congestion are also common. The symptoms of perennial allergic rhinitis are similar to those of hay fever. In addition, nasal congestion and obstruction are likely to become chronic, and may lead to blockage of the Eustachian tubes and hearing difficulties.

Treatment
Both forms of allergic rhinitis benefit from identification and avoidance of specific allergens. Corticosteroids or sodium cromoglycate (BNF

12.2.1) may be administered as both prophylaxis or treatment. Symptoms may be treated with an oral antihistamine (BNF 3.4.1) or a systemic nasal decongestant (BNF 3.10). Topical nasal decongestants (BNF 12.2.2) may be used on a short-term basis, but may cause rebound nasal congestion and obstruction (rhinitis medicamentosa).

Vasomotor rhinitis

Definition and aetiology

Vasomotor rhinitis (non-allergic non-infective rhinitis) is caused by the dilatation of the blood vessels of the nasal mucosa, which may be due to sympathetic nervous system underactivity or parasympathetic nervous system overactivity. Common precipitating factors include emotional disturbances (e.g. anger, anxiety and fatigue), low humidity (e.g. caused by central heating) and sudden changes in temperature (e.g. mild chilling).

Symptoms

Symptoms of vasomotor rhinitis are similar to those of allergic rhinitis, although nasal itching and sneezing are less common. In addition, the nasal mucosa may appear highly coloured, varying from bright red to purplish. Nasal polyposis, asthma and an intolerance to aspirin may also occur.

Treatment

Treatment is similar to that of allergic rhinitis. Intranasal corticosteroids (BNF 12.2.1) may be beneficial in the treatment of nasal polyposis. Humidification of the atmosphere may provide general symptomatic relief. Severe cases may benefit from surgery (e.g. submucosal diathermy) and removal of polyps.

Sinusitis

Definition and aetiology

Sinusitis is inflammation of the paranasal sinuses, affecting primarily the frontal and maxillary sinuses (Figure 12.1). It is usually caused by viral or bacterial infection and often follows an

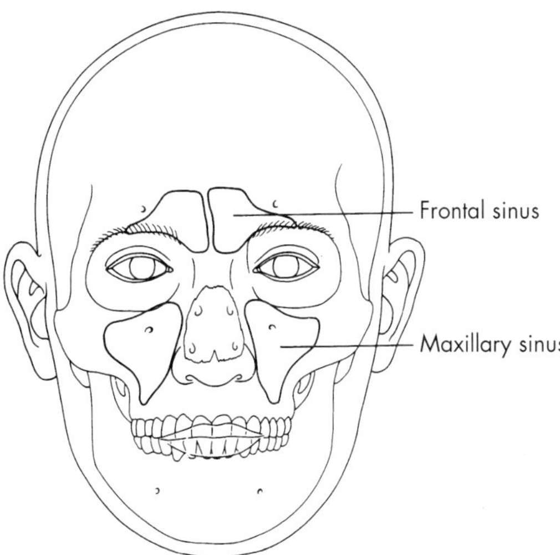

Figure 12.1 Position of the frontal and maxillary sinuses.

attack of the common cold. It may also arise, however, as a result of an underlying dental infection or some anatomical defect (e.g. deviated nasal septum). Sinusitis may be acute or chronic.

Symptoms

Common symptoms include nasal obstruction with purulent rhinorrhoea. Fever may occur, and facial pain over the affected sinus is common and can be exacerbated by bending forwards or coughing. If the frontal sinuses are affected, pain occurs over the eyes as a frontal headache. If the maxillary sinuses are involved, pain occurs under the eyes and may extend into the jaw so as to resemble toothache.

Treatment

Steam inhalations and non-opioid analgesics (BNF 4.7.1) are often helpful. Any primary infection or defect should be treated. Symptoms may be relieved by the administration of a systemic nasal decongestant (BNF 3.10) or by the short-term use of a topical nasal decongestant (BNF 12.2.2). In the presence of bacterial infection, an appropriate antibacterial drug (BNF 5.1) should be given. In unresponsive cases, surgery may be necessary to facilitate drainage of the sinus, which should also be washed out to remove any purulent debris.

12.3 Disorders of the oropharynx

Aphthous stomatitis

Definition and aetiology

Aphthous stomatitis (aphthous ulceration) is a common disorder characterised by the development of small ulcers (i.e. aphthae) on the oral mucosa. The cause is unknown, but a local immune mechanism may be responsible. Contributory factors may include folic acid, iron or vitamin B_{12} deficiencies. Emotional disturbances or physical illnesses may also contribute.

Symptoms

The chief symptom is the appearance of shallow yellow or white ulcers on the tongue or the mucosal surfaces of the cheeks and lips. The ulcers are acutely painful, may occur singly or in groups, and are commonly surrounded by an area of erythema. Although they usually heal spontaneously after about 14 days, recurrence is common. In some severe cases, they may be persistent and can be accompanied by fever and malaise.

Treatment

The use of an antiseptic mouthwash (BNF 12.3.4) may be beneficial in the prevention of secondary bacterial infection. Treatment (BNF 12.3.1) comprises the topical administration of a local anaesthetic or analgesic. A topical protective paste may also be useful and the administration of a corticosteroid lozenge or paste is often effective. A tetracycline mouthwash may be used to treat recurrent ulceration.

Gingivitis

Definition and aetiology

Gingivitis is inflammation of the gums. It is almost always caused by poor oral hygiene, which is characterised by the accumulation of food debris and the formation of dental plaque and calculus. Other causes include dental defects, primary systemic diseases (e.g. diabetes mellitus and leukaemia), and mouth breathing. The administration of phenytoin may result in the development of gingivitis.

Symptoms

The gums become inflamed and swollen and bleed easily, particularly after brushing the teeth or eating. Periodontal disease may develop in the absence of treatment and may result in dental decay or loss. Vincent's infection is a further possible complication.

Treatment

Any underlying dental defect or systemic disease should be corrected. Prophylaxis involves the removal of plaque with dental floss, especially in high-risk individuals. Treatment consists of introducing and maintaining good oral hygiene and regular dental therapy.

Glossitis

Definition and aetiology

Glossitis is a common disorder characterised by inflammation of the tongue. It may be due to infection, mechanical trauma or irritation (e.g. by alcohol, foods and smoking). It may also occur as a result of primary systemic disorders (e.g. anaemia and vitamin deficiencies).

Symptoms

The tongue may become red, swollen and ulcerated. In severe cases, pain may occur and swelling may be such that the tongue protrudes. Subsequent difficulties in eating and speaking may arise.

Treatment

Irritants should be avoided and good oral hygiene encouraged. Any underlying primary disorder should be treated. Treatment of glossitis may include the use of a topical anaesthetic or antiseptic preparation (BNF 12.3.3 and 12.3.4). An appropriate antibacterial drug (BNF 5.1) may be indicated in the presence of infection.

Halitosis

Definition and aetiology

Halitosis (bad breath) is characterised by an offensive unpleasant breath odour. It may be due to dental or gingival disease (e.g. Vincent's infection), respiratory disease or infection, nasopharyngeal disease (e.g. chronic tonsillitis), or simply to the retention of food debris in the mouth. Gastrointestinal disease is not generally thought to be responsible. Although halitosis is often real, it may also be imagined (i.e. psychogenic) and can indicate the presence of anxiety or underlying personality disorders.

Treatment

Any underlying cause should be corrected and good oral hygiene should be encouraged. Reassurance may be beneficial in imagined halitosis.

Laryngitis

Definition and aetiology

Laryngitis is inflammation of the larynx. It is usually caused by viral or bacterial infection and often follows an attack of the common cold. It may also arise, in the absence of infection, as a result of exposure to irritants (e.g. tobacco smoke or alcohol), from excessive use of the voice, or in association with an allergic reaction or respiratory-tract disorders (e.g. bronchitis and influenza). It may be acute or chronic.

Symptoms

The most common symptom is hoarseness, which may progress to complete voice loss. Hoarseness may be accompanied by a sore, dry throat, local oedema, dysphagia and an irritating cough. Fever is uncommon.

Treatment

The voice should be rested and irritants avoided. Steam inhalations are usually beneficial. Although no specific treatment exists for viral laryngitis, an appropriate antibacterial drug (BNF 5.1) may be indicated for the less common bacterial infection.

Oral leucoplakia

Definition and aetiology

Oral leucoplakia is characterised by the development of white thickened patches on the mucosa of the cheeks, tongue and, occasionally, of the gums. It may be due to irritation (e.g. by friction or smoking), infection (e.g. candidiasis or tertiary syphilis), or it may be inherited. In most patients, however, the cause is unknown.

Symptoms

The white patches usually develop over a period of weeks. They may be soft or hard and cover large or small areas of mucosa. The patches cannot be rubbed off. Ulceration may occasionally occur. Recurrence is common; in a small number of patients, malignant changes may develop.

Treatment

Patients should avoid smoking and any sources of friction must be removed, which usually involves dental treatment. In the presence of infection, an appropriate antimicrobial (BNF 5.1 and 5.2) may be indicated. Treatment is often ineffective, and follow-up is essential in order to detect the development of any malignant disease.

Pharyngitis

Definition and aetiology

Pharyngitis (acute sore throat) is an acute inflammation of the pharynx. It is most commonly caused by viral infection. However, group A β-haemolytic streptococcal infections may produce bacterial pharyngitis, particularly in young children which, if untreated, can develop into acute rheumatic fever. In young adults, the causative agent appears to be predominantly *Corynebacterium haemolyticum*. It may also arise as a result of pharyngeal irritation (e.g. by alcohol or smoking).

Symptoms

Pharyngitis is characterised by sore throat, with pain on swallowing and hoarseness. In the presence of infection, fever may occur and the pharynx may develop a membranous covering. A purulent exudate may also be produced. Patients with *C. haemolyticum* infection commonly present with a scarlet fever-like rash.

Treatment

Patients should be encouraged to avoid pharyngeal irritation and to maintain a high-fluid intake. Symptomatic treatment includes the use of antiseptic or anaesthetic gargles, or both, lozenges, or mouthwashes (BNF 12.3.3 and 12.3.4). Non-opioid analgesics (BNF 4.7.1) may be required and, in the presence of bacterial infection, an appropriate antibacterial drug (BNF 5.1) may be indicated.

Sialadenitis

Definition and aetiology

Sialadenitis is inflammation of a salivary gland. It is most often caused by viral (e.g. mumps) or bacterial infection, although it may occasionally arise as a result of an allergic reaction. The obstruction of a salivary duct (*see* Sialolithiasis *below*) may be a contributory factor. Alcoholism and sarcoidosis may also be implicated.

Symptoms

The parotid or submandibular salivary glands may be affected. Common symptoms include pain, which may be acute, and swelling. Local oedema may occur and a purulent discharge may arise from the duct of the affected gland. Fever and malaise may develop. Sialadenitis may be acute, chronic, or recurrent.

Treatment

Good oral hygiene must be encouraged. An appropriate antibacterial drug (BNF 5.1) should be administered in the presence of bacterial infection. Any salivary duct obstruction should be removed, and in chronic or recurrent cases surgical removal of the affected gland may be indicated.

Sialolithiasis

Definition and aetiology

Sialolithiasis is characterised by the formation of salivary stones (i.e. calculi) in the salivary ducts or, less commonly, in the salivary glands. The ducts of the submandibular glands are most often affected. Stones are formed by deposition of calcium carbonate and phosphate from saliva.

Symptoms

Sialolithiasis is most common in adults. It is marked by obstruction of the affected duct or gland, which leads to accumulation of saliva within the gland, particularly when eating. The salivary gland becomes swollen and pain may be experienced. Swelling may persist for several hours.

Treatment

Treatment comprises the removal of the offending stone, usually under local anaesthetic. In recurrent cases, corrective surgery may be necessary.

12.4 Anatomy and physiology of the ear, nose and oropharynx

The ear

The ear (Figure 12.2) is the organ of hearing and balance whose primary centres are located deep within the temporal bone of the skull in fluid-filled chambers. The outer structures are used mainly as a means of channelling sound inward to the hearing receptors. Anatomically, the ear is divided into three distinct, but interconnected, zones.

The outer ear consists of the pinna, the external auditory canal (meatus) and the tympanic membrane (eardrum). The pinna is the external portion of the outer ear, and is of variable size and thickness. It consists of a flap of fixed cartilage contained within thickened skin, and receives and directs sound waves from the environment into the ear. The external auditory canal leads from the pinna to the tympanic membrane. The surface of its outer end is lined with small hairs and ceruminous cells, which secrete cerumen (wax) and serve to minimise the entry of foreign materials into the canal. Sound entering the ear is transmitted along the external auditory canal to the tympanic membrane, which forms the boundary between the outer and middle ear. It is attached by a ring of cartilage to the temporal bone, and is lined by a membrane of thickened skin on its outer surface and a mucous membrane on its inner surface.

The middle ear (tympanic cavity) lies immediately behind the tympanic membrane, and is in an air-filled cavity within the temporal bone. The

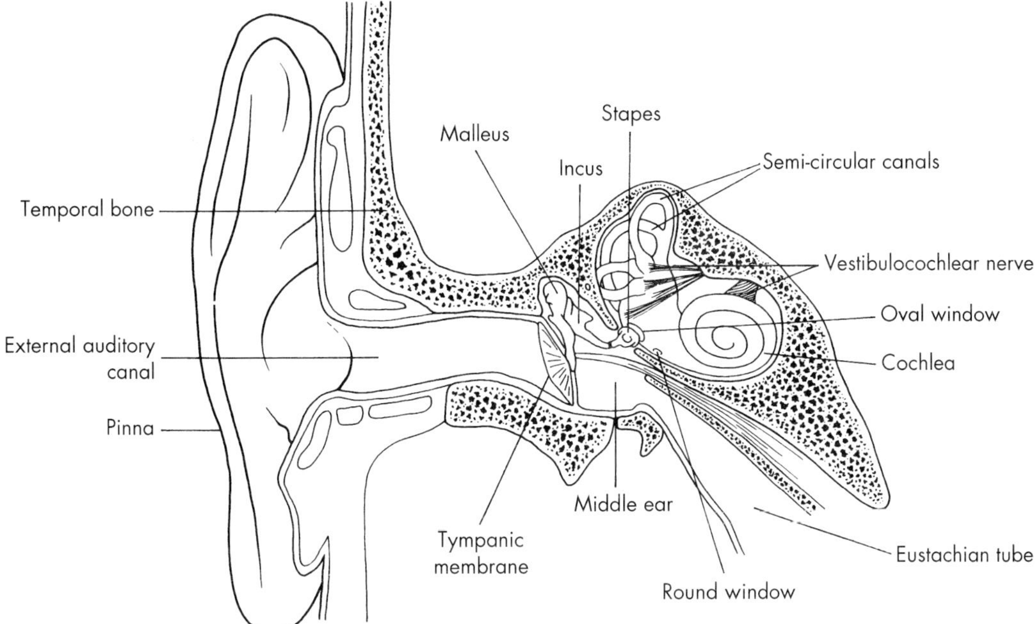

Figure 12.2 The ear in section.

temporal bone lining the rear of the middle-ear compartment is lined by air cells of the mastoid process. The opening to the Eustachian tube is located in the opposite wall of the cavity and connects the middle ear to the nasopharynx. It acts to equalise pressure within the middle ear with that of the external environment, and prevent rupture of the tympanic membrane. The entrance to the Eustachian tube is normally closed except on swallowing, chewing and yawning.

Sound which impinges on the tympanic membrane is transmitted and amplified within the middle ear by the action of the ossicles. These consist of three delicate bones, the malleus (hammer), incus (anvil) and stapes (stirrup). The vibrations created by the action of sound on the tympanic membrane generate an oscillating movement of the tiny bones which subsequently reaches the oval window (fenestra vestibuli). Amplification of sound is produced by the lever-like movement of the ossicles and the concentration of the vibrations at a single focus, the oval window. A second opening to the inner ear is formed by the round window (fenestra cochlea), which lies immediately below the oval window.

The inner ear is the primary centre of hearing and balance. It consists of a fluid-filled membranous labyrinth immersed in a watery fluid, the perilymph, which is itself contained by a bony labyrinth. The inner ear may be divided into the cochlea, the vestibule and the semi-circular canals. The cochlea, a spirally arranged bony tube, consists of three compartments, an upper and lower compartment containing perilymph and a central compartment containing endolymph. Vibrations which reach the oval window set up motions within the perilymph, and are transmitted to fine hairs lining the membrane of the central compartment. The movement of these fine hairs generates a nervous potential which is picked up and transmitted to the brain via the vestibulocochlear nerve (the acoustic eighth cranial nerve).

The vestibule is the central portion of the bony labyrinth, within which the membranous labyrinth is divided into the utricle and the saccule. In conjunction with the three semi-circular canals (arranged at right angles to each other), the vestibule is concerned with maintaining an awareness of orientation of the head and of body position during movements (e.g. rotation).

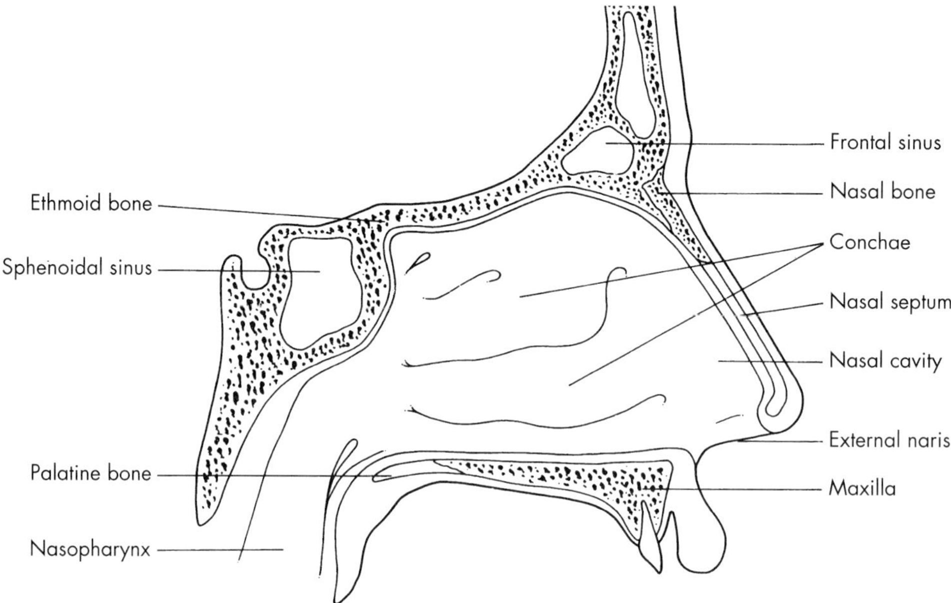

Figure 12.3 Nasal cavity and sinuses.

The nose

The nose is the organ of smell, and the uppermost part of the respiratory tract. The external portion of the nose is formed of bone and cartilage, and contains two openings, the external nares (nostrils). The internal nasal cavity is bordered on its upper surface by the underside of the cranium, and is separated from the oral cavity at its base by the palate (Figure 12.3). The palate is divided into a hard portion at the front of the nasal cavity and a soft portion at the rear. The nasal cavity is divided vertically by a cartilaginous membrane, the nasal septum. The rear of the nasal cavity is marked by two internal nares and the openings of the Eustachian tube from each ear. Pairs of air cavities, which comprise the paranasal sinuses (ethmoidal, frontal, maxillary and sphenoidal sinuses), surround and are linked to the nasal cavity.

The nasal cavity and its internal structures warm and filter the air entering through the nostrils. The internal cavity is divided by bony plates, the conchae, into passages (meatuses), which are lined by hairs contained within a mucous membrane. Olfactory functions are located in cells that lie immediately above the uppermost concha, and are stimulated by the presence of volatile agents in turbulent currents generated by inspired air.

The oropharynx

A detailed description of the structures of the upper respiratory tree may be found in Section 3.4. Only those structures within the oropharynx that have not been previously described will be discussed here.

The oral cavity (Figure 12.4) consists of the cheeks, the hard and soft palates (*see above*), and the tongue. The sides of the mouth are marked by cheeks, which are muscular structures lined internally with squamous epithelium. Movement of the cheeks assists in the mastication of food and in keeping the bolus between the teeth.

The tongue is a highly flexible organ formed of skeletal muscle and covered with a mucous membrane. It plays a fundamental role in the sensation of taste, and assists in mastication, swallowing and the articulation of sounds. The upper surface of the tongue is rough due to the presence of papillae. There are approximately 2000 taste buds found in certain papillae. Additional taste buds are located on the soft palate and in the throat. Particular sensations of taste are highly localised on the surface of the tongue, and may be broadly classified as sour, sweet, salt and bitter.

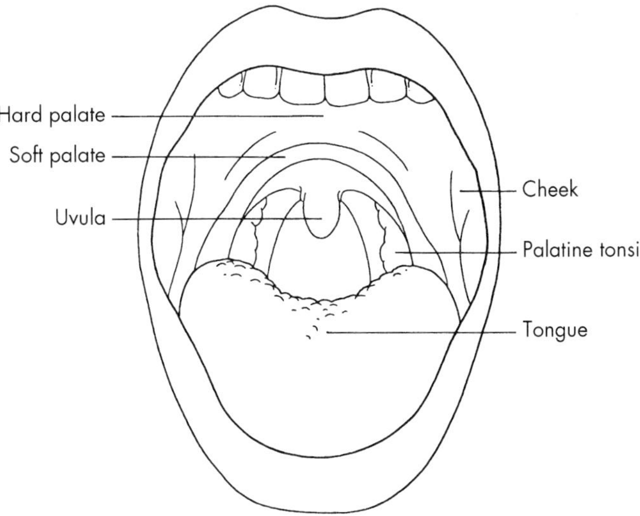

Figure 12.4 The oral cavity.

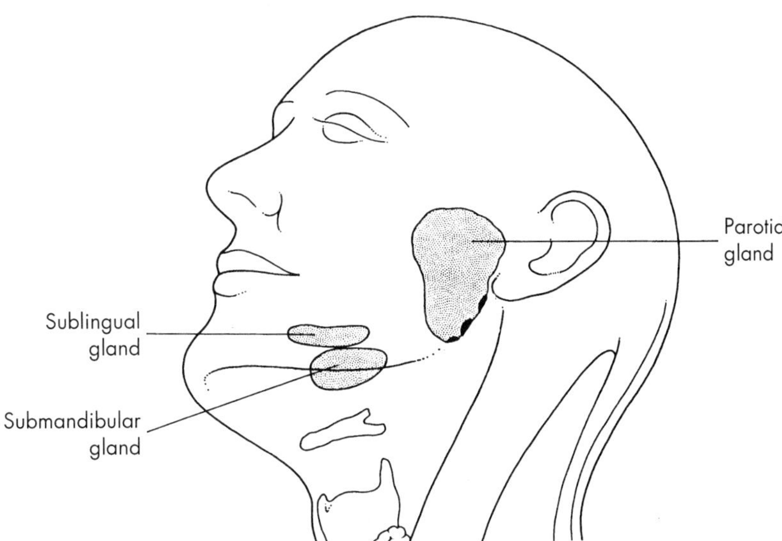

Figure 12.5 Position of the salivary glands.

Three pairs of salivary glands (Figure 12.5) continuously secrete saliva into the oral cavity to keep the mucous membranes moist. The amount secreted increases considerably when food enters the mouth or in anticipation of food. The largest of the salivary glands, the parotid gland, is located immediately in front of each ear. The other two glands are situated below the floor of the oral cavity. The submandibular gland is found near the base of the tongue and immediately behind the sublingual gland, the smallest of the three pairs. The glands secrete fluids of varying composition to constitute saliva which enters the mouth near its roof (parotid duct) and on its floor (submandibular ducts).

13

Skin disorders

13.1 Disorders of the skin

(The diagrammatic representation of a range of common skin lesions is shown in Figure 13.1.)

Acne vulgaris

Definition and aetiology

Acne vulgaris (common acne) is an inflammatory condition of the hair follicle and sebaceous gland (i.e. of the pilosebaceous unit). It commonly occurs at puberty and generally resolves by 30 years of age. It may be caused by increased plasma androgen concentrations or by increased sensitivity of the sebaceous glands to androgens. This results in excessive sebum production and hyperkeratosis. The hair follicles subsequently become blocked with keratin and inflamed, and the sebaceous glands may become infected, often by *Propionibacterium acnes*. Acne may also be precipitated by the administration of drugs (e.g. corticosteroids, oral contraceptives or antiepileptic drugs) or by the use of oily cosmetics. Other contributory factors include emotional disturbance and menstruation. Diet or sexual activity are not thought to play any part in the development of acne.

Symptoms

Acne is characterised by the formation of comedones which may be open (blackheads) or closed (whiteheads). They are usually distributed over the face, neck, chest, shoulders and back. In more severe cases, inflamed papules and cysts may develop. Conglobate and cystic acne are characterised by the formation of inflamed purulent cysts deep in the tissues. Scarring may occur subsequent to healing, particularly after the more severe forms.

Treatment

Patients should be encouraged to wash regularly with water and detergent solutions and avoid picking or squeezing lesions. The value of reassurance and psychological support should not be underestimated. Treatment (BNF 13.6) comprises the topical administration of antiseptic and keratolytic preparations. The prolonged administration of an appropriate antibacterial drug (BNF 5.1, table 1) may be beneficial, particularly in more severe cases. An anti-androgen may be suitable for the treatment of women suffering intractable symptoms. In the presence of severe cystic or conglobate acne, the systemic administration of isotretinoin may be considered, but only under expert supervision. Plastic surgery may be indicated in patients who suffer severe scarring. Ultraviolet radiation can give positive improvement.

Self-help organisation

Acne Support Group

Albinism

Definition and aetiology

Albinism is an autosomal recessive genetic disorder in which there is an absence or malfunction of tyrosinase, an enzyme involved in melanin production. The severity of the condition, which may occur in all races, varies according to the extent of the enzymatic loss.

Symptoms

Albinism is characterised by lack of pigment in the skin, hair and eyes. It may be accompanied by astigmatism, nystagmus, strabismus and photophobia. There is a tendency to sunburn easily and to develop malignant skin disease.

Treatment

There is no treatment available to correct the deficiency. Patients should be encouraged to wear tinted glasses, avoid exposure to sunlight when possible, and apply sunscreening preparations (BNF 13.8.1) to exposed parts regularly. Routine skin examination should be performed to allow early detection of malignant disease.

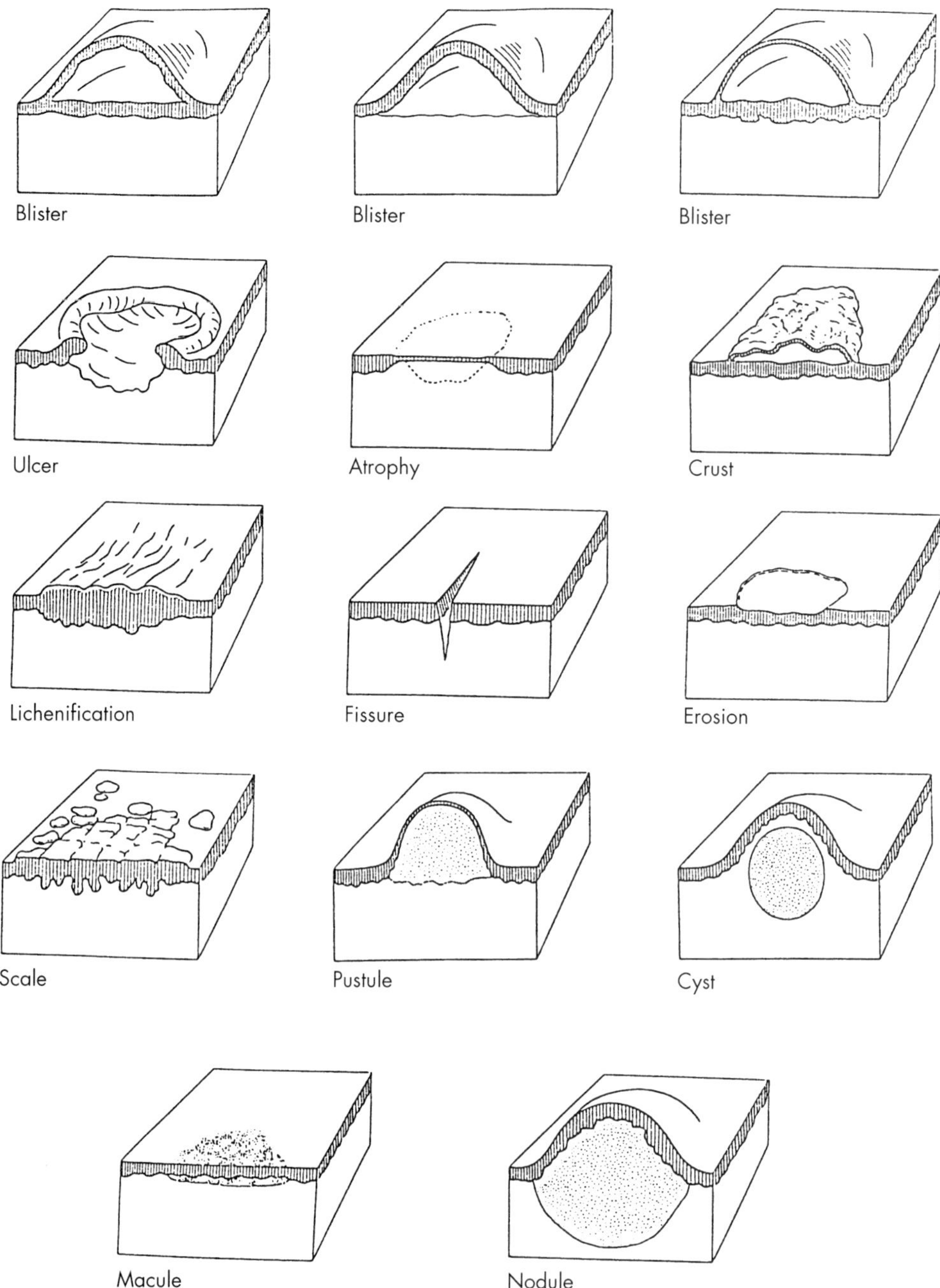

Figure 13.1 Diagrammatic representation of common skin lesions.

Alopecia

Definition and aetiology

Alopecia (Figure 13.2) is the absence or loss of hair, and may be partial or complete. Causes are varied and include physical damage (e.g. excessive traction employed in some hairdressing techniques, vigorous use of stiff hairbrushes and trichotillomania). Toxic alopecia is very often temporary and may be precipitated by chemical

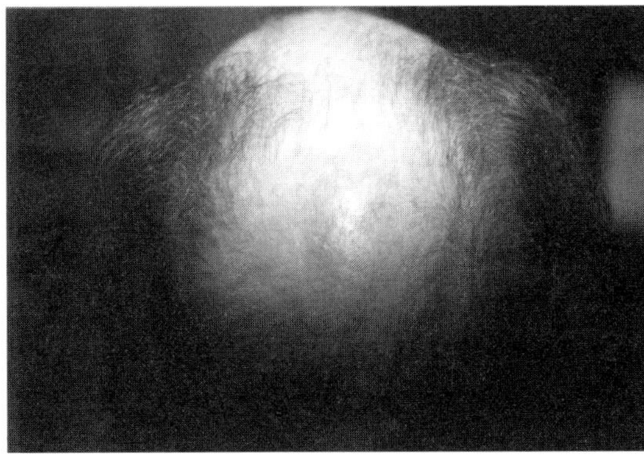

Figure 13.2 Alopecia. (Reproduced with permission from *Pharmaceutical Journal*.)

hair preparations, systemic disease (e.g. myxoedema, severe febrile illness or early syphilis) and drugs (e.g. propranolol, carbimazole, cytotoxic agents, anticoagulants or excessive doses of vitamin A). Injuries to the scalp or diseases resulting in inflammation and tissue damage (e.g. tinea capitis) may lead to permanent alopecia. Alopecia areata is a sudden, and often reversible, patchy hair loss with no apparent cause. Male-pattern alopecia (androgenetic alopecia) occurs as a result of genetically predisposed hair follicles in the scalp responding to stimulation by circulating androgens.

Symptoms

The hair loss due to physical or chemical trauma is generally confined to the areas of damage. Alopecia areata may involve any hairy part of the body and re-growth is characterised by hairs resembling exclamation marks. Male-pattern alopecia usually starts as recession of the hairline in the lateral frontal regions and may be associated with hair loss on the crown. These two areas may, in time, become confluent. The long, coarse pigmented terminal hairs are progressively replaced by short fine colourless vellus hairs. The hair follicles themselves gradually shrink, resulting in a decrease, and eventual cessation, in hair production.

Treatment

Treatment comprises the removal of the cause where appropriate. Systemic or topical corticosteroids may be beneficial in treating some cases of alopecia areata. Minoxidil lotion (BNF 13.9) may be applied to reverse male-pattern alopecia, but treatment must be maintained indefinitely.

Self-help organisation

Hairline International

Angioedema

Definition and aetiology

Angioedema (which should be distinguished from hereditary angioedema, *see below*) is a form of urticaria characterised by large oedematous lesions, involving the dermis and subcutaneous tissues. The causes are as for urticaria.

Symptoms

The sites most commonly affected are the lips, eyelids and genitalia. Other sites include the tongue, and the dorsal surfaces of the hands and feet. The onset is often sudden, marked by single or multiple lesions lasting for 1–2 hours, although occasionally persisting for up to three days. Oedema occurring in the upper respiratory tract may result in potentially fatal respiratory distress.

Treatment

The treatment of angioedema is as for urticaria. Injections of adrenaline (BNF 3.1.1.2), corticosteroids (BNF 6.3.2), antihistamines (BNF 3.4.1) and tracheal intubation may be indicated in severe cases.

Callosities and corns

Definition and aetiology

A callosity (callus) is a hard, circumscribed, thickened area of hyperkeratosis. It is produced by repeated friction or pressure, usually over a bony prominence. It may be caused by a variety of factors (e.g. badly fitting shoes or occupational activities).

A corn is a small, circumscribed area of hyperkeratosis with a central core, always found on the feet. It is produced by repeated pressure or friction over a bony prominence, usually due to badly fitting shoes. Hard corns are usually found on the upper surfaces of toes, while those found between the toes are termed soft corns.

Symptoms

Callosities are commonly found on the toes and soles of feet, and the fingers and palms of hands. They are generally of uniform thickness and colour, with a rough surface, and may cause discomfort, especially on application of pressure. The point of the corn lies in the dermis, and causes pain by pressure on the nerve endings.

Treatment

Treatment of both callosities and corns comprises relieving the pressure where possible using self-adhesive pads. The application of keratolytics (BNF 13.7) may be beneficial in aiding removal of the hard skin. Careful paring of the hard skin with a file or pumice stone (dermabrasion) may also be helpful.

Decubitus ulcer

Definition and aetiology

A decubitus ulcer (bedsore or pressure sore, Figure 13.3) is an area of ulceration caused by ischaemia and subsequent necrosis of tissues exposed to prolonged pressure. It is commonly seen in patients immobilised for a variety of reasons, especially the bedridden and elderly. Other precipitating factors include friction (e.g. due to wrinkled bedding or rough clothing), skin maceration (e.g. due to perspiration, and urine and faecal matter in the incontinent), and dulled or absent perception of sensation. Anaemia, malnutrition, secondary infection, decreased peripheral circulation and any existing cachectic state may accelerate the process.

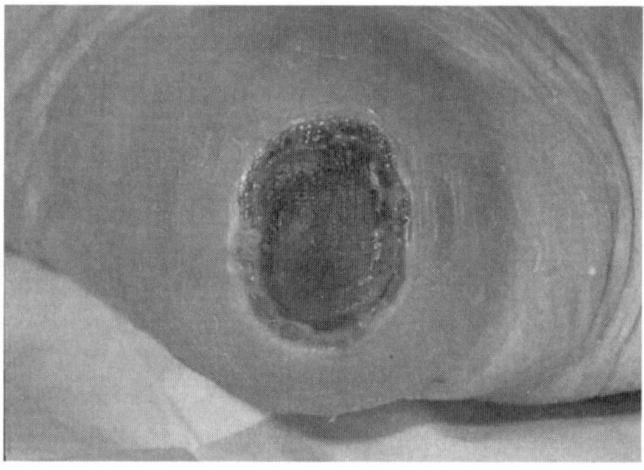

Figure 13.3 Pressure sore of a heel. (Reproduced with permission of Dr P Marazzi/Science Photo Library.)

Symptoms

The initial stages of formation of a bedsore are characterised by erythema, oedema and blister formation. Necrosis follows and may extend through the fatty tissues to muscles and even bone in severe cases.

Treatment

Bedsore formation may be arrested in the early stages by the adoption of preventive measures. These include frequently changing the patient's position, relieving pressure on sensitive areas, regularly inspecting the skin to note any changes, efficient skin cleansing and drying regimes, and encouraging the patient in active movement when possible. Any underlying disorder should be treated and a regular high-protein diet maintained. The treatment of advanced stages consists of debridement using skin disinfecting and cleansing agents or desloughing agents and enzyme preparations (BNF 13.11). Dextranomer beads and gel and colloid dressings (BNF appendix 8) may be beneficial. In severe cases, surgical excision of necrotic tissue and wound closure may be necessary.

Eczema

Definition and aetiology

Eczema (dermatitis) is an inflammatory condition of the skin. It is caused by endogenous factors (e.g. atopic dermatitis) or exogenous factors (e.g. external irritants) as in contact dermatitis and napkin rash.

Symptoms

The acute stage of eczema is characterised by the appearance of vesicles on the skin, formed by the spread of oedema from the dermis into the epidermis. The vesicles may rupture, releasing a clear exudate which dries and forms crusts. Pruritus is a major feature of the condition and is usually accompanied by inflammation and tenderness. During the latter stages, the oedema subsides and the epidermis dries and thickens. Scales may be produced by a fast turnover of cells. Scratching and rubbing of the skin may contribute to the secondary stages and may also cause infection.

Treatment

Any underlying cause should be removed, if possible, and patients should be discouraged from scratching or using topical sensitising agents. Soap substitutes and emollient and barrier preparations (BNF 13.2) may be beneficial for dry lesions. Keratolytics (BNF 13.5) may be required to soften and loosen scales. In some cases, an appropriate topical corticosteroid (BNF 13.4) may be indicated. Wet dressings (BNF appendix 8) and anti-infective skin preparations (BNF 13.10) may be necessary for weeping or infected eczemas. Oral antihistamines (BNF 3.4.1) may be of value in reducing pruritus. Systemic corticosteroids (BNF 6.3.4) may be necessary in severe cases.

Atopic dermatitis

Definition and aetiology

Atopic dermatitis (atopic eczema) is a chronic fluctuating inflammatory condition of the skin. The cause is unknown, although a family history of allergy (e.g. asthma or allergic rhinitis) is common. The age of onset is generally two to six months and it usually resolves spontaneously by 30 years of age. The skin may, however, remain sensitive to physical or chemical irritants.

Symptoms

Atopic dermatitis starts on the face and is characterised by red, weeping, crusted lesions. It spreads to the hands, flexures of the knees, elbows, wrists, ankles and sides of the neck. Pruritus is a major feature and scratching may cause secondary infection. In older children and adults, erythema and lichenification predominate, and the condition is characterised by dry, itching, cracked skin. Contact allergens, emotional disturbances, and changes in temperature or humidity may exacerbate the condition.

Treatment

The treatment of atopic dermatitis is as described under eczema.

Contact dermatitis

Definition and aetiology

Contact dermatitis (contact eczema, Figure 13.4) is an inflammatory skin condition caused by exposure to physical or chemical irritants (i.e. irritant contact dermatitis) or allergens (i.e. allergic contact dermatitis). It may be acute or chronic.

Primary irritants (e.g. acids, alkalis or organic solvents) damage the epidermis, allowing penetration and subsequent inflammation. Atopic dermatitis may predispose an individual to develop irritant dermatitis. Allergens that may cause dermatitis include organic dyes (e.g. hair colorants), topical medicaments (e.g. local anaesthetics and antihistamines), and metal (e.g. nickel fasteners in clothing). Allergic sensitisation may take days, months, or years to develop. Photoallergic and phototoxic contact dermatitis occurs on exposure of the skin to light subsequent to the topical application of sensitising substances (e.g. after-shave lotions and sunscreening agents).

Symptoms

The symptoms of contact dermatitis are as described under eczema. In the acute phase, the

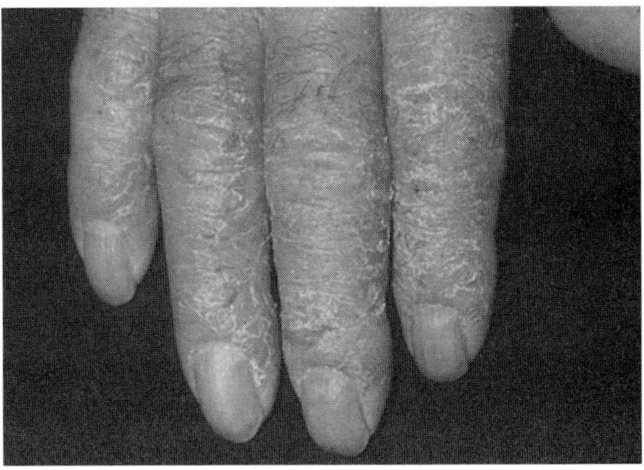

Figure 13.4 Contact dermatitis. (Reproduced with permission of Dr P Marazzi/Science Photo Library.)

site of the lesions caused by primary irritants usually coincides with the point of contact. Chronic cases and allergic reactions may show a more generalised spread.

Treatment

The treatment of contact dermatitis is as described under eczema. The resistance of the skin is lowered for several months after apparently healing, and patients should be encouraged to continue using emollients and barrier creams (BNF 13.2.1) and to avoid sensitising agents.

Exfoliative dermatitis

Definition and aetiology

Exfoliative dermatitis is a severe inflammatory condition of the skin affecting a large proportion of the body surface. The cause is unknown, although it may be precipitated by other skin conditions (e.g. psoriasis and other forms of dermatitis) or drugs (e.g. penicillin, barbiturates or phenytoin).

Symptoms

The onset of exfoliative dermatitis may be sudden, and initial symptoms include widespread erythema, fever, shivering, malaise and sometimes pruritus. Scaling occurs as the condition progresses, and the skin becomes dry and thickened. After some weeks, body and scalp hair, and nails may be shed. Serious metabolic disturbances in chronic cases may be caused by increased blood flow through the skin and the loss of large amounts of exfoliated scale. These include hypothermia, fluid loss, peripheral circulatory failure, hypoproteinaemia and, in susceptible individuals, congestive heart failure. Skin and respiratory-tract infections may occur. The condition may be fatal if not treated promptly.

Treatment

Hospitalisation is usually necessary to monitor protein and electrolyte balance and regulate the environmental temperature. Other measures include the administration of oral corticosteroids (BNF 6.3.2) and the withdrawal of all non-essential medication. Oral antibacterial drugs (BNF 5.1) may be required to treat secondary infection. The application of soothing emollients (BNF 13.2) after bathing may be beneficial.

Napkin rash

Definition and aetiology

Napkin rash (napkin dermatitis, Figure 13.5) is an inflammatory condition of the skin confined to the area in contact with the napkin (i.e. the pubic area, buttocks, genitalia and thighs). Damage to the stratum corneum, resulting from prolonged skin contact with occluded moist napkins, appears to be a precipitating factor. The condition may be further aggravated by ammonia (formed by bacterial degradation of urea), *Candida albicans*, faeces, or residual detergents and antiseptics present in inadequately rinsed napkins.

Symptoms

The onset of napkin rash is rarely seen before the third week of life and resolves spontaneously on discontinuing napkin use. The condition is characterised by erythema in the napkin area, and may be followed by skin peeling. Fine scaling may be apparent in chronic cases. Vesicles and ulcers may be present in severe cases, and dysuria may occur if the genitalia are affected. In some infants, napkin rash can be the first sign of a predisposition to chronic skin disorders (e.g. atopic dermatitis).

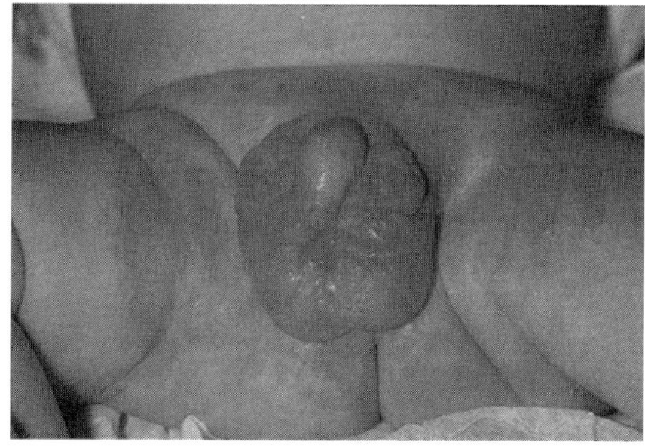

Figure 13.5 Napkin rash. (Reproduced with permission of Dr P Marazzi/Science Photo Library.)

Treatment
Treatment comprises drying the skin surface and reducing the contact time with irritants. Parents should be encouraged to change napkins frequently and be instructed in correct laundering procedures. Exposing the skin to the air for as long as is practical may be beneficial. Mild topical corticosteroids (BNF 13.4) and an appropriate topical antifungal preparation (BNF 13.10.2) may be indicated. Ointment bases should be avoided on a moist skin because of their occlusive action, but may be useful for prophylaxis on unaffected skin. Emollients and barrier creams (BNF 13.2.1) may also help to prevent further outbreaks after healing.

Seborrhoeic dermatitis

Definition and aetiology
Seborrhoeic dermatitis (Figure 13.6) is an inflammatory condition of the skin of unknown cause. It affects areas of the body supplied by sebaceous glands, although the composition and flow of sebum is usually unaltered. Emotional disturbances, fatigue or infection may precipitate the condition in predisposed adults, and a fungal infection has been implicated. It generally occurs between 18 and 40 years of age and is more common in men.

Cradle cap (infantile seborrhoeic dermatitis) is an inflammatory condition of the scalp in infants. It commonly occurs in association with napkin rash, although the cause is unknown. It is often seen in children with a predisposition to develop allergic disorders. The onset of cradle cap occurs during the first three months of life and generally resolves spontaneously within a year.

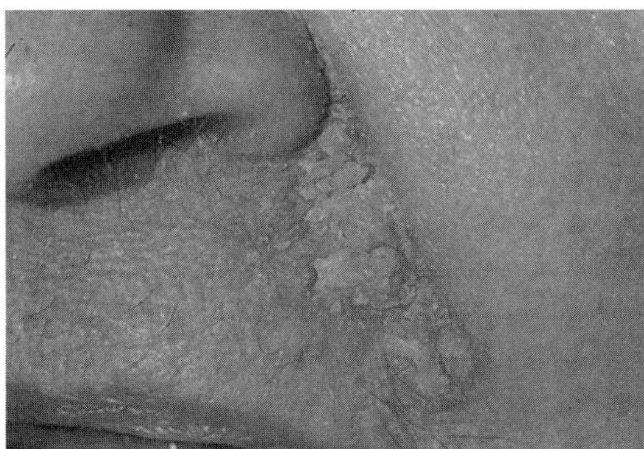

Figure 13.6 Seborrhoeic dermatitis. (Reproduced with permission of Dr P Marazzi/Science Photo Library.)

Symptoms
Seborrhoeic dermatitis is characterised by dry or greasy scales, mild erythema and pruritus. Affected sites include the scalp, hair line, eyebrows, bridge of nose, sternum, external ear canal and the area behind the ears. In severe cases, yellowish-red papules may be present. The distribution may extend to the axillae and inguinal and anal regions, and blepharitis may occur. In some cases, there is an increased susceptibility to infection.

Cradle cap is marked by thick yellow scales on the scalp, extending in some cases to the eyebrows and behind the ears. Other symptoms may include erythema. Small red papules may appear on the face, neck and occasionally the trunk. Secondary infection may occur in severe cases.

Treatment
Treatment consists of medicated shampoos, topical corticosteroid preparations (BNF 13.4), and appropriate anti-infective skin preparations (BNF 13.10) for infected lesions. Keratolytics (BNF 13.5) may be indicated in severe cases.

In cradle cap, the application of olive oil or arachis oil (BNF 13.9) may be useful to loosen scales prior to cleansing with a mild shampoo. The use of potentially sensitising medicated shampoos should be avoided. Mild topical corticosteroids (BNF 13.4) may be indicated in severe cases.

Self-help organisation
National Eczema Society

Erythema multiforme

Definition and aetiology
Erythema multiforme is an acute hypersensitivity reaction occurring in the skin and mucous membranes. It may be precipitated by drugs (e.g. barbiturates, penicillin or sulphonamides), vaccines (e.g. BCG) or viral infections (e.g. herpes simplex

and ionising radiation). In many cases, the cause is unknown.

Symptoms
The onset is generally sudden and marked by erythematous lesions, often with a purple centre. They are symmetrically distributed over the extremities and, less often, the trunk and face. The lesions may be macules or slightly raised papules, gradually fading in one to two weeks. Vesicles may occur in similar sites and on the mucous membranes. The condition is often recurrent. The Stevens–Johnson syndrome is a very severe form characterised by bulla formation involving the eyes, genitalia, oral mucosa and skin. Accompanying symptoms may include arthralgia, fever and malaise. If left untreated, it may prove fatal.

Treatment
The causative agent should be identified and avoided where possible. Milder forms resolve spontaneously and may only need symptomatic treatment such as antipruritic preparations (BNF 13.3). Oral corticosteroids (BNF 6.3.4) may be indicated in severe cases, and antibacterial drugs (BNF 5.1) may be necessary to treat or prevent secondary infection.

Erythema nodosum

Definition and aetiology
Erythema nodosum is an acute inflammatory skin reaction characterised by erythematous nodules. It is most commonly caused by underlying streptococcal infections or sarcoidosis. Other causes include mycotic and viral infections, tuberculosis, leprosy, psittacosis and ulcerative colitis. Some drugs (e.g. sulphonamides, iodides and oral contraceptives) may also precipitate this condition. The incidence of erythema nodosum is greater in females and is most frequently seen between 20 and 45 years of age.

Symptoms
The onset of erythema nodosum is often sudden and is characterised by red, painful, tender nodules appearing on the lower legs. Occasionally, the thighs, arms or face may be affected. Characteristic nodular colour changes occur, from bluish-purple to yellowish-green, finally resembling a bruise. It is generally accompanied by arthralgia, fever and malaise. Spontaneous resolution usually occurs in about three to six weeks. The condition may be recurrent on subsequent challenge by an offending agent or infection.

Treatment
Treatment of the underlying disorder and bed rest may be all that is required. In some cases, administration of aspirin or other non-steroidal anti-inflammatory drugs (BNF 10.1.1) may also be helpful. Ambulant patients should be encouraged to wear support bandages or stockings.

Folliculitis

Definition and aetiology
Folliculitis is a superficial inflammation of the upper part of the hair follicle, often caused by infection with *Staphylococcus aureus*. Folliculitis of a non-infective origin may arise as a result of chemical or physical trauma (e.g. contact with mineral oils, tar products or adhesive dressings). Re-penetration of the skin by sharp shaved hairs results in the inflammatory condition pseudofolliculitis.

Symptoms
Folliculitis commonly occurs on the face and is marked by small papules or pustules at the point of emergence of the hairs. The condition may become chronic (*see* Sycosis barbae).

Treatment
Suspected irritants should be avoided where possible. The use of a suitable skin disinfecting and cleansing agent (BNF 13.11) may be of value and the application of an appropriate anti-infective skin preparation (BNF 13.10) may be necessary in severe cases. In many instances, however, no treatment is required. Pseudofolliculitis may be prevented by altering shaving technique to leave hairs a little longer, or by not shaving at all.

Haemangiomas

Definition and aetiology
Haemangiomas are benign, vascular tumours arising as a result of hyperplasia of blood vessels.

Most are congenital or develop shortly after birth, and may be due to part of the angioderm remaining isolated as the vascular system develops. They may be superficial, subcutaneous or a combination of the two. Superficial haemangiomas are more likely to be of the capillary type in which localised hyperplasia of the angioderm has taken place. Subcutaneous lesions are generally of the cavernous type which consist of irregular vascular spaces.

Strawberry naevus

Definition and aetiology
A strawberry naevus is a superficial capillary haemangioma, which may develop subcutaneous components as it enlarges. It is usually not present at birth, but develops shortly afterwards.

Symptoms
Growth commences shortly after birth and progresses rapidly for a few weeks. The lesion then continues to enlarge slowly, generally reaching maximum size within six months. It appears as a soft, scarlet, well-defined swelling with a lobulated surface of variable size. Any part of the body may be affected, but it occurs most frequently on the head and neck. Other sites include the trunk and anogenital region. The lesion may ulcerate, especially if near the mouth or in the nappy area. Bleeding may also occur although this is not usually serious. Lesions close to the eye may result in visual impairment. Spontaneous and complete regression occurs in most cases after two to five years, although some individuals may be left with a brown pigmentation, telangiectases, wrinkling or scarring in the affected area.

Treatment
Reassurance is all that is required for most patients. Treatment is necessary only if there are complications or a poor cosmetic appearance is predicted subsequent to regression (i.e. ulcerative lesions or those with a deep subcutaneous component). Intralesional injections of corticosteroids or oral corticosteroids may facilitate shrinkage. Local injections of sclerosants may be necessary in those cases where regression is incomplete, or surgical excision may be required to remove any excess skin folds remaining.

Cavernous haemangioma

Definition and aetiology
A cavernous haemangioma is subcutaneous but may be overlaid in some cases by a strawberry naevus.

Symptoms
It may be seen as a soft, bluish, ill-defined swelling beneath the skin, generally present at birth. It may occur at any site and regresses less readily than superficial haemangiomas.

Treatment
Treatment is as for a strawberry naevus, although it may be less successful.

Port wine stain

Definition and aetiology
This is a capillary haemangioma present in most cases at birth.

Symptoms
It occurs as a pink, red or purple lesion of variable size, generally unilateral and appearing most commonly on the head. It is initially flat, but may gradually become raised and of a deeper colour. Most cases persist for life.

Treatment
Camouflaging preparations (BNF 13.8.2 and appendix 7) may be of value in cases where the cosmetic appearance causes the patient psychological distress. Laser therapy has been used with success in some cases.

Hereditary angioedema

Definition and aetiology
Hereditary angioedema (which should be distinguished from angioedema, *see above*) is the result of an autosomally dominant inherited deficiency or, in some cases, malfunction of C1 esterase inhibitor. The result is the continuous activation of C1, the first component of complement. Attacks may be precipitated by emotional disturbances, viral infection or trauma.

Symptoms

The condition is characterised by recurrent, hardened, painful swellings of the skin and mucous membranes. If the gastrointestinal tract is affected, accompanying symptoms may include nausea and vomiting, colic, and occasionally obstruction. Common symptoms of urticaria are not present. Obstruction in the upper respiratory tract causes the death of about 20% of all cases before middle age.

Treatment

Hereditary angioedema does not readily respond to the treatment used for urticaria. Fresh frozen plasma administered in the early stages of a severe attack may be beneficial in temporarily replacing the deficient enzyme inhibitor. Tranexamic acid (BNF 2.11) and danazol (BNF 6.7.2) are of value in long-term management, and stanozolol (BNF 6.4.3) may be used for preventing attacks.

Hyperhidrosis

Definition and aetiology

Hyperhidrosis is characterised by overactivity of the sweat glands, resulting in excessive perspiration. It may be precipitated by an underlying systemic disorder (e.g. febrile illness, hyperthyroidism, an infection, malignant disease or the menopause). Other causes include alcoholic intoxication, lesions in the sympathetic nervous system, obesity and psychogenic factors.

Symptoms

Hyperhidrosis may be generalised or localised, common sites being the axillae, palms and soles. The skin often appears pink and in severe cases may become macerated, fissured or scaly. Decomposition of the sweat by bacteria and yeasts may result in an unpleasant odour (bromhidrosis).

Treatment

Any underlying systemic disorder should be treated, where possible. Sweat production in the feet may be reduced by soaking them in solutions of formaldehyde or glutaraldehyde. The local application of aluminium chloride salts (BNF 13.12) to the axillae may be beneficial. In severe cases, sympathectomy or excision of portions of axillary skin may be necessary.

Ichthyosis

Definition and aetiology

Ichthyosis is a generalised non-inflammatory skin disorder, characterised by abnormal scalings. This may be caused by overproduction of keratin or abnormalities in desquamation. It is inherited (e.g. ichthyosis vulgaris) or acquired following systemic diseases (e.g. carcinoma, Hodgkin's disease, hypothyroidism and leprosy).

Symptoms

Ichthyosis is characterised by a rough and scaly skin surface which affects all parts of the body, although it is usually most severe on the lower legs. There is often reduced secretion from the sebaceous and sweat glands, which exacerbates the condition. The symptoms may worsen during the winter months.

Treatment

Treatment is palliative and consists of the topical administration of emollients (BNF 13.2.1). Patients should be discouraged from excessive bathing and use of degreasing agents (e.g. soap). Removal of scale in severe cases may be assisted by the use of keratolytics (BNF 13.5). Etretinate may be indicated in severe cases under hospital supervision.

Keloid

Definition and aetiology

A keloid is a raised nodule formed in the skin as a result of excessive amounts of collagen laid down during repair of connective tissue (e.g. after trauma). It may also arise spontaneously. The cause is unknown, although precipitating factors include burns, infections, surgical incisions, tension on a wound and the presence of foreign bodies (e.g. surgical sutures). Keloid formation is rare in infancy and the elderly, occurring most commonly between puberty and 30 years of age. There is a genetic tendency and keloids occur more frequently in black people and in women; pregnancy appears to increase the incidence.

Symptoms

Commonest sites of keloids include the chest, ear lobes, neck and shoulders. A keloid is generally shiny, smooth, firm, and pink or red.

Treatment

Local corticosteroid injections (BNF 10.1.2.2), radiotherapy and compression therapy may each be of value alone, or as an adjuvant to surgical excision, to prevent reformation. Keloid formation may be prevented by avoiding all non-essential surgery in predisposed individuals. Where surgery is necessary, measures should be taken to prevent secondary infection and reduce the tension on wounds.

Lichen planus

Definition and aetiology

Lichen planus is an inflammatory skin disorder characterised by collections of papules (lichen) which are small, shiny and violet-coloured with angular borders. It appears to be idiopathic, although it may be associated with an altered state of immunity. It often occurs in conjunction with myasthenia gravis, thymoma, ulcerative colitis and vitiligo. Drugs (e.g. antimalarials or gold) and chemicals (e.g. dyes used as developers in colour photography) may cause similar lichenoid eruptions. The onset of lichen planus is often insidious and generally occurs between 30 and 60 years of age, affecting more women than men. It is usually self-limiting and will regress spontaneously within 6–18 months, although it may recur.

Symptoms

The condition may be acute or chronic, the acute form showing a sudden onset, a more generalised distribution of lesions over the whole body, and a shorter course. The characteristic lesions are often distributed symmetrically and may occur at any site. They appear most commonly on the wrists, ankles and trunk. They may be separate or confluent, linear or annular, and may exhibit white lines (Wickham's striae) on the surface of the papule. The area may show increased pigmentation subsequent to healing. Hypertrophic lesions may form, usually on the lower legs, if the papules increase in size and thickness, and these may result in atrophy and scarring. Papules are rarely seen on the scalp, but an associated complication for some patients is permanent patchy hair loss. Pruritus of varying degree occurs in most cases of lichen planus. Some patients have bluish-white linear lesions on mucosal surfaces, especially the mouth, but also arising in the anogenital region, the larynx and nails. Oral lesions may become eroded and painful.

Treatment

Treatment is symptomatic and may include the application of topical fluorinated corticosteroid preparations (BNF 13.4) and oral antihistamines (BNF 3.4.1) to relieve pruritus. Corticosteroids in lozenges or in dental paste (BNF 12.3.1) may be indicated in cases of erosive oral lesions. Systemic corticosteroids (BNF 6.3.2) may be necessary in severe cases.

Mole

Definition and aetiology

A mole (melanocytic naevus or naevocytic naevus) is a benign pigmented circumscribed growth of the skin. It is idiopathic and formed by proliferation of melanocytes at the junction between the dermis and epidermis. Moles are common and occur in all races. Their development is greatest in children and adolescents, decreasing with advancing age.

Symptoms

There are several different forms which are classified histologically. Most are small (<15 mm diameter) and vary in colour from flesh-tinted to yellow or light brown through to dark brownish-black. They may be flat, raised or pedunculated, and with a smooth or rough surface. They can arise at any site on the body and may be hairy. Occasionally, melanomas may arise from the melanocytes in a mole.

Treatment

Excision and biopsy may be necessary in cases where a mole has shown a sudden increase in size, changed in colour, become inflamed, painful or pruritic, or started to bleed or ulcerate. In most cases, however, treatment is unnecessary and the patient should be reassured that moles are generally quite harmless.

Pemphigus

Definition and aetiology

Pemphigus (Figure 13.7) is a group of skin diseases characterised by severe and chronic blistering. It is thought to be due to an autoimmune reaction. It is often associated with myasthenia gravis and thymoma, and may be precipitated by drugs (e.g. captopril, penicillamine or rifampicin). Pemphigus tends to occur in middle or old age and is rarely seen in children. The incidence is greater in specific populations (e.g. the Brazilian, Indian and Jewish races).

Symptoms

The initial stage is characterised by bullae on the oral mucosa, formed as a result of the destruction of intercellular bonds between epidermal cells (acantholysis). The lesions are painful and slow to heal. Other mucous membranes may be affected, including the conjunctiva, upper oesophagus and vulva. Similar eruptions occur on the skin several months later, and commonly affect the face, trunk, groin and axillae. Secondary skin infection and septicaemia may be further complications. The condition may be fatal if left untreated.

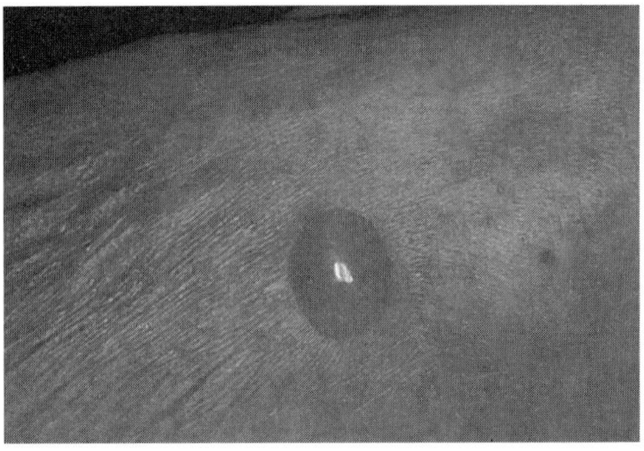

Figure 13.7 Tense blister of pemphigoid. (Reproduced with permission of Mike Wyndham.)

Treatment

Treatment consists of the oral administration of very high doses of corticosteroids (BNF 6.3.2). Immunosuppressants (BNF 8.2) may be indicated in cases where a reduced corticosteroid dose is necessary. An appropriate antibacterial drug (BNF 5.1) may be necessary to treat secondary infection.

Photosensitivity

Definition and aetiology

Photosensitivity is an abnormal reaction of the skin to ultraviolet radiation. Sunburn is caused by excessive exposure to UVB light (wavelength 290–320 nm). It should be distinguished from phototoxicity, which can develop from exposure to normal amounts of sunlight in sensitive or sensitised individuals. Precipitating factors of photosensitivity caused by phototoxicity include contact with perfumes, plants and preparations containing coal tar, or ingestion of drugs (e.g. griseofulvin, nalidixic acid, sulphonamides, tetracyclines or thiazides). It may be caused or aggravated by disease (e.g. porphyria or systemic lupus erythematosus).

Symptoms

Symptoms are of varying intensity and include erythema, oedema, urticaria, eruptions of vesicles or bullae and, in chronic cases, thickened scales. Herpes labialis often results from exposure of the latent herpes simplex virus to strong sunlight.

Treatment

Treatment of any underlying disorder or the removal of precipitating substances will be effective in many cases. Where this is not possible, preventive measures include avoiding exposure to sunlight or covering exposed areas. The application of sunscreening preparations (BNF 13.8.1) may be of value, particularly the reflectant barrier-type such as titanium dioxide paste. Topical corticosteroids (BNF 13.4) may be beneficial in treating severe reactions.

Pilonidal disease

Definition and aetiology
Pilonidal disease is characterised by the formation of a cyst or sinus in the midline of the sacrococcygeal area. This condition occurs most commonly in young hirsute males.

Symptoms
The lesion may be pigmented and contain hair, and is asymptomatic unless infected, in which case abscesses may form.

Treatment
Acute abscesses may be treated by incision and drainage. Chronic sinuses must be completely removed by surgical excision followed by closure.

Pityriasis

Definition
Pityriasis is a term applied to disorders of the skin in which fine, branny scales are formed.

Pityriasis alba

Definition and aetiology
Pityriasis alba is a common non-specific eczema of unknown cause, although impetigo, exposure to sunlight and soap have been suggested as aggravating factors.

Symptoms
The condition generally occurs in children and adolescents. It most commonly affects the face, particularly the cheeks and chin, but other sites include the neck, shoulders and upper arms. The lesions are well-defined, round or oval; they may be skin-coloured (and barely visible) or erythematous. They may become depigmented with persistent fine scaling. It may last for a year or more and is often recurrent, although it usually clears completely by puberty.

Treatment
There is little effective treatment. Application of emollient creams (BNF 13.2.1) may facilitate removal of scales and prevent dryness.

Pityriasis capitis

Definition and aetiology
Pityriasis capitis (dandruff) is a chronic non-inflammatory condition of the scalp characterised by the excessive production of scales. The cause is unknown, although it may arise as a result of increased sebaceous activity and hormonal changes occurring at puberty. The incidence of dandruff peaks between 10 and 20 years of age and is rarely seen in children.

Symptoms
The condition is marked by greyish-white scales which may be dry or greasy. They can occur in small patches or involve the entire scalp.

Treatment
The frequent use of mild shampoos may be beneficial in removing scales. Shampoos containing cytostatic agents (BNF 13.9) may help to slow down the rate of production of epidermal cells. Keratolytic agents (BNF 13.6) may be useful, and topical corticosteroids (BNF 13.4) may be indicated in severe cases.

Pityriasis lichenoides

Definition and aetiology
Pityriasis lichenoides resembles psoriasis in some of its features, and occurs mainly in adolescents and young adults. The cause is unknown.

Symptoms
The chronic form is characterised by small reddish-brown papules, each with an adherent but detachable scale, distributed over the trunk and limbs. Individual lesions generally disappear in three to four weeks, but new crops continually form and the condition may persist for years before completely resolving. An acute form exists and has a shorter course, often resolving within six months. It may be preceded or accompanied by mild symptoms of fever, headache, and malaise. The lesions are oedematous and may become haemorrhagic, resulting in scarring on healing. Transient depigmented areas may be a consequence of both acute and chronic forms.

Treatment

There is little effective treatment, although psoralens and ultraviolet A (PUVA) (BNF 13.5) has been beneficial in some cases.

Pityriasis rosea

Definition and aetiology

Pityriasis rosea (Figure 13.8) is an acute, self-limiting, common skin disorder, possibly of viral origin. It occurs mainly between 10 and 30 years of age, and is less common during the summer months.

Symptoms

It is characterised by a single, red, scaly, round or oval macule (the herald patch) appearing on the trunk or upper limbs. Smaller red papules and pink oval macules covered with silvery grey scales appear a few days later. The macules lose their pink colour, wrinkle in the centre, and peel outwards to form a collarette of scale around the margins. Pruritus may be present, but constitutional symptoms are usually absent and the condition generally resolves in six to eight weeks without further recurrence.

Treatment

Most cases require no treatment. Soap, water and wool may irritate the lesions and contact should be minimised. Application of calamine cream or lotion (BNF 13.3) or topical corticosteroid preparations (BNF 13.4) may be beneficial in relieving irritation.

Figure 13.8 Close-up of skin lesion of pityriasis rosea showing centripetal scaling. (Reproduced with permission of Mike Wyndham.)

Pruritus

Definition and aetiology

Pruritus (itching) is a cutaneous sensation from which relief is sought by scratching or rubbing the skin. Localised pruritus may arise as a result of an allergic reaction or may be caused by eczema, insect bites or infections (e.g. intestinal worms, which cause pruritus ani). Factors contributing to generalised pruritus include dry skin, atopic and contact dermatitis, lichen planus, urticaria and psoriasis. Systemic disorders (e.g. diabetes mellitus), hepatic, renal or malignant disease, and polycythaemia may also be responsible. Many drugs (e.g. antidepressants, barbiturates, chloroquine and opioid analgesics) produce pruritus. Emotional disturbances may precipitate or exacerbate the condition. In some individuals, essential pruritus occurs without any apparent cause.

Symptoms

The symptoms are due to self-inflicted skin damage and include varying degrees of erythema, urticarial eruptions, excoriation, fissures and crusting. Lichenification and changes in pigmentation may occur after prolonged scratching and rubbing.

Treatment

The cause should be identified and avoided where possible, and any underlying disorder treated. Patients should be encouraged to avoid dry atmospheres, the intake of vasodilators (e.g. alcohol), wearing rough or irritating clothing, and becoming overheated. Oral antihistamines (BNF 3.4.1) may be beneficial, especially the sedative type if pruritus at night is a problem. Local applications containing calamine or crotamiton (BNF 13.3), and emollients (BNF 13.2.1) may also be of value. Local corticosteroid preparations (BNF 13.4) may provide relief in some cases, but should not be used indiscriminately.

Psoriasis

Definition and aetiology

Psoriasis (Figure 13.9) is a common chronic recurrent skin disorder of unknown cause. There is a genetic predisposition to develop the condition, although individual attacks may be precipitated

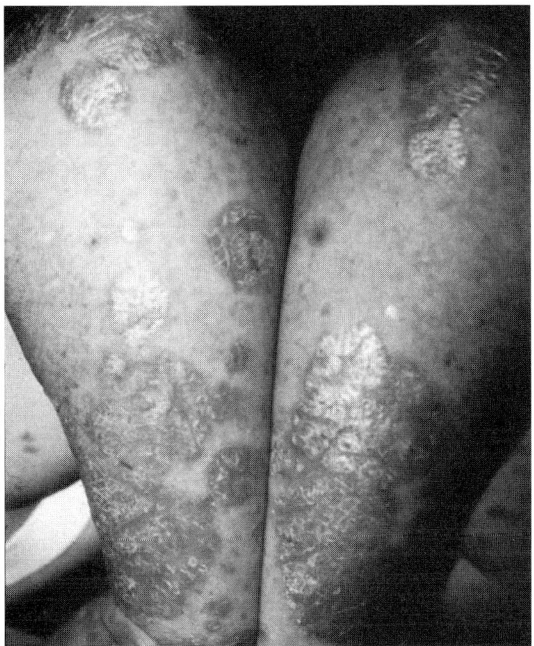

Figure 13.9 Psoriasis. (Reproduced with permission from *Pharmaceutical Journal*.)

by a variety of factors. These include emotional disturbances, hormonal changes, strong sunlight, streptococcal infection of the throat, local trauma, topical irritants and drugs (e.g. chloroquine or lithium). A resistant form of psoriasis often develops following withdrawal of systemic corticosteroids.

Symptoms

The onset is gradual and usually occurs in young adults. An increase in the rate of proliferation of epidermal cells results in well-defined, slightly raised, dry, vivid-red lesions covered with silvery scales. Common sites include the scalp, elbows, knees and lower back, and less commonly the axillae, anogenital region, eyebrows and nails. There may be remissions and relapses throughout life. It rarely affects the patient's general health, although psoriatic arthritis and generalised exfoliation are serious complications which may occasionally arise.

Treatment

In many cases, the removal of any precipitating factors, reassurance and simple remedies such as emollients (BNF 13.2.1) are all that is required. Topical preparations containing keratolytics (BNF 13.5) to facilitate scale removal may be of value. Psoralens and ultraviolet A (PUVA) (BNF 13.5) in controlled doses may be beneficial in severe cases. Antimetabolites (BNF 8.1.3) and etretinate (BNF 13.5.2) may be used under expert supervision to treat resistant lesions.

Self-help organisations

Psoriasis Association
Psoriatic Athropathy Alliance

Pyoderma gangrenosum

Definition and aetiology

Pyoderma gangrenosum is a non-infective necrosis of the cutaneous tissues. The exact cause is unknown, although it may be caused by a disorder of the immune system. It is often associated with Crohn's disease, rheumatoid arthritis and ulcerative colitis. Lesions may also arise in the presence of existing skin disease (e.g. acne) or at a site of trauma.

Symptoms

The condition is characterised by two different types of lesion, which may be present simultaneously or sequentially. Both are painful and rapidly ulcerate. Tender erythematous nodules, which become blue in the centre before ulcerating, may develop on any part of the body, but most commonly occur on the face, calves, thighs and buttocks. A scar often remains after healing. Pustular vesicles can also occur at any of the above sites and on the eyelids, lips and oral mucosa. Haemorrhagic bullae may occur in the presence of leukaemia.

Treatment

Treatment consists of the oral administration of very high doses of corticosteroids (BNF 6.3.2). In addition, any underlying disorder should be treated.

Sebaceous cyst

Definition and aetiology

Cysts, commonly referred to as sebaceous cysts, are more correctly termed epidermoid cysts. The contents consist primarily of keratin and its breakdown products, although follicular and sebaceous materials may also be present. They arise in damaged or blocked pilosebaceous follicles. Cysts containing sebum as their main component are called steatocystoma multiplex and are relatively uncommon.

Symptoms

Sebaceous cysts are common in adults, and frequently occur on the face, ears, scalp, neck, upper trunk and scrotum. They are pale, firm, globular swellings of variable size, and may be single or multiple. They enlarge slowly, and are usually painless and harmless unless they become infected and result in abscess formation and suppuration.

Treatment

Removal is unnecessary unless a cyst is infected or cosmetically unacceptable. Infections may be treated using an appropriate oral antibacterial drug, and the cyst drained through an incision. Larger cysts may require surgical excision. The cyst wall must be removed to prevent recurrence.

Sunburn

Definition and aetiology

Sunburn is an inflammatory skin condition resulting from excessive exposure to ultraviolet radiation, in particular to the shorter wavelengths of 290 nm to 320 nm (i.e. UVB).

Symptoms

The extent of the reaction varies between individuals, the most susceptible being pale-skinned people. Erythema usually appears 2–8 hours after exposure and fades within 36 hours. Symptoms of heavier doses include bullae, oedema, pain and tenderness, which generally reach a peak on the second day. Extensive areas of sunburnt skin may result in constitutional symptoms (e.g. fever, malaise and headache). Hyperpigmentation and epidermal thickening occur in varying degrees a few days later, and constitute an attempt to protect the skin against further doses of radiation. Prolonged and repeated exposure may in time cause premature ageing of the skin and the development of malignant disease (e.g. melanoma and rodent ulcer).

Treatment

Further exposure should be avoided until successful treatment has been completed. The skin should be cooled by cold-water compresses or sponging. Topical corticosteroid preparations (BNF 13.4) may be prescribed to reduce minor inflammation, and non-opioid analgesics (BNF 4.7.1) may be indicated for pain. Systemic corticosteroids (BNF 6.3.2) may be necessary in severe cases. The patient should be counselled on preventive measures, which include using sunscreening preparations (BNF 13.8.1) and gradual suntanning to allow the skin to acclimatise.

Telangiectasia

Definition and aetiology

A telangiectasia is a lesion on the skin or mucous membranes formed by a group of permanently dilated, superficial blood vessels. Contributory factors include the prolonged topical administration of fluorinated corticosteroids, prolonged vasodilatation (e.g. in rosacea and varicose veins), or atrophy of local supporting tissue caused by ageing, excessive exposure to sunlight, trauma or X-ray therapy. Telangiectases may also accompany systemic diseases (e.g. dermatomyositis, systemic lupus erythematosus and systemic sclerosis). Some forms may be genetically inherited, although in many cases the cause is unknown.

Symptoms

Lesions may be linear, punctate, spider-like or stellate and can be accompanied by increased melanin pigmentation. They are generally small and dull-red in colour, and blanch temporarily on the application of pressure.

Treatment

In many cases no treatment is required, although camouflaging preparations (BNF 13.8.2 and appendix 7) may be used to conceal cosmetically unacceptable lesions. Where appropriate, small telangiectases may be destroyed by cauterisation, cryotherapy or electrolysis.

Toxic epidermal necrolysis

Definition and aetiology

Toxic epidermal necrolysis (scalded skin syndrome or Ritter–Lyell syndrome) is a serious skin disorder characterised by exfoliation of extensive areas of necrotic epidermis. The cause is unknown, although it may arise as a reaction to drugs (e.g. barbiturates, ethambutol, phenolphthalein, phenytoin or sulphonamides). It may also be associated with viral infections, leukaemia and radiotherapy. In infants, it usually occurs as a result of staphylococcal infection.

Symptoms

The onset is rapid and initial symptoms include erythema and tenderness, often accompanied by anorexia, fever and malaise. In addition, flaccid bullae may be present. Desquamation of the skin, which may be localised or extensive, occurs after 36–48 hours and leaves raw, painful areas. The prognosis in adults is poor due to possible complications (e.g. secondary infection, and fluid and electrolyte imbalance). Scarring, and loss of hair and nails may follow healing. The prognosis is more favourable in the staphylococcal-induced form because the damage to the epidermis does not extend to as great a depth.

Treatment

Any underlying infection or disorder should be treated and causative agents withdrawn or changed. Other measures include hospitalisation, correction of fluid and electrolyte imbalance, and minimal physical handling to reduce the degree of skin loss. Careful application of anti-infective skin preparations (BNF 13.10) may be necessary. Infants may require isolation to prevent contagion.

Ulcers

Definition and aetiology

The formation of an ulcer in the skin is caused by local destruction of the epidermis and part of the underlying dermis. It may be simple and without further complications, or chronic and unresponsive to treatment.

Varicose (venous) ulcers are caused by venous stasis, which may be a consequence of deep vein thrombosis, varicose veins or peripheral vascular disease (e.g. in diabetes mellitus). Ischaemic (arterial) ulcers are caused by a diminished arterial blood supply to the skin, which may be a consequence of atherosclerosis, hypertension or scar tissue. Decubitus ulcers occur at sites exposed to prolonged pressure. Infections, malnutrition or trauma may precipitate ulceration in predisposed individuals, or complicate existing ulcers.

Symptoms

Venous ulcers (Figure 13.10) occur most commonly in the elderly, particularly in women. They generally occur on the lower leg and are of variable size, encircling the whole leg in severe cases. There is an initial erythema which progresses to a bluish-red discoloration and finally to

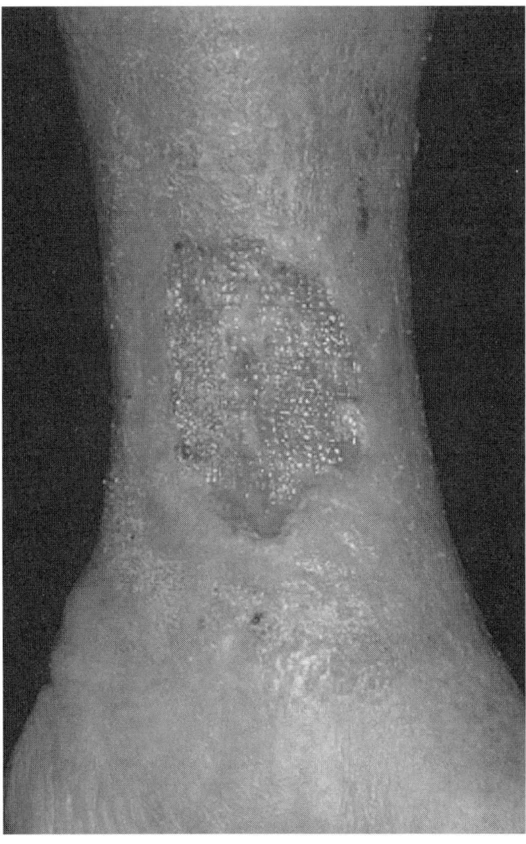

Figure 13.10 Varicose ulcer surrounded by varicose eczema. (Reproduced with permission of Mike Wyndham.)

necrosis. The edge is often irregular in outline and may be indurated. The skin around the ulcer may show deposits of haemosiderin. Ischaemic ulcers are more painful than venous ulcers, have less pigmentation in the surrounding skin, and have well-defined margins. They frequently occur on the front of the tibia. There is little exudate and healing is generally slow.

Treatment

Any underlying disorder should be treated. Patients should also be encouraged to exercise when possible to improve the circulation. Successful treatment of venous ulcers may be promoted by improving venous drainage by the use of compression bandages and support stockings. Non-ambulant patients should spend part of each day with their legs in an elevated position. Treatment of the ulcer itself consists of debridement using various skin cleansing or desloughing agents and enzyme preparations (BNF 13.11). Dextranomer beads and gel and colloid dressings (BNF appendix 8) may be beneficial. The use of anti-infective skin preparations should be avoided unless absolutely necessary, as these can be sensitising.

Urticaria

Definition and aetiology

Urticaria (Figure 13.11) is characterised by transient erythema and wheals in the dermis. It is the result of localised oedema caused by increased permeability of the small blood vessel walls due to the release of mediators (e.g. histamine, kinins or prostaglandins). Acute urticaria may be precipitated by a variety of stimulants (e.g. drugs, foods or food additives, and underlying systemic infections or disorders). The cause is unknown in 50% of chronic cases, but psychogenic or physical factors (e.g. heat, cold or sunlight) may be important.

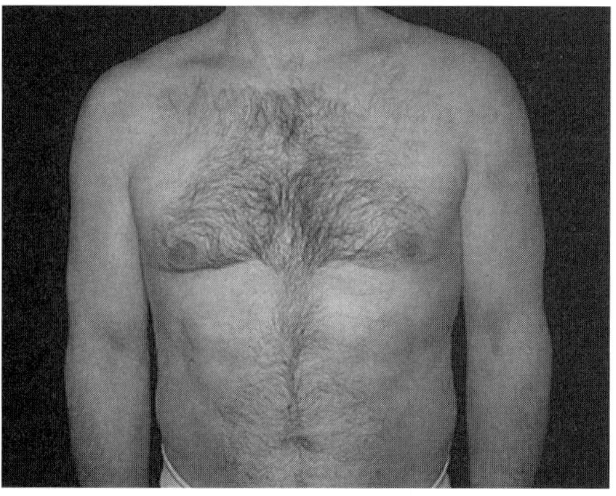

Figure 13.11 Urticaria. (Reproduced with permission of Mike Wyndham.)

Symptoms

The first common symptom is pruritus. It is followed by large or small wheals, which may occur at any site, and disappear after a few hours. The larger wheals characteristically show a white centre surrounded by a ring of erythema. In some cases, erythema occurs without wheals, and occasionally bullae may be present. Larger swellings occur more diffusely and may be characteristic of angioedema. The condition is often self-limiting. Acute urticaria generally disappears within one to seven days, while chronic cases may take up to two years to regress.

Treatment

Where possible, the cause should be identified and avoided, and any underlying disorder treated. The patient should be counselled to avoid potentially sensitising agents (e.g. azo colouring agents and benzoates used as food additives, and salicylates). Oral antihistamines (BNF 3.4.1) may be of value in relieving symptoms, and oral corticosteroids (BNF 6.3.2) may be indicated in severe cases. Adrenaline (BNF 3.4.3) may be required in severe acute attacks.

Vitiligo

Definition and aetiology

Vitiligo (Figure 13.12) is an acquired condition characterised by lesions devoid of pigment, possibly caused by a toxin or an autoimmune reaction which destroys melanocytes. It often arises in association with Addison's disease, diabetes mellitus, melanoma, myasthenia gravis, pernicious anaemia and thyroid disorders. It may be idiopathic or inherited.

Symptoms

The condition affects all races and generally develops before 20 years of age. Common sites

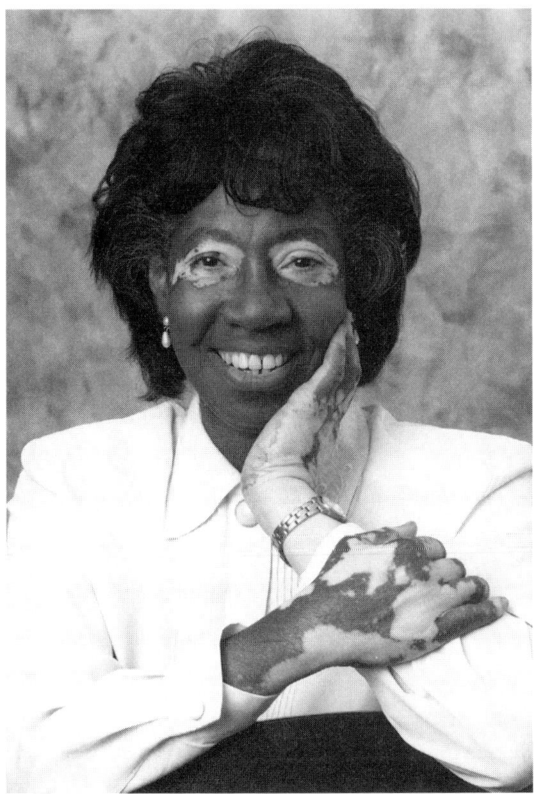

Figure 13.12 Vitiligo. (Reproduced with permission from *Pharmaceutical Journal*.)

initially affected include the face and neck, and areas exposed to trauma (e.g. knuckles, hands, elbows, knees, ankles and feet). It spreads gradually, and in rare cases may affect the entire skin surface. The lesions, which generally show a symmetrical distribution, have well-defined and often hyperpigmented margins. The melanocytes of the hair follicles are usually unaffected, although hairs in older lesions may become white. Spontaneous repigmentation, commencing at the hair follicles, occurs in a small proportion of cases but is rarely complete. The condition does not affect general health, although there is an increased tendency to sunburn in the depigmented areas.

Treatment

Cosmetic camouflage preparations (BNF 13.8.2 and appendix 7) may be of value, and sunscreening preparations (BNF 13.8.1) should be applied to exposed lesions. Skin bleaching agents may be used to remove the few remaining pigmented areas in cases of extensive vitiligo.

13.2 Anatomy and physiology of the skin

The skin

The skin is one component of the integumentary system, which also includes the nails, hair, sebaceous and sudoriferous glands, and ceruminous glands. It is the single largest system in the body, and provides one of the major routes through which the external environment is monitored and experienced. It is an organ which is being continuously replenished to replace cells lost or damaged.

The skin may be considered to consist of a layer of dermis supporting an outer layer of epidermis and padded from within by a layer of fat (Figure 13.13). The microscopic structure, however, is considerably more complex, reflecting the diverse roles that the skin plays.

The outermost layer of the skin is composed of the epidermis. It consists of four types of cells of which the bulk are the keratinocytes. Keratinocytes are formed from the deepest layer of the epidermis, the stratum basale (stratum germinativum), and migrate upwards to the surface. In their passage towards the surface, the cells are responsible for the formation of a protein, keratin. The waterproof keratin resides in the outermost layer of the epidermis, the stratum corneum, within denucleated dead keratinocytes. The cells of the stratum corneum also provide a barrier to other potentially harmful agents (e.g. bacteria, heat and light waves). Dead cells are eventually sloughed off the surface of the epidermis and continually replaced by new cells from below. The period between their formation in the basal layer and their loss is approximately two to four weeks.

The epidermis also contains melanocytes, Langerhans cells and Granstein cells. Melanocytes synthesise the pigment melanin from the amino acid tyrosine, and the rate of melanin synthesis, rather than the number of melanocytes, determines the darkness of the skin. Increased production is induced by exposure to ultraviolet

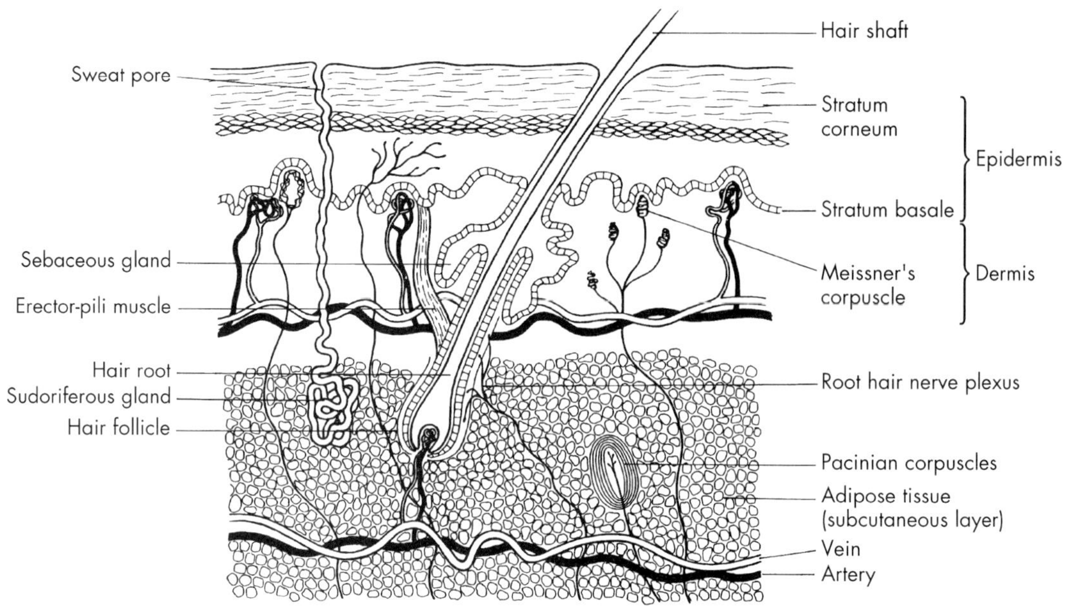

Figure 13.13 Skin section.

radiation. As a result, the degree of skin tanning is increased, and the underlying dermis is protected from the harmful effects of further irradiation. The rate of synthesis and distribution of melanin is also affected by an anterior pituitary hormone, melanocyte-stimulating hormone. The Langerhans cells are similar to melanocytes but are derived from the bone marrow. Both the Langerhans cells and the Granstein cells play an active role in the immune system. They are responsible for rendering T-cells aware of the presence of antigens that penetrate the upper layers of the epidermis.

Immediately below the epidermis is the dermis. This layer of the skin is highly vascularised and innervated, and contains hair follicles and sebaceous glands. The bulk of the dermis comprises a network of elastic and collagen fibres throughout a bed of connective tissue, which imparts extensibility, elasticity and strength to the skin.

The sensation of touch is provided by the presence of Meissner's corpuscles in dermal projections into the epidermis, and by epidermal tactile discs. Root hair nerve plexuses, which surround hair follicles, transmit sensations induced by the movement of the hair. Naked nerve endings are also widely distributed over the surface of the skin. Pressure on the surface is monitored by Pacinian (lamellated) corpuscles located within the dermal projections into the subcutaneous fat layer.

The sensation of pain is monitored by pain receptors (nociceptors) distributed throughout the skin. An awareness of pain in the skin is described as superficial somatic pain, whilst pain arising in deeper structural tissues (e.g. tendons and muscles) is described as deep somatic pain. The nerve impulse generated by stimulation of the nociceptors is transmitted to the central nervous system via the spinal and cranial nerves.

Hair

One of the most distinctive features of the skin is the presence of hair. Each hair consists of a shaft, the majority of which lies above the surface of the skin, and a root, which lies within the dermis. In dark hair, the central layer of the shaft contains pigmented cells, whereas the same cells in white hair are filled with air. The root of the hair is contained within a follicle whose base is enlarged to form a bulbar structure. This swelling contains the blood supply to nourish the hair, and the germinal cells to produce a new hair when the old one is shed.

The primary function of hair is protection (e.g. prevention of the effects of harmful radiation on the scalp and entry of objects into cavities). Hair grows at the rate of approximately 1 cm per month and has an average life of three years. Although the numbers vary considerably, there may be about 300 000 hairs on the scalp, and of these about 50–100 are shed each day.

Glands of the skin

The majority of the sebaceous glands, which secrete sebum, are closely associated with the hair follicles (forming the pilosebaceous unit). Sebaceous glands are widely distributed over most of the body with the exception of the soles of the feet and the palms of the hands. Glands not associated with hair follicles, and which secrete sebum directly onto the surface of the skin, may be found in the tarsal glands of the eyelid, the lips and in genital regions. The activity of these glands is stimulated by androgens and inhibited by oestrogens. Sebum is an oily fluid containing wax esters, triglycerides, squalene and sterol esters and serves to moisturise the skin and hair, limit the evaporation of water from the surface of the skin; it is bacteriostatic.

Sudoriferous (sweat) glands, which may be classified as apocrine or eccrine, occur all over the body. Apocrine glands are localised to the pigmented areas of the breast, the axillae, and the pubic area, and only become active at puberty. Body odour is produced by the bacterial decomposition of the sweat from apocrine glands. Eccrine glands are more widely distributed than apocrine glands. About 500 mL of sweat may be normally produced by the three or four million eccrine glands each day. Sweat comprises a mixture of components (e.g. inorganic salts, urea, ammonia and lactic acid), but eccrine sweat is less viscous than apocrine sweat. The production of sweat is a major component of thermoregulation, and only a minor contributor to the excretion of body waste. The activity of the glands is regulated by cholinergic neurons, which are controlled by the hypothalamus. Increased activity, particularly of glands of the hands and feet, may occur in response to anxiety and stress.

Nails

A nail is a plate of flattened, keratinised, epithelial scales located on the upper portion of the end of each digit (Figure 13.14). The fingernails are used primarily to assist in picking up small objects and for scratching. Growth of a nail occurs by the conversion of epithelial cells in the nail matrix (nail bed) into nail cells at the root of the nail. The growth of the nail from its root forces the nail body forward to the tip of the digit. Toenails grow at a slower rate (approximately 1 cm in 9–24 months) than fingernails (1 cm in three months).

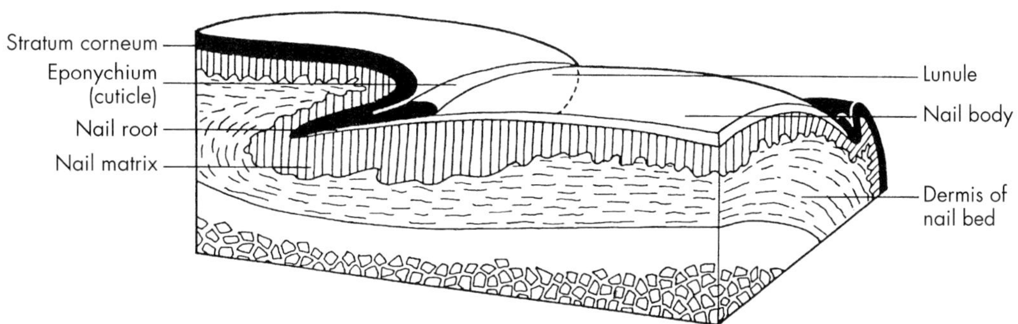

Figure 13.14 Longitudinal section showing structure of a nail.

Part B

Patient advice

Introduction

The ability of pharmacists to be able to relate to patients and to perceive their needs is one of the major requirements of successful pharmacy practice (and indeed of all healthcare). No amount of knowledge about diseases and drugs is sufficient in itself unless pharmacists can communicate with patients and medical personnel, and can recognise the special problems that individuals face. Patients should be the focus of all the care provided by pharmacists.

With these factors in mind, two main components of Part B of the *Handbook of Pharmacy Healthcare* have been devised. First, it provides information on those groups of the population whose circumstances may require special skills, and outlines the most appropriate means by which information and advice may be imparted. Secondly, it emphasises the increasingly important concept of personal responsibility for health by identifying the benefits and problems of self-medication, and highlighting how pharmacists can contribute to self-determination in minor illness. The importance of self-help groups must also be recognised and detailed information on a wide range of organisations is listed.

Pregnant women frequently visit pharmacies and often have questions in relation to what they should and should not do during pregnancy. There is so much advice and information available to the pregnant woman that she may become confused and pharmacists should be a source of clear, unbiased information in this area. Pharmacists therefore need to be aware of the nutritional requirements of pregnant women and be able to advise on healthy eating during pregnancy. Food hygiene is important at all times, but particularly so during pregnancy when the woman's immune response may be compromised and there is a risk of passing on infection to the unborn child. Other lifestyle factors such as smoking, exercise and alcohol are also important. The use of medicines, both prescribed and over the counter, as well as vitamin and mineral supplements and herbal and homeopathic remedies, is another area where pregnant women value clear guidance. Pharmacists are well placed to provide advice to pregnant women on all these matters and **Chapter 14** covers the main areas where pharmacists are likely to receive questions.

The speciality of child health has always been one in which pharmacists, particularly those within the community, have been intimately involved. Many of the regular visitors to pharmacies are mothers accompanied by infants and young children. The bewildering array of milk products, first foods and feeding equipment can frequently confuse parents. It is therefore vital that pharmacists possess adequate knowledge of the types of products available and the rationale for their use. Awareness of the current recommendations concerning breast and bottle feeding, the advantages and disadvantages of each, and the most appropriate means by which bottle feeding can be carried out, may seem relatively straightforward to the pharmacist who has reared her own children, but can appear an intimidating minefield to newly qualified pharmacists of both sexes. **Chapter 15** provides information which is intended to be of use to both experienced and less experienced pharmacists, enabling them to advise parents informatively and confidently.

The occurrence of minor illness in infants and young children, and in particular illnesses associated with feeding difficulties, can pose special management problems. The ability to distinguish minor causes of feeding problems from those of a serious nature is essential, and guidance is provided to assist pharmacists in this task.

An awareness of the importance of contributing towards the healthy development of children is often enhanced within the pharmacy by the prominent display of weighing scales and height charts. By themselves, they are of little value; but in conjunction with explanation of their purpose, and suggestion as to when it may be necessary to seek further advice, pharmacists can contribute to the early identification of developmental abnormalities. Advice is also given in Chapter 15 on the vexed questions of fluoride supplementation, use of sugar-free medicines and immunisation. The emphasis within each of these sections is on providing detailed information for pharmacists so that they may make constructive suggestions to parents on each of these matters.

At the opposite end of the spectrum of life, recognition of the needs of older people has become increasingly important for all personnel in the healthcare professions and many of these special needs are discussed in **Chapter 16**. The multidisciplinary (e.g. involving health visitors, district nurses, home helps) and multifaceted (e.g. involving family practitioner services, hospital services and social services) approaches to the care of this ever increasing group is highly complex, but pharmacists can play an important role in promoting health in this population group, where polypharmacy is very common. In the UK, government recognition of the importance of input from pharmacists has been attained by the introduction of payment to pharmacists providing services to residential homes.

It is vital to recognise that the numbers of elderly people, and by implication the incidence of problems that pharmacists will encounter, is bound to increase. In the UK, since the early 1930s the number of people aged over 65 has more than doubled and today a fifth of the population is over 60. Between 1995 and 2025 the number of people over 80 is set to increase by almost half and the number of people over 90 will double.

Identifying regular visitors to the pharmacy and assisting the elderly in their use of medicines can provide an invaluable and rewarding service. Four in five people over 75 take at least one prescribed medicine, with 36% taking four or more medicines, and it is important to ensure that medicines are prescribed and used effectively.

The possession of a specialist knowledge in any area of expertise is useless unless that information can be imparted to others. In the healthcare professions, the ability to communicate effectively with patients and other health workers is essential. Various aspects of the social and behavioural skills required for the effective practice of pharmacy (including a knowledge of the means of achieving effective communication, and applying that knowledge in counselling) are explained in **Chapter 17**. Patients' perceptions of pharmacy and pharmacists are significantly influenced by the way in which they, the patients, are dealt with. Do pharmacists make themselves available for members of the public to make direct contact? Is the environment in which the 'consultation' takes place conducive to personal exchange of information? Do pharmacists make a pro-active attempt to talk with patients, or is communication nearly always initiated by patients? Are opportunities taken to offer general health advice at the same time as responding to patients' specific enquiries?

One of the most important ways in which pharmacists can contribute towards healthcare is by discussing the appropriate use of drugs and medicines, and encouraging patients to comply with their dosage regimens.

Many patients are reluctant to consult their doctors about symptoms which they themselves consider trivial. In fact, it has been estimated that only about one in three symptoms experienced by patients are referred to doctors. Many of the symptoms that are not referred to doctors are brought to the attention of pharmacists; the ability to screen out minor illnesses by pharmacists is an important element in maintaining the viability of the health services, and is discussed in **Chapter 18**. Many of the symptoms reported to pharmacists require no medical treatment, often only requiring advice on lifestyle matters (e.g. diet or exercise) or reassurance. Guidance on self-medication can be usefully given for those minor symptoms which might benefit from the use of non-prescription medicines. At all times, however, pharmacists should be alert to the possibility of reported symptoms being one manifestation of more serious disease, and in such cases, the importance of seeking immediate medical advice should be stressed to patients.

Many patients require diagnostic tests from time to time. These can range from relatively simple blood tests to the more complex examinations such as ultrasound and computed tomography. Sometimes patients will have been given the name of the test for which they are booked, but they may have little information on what the procedure involves, why it is being used and what the results might mean. Such lack of information may result in undue concern for the patient.

Chapter 19 describes a range of commonly used diagnostic procedures to help pharmacists explain their rationale and allay patients' concerns. This chapter also provides information on indices for various test procedures with ranges and their interpretation.

Every individual ultimately has the right to self-determination in matters of health, and, whenever possible, pharmacists should be encouraging patients to take full responsibility for their own health. Equally it is important that patients participate in decisions taken about their health so that they can develop this self-determination and autonomy. It should be recognised that compliance with a particular course of action (e.g. taking medicines or adopting a healthier lifestyle) is considerably easier to achieve if patients have been intimately involved in the decision process. One potent manifestation of the desire by patients to participate in maintaining their own health is the proliferation of self-help organisations (**Chapter 20**), which operate in parallel to the 'official' health services. Pharmacists are frequently approached by members of the public for information on specific groups, or for advice about whether other patients in a similar predicament can be contacted. Pharmacists should recognise the importance of such groups; referring patients to them can be just as important in the overall care of patients as handing out prescription and non-prescription medicines.

All cross-references specified within Part B are to the BNF.

14

Pregnancy

14.1 Introduction

Pregnancy is a time when many women tend to become more receptive to advice about health than at other times. Pharmacists can make the most of this opportunity as well as answering questions and providing information on issues that women might have before becoming pregnant and once their pregnancy has been confirmed.

Before pregnancy, women may need advice on folic acid supplementation, smoking and alcohol. Pre-conceptually women should be encouraged to think about their diet, making any appropriate adjustments such as increasing intake of fruit and vegetables and reducing fatty and sugary foods. During pregnancy, they may need further dietary information, guidance on food hygiene and advice on the management of common ailments. Pharmacists can encourage pregnant women in appropriate self-care, including the importance of having a dental check-up early in pregnancy.

The use of medicines in women who are pregnant is often a difficult issue for pharmacists and is a question of fine balance. The benefits of treatment should always be weighed against the risk, but all medicines should be avoided in pregnancy unless they are essential. Pharmacists therefore have an important role in encouraging women to use other approaches, particularly to common ailments such as sickness and constipation, where dietary and lifestyle changes can sometimes be of considerable help.

14.2 Nutrition and lifestyle issues in pregnancy

Nutrition

Eating a well-balanced diet is beneficial to both mother and infant, both before conception and throughout pregnancy. Dietary advice is aimed at reducing the risk of birth defects and of having an infant of low birth weight. Low-birth-weight infants are at risk of poor health during infancy and possibly also in adulthood. Low birth weight may exacerbate the predisposition to conditions such as hypertension, coronary heart disease and diabetes mellitus in middle and older age.

Nutrition has different implications at different stages of pregnancy. Before the formation of the placenta, the embryo is directly exposed to the maternal blood circulation and hence is vulnerable to excesses or deficiencies of nutrients and to the toxic effects of drugs, alcohol or other toxic substances. As the placenta develops, the embryo is increasingly protected from harm, and as the pregnancy progresses the nutritional needs of the fetus start to take precedence over those of the mother. The placenta becomes increasingly efficient at extracting nutrients from the mother's blood, and during later pregnancy, if there is a shortage of, say, vitamins and minerals, it is the mother rather than the infant who will suffer.

The nutritional requirements for the pregnant and non-pregnant woman are shown in Table 14.1. Given that the demand for nutrients during pregnancy is known to be relatively high, the fact that no increases are recommended for some nutrients (e.g. calcium, iron, magnesium, zinc, vitamin B_6 and vitamin B_{12}) may seem surprising. However, various adaptive mechanisms occur in the mother during the early weeks of pregnancy, such that absorption of vitamins and minerals is increased, excretion reduced and metabolism made more efficient.

The metabolism of energy and protein also becomes increasingly efficient, and the traditional idea that the mother has 'to eat for two' no longer holds. Even during the last trimester, average energy requirements increase by only about 200 kcal per day.

Folic acid

Folic acid is a B vitamin that is essential for cell division. Adequate intake is important throughout pregnancy to prevent the development of megaloblastic anaemia, but folic acid seems to be particularly crucial in early pregnancy when inadequate intake has been shown to increase the risk of neural tube defects (NTDs), such as spina bifida. An Expert Advisory Group from the Department of Health has therefore issued recommendations on folate intake before and during pregnancy as follows:

- Women with no history of NTD who are planning a pregnancy should be advised to take a folic acid supplement at a dose of 400 µg per day before conception and during the first 12 weeks of pregnancy. Women who have not been taking supplements and who suspect they are pregnant should start a supplement at once and continue until week 12 of pregnancy.
- Women with a history of NTD in a previous child (or if she or her partner has spina bifida) who are planning a pregnancy or at risk of becoming pregnant should be prescribed a folic acid supplement in a dose of 5 mg per day. Women receiving antiepileptic therapy need individual counselling by their doctor before starting on folic acid (BNF 9.1.2).

In addition, foods rich in folate (e.g. fortified breakfast cereals, fortified breads, green leafy vegetables, oranges and pulses) should be emphasised.

Recent surveys suggest that awareness of the importance of folic acid in pregnancy is not all it could be. Pharmacists have an important educational role, particularly since they sell ovulation and pregnancy test kits and have opportunities on these occasions to discuss folic acid.

Interestingly, a recent study in Sweden indicated that pregnant women who take folic acid supplements might be more likely to have twins. While supplements reduce the risk of birth defects, twins have their own problems in that they are more likely to be premature, have low birth weights and cerebral palsy. The reasons for the link with folic acid are not clear, and there is a need for much more research to establish whether the link is genuine.

Iron

Iron is an essential nutrient and additional amounts are required during pregnancy for development of the fetus and expansion of blood

Table 14.1 Reference nutrient intakes (per day) for pregnant and non-pregnant women[1] for energy and nutrients

	Non-pregnant	Pregnant
Energy MJ (kcal)[2]	8.10 (1940)	+0.8 (+200)[3]
Protein (g)	45	+6
Vitamins		
A (μg)	600	+100
D (μg)	–	10
E (mg)	>3[4]	*
K (μg)	1 μg/kg[4]	*
Thiamine (mg)	0.8	+0.2[3]
Riboflavine (mg)	1.1	+0.3
Niacin (mg)	13	*
Vitamin B_6 (mg)	1.2	*
Vitamin B_{12} (μg)	1.5	*
Folate (μg)	200	+100[5]
Pantothenic acid (mg)	3–7	*
Biotin (μg)	10–200[4]	*
Vitamin C (mg)	40	+10
Minerals		
Sodium (mg)	1600	*
Potassium (mg)	3500	*
Chloride (mg)	2500	*
Calcium (mg)	700	*
Phosphorus (mg)	550	*
Magnesium (mg)	270	*
Iron (mg)	14.8	*
Copper (mg)	1.2	*
Zinc (mg)	7.0	*
Manganese (mg)	1.4[4]	*
Chromium (μg)	25	*
Selenium (μg)	60	*
Iodine (μg)	140	*
Molybdenum (μg)	50–400[4]	*

* No increment.
[1] RNI for women 19–50 years.
[2] Estimated Average Requirement (EAR).
[3] For the last trimester only.
[4] Safe intake.
[5] A 400 μg per day supplement should be taken from conception to the 12th week of pregnancy.

volume. However, these extra needs can normally be met by adaptive mechanisms in the mother such as increased intestinal absorption, mobilisation of maternal iron stores and the reduction in iron loss due to cessation of menstruation. The need for routine iron supplementation in pregnancy has therefore been questioned, and even though haemoglobin levels fall, this is normally a haemodilution effect rather than anaemia. Because iron is associated with gastrointestinal side-effects and it can also reduce the absorption of other minerals (e.g. zinc), unnecessary supplementation is probably best avoided.

However, consideration of iron status in pregnancy remains important since anaemia increases the risk of having an infant with low birth weight as well as premature delivery, not to mention poor health in the mother. Where iron status is poor, iron supplementation may therefore be required.

When discussing diet with pregnant women, pharmacists should emphasise iron. Iron-rich foods include red meat, green vegetables, dried fruit, fortified breakfast cereals and sardines. Vitamin C improves the absorption of iron from non-animal sources, so a glass of fruit juice, a tomato or a piece of citrus fruit with each meal or snack is beneficial, particularly for vegetarians. Tannins and caffeine, found in tea and coffee, inhibit iron absorption, and are best avoided at mealtimes.

Calcium

Calcium requirements double during pregnancy, but no dietary increase is recommended because the mother's body adapts by absorbing more. However, calcium should still be emphasised because the increased requirement can only be met if the mother's stores are adequate.

Dairy foods are the most concentrated and highly bioavailable source of calcium, and the 700 mg a day requirement can be met by consuming, for example a large glass of skimmed milk, a pot of yoghurt and a small piece of cheese (i.e. about the size of a matchbox). Non-dairy sources include fortified soya milk, tofu, fish with small bones (e.g. sardines), white bread, sesame seeds and green vegetables, but in some cases, huge quantities have to be consumed to obtain the Reference Nutrient Intake (RNI) for calcium. For example, three slices of white bread, 25 g sesame seeds or a large portion of curly kale, spinach or watercress contains only around 150 mg calcium.

Vitamin D

Vitamin D helps the absorption of calcium. Most of the requirement is obtained by the action of sunlight on the skin, but in northern climates and in darker skinned people, this is not always a reliable source, and dietary intake should be emphasised. Oily fish, milk, eggs, butter, margarine and fortified spreads are good sources, but not normally consumed frequently or in sufficient amounts to meet the vitamin D requirement in pregnancy. A 10 μg daily supplement should therefore be recommended, particularly for women with little exposure to sunlight.

Vitamin A

Vitamin A is required during pregnancy as at any other time of life for normal vision and for cell growth and bone development. However, excessive ingestion of vitamin A (in the form of retinol) in pregnancy has been linked with birth defects, and daily doses of 15 000 IU or more are potentially harmful. The Department of Health advises the avoidance of liver and foods made from it (e.g. liver pate, liver sausage) because liver may contain high concentrations of vitamin A. However, other less concentrated sources of retinol such as dairy produce are safe in terms of vitamin A content, as are foods containing vitamin A in the form of carotene (e.g. fruits and vegetables).

The Department of Health recommends that dietary supplements containing vitamin A (including fish liver oils) should not be taken in pregnancy. However, provided the diet does not contain excessive amounts of the vitamin, supplements containing no more than the recommended daily amount are likely to be safe. Moreover, supplements containing vitamin A in the form of beta-carotene are also considered to be safe, but in the majority of women are probably unnecessary.

Omega-3 fatty acids

Omega-3 fatty acids are a particular group of polyunsaturated fats that have a role in ensuring optimal brain and nerve development in the unborn child. The best source is oily fish (e.g. mackerel, herring, sardines, salmon). Linseed or flaxseed oil is an alternative for vegetarian women.

Weight

If possible, 'ideal' weight (i.e. Body Mass Index of 20–25), or as near to it as is practicable, should be attained before pregnancy begins. Being overweight increases the chance of the mother having gestational diabetes and hypertension as well as having an infant that is too heavy.

However, once pregnancy is confirmed, women should be discouraged from trying to lose weight. Low energy intake increases the risk of having a low-birth-weight infant as well as restricting the intake of essential nutrients.

On average a woman gains 10–12 kg during pregnancy, but blanket recommendations for weight gain are no longer made as they were in the past. Thus if a woman is underweight at the start of pregnancy, she should gain more than the average (e.g. about 13.5 kg), while those who are overweight or obese should gain less (e.g. about 7.5 kg).

Dietary advice for pregnancy

In general, the same healthy eating guidelines apply pre-conceptually and during pregnancy as at any other time, and most women can achieve their own nutritional needs and those of their infant by eating regular balanced meals and snacks based on the following food groups:

- Starchy carbohydrates such as bread, potatoes, breakfast cereals, pasta and rice. These foods should make up the main part of every meal and snack. They are good sources of carbohydrate, protein and B vitamins and low in fat. Wholemeal and high-fibre varieties should be emphasised because they tend to contain more vitamins and minerals than their lower fibre equivalents.
- Fruit and vegetables. This includes fresh, frozen and tinned varieties, as well as fruit and vegetable juices. Fruit and vegetables provide vitamin C, carotenoids and some of the B vitamins, but to retain these vitamins, fresh fruit and vegetables should not be stored for long, should be cooked quickly and in a minimum amount of water, or steamed or microwaved. In addition, they should be eaten as soon as possible after cooking.
- Meat, fish and alternatives, such as eggs, nuts and pulses (e.g. beans, lentils, chickpeas). These are a good source of protein, B vitamins, iron and zinc. They should be consumed in moderation and lower fat versions chosen whenever possible.
- Milk and dairy foods. These foods are particularly high in calcium and good sources of protein and some B vitamins. Lower fat versions should be chosen whenever possible, and women reminded that skimmed and semi-skimmed milk contain just as much calcium and protein as full fat milk.
- Foods containing fat and sugar. Foods such as chocolate, sweets, cakes, biscuits, pastries, crisps and fried foods should be eaten in only small amounts and/or infrequently.

Alcohol

Excessive alcohol intake should be avoided throughout pregnancy and during the first trimester alcohol is best avoided altogether. During later pregnancy it is best to limit alcohol as much as possible, not exceeding an intake of one to two units a week.

Caffeine

Caffeine is found in coffee, tea and cola drinks. These drinks should be consumed in moderation and the UK Food Standards Agency (FSA) Committee on Toxicity of Chemicals in Food, Consumer Products and the Environment (COT) has recommended that the intake of caffeine should not exceed 300 mg daily during pregnancy. This is roughly equivalent to three average size mugs of instant coffee. The caffeine content of various drinks and foods is found in Table 14.2. Caffeine is also found in various cold and flu remedies.

Table 14.2 Caffeine content of various beverages and foods

Average cup of instant coffee	75 mg
Average mug of coffee	100 mg
Average cup of brewed coffee	100 mg
Average cup of tea	50 mg
Regular cola drink	up to 40 mg
Small bar of chocolate	up to 50 mg

Food hygiene

Food hygiene is important at all times, but particularly during pregnancy when there are particular risks from foodborne infections.

Common sense preventive measures include:

- Washing hands before and after food preparation
- Defrosting and cooking food thoroughly
- Ensuring all reheated food is piping hot
- Not storing or preparing raw meat near to other food (e.g. place raw meat on the bottom shelf of the fridge, not above other food)
- Discarding food which is past its use-by date.

In addition, pets are best kept out of the kitchen if possible, and hands should always be washed after handling animals and before preparing or eating food. Different utensils and bowls should be used for pets and washed separately.

Salmonellosis

Salmonella can cause severe gastroenteritis, and the risk is increased particularly during the first trimester when resistance to any infection may be reduced. Although salmonellosis cannot be passed onto the unborn child, it is wise to avoid any infection during pregnancy.

The most likely food culprits are raw eggs consumed in homemade mayonnaise or desserts. Pregnant women should be advised to ensure that all the eggs they consume are bought fresh, stored in the fridge and cooked until the yolk is set. All egg dishes should be thoroughly cooked. Raw or undercooked meat also carries a risk of salmonellosis and should be avoided.

Listeriosis

Listeriosis is a rare infection (affecting about 1 in 20 000 pregnancies), causing a mild flu-like illness in the mother, but which can cause miscarriage or stillbirth. Unpasteurised milk, pates, blue-veined cheese (e.g. Danish blue, Gorgonzola, Roquefort, Stilton, Blue Brie) and soft unpasteurised cheese (e.g. Brie, Cambozola, Camembert) are the main culprits. Cheese which is safe includes all hard cheese and soft cheese that is processed (e.g. cottage cheese, Philadelphia, Quark, Ricotta, cheese spreads).

Toxoplasmosis

Toxoplasmosis is an infection (affecting 1 in 50 000 pregnancies) caused by a parasite in cats' faeces, soil, raw meat and unpasteurised milk. Anyone is at risk of this infection, but if acquired during pregnancy it can cause severe fetal abnormalities. To reduce the risk, women should be advised to avoid raw meat and eggs, ensure all meat is properly cooked and only use milk that has been pasteurised. Vegetables should be washed thoroughly before consumption.

It is also important to avoid cat litter, but if this is not possible, protective gloves should be worn. In addition, gloves should always be worn when gardening. Moreover, it is best to avoid contact with lambs and sheep that have just given birth (because of the risk of toxoplasmosis, listeriosis and chlamydiosis).

Smoking

Women should be encouraged to stop smoking before conception if possible. Smoking during pregnancy is linked with miscarriages, low birth weight, birth defects and possibly increased postnatal complications.

Currently, there is controversy about the use of nicotine replacement therapy (NRT) during pregnancy. Although cigarette smoking is a preventable cause of fetal morbidity and mortality, currently available NRT preparations are contraindicated during pregnancy.

Exercise

Exercise is important at all times, including pregnancy, although some types (e.g. horse riding, skating, step aerobics, skiing, scuba diving) are best avoided. Swimming and walking are ideal. Exercise should be encouraged at least three times a week, but at a level and duration that feels comfortable for the woman.

Useful advice on nutrition and lifestyle for women pre-conceptually and during pregnancy can be summarised as follows:

- Consume a varied diet with plenty of starchy, high-fibre carbohydrates, fruit and vegetables, moderate amounts of meat, fish, eggs or pulses, milk and dairy produce (preferably low-fat varieties), with limited amounts of fatty and sugary foods.
- Take a folic acid supplement (400 μg daily) from the time when pregnancy is planned until the 12th week of pregnancy.
- Be aware of the importance of foods rich in folate, iron, calcium and vitamin D.
- If excessive weight is gained during pregnancy, reduce the intake of fatty and sugary foods.
- Avoid or restrict the intake of alcohol to two units a week.
- Avoid supplements containing doses of vitamin A in excess of the RDA.
- Avoid liver and products containing it.
- Take regular exercise.
- If a smoker, make every effort to quit.

14.3 Use of medication during pregnancy

Pharmacists have an important role in advising on the use of medication during pregnancy, although questions in relation to drug safety are often very difficult to answer. Information on the safe and effective use of medicines in pregnancy has not kept pace with that in other areas of therapeutics. This is because systematic research on drugs in pregnancy is difficult for a whole range of ethical, legal, practical and emotional reasons, yet to prove or disprove that a drug is safe demands randomised controlled studies involving large numbers of women and fetuses. Because such studies are not conducted, knowledge is based on much smaller studies or anecdote and for this reason, no drug can be said with certainty to be safe during early pregnancy.

All medicines should therefore be avoided in pregnancy unless they are essential. This includes both prescribed and over-the-counter medicines as well as vitamin and mineral supplements, herbal, homeopathic and other complementary medicines. In the case of herbal remedies, there are no convincing data to indicate they are safe. In addition, aromatherapy, which involves the use of oils applied to the skin, cannot be assumed to be safe because these highly concentrated oils may be absorbed through the skin and enter the bloodstream.

Deciding what is an essential medicine, however, can be fraught with difficulty and a balanced approach is important. The benefits of giving a medicine should always be weighed against the risks of not giving a medicine. For example, in a woman with epilepsy, it might be more hazardous not to give medication because of the risk to the mother and fetus from poor seizure control. However, for a woman with acne taking long-term antibiotics, the risks of stopping treatment will be minimal.

The risk to the fetus depends to some extent on the timing of drug therapy. Thus during the pre-embryonic period, which lasts until 14 days after conception, exposure to a teratogenic drug seems to be an all or nothing response. A drug may cause death of most or all the embryonic cells resulting in death of the conceptus or it may cause death of just a few cells in which case normal fetal development may ensue. Thus, women who have used medication during the month or so following the last menstrual period can often be reassured, but only if the drug has been completely eliminated in this time. Clearly, this does not apply if the drug has a long half-life or if the time of conception is uncertain.

The period of greatest risk for the fetus is from the third to the eleventh week of pregnancy when the major organ systems are developing. During the second and third trimesters the fetus is less susceptible, although some organs (e.g. the cerebellum, the genito-urinary structures) continue to be formed during this period. The problems caused by drugs during this period tend to be related to growth or functional development in the fetus, although drugs given near to term or during labour may have adverse effects on the infant after delivery. Moreover, adverse effects in relation to drug exposure can sometimes be delayed. For example, diethylstilbestrol is a synthetic oestrogen which was used in the treatment of threatened abortion, and several female fetuses exposed before the ninth week of pregnancy developed vaginal or cervical cancer later in life.

A list of drugs to be avoided or used with caution in pregnancy can be found in the BNF (appendix 4). This contains brief information on drugs which may have harmful effects in pregnancy, together with the trimester of risk. However, just because a drug is not listed it cannot be assumed to be safe.

14.4 Common ailments during pregnancy

The body undergoes an enormous number of changes during pregnancy, and it is not uncommon for women to suffer from a range of health problems and ailments, such as nausea, cravings, heartburn, constipation, haemorrhoids, gingivitis and so on. Pharmacists will often be asked for advice about such problems and are ideally placed to encourage appropriate self-care during pregnancy.

Nausea and vomiting

Nausea and vomiting are common, particularly during early pregnancy. Such symptoms usually start soon after the first missed menstrual period and subside by the 16th week, but occasionally can continue throughout pregnancy. Commonly known as morning sickness, symptoms can actually occur at any time of day. The causes of nausea and sickness in pregnancy are still unclear, although human chorionic gonadotrophin (HCG) and raised thyroxine levels have been implicated. Provided weight gain falls within the desirable range, it is unlikely, however, that sickness will harm the fetus. Indeed, pregnancies in which mild to moderate vomiting occur seem to be less likely to end in miscarriage or lead to fetal malformation. Nevertheless, such symptoms will often cause severe discomfort for the prospective mother. Moreover, if a pregnant woman vomits heavily and frequently, she may lose so much fluid that she becomes dehydrated. If this occurs and she cannot keep fluids down at all, she is said to be suffering from hyperemesis gravidarum, and she will need to be admitted to hospital for evaluation and fluids may need to be administered intravenously.

Most cases can generally be managed without drug treatments and the following advice may be helpful:

- If nausea is severe first thing in the morning, eat a small snack (e.g. plain biscuits or crackers) at the time of waking and before getting out of bed.
- Eat little and often (i.e. every 2–3 hours) whether hungry or not and also eat just before going to bed.
- Suitable snacks include bread, toast, plain biscuits, crackers, cereals, soup, milk drinks, jacket potatoes.
- Fatty and spicy foods are best avoided.
- Drink plenty (10–12 glasses) of liquid (e.g. water, fruit teas, fruit juice) each day, but avoid or limit the intake of caffeine and alcohol.
- Avoid smells that aggravate nausea and take as much rest as practicable.

Plain ginger might also be worth considering. There is no officially recommended dosage, but several proprietary preparations are now available as well as ginger tea. Elastic wristbands (e.g. Seabands), sold mainly for travel sickness, which apply pressure to a defined point on the inside of the wrists, are now also available. There is limited evidence of clinical effectiveness for such products, but again they might be worth a try in pregnant women. They are unlikely to be harmful.

Where symptoms of sickness are severe, referral is necessary and specialist opinion should be sought (BNF 4.6).

Cravings

Several women experience cravings and taste alterations during pregnancy. Provided that the diet is not substantially altered, there is little danger to either the mother or the infant. Going off tea and coffee, for example, which is very common, will do no harm at all, although craving for sweet fatty foods may encourage excessive weight gain and discourage consumption of more nutritious foods.

Heartburn and indigestion

About 70% of women suffer from heartburn during pregnancy, particularly in the last trimester. This is due partly to pressure caused by the growing uterus on the abdomen and also incompetence of the lower oesophageal sphincter.

The following advice may be helpful:

- Eat little and often, eat slowly and avoid any foods, which in the woman's experience seem to exacerbate the problem. Eating near to bedtime is best avoided.
- Sleep with extra pillows and try to avoid stooping as much as possible.

Antacids and alginates may be recommended if the above measures fail to work. These medicines have not been shown to produce teratogenic effects and are generally considered to be safe during pregnancy as long as chronic high doses are avoided. However, aluminium-containing antacids may worsen constipation, where this is a problem. Preparations containing sodium bicarbonate are best avoided because of the risk of systemic alkalosis and sodium load, which may lead to oedema. Histamine H_2-receptor antagonists (e.g. cimetidine, ranitidine) and proton pump inhibitors (e.g. omeprazole) should not be used for relief of heartburn because their safety in pregnancy has not been established.

Constipation

During pregnancy, particularly in the second and third trimesters, gastrointestinal motility slows as a result of an increased amount of circulating progesterone. This together with the physical compression of the bowel by the growing uterus, may lead to constipation. Iron therapy may exacerbate the problem. Other lifestyle changes that may occur in pregnancy such as reduced exercise and changes in eating habits may also be contributory factors, and it has been estimated that one in three women suffer from constipation in pregnancy.

Dietary measures (i.e. increasing fibre and fluid intake) should be advised in the first instance. Exercise also helps in that it stimulates the bowel and improves digestion. However, if these measures are not effective, bulking agents such as ispaghula, methylcellulose and sterculia may be recommended, although these may cause abdominal discomfort to women when used in late pregnancy. Docusate sodium and lactulose have been used in pregnancy with no evidence of adverse effects, but stimulant laxatives such as senna and bisacodyl are systemically absorbed, so are best avoided. Saline laxatives (e.g. magnesium and sodium salts) and liquid paraffin should be avoided.

Haemorrhoids (piles)

Pregnant women have a higher incidence of haemorrhoids than non-pregnant women. This is thought to be due to the pressure of the growing uterus on the haemorrhoidal vessels. Constipation can exacerbate symptoms of haemorrhoids, so efforts should be directed towards preventing constipation. This can best be achieved by dietary adjustment (i.e. increasing fibre and fluid intake). If the haemorrhoids are swollen and painful, application of an ice pack (e.g. a bag of frozen peas) may bring relief. A bland astringent cream (BNF 1.7.1) may be recommended for symptomatic relief if necessary.

Diarrhoea

Diarrhoea can occur in pregnancy as at any other time and is usually self-limiting. Treatment should be aimed at maintaining hydration, recommending oral rehydration therapy if necessary (BNF 9.2.1.2). Use of anti-diarrhoeal drugs should be avoided as their safety has not been established.

Threadworms

Threadworm infestation is common in pregnancy and should be managed by paying strict attention to hygiene. Daily changing of bed linen, nightwear and towels, together with thorough scrubbing of the hands and nails after going to the toilet and avoiding scratching of the perianal area should ensure that the condition clears within a couple of weeks. None of the available threadworm treatments has been proved to be safe, and drugs should be avoided in this condition.

Colds and coughs

Remedies for colds tend to contain a diversity of ingredients including antihistamines, decongestants, caffeine and analgesics. All such preparations are best avoided in pregnancy and women should be encouraged to have hot soothing drinks such as lemon and honey or blackcurrant. Paracetamol alone is probably the safest option if a medicine for pyrexia is required.

Cough preparations tend to contain either cough suppressants (e.g. codeine, pholcodine, dextromethorphan) or expectorants, often with additional ingredients. There is a paucity of data on the safety of all these ingredients and their efficacy is in many cases questionable. As with colds, it is best to recommend hot drinks and soothing demulcent mixtures or lozenges containing honey and/or glycerol to coat the throat.

Pain

Pain such as headaches or backache can occur at any time, but women who suffer during pregnancy may ask for advice on what is safe to take. Paracetamol has been widely used in pregnancy and is not known to be unsafe, but aspirin and non-steroidal anti-inflammatory drugs (NSAIDs) should not generally be recommended during pregnancy without referral to a doctor.

Aspirin can have a number of adverse effects in the pregnant woman, particularly in late pregnancy. In the usual analgesic doses it increases the risk of maternal and neonatal bleeding by virtue of its anti-platelet effect, and it may delay the onset of labour and increase its duration.

NSAIDs have been linked with a number of undesirable effects in newborn infants, such as intracerebral haemorrhage and renal dysfunction if given after 24 weeks gestation. In addition, their use may lead to premature closure of the ductus arteriosus at term.

Sleeping problems

Women often have problems sleeping, particularly during the last three months of pregnancy, because of the physical changes taking place. They may feel uncomfortable, suffer from leg cramps, need to get up to pass urine or be troubled by unpleasant dreams.

The best bed resting position during pregnancy is for the woman to lie on her side, and if backache is a problem, it can be helpful to experiment with pillows, for example under the abdomen, between the legs, behind the back, as well as additional pillows under the head.

Cramp can be eased by pressing the legs against the wall or standing up and stretching the legs. Lack of calcium can sometimes make cramp worse, so it is important to emphasise calcium in the diet.

Needing to pass urine more frequently is probably unavoidable but can be minimised by not drinking just before going to bed, and limiting the intake of coffee and tea because these act as mild diuretics.

Vaginal candidiasis

About one in five women will suffer an episode of vaginal thrush during pregnancy. Hormonal changes and the consequent alteration of the vaginal environment leading to increased glycogen production is thought to be the main contributory factor. Women suffering from this condition in pregnancy should be referred to the doctor. Treatments such as topical clotrimazole and oral fluconazole are prohibited by their licenses for over-the-counter sale during pregnancy.

Cystitis

Pregnant women often develop cystitis. This may be the result of pressure from an enlarging uterus, and the symptoms will often resolve spontaneously. However, symptoms persisting or worsening over a couple of days should be investigated because bacteria in the urine can lead to kidney infection and other problems.

Gingivitis

Pregnant women are more susceptible to gingivitis than non-pregnant women. Hormonal changes during pregnancy may contribute to changes in the soft oral tissues, making them more sensitive to bacterial dental plaque and resulting in an increased incidence and severity of gingivitis. Careful attention to brushing and flossing and rinsing the mouth help to prevent all oral health complications.

Skin complaints

Skin disorders are not uncommon during pregnancy, particularly itching, which affects one in six pregnant women. There are many causes of itching skin, and women should be advised to seek their doctor's advice, because it is important to exclude those conditions, which although fairly rare, can have undesirable effects on the pregnancy (e.g. prurigo gestationis, impetigo herpetiformis). Once such conditions have been excluded, the woman may be advised to use simple moisturising preparations (e.g. aqueous cream) or soothing preparations such as calamine lotion.

Hair loss

Hair loss is common both during and after pregnancy due to hormonal changes. Although this can be distressing, pharmacists should reassure pregnant women that its occurrence is normal and that the hair will grow again. Treatment is not appropriate.

Scabies and headlice

There is a lack of data on the safety of treatments for scabies and headlice. However, there has been more experience with the use of malathion than with the newer preparations, such as permethrin and phenothrin. In addition, malathion is poorly absorbed from the skin. Malathion is therefore first choice for both conditions during pregnancy, although headlice should if possible be managed without recourse to topical treatment (i.e. by use of a fine-toothed comb) if possible. If topical treatments are used, an aqueous rather than an alcoholic solution should be recommended, and women should be advised not to exceed the recommended dose.

15

Child health and immunisation

15.1 Introduction

As emphasised in Chapter 17, the pharmacist is a readily accessible healthcare professional, a fact confirmed by the approximately six million visitors to pharmacies each day in the UK. A large number of these visitors are mothers accompanied by infants and young children. Pharmacists can be a valuable source of information for parents who may be concerned about the health of their children, by providing advice on a wide range of paediatric issues (e.g. feeding), and recommending an appropriate course of action.

It is vital that pharmacists can distinguish between minor ailments and potentially serious childhood conditions. In determining the potential severity of the symptoms, it is essential that pharmacists listen to what parents tell them, and in particular what form of treatment (if any) has already been tried. In this respect, there is little difference between the range of questions which should be asked for an adult illness (*see* Section 18.3) and one occurring in a child. What may be more important is the fact that the child may be causing the parent emotional stress and distress. Pharmacists should therefore be capable of reassuring the parent with a calm confident manner that recognises the parent's concern but confirms the best course of action.

Many community pharmacies also stock a wide range of babycare products, and pharmacists should be prepared to assist the parent in the selection of foods, feeding utensils and sterilisation equipment, especially for the mother of a first-born child.

This chapter will detail some of the problems most commonly presented to the pharmacist and outline the action to be taken in each case. The terms infant and baby are used here to define a child under one year of age, and a young child is classed as between one and three years of age.

15.2 Infant feeding

Breast versus bottle feeding

The vital importance of adequate nutrition during the first 12 months of life is highlighted by the fact that a baby trebles its weight and that 50% of postnatal brain growth takes place during this time. Breast feeding is considered to be the best form of feeding for almost all infants, but until recent years it was diminishing, particularly in developed countries through increased wealth, changes in maternal lifestyle (e.g. returning to work immediately after a baby has been born) and a reluctance to feel tied to the baby for long periods. Many more women have elected to bottle feed the baby at the earliest opportunity, although active education campaigns have now marginally increased the proportion of breast-feeding women in developed countries at different stages after the birth. Between 1995 and 2000 all countries in the UK showed an increase in the incidence of breast feeding, as had been the case between 1990 and 1995. The rate for England and Wales increased from 64% in 1990 to 68% in 1995 to 70% in 2000. In Scotland the corresponding increases were from 50% to 55% to 53%, while in Northern Ireland the incidence was 36% in 1990, rising to 45% in 1995 and 54% in 2000. There is a strong correlation between the incidence of breast feeding and mothers of first rather than later babies, continued education after 18 years of age, a high social class grading (i.e. professional and managerial as opposed to unskilled women), and living in more affluent parts of a country. Conversely, unhappy experiences or difficulties with breast feeding a first-born child reduce the likelihood of subsequent children being put to breast.

The characteristics of human milk

The structure of the breast and a description of the secretion of milk is given in Section 7.6. Immediately after birth, the initial secretion from the mammary gland is a thin yellow fluid, colostrum, which is high in protein, vitamin A and cyanocobalamin, lymphocytes and macrophages but low in fat content. Colostrum also contains a polypeptide (the mucosal growth factor) specific for intestinal mucosa, and this stimulates DNA synthesis and activates cell division. The presence of the polypeptide leads to the rapid growth of the jejunum and ileum necessary for the adaptation of the infant's intestine to milk feeding. Colostrum also contains a high concentration of immunoglobulins, and in particular immunoglobulin A (IgA), which retard the multiplication of bacteria and viruses within the gastrointestinal tract. Early suckling by the baby increases the secretion of colostrum, but within 72–96 hours the thin fluid is gradually replaced by milk. The term mature milk is used for the milk produced by about the tenth postnatal day.

Breast milk contains all the ingredients necessary to sustain the baby during the early months of its life (Table 15.1). Carbohydrate is present predominantly in the form of the disaccharide lactose, which is broken down in the intestine into galactose and glucose by the enzyme lactase (*see* Lactose intolerance, Section 9.2.2). About half of the baby's energy requirements are provided by fat (predominantly triglycerides surrounded by lipoprotein) and approximately one quarter by saturated fatty acids. The fatty acid content of breast milk largely reflects the content in the maternal diet. By comparison, the protein content of breast milk is low and about 60% of this is comprised of easily digestible whey rather than relatively indigestible curds (casein). The benefits of whey are that it also supplies albumin, lactoferrin (a protein which binds iron and makes it unavailable for bacterial multiplication), lysozyme and IgA. Other constituents include minerals, enzymes (e.g. lipase) and cellular components (e.g. macrophages) which help to resist the development of infection in the milk ducts and in the infant's intestine. The vitamin content of a healthy and well-nourished mother's milk should be adequate to supply all of the infant's requirements. However, if the vitamin D and vitamin K status of the mother is low, there is a risk of the development of rickets and late haemorrhagic disease.

Other forms of milk

It is also useful at this stage to briefly consider the different types of milks that are available for

Table 15.1 Mean composition of mature mother's milk per 100 mL

Energy (kcal)	70
(kJ)	293
Protein (g)	1.3
Lactose (g)	7
Fat (g)	4.2
Vitamins	
A (μg)	60
D (μg)	0.01
E (mg)	0.35
K (μg)	0.21
Thiamine (μg)	16
Riboflavine (μg)	30
Nicotinic acid (μg)	230
Pyridoxine (μg)	6
Cyanocobalamin (μg)	0.01
Total folate (μg)	5.2
Pantothenic acid (μg)	260
Biotin (μg)	0.76
Ascorbic acid (mg)	3.8
Minerals	
Sodium (mg	15
Potassium (mg)	60
Chloride (mg)	43
Calcium (mg)	35
Phosphorus (mg)	15
Magnesium (mg)	2.8
Iron (μg)	76
Copper (μg)	39
Zinc (μg)	295
Manganese (μg)	1.2
Chromium (μg)	0.6
Selenium (μg)	1.4
Iodine (μg)	7
Fluorine (μg)	7.7

purchase. Pasteurised (household or doorstep) milk is whole cow's milk which has been heat treated to remove potentially pathogenic microorganisms (e.g. *Brucella melitensis* and *B. abortus*, *see* Brucellosis, Section 5.2). Cow's milk is unsuitable as a main drink for children under 12 months of age, but can be used in custard and consumed as yoghurt from the age of six months. If the milk is not pasteurised or there is no refrigerator in the home, the milk should be given to children under 12 months of age only after it has been boiled. The main disadvantage of heat treatment of cow's milk is that destruction of its useful components (e.g. lactoferrin and IgA) also takes place. Almost all infant feeding with cow's milk has now been replaced with modified formula dried milk powders or evaporated milk. Whole cow's milk should be a staple component of the diet in all children over one year of age.

Homogenised milk is a form of pasteurised milk which has been further treated to evenly distribute the fat throughout the milk. Sterilised milk is homogenised milk that has been further treated, and has a thickened texture. The partial removal of water from pasteurised milk by evaporation forms evaporated milk, and the addition of sugar to evaporated milk produces condensed milk. The content of all of these milks is essentially the same as cow's milk, and the same limitations on its use in children under one year of age apply.

Other milks are available in which the nutritional content can vary significantly from its original value. Skimmed and semi-skimmed milk are by-products of the butter- and cream-producing industries which utilise the fat in milk. Almost all of the fat has been removed from skimmed milk, while about half is removed to produce the semi-skimmed form. Although these milks contain a high proportion of proteins and calcium, the lack of fat and fat-soluble vitamins may lead to energy and vitamin deficiencies. Skimmed and semi-skimmed milk should not be given to children under 12 months of age and are not recommended for those under five years of age. Of course, semi-skimmed milk is commonly used in many households these days and for the sake of convenience it may therefore be introduced from two years of age provided the overall nutritional status can be assured.

Dried milks may provide a convenient form of milk in situations where refrigeration is lacking or ineffective. Low-fat milks and many of the infant formulas are available in this form. They are reconstituted by the addition of water, although the manufacturer's instructions must be closely followed.

Ultra heat-treated (UHT) milk has been subjected to higher temperatures than pasteurised milk and, when it is aseptically packed, it may remain drinkable without refrigeration for up to three months.

Goat's milk is of a similar composition to cow's milk and has been used in an attempt to overcome allergy to cow's milk. However, like cow's milk, its use is not recommended for babies under six months of age as it is deficient in many vitamins and pasteurisation cannot be guaranteed.

Advantages of breast feeding

It is recognised that breast milk is the best source of nourishment for the newborn baby and for the first six months of life. Most mothers can provide adequate nutrition from the breast to nourish their infant for the initial four to six months of life. It also encourages the development of a close maternal–child bond and allows the mother the opportunity to rest and relax. Mother's milk provides an excellent source of nutrition, it is sterile, and is normally readily available at the correct temperature. The presence of breast milk in the infant's intestine encourages the growth of *Lactobacillus bifidus* which promotes the absorption of nutrients (the bifidus factor). The resultant intestinal acidification limits the growth of *Escherichia coli* and reduces the incidence of gastroenteritis.

Equally important is the protective role afforded by the transfer of immunoglobulins in the milk which are recognised by the infant as 'self', and this may reduce the risk of eczema in infancy and asthma in later life. There is also a decreased tendency to obesity in breast-fed infants and this is important as obese babies are liable to grow into obese adults. One consequence of breast feeding is reduced fertility in the mother, which results in ovulation in only about 10% of women, although breast-feeding mothers should be warned that this is not an efficient means of contraception. The choice of contraception after the birth of the child may be determined by the reduced inhibitory effect that progestogen-only contraceptives have on milk flow in comparison to combined oral preparations.

The reasons for not breast feeding

Social and domestic reasons are commonly cited for the reluctance to start or continue breast feeding. Bottle feeding allows the mother to return to work and may also be carried out in public places (e.g. at work or in shopping centres) where breast feeding can be unwelcome and inconvenient. The mother may also be uncertain whether the infant is getting sufficient nourishment and have greater confidence once a bottle of milk has been seen to be taken.

Insufficient milk is often stated as a cause of stopping breast feeding at an early stage after the birth. Mothers should be advised that the hormonal stimulation of milk flow will only occur if attempts to breast feed are continued, perhaps with decreasing intervals between attempts. If bottle feeding is introduced at the first sign of limited flow, the lack of demand for breast milk will aggravate the situation.

Medical reasons which preclude breast feeding are rare. They include the presence of galactosaemia and phenylketonuria in the infant, serious maternal diseases (e.g. heart disease, depressive disorders and glomerulonephritis) which inhibit lactation, and the presence of the human immunodeficiency virus (HIV) in the mother. However, maternal infection with hepatitis B virus is not a contraindication, with appropriate immunisation of the infant. Difficulties in breast feeding are compounded with twins and multiple births, as the demand for milk cannot always be met. Some women may develop painful engorged breasts, particularly in the first days after birth, because the supply is greater than demand. The pressure and pain generated further reduces the flow of milk and the swollen nipple limits the infant's ability to suckle. The milk may be expressed using a breast pump (*see below*) following warm bathing of the breast, or gentle palpation to reduce the build-up and relieve symptoms. Sore or cracked nipples may arise through incorrect positioning of the infant at the nipple. Application of a skin disinfectant or cleansing agent (BNF 13.11) may be beneficial, in conjunction with avoidance of the affected breast.

Accessories for breast feeding

Breast pumps

One method of overcoming some of the social problems cited as reasons for stopping breast feeding, and which may be particularly useful for the mother who wishes to return to work, is to express the milk so that it may be given at a later time, possibly by someone other than the mother. Milk may be expressed manually or with a breast pump. The manual method will be demonstrated to the mother by the midwife or a nurse. Breast pumps can be purchased from a pharmacy and it is important that pharmacists should be aware of their mode of action in the event of queries from the mother.

Milk should ideally be expressed in the early morning or, if night-time feeds have ceased, in the evening. The two most common types of breast pump are the bulb pump and the syringe pump. The bulb pump consists of a plastic or rubber bulb which is gently squeezed to draw milk from the breast into a reservoir. In the syringe pump, the suction necessary to draw milk from the breast is provided by the downward movement of a piston, and milk is drained into the body of the syringe. Cleanliness in the use of both types of pump is essential. Hands should be washed, and the pump and receiving containers washed and sterilised. Once the milk has been collected, it can be stored for up to 48 hours in a refrigerator. The milk can also be frozen and kept for up to six months.

Nipple shields

The presence of a prominent nipple is obviously essential for successful breast feeding. If the nipple sits within a pit, or retracts into a depression when the areola is gently squeezed, the nipple is described as inverted or pseudo-inverted respectively. This may be corrected by the use of a nipple shield, which consists of a saucer with a central orifice through which the nipple is inserted. A plastic cup fits over the saucer and the complete assembly is worn inside the bra to exert continuous pressure on the areola and encourage the nipple to stand proud within the shield. Women should be advised to wear the shields for short periods initially from about half way through the pregnancy, and gradually increase the wearing period until they can be tolerated throughout the day. They should not be worn at night.

Nipple shields may also be worn if the nipple is cracked or sore. In this case, the shield may be positioned over the nipple and held in place whilst the infant feeds through it.

Bottle feeding and infant formula milks

Infant formula products are manufactured so as to approximate the composition of mother's milk. Most products are based on cow's milk, even though cow's milk has a different composition to human milk. Some formulas are based on other proteins (e.g. soya protein) for infants with special nutritional requirements (*see below*). Energy values, the ratio of saturated to unsaturated fatty acids, and the levels of carbohydrates, essential fatty acids, and most major minerals and trace elements are similar in breast milk and infant formula products. The main differences in composition of manufactured milks occur in the increased energy content derived from protein; the absence of immunoglobulins, lymphocytes and macrophages; the lack of non-protein nitrogen (e.g. urea, creatinine, uric acid and free amino acids); and increased concentrations of vitamins and iron.

Modifications to cow's milk

The modifications to cow's milk involve changes to carbohydrate, fat, or protein content (*see* Table 15.2).

Added carbohydrate, substituted fat, or both
Cow's milk contains considerably less carbohydrate, more protein, and slightly less fat and provides roughly the same energy value as human milk. The addition of carbohydrate is the simplest modification made to cow's milk in the preparation of infant formula milks. Dilution with carbohydrate reduces the overall concentration of protein and minerals, and reduces the risk of renal overload produced by excess protein (*see also below*). Lactose is not used as the sole diluent, as overloading the infant's intestine with this carbohydrate may lead to frothy diarrhoea and reduced absorption. Instead, maltodextrins, singly or in combination with sucrose, are used to supplement the additional lactose.

Another alternative is to substitute cow's milk fat by vegetable and animal fats that are more

Table 15.2 Comparison of the two main types of infant milk formulas used in the UK, derived from cow's milk

	Added carbohydrate and substituted fat (less highly modified formulas)	Demineralised whey (highly modified formulas)
Protein (whey:casein ratio)	20:80	60/70:40/30
Carbohydrate	Lactose, often with maltodextrins and sucrose	100% lactose
Fat	(Blend of vegetable oils, cow's milk fat, and occasionally animal fat (e.g. butterfat))	
Examples in the UK	Cow and Gate Plus SMA White Cap Farley's Second Milk Milumil	Cow and Gate Premium SMA Gold Cap Farley's First Milk Aptamil

easily digested. This modification is in addition to the extra lactose. Examples of substituted fat and added carbohydrate products (also described as less highly modified formulas) available in the UK are SMA White, Farley's Second Milk, Milumil, and Cow and Gate Plus.

Demineralised whey formulas Cow's milk contains more protein than human milk, and a much higher percentage of the protein is curds. Milk in which the fat and the curd protein has been removed is referred to as whey. It consists of water-soluble whey proteins, lactose (which constitutes all the carbohydrate content) and minerals. Demineralised whey is formed when the mineral content of whey is reduced by ion exchange, electrodialysis (the passage of an electrical current through whey) or ultrafiltration (the total mineral content is not eliminated completely).

Demineralised whey formulas are prepared by the addition of skimmed or semi-skimmed milk (which re-introduces curd protein but in a smaller concentration, lactose and minerals), a blend of butterfat (or modified beef fat) and vegetable oils to provide a fat content similar to breast milk, and vitamins. Examples, which are also referred to as highly modified formulas, available in the UK are SMA Gold, Cow and Gate Premium, Aptamil, and Farley's First Milk.

Infant formula milks are manufactured as ready-to-use preparations or as powders to which water must be added. It is essential that the manufacturer's guidelines for preparing feeds are rigidly followed. Some preparations are reconstituted by the addition of a stated volume of water, while others must be made up to the required volume by adding a sufficient quantity of water. Incorrect preparation (e.g. adding too much powder by compressing or not levelling off the powder in the scoop) is potentially harmful and carries the risks of hypernatraemia and obesity. Hypernatraemia can arise because the sodium content of cow's milk is about three times that of mother's milk. Obesity may be more common in bottle-fed babies because the mother may not respond to the baby's satiety when given a bottle, whereas on the breast the baby will determine its own degree of satiety. Parents should also be reminded that scoops are invariably *not* interchangeable between different product manufacturers, and the use of an inappropriate scoop may also lead to errors in quantities given.

The water used to reconstitute feeds should be boiled and allowed to cool to about 60°C. Water should be used direct from the mains and not from a water-softened supply, as the sodium content may be significantly increased in the latter. Water from a kettle which has been repeatedly boiled should not be used as repeated evaporation can lead to concentration of minerals.

The different characteristics of whey proteins and curd proteins have already been mentioned. In addition to the classifications mentioned above, infant formula milks may also be termed whey-based milks and curd-based milks (in which

Table 15.3 Quick reference guide to the use of milks in infants and young children

	Under 6 months	6–12 months	Over one year
Breast milk	Ideal, for at least four months	May suffice in conjunction with other foods	Not suitable as a sole source of nutrition
Whole cow's milk	Unsuitable	Pasteurised milk may be given but not as a main drink; non-pasteurised only if boiled and cooled	Essential component of diet
Skimmed milk	Unsuitable	Unsuitable	Not recommended for under-fives
Semi-skimmed milk	Unsuitable	Unsuitable	Not recommended for under-twos
Infant formula milks	Suitable	Suitable on their own or to supplement breast milk	A useful adjunct to solids
Follow-on milks	Unsuitable	Suitable on their own or to supplement breast milk	A useful adjunct to solids

the dominant protein is casein), the latter containing higher concentrations of protein and minerals. The curd-based milks correspond to the added carbohydrate and substituted fat (less highly modified) milks, and the whey-based milks to the demineralised (highly modified) products. It is common for mothers to change from one milk formula to another, sometimes more than once, usually on the basis that the infant does not appear to be satisfied on the current product. The proportion of babies receiving curd-based milks increases with age, on the basis that the relatively indigestible curds provide an increased sense of satisfaction within the intestine, although there appears to be little nutritional difference between the two types nor any hard evidence that curd-based milks do increase satiety.

Follow-on milks

A follow-on milk is one which can be used to satisfy the nutritional requirements of an older infant (over six months of age) and the young child. These milks differ from the infant formula milks described above in that they contain a higher concentration of electrolytes and protein, although the content is still less than that of cow's milk. Iron and vitamin D levels are greater than in infant formulas and cow's milk and this may be of particular benefit to Asian children and to children from low-income families who are often found to have these specific deficiencies.

It is doubtful whether there is significant benefit of changing an infant to a follow-on milk if the child is satisfied with its current feed. Breast milk or infant formula milk, supplemented as required by intermittent solids, should provide all the nutritional requirements. If the mother insists on a change, follow-on milk is certainly preferable to cow's milk.

A reference guide to the suitability of different milks in infants and young children is given in Table 15.3.

Cow's milk substitutes

Some infants may develop sensitivity to the protein of cow's milk present in infant formula products or be intolerant to lactose. Allergy to cow's milk is relatively rare (with an incidence of about 2%) and although it should not be dismissed as unimportant, efforts should be made to dissuade mothers from choosing cow's milk substitute products in the absence of appropriate medical diagnosis.

Other conditions may also benefit from the temporary or more prolonged withdrawal of cow's milk protein, although all indications must be medically supervised by the child's doctor or dietitian, or both. The most common indications for the use of cow's milk substitutes are:

- atopic disease with suspected food allergy
- cow's milk-protein intolerance
- following gastrointestinal surgery
- galactosaemia
- intractable diarrhoea in infancy
- lactose intolerance.

Gastrointestinal symptoms of cow's milk-protein intolerance include diarrhoea (which may be bloody and accompanied by mucus), vomiting and colic. The presence of atopy may be characterised by eczema, urticaria, erythema and rhinitis.

Cow's milk substitute preparations contain casein hydrolysate or soya protein. They contain no lactose, and reduced absorption of minerals from these formulas has been reported. Methionine, vitamin K and iodine are additions made during manufacture. Casein hydrolysate preparations are hypoallergenic and are preferable to soya products for the treatment of gastroenteritis, as the intestinal mucosa may also be sensitised to soya protein. Cow's milk substitutes should not be used in an attempt to prevent the development of atopic disease in a child who may be at increased risk of hypersensitivity (e.g. an infant with one or both parents known to have a history of atopic disease). Additionally, it is essential to ensure that the product is suitable as a sole source of nutrition for an infant (e.g. comminuted chicken meat must be supplemented with carbohydrate, fat, vitamins and minerals, whereas other sources are nutritionally complete). The consumer should also be aware of the wide variety of other soya liquids and powders available. These must under no circumstances be used instead of nutritionally complete soya preparations for infants. Soya milk drinks are also inadequate substitutes for cow's milk for infants under five years of age and should not be recommended.

Parents of infants with cow's milk-protein intolerance may require special guidance on the purchase of other nutritional products for their child, especially once weaning starts. Beef (which possesses a range of antigens similar to milk), milk and milk products must be avoided, and it is essential that the labels of all products are carefully scrutinised. Many manufacturers have increased the range of information on labels to assist in appropriate choice.

Feeding equipment

The basic feeding equipment necessary for non-breast milk feeding is a bottle and a teat. However, there is a bewildering array of shapes and sizes of these items and many mothers may be confused about the differing claims made by manufacturers. Pharmacists should be familiar with the range of equipment (a complete list is given in Table 15.4) and act on their own experiences as parents or, equally importantly, listen to others with experience so they can form an opinion about its suitability.

Bottles should be wide-necked to allow easy cleaning and made of unbreakable plastic. Graduation marks are often included on the outer surface but their accuracy cannot always be guaranteed, especially on bottles without straight sides. The bottle should have a cap to allow the teat to be inverted and covered during travelling.

The selection of the correct size of teat and teat hole is more critical. If the teat hole is too small, the infant will swallow air and develop gastric distension which can cause underfeeding. The child will also become frustrated because of the effort necessary to take milk, and feeds can take as long as 60 minutes. Ideally, the milk should drip out of the teat in a fine, steady stream at the rate of about one drop per second, and feeds should take no longer than 30 minutes. Teat holes which are too small may be enlarged by using a red-hot needle. One end of the needle

Table 15.4 The range of equipment necessary for bottle feeding

Bottles (6–8)
Teats (the same number as bottles +1)
Bottle-cleaning brush
Sterilising solution/tablets
Sterilising vessel
Flat-edged knife (for levelling off powder scoop)
Salt
Graduated measuring jug (if feeds are not prepared in the bottle)

should be placed in a cork which is held while inserting the other end of the needle into the blue part of a flame. When the tip of the needle glows it should be pushed through the rubber teat.

Repeated washing and sterilising of teats will cause their gradual deterioration and softening. Conversely, a new teat can be firm and relatively inflexible and may benefit from gentle squeezing in warm water to soften it.

Sterilising feeding equipment

It is essential to ensure impeccable standards of hygiene during the preparation of bottle feeds for infants and young children. The ability of the child to counteract the accidental introduction of microorganisms is poorly developed, and gastroenteritis can easily result from poor hygiene. Before feeding utensils are sterilised, it is important to remove any remnants of dried milk as these can inactivate sterilising solutions. Bottles and teats should ideally be rinsed in cold water immediately after a feed to prevent the deposition of a thin film of dried milk on their inner surfaces. At a later convenient time, the bottle should be cleaned with washing-up liquid and warm water using a brush kept exclusively for this purpose. Thorough cleaning of the teat can be ensured by everting it, sprinkling the inner and outer surfaces with salt, and rubbing between the fingers. Teats and bottles should be rinsed after cleaning.

Equipment used to give the feed must be sterilised by chemicals (e.g. dichloroisocyanurate and sodium hypochlorite) which release chlorine, or by boiling. Sterilising agents may be purchased as a solution or tablets and made up according to the manufacturers' instructions. Fresh solutions must be made up every 24 hours. A large plastic container (of capacity sufficient to hold at least two feeding bottles) is filled with water and the sterilising agent added according to the manufacturers' instructions. Bottles and teats must be completely submerged within the sterilising solution. Pinching teats to release trapped air bubbles helps to prevent them from floating to the top of the solution. The time taken to achieve sterilisation with chemical agents varies, and the utensils should be left in the solution until they are required. The manufacturers' instructions about rinsing before use with boiled and freshly cooled water must be followed.

An alternative form of sterilisation is to boil the feeding equipment. The bottles should be immersed completely in water in a large saucepan used exclusively for this purpose. The water should be heated to boiling point, the saucepan covered, and teats added once the water has started boiling. Teats and bottles should remain in the boiling water for at least 5 minutes, after which time the teats should be transferred to a sterile lidded jar. The bottles may be left in the covered saucepan until required.

Microwave ovens should not be used to sterilise feeding equipment immersed in water or in sterilising solutions.

Introducing solids

The gradual introduction of semi-solids to a milk diet is termed weaning. This should not be attempted until the infant is at least four months of age, and ideally not later than six months of age. Before four months of age, the intestine of the infant is immature and has an increased permeability, especially to protein. Excessive absorption of protein may trigger allergic reactions in susceptible individuals, and the lack of maternal IgA in infants who have been bottle fed almost from birth may render them more vulnerable to this effect. Solids also contain a higher electrolyte (e.g. sodium) concentration than breast milk. The concentrating ability of the infant's kidneys is not fully developed in the early months of life and therefore high levels of fluid intake are essential to allow the complete excretion of excess dietary electrolytes. Although the kidneys of most infants may adapt satisfactorily in health, any degree of dehydration (e.g. caused by infection, diarrhoea or vomiting) will considerably overstress their function and lead to hypernatraemia. A third reason to delay the introduction of solids for as long as is practical is that the presence of baby foods may have a deleterious effect on the absorption of iron from breast milk.

The earliest foods given during weaning include rusks, non-wheat cereals or commercial weaning foods. Cereals such as baby rice are popular as they provide a soft texture and familiar flavour when mixed with milk. Alternatively, cooked and puréed vegetables and non-citrus fruits may be equally appropriate. However, infants should not be fed on fruits and vegetables alone because their bulk can induce satiety at a level of energy intake which is too low to satisfy the demands for growth in a young child. The introduction of puréed home-prepared meals may be a useful means of familiarising the baby with the family's diet. Small amounts only (e.g. one to two teaspoonfuls) should be given initially and limited to one meal a day. The quantity may be gradually increased to about three to five teaspoonfuls within two weeks (although individual requirements may vary significantly), and subsequently to two to three meals a day by six to eight months. Foods containing wheat, eggs and citrus fruits should not be introduced under the age of six months because of the risk of allergic reactions.

Most pharmacies offer a wide range of strained or homogenised foods specially manufactured as 'first foods', and these offer a wide variety of choice (e.g. from beef broth with vegetables to fish in cheese sauce) and flavours (e.g. bland and savoury). Manufactured products are also available as gluten-free, milk-free, egg-free, vegetarian and sugar-free (e.g. all savoury foods). Many are also advertised as free of preservatives, colourings and artificial flavourings. Their use can be ideal for busy mothers, in situations where adequate hygiene may be lacking, or as temporary measures (e.g. on holiday), but it is preferable to recommend that mothers introduce a puréed form of the rest of the family's food at the earliest opportunity. Although high standards of cleanliness and hygiene must be maintained, sterilisation of feeding equipment is not necessary once weaning has started.

15.3 Feeding and gastrointestinal problems

An infant who appears to be healthy may suffer from a variety of gastrointestinal problems. These problems may be related to the intake of food or they may be a consequence of underlying illness. It is important that pharmacists can recognise the possible cause and suggest appropriate action.

Food allergy and intolerance

There is growing concern among parents about food allergy in their infants and children, with many parents believing their child is allergic to something they eat or drink. The term allergy here is used to mean a reaction to food that is immune mediated. This should be distinguished from food intolerance, a term which includes allergy, but which is used to describe a range of other reactions as well, such as adverse effects arising from enzyme deficiencies (e.g. lactose intolerance), pharmacological effects and other poorly defined idiosyncratic responses.

The true magnitude of food allergy and intolerance is not known due to the paucity of robust data in this field, but it appears that food allergy has increased in the last 30 years and will probably continue to do so in the foreseeable future. Estimates suggest, however, that the current prevalence is not as high as many people believe. Thus, about 1–2% of children suffer from allergy and about 5–8% from food intolerance. The prevalence in adults is less, but overall as many as 20% of people believe themselves to be allergic or intolerant to certain foods. Nevertheless, although the numbers of children who truly have food allergies and intolerances may be small, these conditions should not be dismissed of no importance, because for the sufferer, the consequences in terms of ill-health may be considerable, and in some cases, life threatening.

Both genetic and environmental factors influence susceptibility, but the most potent risk factor for food allergy in infancy and childhood appears to be a history of atopy in the family. Exclusive breast feeding for the first three to four months may reduce the risk of developing allergic disease in a susceptible child and should in any case be encouraged for many other reasons in addition to reducing the risk of atopy. There is some evidence that exclusive breast feeding for four to six months may be particularly important for infants at high risk of atopy, although benefits beyond six months are unclear. Avoidance of dietary allergens during pregnancy is sometimes suggested to protect the unborn child, but evidence for any benefit from this practice in relation to development of allergy in the infant is also unclear, and it should not be recommended without reference to a dietitian.

Common foods that can cause allergic reactions include cow's milk, eggs, peanuts, soya beans, fish, shellfish and wheat. A variety of fruits and vegetables can also cause allergic reactions. Cow's milk is the most common culprit and a cow's milk substitute may be prescribed where allergy has been properly diagnosed (*see* Section 15.1). Treatment of all food allergies depends on appropriate diagnosis and the use of a nutritionally balanced diet that excludes the offending food. Achieving such a diet can be quite difficult and whenever substantial dietary restriction is envisaged, the best advice for the parent is to seek the advice of a dietitian. Sticking to an exclusion diet can be a challenge particularly for older children once the parents have less control over what the child eats. Another challenge is the need to read food labels carefully for the offending substance, and if in any doubt, parents should speak to manufacturers directly.

Although there is a tendency for food allergy to decrease or disappear with time, allergies to milk, egg and wheat and particularly peanuts are more resistant, and there is less of a tendency for them to remit in the older child. In the most severe cases of childhood food allergy, where, for example, the child is at risk of anaphylaxis or has asthma, it is important that the child and/or a carer (e.g. a school teacher) should have access to adrenaline and know how to use it. In addition, information concerning the child's allergy should be available to others at all times, for example, through the wearing of a Medic-Alert bracelet.

Colic

Incessant crying by an infant, especially in the early evening, can often be attributed to colic. The infant may cry and even scream at the same time as drawing the knees up to the chin and going red in the face. The phenomenon occurs commonly in infants of between one and four months of age without any outward signs of accompanying illness or distress. Cuddling and picking up the child may produce little improvement and many parents become considerably upset at its daily recurrence.

A wide range of factors have been linked to the development of colic (e.g. under- and overfeeding, tension, allergy, and under- and overcossetting), but the pathophysiology is unknown. Gripe waters containing carminatives (e.g. dill) are traditional remedies, and preparations containing simethicone may be useful, but reassurance and checking the suitability of feeding teats may be more constructive advice.

Regurgitation and acute vomiting

After a feed, many babies will regurgitate small quantities of food, especially if winding is encouraged. This is described as posseting and may be due to aerophagia caused by inappropriately sized teats (*see* Section 15.2). If the regurgitation is more voluminous, it may be caused by over-zealous feeding, which should be discouraged to minimise the likelihood of obesity. Positive action which may be taken to encourage the retention of feeds is to thicken the milk (e.g. with carob flour) and to feed the child lying down but tilted up at an angle of 10–20 degrees. Frequent small-volume drinks can also help to prevent the risk of dehydration caused by regurgitation.

Vomiting which is more persistent and forceful and stained with blood or bile, but not always directly related to the intake of food, may indicate a more serious problem and should be referred. Common causes include a mild infection (e.g. upper respiratory-tract infection or gastroenteritis) or, more rarely, a serious infection (e.g. meningitis), gastrointestinal obstruction (e.g. pyloric stenosis) and metabolic disease (e.g. galactosaemia). Other conditions which may produce vomiting include intolerance to the feed and concomitant drug administration. Infants suffering from any of these conditions will be clearly less well than those who are posseting.

Diarrhoea and constipation

As in adults, definitions of diarrhoea and constipation are only valid when an individual's normal bowel movements are considered (*see* Section 18.3). Like adults, there is a wide range of frequency of bowel movements, although, in general, there is a gradual decrease as the neonate progresses through the first few weeks of life. When the infant is fed solely on breast milk, the stools are light yellow and pasty, and may be passed as frequently as after every feed or as infrequently as once every three days. Bottle-fed infants tend to have more frequent and malodorous stools which are firmer and more brown than those of breast-fed infants. If the stools appear too compacted, extra water may be advisable between feeds.

On the rare occasions when mothers seek advice from pharmacists about diarrhoea in infants under three months of age, the child should be immediately referred to the doctor or to the local casualty department. The loss of fluid and electrolytes at this age can be potentially fatal. Similar action should be taken with older infants with diarrhoea who appear listless, or who are excessively irritable and display a cold grey skin that is dry or clammy. These are the cardinal signs of dehydration.

Acute diarrhoea may be treated by the administration of an oral rehydration solution (BNF 9.2.1.2). Instructions issued with proprietary preparations should be followed, but pharmacists may usefully give additional advice. About 50–100 mL of oral rehydration solution should be given for each loose stool for initial rehydration. Breast-fed infants will derive an adequate volume of fluid from the mother's milk, but it is important to supplement the fluid intake of non-breast-fed infants with water, giving a volume equal to about half the volume of rehydration solution administered. This supplement should be given about 2–3 hours after administration of the rehydration solution. Older children may prefer weak tea or dilute fruit juice and they should be encouraged to drink as much as they want.

Both breast and bottle feeding can be continued during the period of diarrhoea. Young children who have been weaned onto solids should be starved for only as long as they refuse food, after which time mild bland foods may be gradually re-introduced. Extra foods should be given in the convalescent period following diarrhoea to allow growth catch-up. Preparations containing kaolin should be avoided in infants in deference to the prime objective of rehydration. If diarrhoea is persistent but relatively mild, the child should be referred to investigate possible causes (e.g. coeliac disease, cystic fibrosis, lactose intolerance and milk-protein intolerance).

Constipation in infants and young children is rare and is commonly caused by inappropriate fluid or dietary intake or by changing from breast to bottle milk, and less commonly to disease (e.g. megacolon and Hirschsprung's disease). Treatment should be directed to the underlying pathology, or at modifying fluid or dietary intake. In the young child who has been weaned, constipation may be rectified by an increase in the intake of fibre, fresh fruit and vegetables. If no significant improvement is seen following these measures, the child should be referred.

15.4 Growth, development and failure to thrive

Height and weight

Some pharmacies offer public use of weighing scales and devices for measuring height. However, all pharmacists must be prepared to respond to queries from mothers about the 'normal' and 'abnormal' weight and height for an infant of a particular age.

Growth is measured in terms of height and weight. In a child under two years of age height is measured with the child lying down, although at this age weight is a more useful (and more accurately taken) measure of growth. Growth is most rapid during the first six months of life and gradually slows towards 12 months of age.

Many mothers plot the infant growth on height and weight (anthropometric) charts and compare progress with average charts. Average charts display the height and weight of the average (50th percentile), and the normal range of weight and height (which extends from the

Table 15.5 Major milestones during the first 12 months of life

1–2 months	Responds to speech by smiling and, when placed on his stomach, can lift and maintain head in the same plane as the body for a brief period. Reflex grasping will be gradually replaced by more voluntary holding.
3 months	Will grasp hands for short periods and, when lifted upright from a horizontal position, can support his head. A rattle can be held when placed in the hand and there will be a directional response to noise.
4 months	When placed on his stomach, the infant will be capable of lifting up his head and chest by propping himself up on his arms. He will also be capable of sitting when supported.
5–6 months	Capable of rolling from his back to his side and can successfully reach for an object. Will grasp items between both hands (e.g. often suck his own toes).
7 months	Can sit upright briefly when unsupported, although is dependent on his hands for support. Can feed himself by holding a biscuit.
8 months	Can sit upright without support, although cushions should be placed around the child as a precautionary measure. Larger items (e.g. play-bricks) can be picked up and grasped.
9 months	Crawling may be attempted when the child can support himself on his hands and knees. He can also pull himself to a standing position, hold his feeding bottle, and be capable of imitating words such as 'mama' and 'dada'.
12 months	May be able to walk when supported (although walking can start anytime between 10 and 18 months of age), say several words, feed himself, accept and give objects, and speak two or three meaningful words.

3rd to the 97th percentile, i.e. 3% of children fall above or below the normal range). If the mother queries the growth of her child when plotted on such a graph, it is important to remember that individual measurements are of little value and that all charts are constructed for the average normal child. A non-average child is not necessarily abnormal. The greater importance of trends in growth rather than individual measurements should be stressed, but if the mother requires further reassurance she should be referred to her health visitor or doctor.

Developmental milestones

Although timing may be subject to wide variations, an infant will reach different milestones in development in a well-defined sequence. It is important to remember that development always proceeds from head to toe. The earliest milestones reflect the control gained in posture and movement of the head, followed by increased grasping and manipulative control of the hands, and culminating in the ability to crawl, stand and eventually walk. The major milestones during the first 12 months of life are outlined in Table 15.5.

Failure to thrive

A child who is healthy looking, alert and responsive is thriving and should give no cause for concern. However, one who is continually crying, lethargic, who consistently falls outside the third percentile on the growth chart, or who develops a sudden decline in a previously acceptable pattern of growth, is described by the term 'failure to thrive'. Other indications of illness in infants and young children are an inability to attract or maintain the child's attention, irritability or restlessness.

Prenatal causes of failure to thrive may be a consequence of maternal intake of drugs and alcohol, smoking or viral infection. After birth, it may be caused by inadequate food offered or taken (*see* Section 15.2), chronic infection (e.g. of the urinary tract), or malabsorption (e.g. caused by coeliac disease or cystic fibrosis). Rarer causes include milk-protein intolerance, congenital heart disease, cirrhosis or renal insufficiency.

Occasionally, rejection of the child by one or both parents, or marital discord, may contribute to the condition. In all cases of failure to thrive, the mother should be referred to the doctor.

Teething and fluoride supplementation

Teething

In child health, the eruption of the deciduous (milk or baby) teeth commonly starts at six months of age and is generally completed by two years of age, although there can be wide variations in timing. The earliest signs of the gradual movement of the teeth from their prenatal position beneath the gums are increased salivation and crying.

The first teeth to appear are commonly a pair of central lower (mandibular) incisors followed after about six to eight weeks by the corresponding upper (maxillar) incisors. In all subsequent eruptions, the upper usually precede the lower teeth. A further pair of lateral incisors subsequently erupts, one on each side of the initial pair. The first pair of molars appear on the upper jaw at between 12 and 15 months, and the spaces between these and the incisors are filled by the canine (eye) teeth at 16–20 months of age. Finally, the four second molars penetrate the gums to the rear of the first molars at about two years of age, with one on each side and on each upper and lower surface. The 20 deciduous teeth are lost steadily between 6 and 12 years of age and replaced by 32 permanent, slightly larger teeth.

Teething can be a traumatic period for children and their parents. In addition to the symptoms described above, the cheeks and gums may become inflamed and reddened and there may be pyrexia, loss of appetite and disturbed sleep patterns. Although dribbling may occur, particularly during eruption of the front teeth, other symptoms may be worse when the rear teeth push through. General measures which may help relieve discomfort include providing a firm object to chew (e.g. a teething ring, rusk or raw carrot) and gentle rubbing of the surface of the gums by the parent with a washed finger.

Fluoride supplementation

Pharmacists are often asked about the fluoride content of the drinking water in their locality, and to advise on the necessity of dietary supplementation in infants. If doubt exists as to whether the local water supply is supplemented with fluoride, the local water authority should be contacted. Fluoride has been shown to significantly reduce the incidence of dental caries by reducing the solubility of enamel, remineralising any early lesions of dental caries, and directly inhibiting plaque bacteria. Daily administration of tablets or drops may be beneficial where the fluoride content of drinking water is less than 0.3 parts per million (300 μg/L) (Table 15.6). The importance of the local action of fluoride at the site of application is emphasised by the greater benefits which are conferred by dropping the fluoride onto the tongue or sucking the tablets, rather than swallowing. Pharmacists should

Table 15.6 Dosage recommendations for administration of fluoride supplements to infants (BNF 9.5.3)

Fluorine content of water (μ/L or parts per million)	Age of infant	Dose of fluoride ion daily (μg)
Less than 300	under 6 months	none
	6 months to 3 years	250
	3–6 years	500
	over 6 years	1000
300–700	under 3 years	none
	3–6 years	250
	over 6 years	500
More than 700	all ages	not recommended

advise that fluoride supplementation should not be given to infants less than six months of age (BNF 9.5.3). No benefit in the prevention of dental caries in children has been demonstrated from the mother taking fluoride supplements during pregnancy.

If the water supply is fluoridated, parents must be warned that additional fluoride administration is unnecessary. Excess fluoride can lead to dental fluorosis, in which the enamel becomes demineralised, pitted and has a white mottled appearance on the surface of permanent teeth (which start to develop within the gums from birth).

Pharmacists should be prepared to advise parents on the supply of fluoridated toothpastes which comprise almost all sales of dentrifices. Most young children start to use toothpaste by 18 months of age, although appreciable quantities may be swallowed by children up to three years of age. To prevent ingestion of excessive quantities of fluoride and the resultant dental fluorosis, the amount of toothpaste used by a child living in an area where the water is fluoridated should be limited to the size of a small pea. Once a child has reached six years of age, effective spitting out after teeth-cleaning is possible and the amounts ingested are minimal. Fluoride is present in toothpaste at a concentration of 1000 parts per million as sodium monofluorophosphate (0.8%), stannous fluoride (0.4%) or sodium fluoride (0.25%). Mouthwashes and topical applications (e.g. gels, varnishes or solutions) may also be applied by dentists. However, because they are packaged in large volumes (e.g. 250 mL) and contain a lethal quantity of fluoride, they are not recommended for home use.

Sugar-free medicines for children

A greater public awareness of the potential cariogenic effects of regular intake of glucose, sucrose and fructose has led to the increased introduction of sugar-free formulations of medicines for children. While any attempts to reduce the dietary intake of sugars is to be welcomed, it must also be borne in mind that many of the preparations for children are given for short-term treatment only. The presence of potentially cariogenic carbohydrates will have little effect on the overall development of dental decay. Reformulated preparations must retain the properties conveyed by the sugar-containing ingredient (e.g. syrup), which may include preservation, viscosity and sweetening.

The greatest benefit of the use of sugar-free formulations is for the chronic administration of medicines to children (e.g. in the treatment of epilepsy, cystic fibrosis and asthma) or in giving those which are to remain in contact with the teeth (e.g. teething gels). The replacement of syrup BP by an alternative vehicle for preparations in chronic use has been encouraged by the BP Commission, although sugar-based extemporaneous preparations have not been subject to amendment. It is obviously essential that pharmacists are aware of the correct diluent for reformulated products.

The BNF includes information on those preparations which are sugar-free.

15.5 Immunisation of infants and young children

Pharmacists can play a vital role in advising parents of the importance of immunising their children against infectious diseases. Parents may be concerned about the relative merits and potential drawbacks of immunisation (e.g. to protect against pertussis and the MMR vaccine) and may ask pharmacists, as readily accessible healthcare professionals, for advice. Pharmacists should be familiar with immunisation schedules and, in particular, be prepared to respond to items in the local and national press about the use of vaccines. They should also be aware of the contraindications to immunisation and the possible reactions which may be caused by the administration of a vaccine.

This section will not detail the causes and symptoms of the diseases for which childhood immunisation is recommended. These may be found in the relevant monographs in Chapter 5. Detailed information on the preparations available and their administration is given in BNF, chapter 14.

The importance of immunisation

At birth, an infant is protected initially from pathogenic microorganisms by the transfer of maternal IgG antibodies across the placenta. Consequently, the infant may be passively immunised against a range of infections (e.g. chickenpox, measles and mumps), although significant by its absence from this category is pertussis. However, antibodies derived from the mother gradually decline during the first six months of life and are replaced by the infant's own antibodies produced in response to antigenic challenge. This explains why infants of under six months of age rarely contract infectious illnesses but the incidence gradually increases with age. An infant below six months of age which the mother considers is showing signs of an infectious disease must always be referred, particularly as severe complications may develop in very young babies.

Active immunity is promoted in the young child by the administration of inactivated or live attenuated microorganisms or their products (e.g. toxoids) (Table 15.7). The administration of these products stimulates a primary response, the production of predominantly IgM antibodies. Subsequent injections cause an accelerated response, resulting in high levels of IgG antibodies which can remain in the circulation for months or years. Even if the levels fall off, the mechanism for their production has been sensitised and a rapid increase in antibody levels will follow re-inforcement (booster) vaccination.

The concept of herd immunity is important in immunisation programmes. Herd immunity is the immunological status of the community against a particular infectious disease. It is desirable to ensure that the uptake of vaccination is as high as possible. This helps to ensure that protection is afforded not only to those who have been immunised, but that the overall reduced incidence of the disease in the population significantly lowers the risks of infection to those who cannot, or will not, be immunised. Additionally, most infectious diseases are rarely completely eradicated from the environment or healthy carriers and, if the level of herd immunity falls, epidemic outbreaks quickly develop.

The role of pharmacists

Pharmacists can play an important role in advising parents on the importance of immunisation and help increase the uptake of vaccine use. However, in order to be capable of responding to enquiries from parents, pharmacists must be aware of current information on the relative risks and benefits associated with individual vaccines. In particular, they should bear in mind that sensationalised media reports (which commonly provoke enquiries by anxious parents) are invariably unbalanced and stress only the rare adverse reactions to a vaccine.

The positive contribution to health of the immunisation programme has meant that many young parents are happily unaware of the dangers to their children of infectious diseases. They may not have witnessed the trauma undergone by a child with pertussis and are ignorant of the congenital malformations (e.g. deafness, cataracts and heart problems) that may result from an attack of rubella in the mother during pregnancy (*see below*). Similarly, the perception of measles as a minor illness (despite the associated risks of permanent brain damage which may be fatal) may contribute to parents' belief that

Table 15.7 Types of vaccines

Live attenuated	Inactivated	Toxoid
Measles, mumps, rubella (MMR)	Pertussis	Tetanus
Polio (oral form)	Polio (parenteral form)	Diphtheria
Rubella		
BCG (tuberculosis)		

the risks of vaccination are greater than the condition itself.

In immunisation, perhaps more than any other health topic, it is important that all health professionals give uniform advice to parents. Conflicting advice (e.g. from pharmacists, health visitors and doctors) confuses parents and can undermine their confidence in the healthcare team. The importance of uniform advice illustrates the benefits of maintaining good relations and communications between professionals at all times. Pharmacists could usefully be encouraged to contact other members of the team to clarify what advice they are giving.

A brief description of some of the facts concerning the use of specific vaccines is presented below.

The use of specific vaccines

The contraindications to vaccination are specified in the BNF and pharmacists should consult this source for current information. Parents may ask a range of questions about other aspects of childhood vaccination and some of the following points have been confirmed by the Joint Committee on Vaccination and Immunisation. All children with asthma, eczema, allergic rhinitis and any history of allergy or minor upper respiratory-tract infections should follow the standard vaccination schedule. Treatment with antimicrobials, topical or inhaled steroids, and breast feeding are also not contraindications. Adherence to the immunisation schedule is preferable, but a child over a particular age will still be immunised. No allowance is necessary for premature infants, who should be immunised at three months of age and not three months after the expected date of delivery. Mothers who report that the child has already had pertussis, measles or rubella should be advised that immunisation for these diseases is still necessary. A child who has missed one dose in a course of vaccination should continue the course immediately with the previously missed dose and subsequent recommended dose intervals. No attempt should be made to 'catch up' on the original dosage schedule by increasing the dose or reducing the dosage interval.

Pertussis

Although concern had been previously expressed, the publication of and widespread publicity given to a paper in 1974 which linked pertussis vaccination and neurological damage had a dramatic effect on the uptake of the vaccine. Vaccination rates dropped from 80% in 1968 to 30% in 1976, but have since regained some ground. Parental fears, however, of the production of convulsions, cerebral palsy and mental retardation can be countered by an incidence of less than 1 in 100 000 injections. In the UK, the Joint Committee on Vaccination and Immunisation has advised that absolute contraindications to pertussis vaccine are any severe local or general reaction to a preceding dose. In cases of a history of cerebral irritation or damage in the neonatal period, a history of convulsions, or children with parents or siblings that have a history of idiopathic epilepsy, special care must be taken in the administration of the vaccine. In each of these cases there may be an increased risk from vaccination, but this must be balanced against the potentially greater risks from an attack of the disease. Vaccination may be postponed if the child has an acute febrile, and particularly respiratory, illness but these are not contraindications.

Measles

Although measles has the reputation of a minor illness, it can produce a range of complications (e.g. otitis media, respiratory-tract conditions and, rarely, encephalitis) which warrant strict attention to its prevention. An attack of measles has particularly high mortality in children with malignant disease (e.g. acute lymphoblastic leukaemia), even during remission. This can be an especial problem as these children cannot be given live vaccines.

The single measles vaccine which was introduced in 1968 is no longer available in the UK, and has been replaced by a trivalent vaccine for measles, mumps and rubella (MMR). Since the introduction of these vaccines, measles, mumps and rubella have become rare diseases. However, on the basis of research, primarily from one unit, which suggested that vaccination predisposed children to inflammatory bowel disease and autism, some parents and health professionals have become concerned about the safety of MMR vaccine. This has led to a decline in uptake and fears of impending outbreaks. However, research showing these links has been criticised for being flawed, and many experts say there is no good scientific evidence to support a link between MMR vaccine and autism or inflammatory bowel disease. Moreover, the use of separate vaccines is untried and untested. There is also considerable evidence for the safety and efficacy of MMR vaccine, and while the final decision rests with the parents, pharmacists should not be concerned about recommending its use (*see* BNF, chapter 14 and www.immunisation.org for up-to-date information).

Rubella

Rubella in a young child is itself a relatively minor illness and would not be a case for urgent and effective immunisation programmes. However, rubella contracted during pregnancy can have devastating effects on the health of the unborn child, as characterised by the congenital rubella syndrome.

The policy of protecting women of childbearing age from the risks of rubella in pregnancy has been replaced by a policy of eliminating rubella in children. The single antigen rubella immunisation programme for 10–14-year-old girls has been discontinued and replaced by the MMR vaccine, which is given during childhood.

However, some women of childbearing age may not have been immunised and every effort should be made to identify and immunise all those who are seronegative. This also applies to those who might put pregnant women at risk of rubella infection (e.g., doctors and nurses in obstetric units). A single antigen vaccine is still available for these purposes. Active immunisation is also offered to seronegative women after pregnancy, although strict contraceptive cover must be ensured for at least three months after vaccination.

Poliomyelitis

The risks of paralysis produced by poliomyelitis have been almost completely eradicated through effective immunisation programmes introduced at the end of the 1950s. Protection can be given by an oral live attenuated vaccine (the Sabin vaccine), or a slightly less vigorous response may be obtained by an inactivated vaccine (the Salk vaccine), given parenterally. In the UK, the injectable form is given only if the patient requiring protection is pregnant or immunocompromised. There is a very small risk of developing poliomyelitis following oral vaccination, and there is also a risk that the disease can be passed on from an individual who has been recently immunised to an unprotected person. Theoretically, the virus can become strengthened on transmission and may lead to full-blown poliomyelitis, although this occurs in only about 1 in 5 million immunisations. To minimise this risk, parents who are uncertain of their immune status should also receive vaccination at the same time as their children. The household contacts (e.g. parents and siblings) of immunosuppressed children should, therefore, receive only the injectable form.

Mumps

Mumps immunisation is given as part of the vaccine for mumps, rubella and measles (MMR). A similar triple vaccine is given to infants in the USA at 15 months of age. It may be effective for up to 12 years.

Meningitis

Since 1999 meningitis (for protection against infection by sero-group C of *Neisseria meningitidis*) has been a component of the primary course of childhood immunisation.

Haemophilus influenzae type B

Children under the age of 13 months are at high risk of *Haemophilus influenzae* type B infection and the vaccine is a component of the primary course of childhood immunisation.

Diphtheria

In the UK, diphtheria vaccination has resulted in the virtual elimination of the infection. Natural

Table 15.8 Characteristics of common infectious illnesses in children

Infection	Incubation period (days)	Distinguishing features	Degree of infectivity	Isolation required?
A. Bacterial infections				
Diphtheria	2–5	Wide range of symptoms from mild pyrexia, headache, and fatigue to difficulty in swallowing caused by a greyish-white membrane over the tonsils. In severe cases the membrane may spread to the trachea and bronchi, and may cause death if breathing is obstructed.	Very	Yes
Erysipelas	2–5	Tender red swollen areas over the face, arms, and legs preceded by headache, fever, malaise and vomiting.	Rendered non-infective if treated	Necessary until treated
Meningococcal meningitis	1–5	Upper respiratory-tract infection may occur 2–3 days before severe symptoms. Early signs include fever, lethargy, drowsiness, crying, irritability, neck stiffness and dislike of bright lights. Confusion and coma can follow within 12–24 hours. A macular rash occurs in about 50% and can develop into petechiae.	As long as microorganisms are in the throat and nose	During initial 24 hours
Pertussis	7–10	Catarrhal stage of 7–14 days characterised by symptoms of an upper respiratory-tract infection followed by a dry cough. In the paroxysmal stage, cough becomes more severe and spasmodic and is terminated by a whoop. It may be accompanied by vomiting and convulsions.	Mainly during catarrhal stage	Avoid contact with babies
Scarlet fever	2–3	Sudden onset with sore throat, fever, malaise, vomiting, and 'strawberry tongue'. Rash appears after 24–36 hours on chest, neck, and arms and spreads to rest of body. The rash is formed of red dots on pink skin. The tongue is white but peels to leave a red raw surface. The skin may peel after three days.	Non-infective after starting antibiotic treatment	Until treatment
Tetanus	1–14	Muscular rigidity of jaw and face, and stiffness of neck, back muscles, and abdomen. Spasms may occur on external stimuli.	None	None
B. Viral				
Chickenpox	14–16	Early signs are fever, malaise, and anorexia. Macular rash develops into fluid-filled blisters in crops over the trunk, face, and scalp. Limbs are rarely affected. Blisters encrust and the scabs formed gradually fall off.	Highly infectious before rash appears – less so later	No

Table 15.8 Continued

Infection	Incubation period (days)	Distinguishing features	Degree of infectivity	Isolation required?
Infectious mononucleosis	28–49	Early signs of headache, fatigue, and malaise are followed by sore throat, fever, and lymphadenitis usually in the neck. Faint rash may occur.	Low	No
Measles	8 to 14	Prodromal symptoms include fever, sneezing, cough, catarrh, and conjunctivitis. White spots surrounded by a red ring (Koplik's spots) occur on the buccal mucosa. Fever declines, spots disappear, and are replaced by a rash starting on the neck (behind the ears) and face and spreading to the rest of the body. Fever rises again with the rash.	Catarrhal stage is very infectious	No
Mumps	14–18	Pain and swelling of the salivary (and especially parotid) glands. Dry mouth, malaise, fever and chills.	14–21 days	No
Roseola infantum	5–15	Abrupt onset fever with lethargy and occasionally convulsions. Fever abates on appearance of macular rose-pink rash on trunk. The rash fades on pressure and may last a few hours or several days.	Unknown	No
Rubella	14–21	Tender lymph nodes in the neck with malaise, headache, slight fever, sore throat, and conjunctivitis. A fine red rash starts on the face and trunk and fades as the areas of erythema merge over the rest of the body. The rash fades within three days.	Until the rash fades within three days	No

immunisation, therefore, cannot occur and the high acceptance rate must be maintained to protect the population from a resurgence of the disease. This may occur especially following introduction from overseas.

Tetanus

Tetanus vaccination, since its introduction in the UK in 1961, has resulted in a sharp decline in the incidence of children developing tetanus. However, adults continue to be affected at a higher rate because of the lack of vaccination in their childhood. This emphasises the need to maintain a high acceptance rate.

Tuberculosis

The incidence of tuberculosis declined after 1950 but has increased in recent years, and fatalities still occur in the UK. In addition to the recommended schedule for vaccination against tuberculosis, BCG vaccination may be offered when an infant is known to be in contact with a case of active respiratory tuberculosis, to children in immigrant communities who exhibit a higher incidence of tuberculosis, and if an infant is to travel to a high-risk area or where crowded conditions prevail. Vaccination is also offered to children between 10 and 14 years of age.

15.6 Other common infectious illnesses in children

The information in Table 15.8 summarises the characteristics of common infectious illnesses in children and is intended to act as an *aide-mémoire* for pharmacists. More detailed information on the individual diseases can be found in the relevant monographs in Chapter 5.

16

Care of older people

16.1 Concepts in ageing

Ageing is an inescapable fact of life. The inevitable sequel to ageing is death, which is necessary for the prolonged vigour and health of the species. Death prevents a population explosion and allows youth to develop its full potential.

The process of ageing may be described as either primary or secondary. Primary ageing represents a natural decline in efficiency characterised by loss of homeostasis and weakening of physical structure. Both effects eventually lead to a breakdown in health, followed by death. Secondary ageing results from disease and trauma, causing irreversible degeneration. Although it is impossible to slow the rate of primary ageing, the incidence of disease, and by inference longevity, can be influenced by lifestyle and medical care.

It has been suggested that ageing arises from an accumulation of errors of metabolism throughout life. Essential biological materials (e.g. RNA and DNA) may be damaged by environmental and chemical factors (e.g. radiation and drugs). If the number of accumulated errors exceeds a predefined level, cells and tissues may lose their functional capacity and perish.

Why has the elderly population increased?

The average life expectancy at birth in the UK has risen by more than 20 years since the beginning of the twentieth century. The infant mortality rate has dropped radically from 200 per 1000 live births in the nineteenth century to the present rate of approximately 15 per 1000. This upsurge in survival rate can largely be attributed to better environmental and health conditions. The net result of these changes is that there has been a shift in the population distribution, with considerably greater numbers of people over 65 years of age. In the UK, since the early 1930s, the number of people aged over 65 has more than doubled and today a fifth of the population is over 60. Between 1995 and 2025 the number of people over the age of 80 is set to increase by almost a half and the number of people over 90 will double.

Why does care of older people create special problems?

Older people are a diverse group with a wide range of needs, and this should be taken into account when care is being provided. Some are as fit and active as people many years younger, while others are frail and require a high level of care. Moreover, in recent years attitudes to ageing have changed somewhat and retirement is no longer seen as a preparation for decline. Respect for older people, although not as great as it was during the early years of the twentieth century, say, is increasing again, and older people should not be viewed as a burden on society.

Many problems of older people are socio-economic as well as medical. The background to such problems should be borne in mind by pharmacists in their day-to-day contact with older people. Lack of status and loneliness contribute to undermine the confidence of old people. Almost half the over-75s live alone. Nearly one-third of this group have never had children, and of those that have, nearly 40% have outlived their progeny. Many therefore may have little family contact or support, relying on friends, neighbours and other members of the local community for their social contacts. The support of health and welfare organisations, either directly or through families, friends and neighbours, provides a tremendous asset in promoting happiness.

The problems caused through inadequate social contacts are increased when considerable age is attained. It has been estimated that 80% of the over-85s need assistance with everyday living. Other elderly, but perhaps slightly younger, groups who may be equally dependent include the recently bereaved, and those discharged from hospital who must re-adapt quickly to their home environment if they are to survive.

About 6% of older people live in care homes and the numbers are increasing. Hospitalised patients are located either in geriatric wards, psychiatric hospitals or in acute services. Almost two-thirds of general and acute hospital beds are used by people over 65. A new layer of care, between primary and secondary care, is being developed to help prevent unnecessary hospital admissions, support early discharge and reduce or delay the need for long-term residential care, and older people will be the main users of these services.

A significant majority of older people live in the community, either coping independently, living with relatives, or relying on the social, welfare and health services. The pharmacist, in providing a vital link in the healthcare team, can make a significant contribution to the health and quality of life of this ever-increasing group, mainly in helping to ensure that medicines are appropriately prescribed and appropriately used, but also in helping older people to maintain a healthy lifestyle.

16.2 How does ageing affect body systems?

Ageing comprises many physiological changes which are reflected by alterations to body composition from 40 years of age. These changes occur in the absence of any associated pathology. Table 16.1 lists the common diseases of the elderly by physiological system.

Table 16.1 Common disorders of older people

Classification	Example
Gastrointestinal tract disorders	Cholestatic jaundice
	Constipation
	Crohn's disease
	Diverticular disease
	Dysphagia
	Gallstones
	Malabsorption syndromes
	Peptic ulceration
	Pyloric stenosis
	Reflux oesophagitis
	Ulcerative colitis
Cardiovascular system disorders	Arrhythmias
	Arteriosclerosis
	Hypertension
	Ischaemic heart disease
Respiratory system disorders	Chronic bronchitis and emphysema
Nervous system disorders	Depressive disorders
	Insomnia
	Parkinsonism
	Stroke
	Transient ischaemic attacks
Infections	
Bacterial	Infective endocarditis
	Pneumonia
	Pulmonary tuberculosis
Viral	Herpesvirus infections
	Influenza
Endocrine system disorders	Diabetes mellitus
	Hyperthyroidism
	Hypothyroidism
Genito-urinary system disorders	Renal failure
	Urinary incontinence
	Urinary-tract infection
Malignant diseases	Bladder cancer
	Breast cancer
	Gastro-intestinal tract tumours
	Gynaecological tumours
	Haematological malignant tumours
	Lung cancer
	Prostate cancer
Blood disorders	Anaemias
	Thrombocytopenia
Musculoskeletal and connective tissue disorders	Giant cell arteritis
	Gout
	Osteitis deformans
	Osteomalacia
	Osteoporosis
	Polymyalgia rheumatica
	Rheumatoid arthritis
Eye disorders	Cataract
	Glaucoma
Ear, nose and oropharynx disorders	Impacted wax
	Otosclerosis
	Speech disorders
Skin disorders	Decubitus ulcer
	Eczema
	Pruritus
	Psoriasis

Gastrointestinal tract

Salivary secretion is reduced, causing dry mouth and difficulty in swallowing. Gastric acid secretion is also decreased, and may be associated with atrophy. Malabsorption may develop, affecting particularly iron and calcium absorption.

Intestinal motility can become disorganised, causing constipation, and this may be aggravated if the elderly person is immobile.

Cardiovascular system

Reduced lean body-mass decreases metabolic demands, which in turn reduces cardiac ouput. Consequently, regional blood-flow is altered, with a greater proportion of the available supply going to the heart and brain at the expense of the kidneys and muscle.

Fibrosis occurs everywhere, producing increased rigidity and decreased elasticity. The pressure within the system, and hence the work required by the heart to eject the stroke volume, is raised.

The heart is less able to respond to stress because the cardiac reserve capacity is reduced.

The older person will notice this particularly during exercise.

Respiratory system

Atrophy of lung tissue produces an increase in the size of the alveoli, thinning of their walls and loss of elasticity. Chest diameter may increase while residual volume and vital capacity are reduced. The risks of respiratory infection are increased due to unsatisfactory functioning of the cilia, reduced cough efficiency and increased dead space.

Nervous system

The effects of ageing on the nervous system are amongst the most important in considering the care of older people.

Manifestations of degenerative CNS changes (e.g. forgetfulness and movement disorders) are due primarily to faulty neurotransmitter metabolism rather than loss of neurons. Increased confusion may be related to decreased cerebral blood-flow. Sleep disorders increase in frequency, particularly the incidence of awakening during the night.

Changes in autonomic function cause bradycardia and a significant incidence of thermoregulatory disorders. The failure of vasoconstriction during cold weather can produce hypothermia, while inefficient vasodilatation or sweating in hot conditions produces overheating.

Endocrine system

Plasma thyroid hormone concentrations are marginally reduced in older people. The rate of secretion of insulin in response to glucose loading is also decreased. Normal fluid intake should be maintained to prevent dehydration because the ability of the kidney to respond to the secretion of vasopressin is reduced. Conversely, compensatory thirst mechanisms are impaired as a result of ageing.

In general, other endocrine functions are not significantly affected by ageing.

Renal function

There is an age-related decline in kidney function even in the absence of disease. The kidneys lose approximately 20% of their weight and 30% of their functioning glomeruli between 40 and 80 years of age. Despite compensatory hypertrophy, renal function decreases by up to 50% by 80 years of age. Such changes are particularly important in the pharmacokinetic assessment of drug administration (*see* Section 16.3 *below*).

Reproductive system

In the female the decline of ovarian function at the menopause is one of the most dramatic indications of ageing. This change is accompanied by variable degrees of atrophy of the hormone-dependent organs (i.e. the vulva, vagina, cervix, corpus uteri, Fallopian tubes and ovaries).

In the male, gonadal function may remain intact or decrease only slowly with age.

Blood

Blood elements are remarkably durable. Age-related degeneration does not occur unless it is a consequence of associated pathology (e.g. iron depletion).

Any increased tendency towards thrombus formation is usually due to the effects of arteriosclerosis rather than an increased platelet count. This tendency is further increased with lack of mobility.

Musculoskeletal system and connective tissue

A progressive reduction in muscle strength results from cell loss and disorganisation. Lost muscle is replaced by fat and connective tissue, maintaining or even increasing total body weight.

The effects of ageing on connective tissue are widespread. Cross-linkages are formed within the collagen macromolecule, causing loss of elasticity of blood vessels, muscle and joints. Damaged cartilage has little capacity for repair, resulting in osteoarthritis.

Changes in the skeletal structure can be profound. Reabsorption of bone exceeds its formation, especially in postmenopausal women and, as a result, osteoporosis develops, which may lead to fracture (e.g. in the hip).

Skin

The appearance of the skin is one of the most obvious indicators of increasing age. It sags, thins and becomes wrinkled. Loss of melanin may produce skin with a white translucent look, or of a yellow appearance with blotches. Subcutaneous fat and vascularisation are reduced, increasing the likelihood of the development of decubitus ulcer.

Eye

Symptomatic visual changes develop from middle age. Presbyopia, due to hardening of the lens, is one of the most common. It renders accommodation for reading small print and other forms of close work more difficult. The symptoms of this degenerative process, which is normally complete by 65 years of age, can benefit from the use of appropriate spectacles.

After this age, visual changes are more subtle and increasingly occur as a consequence of associated degenerative and pathological processes. Examples of such changes include increased opacity of the lens, and pupillary deterioration. The size of the pupil and its ability to react to alterations in light intensity are reduced. Changing glasses at this stage is not usually of significant benefit.

Ear

Presbyacusis is a natural consequence of ageing. It is characterised by high-tone deafness, and affects mainly those over 60 years of age, especially men.

Although wax volume is not increased, its consistency is changed. It thickens and impacts as it dries, resulting in hearing difficulties.

16.3 How does ageing affect drug handling?

Even in the absence of disease, age-related changes occur in the absorption, distribution, metabolism and excretion of drugs. The existence of multiple pathologies further complicates these pharmacokinetic parameters. Exaggerated drug action and side-effects are examples of resulting pharmacodynamic changes.

Absorption

The oral route is the most common route for drug administration. However, impaired drug absorption may occur in older people due to a reduction in the volume of secretions, blood-flow to intestinal tissue, and the number of absorbing cells. Delayed gastric emptying also occurs.

Drugs actively transported from the gut (e.g. calcium, thiamine and iron) are more susceptible to these changes than those which enter the circulation by passive diffusion (e.g. aspirin and paracetamol).

In common with patients of any age, older people with renal disease may suffer from nausea, vomiting and diarrhoea. Cardiac disease causes poor tissue perfusion. In both instances, drug absorption will be reduced.

Distribution

The distribution of drugs is influenced by plasma protein binding, blood-flow rate, and tissue fat content. Circulating drugs are bound largely to the plasma protein, albumin. Plasma-albumin concentrations decrease with age, particularly in patients with chronic liver and renal disease. As a result, the amount of free (and therefore active) drug is increased, resulting in enhanced therapeutic effects.

The blood-flow rate is an important determinant of drug uptake by tissues. The total systemic perfusion and cardiac output decrease with age. As a result, the proportion of blood entering the liver and kidneys is reduced, significantly affecting drug kinetics.

The amount of body fat increases with age, while body water, intracellular water and lean body mass decrease. This may be significant in drug kinetics, producing an increase in the half-life of highly lipid-soluble drugs (e.g. benzodiazepines). When great age is attained (>85 years of age), the increased amount of body fat reverts to normal.

Metabolism

In the aged, the capacity of the liver to metabolise drugs is reduced by up to two-thirds of the normal adult capacity. Consequently drugs for which the liver is the major site of metabolism (e.g. non-steroidal anti-inflammatory drugs, antiepileptics and analgesics) exhibit increased plasma concentrations and a longer half-life.

The rate at which drugs are delivered to the liver is an important factor in metabolic capacity. In older people, liver perfusion can fall by 40–45%, and this significantly affects the metabolism of hypnotics (e.g. chlormethiazole) and antipsychotic drugs (e.g. chlorpromazine).

The effects of microsomal enzyme induction are reduced by ageing, possibly causing toxic effects through increased plasma concentrations. Alternatively, enzyme inhibition may be reduced, thus increasing the rate of metabolism of a second drug, and rendering the dose ineffective. Such considerations emphasise the problems of polypharmacy in older people.

Excretion

As a result of the decline in renal function with age, the excretion of many drugs and metabolites is significantly impaired. However, the use of creatinine clearance values as an indicator of the glomerular filtration rate may be misleading in older people as creatinine production decreases with age. In conjunction with decreased kidney function, almost normal plasma creatinine concentrations may be measured even in the presence of considerable kidney disease.

Pharmacodynamics

Many older patients exhibit altered responsiveness to medicines. The brain shows particularly increased sensitivity, and patients become confused and disorientated at doses normally well tolerated by younger patients. Medicines which cause particular problems are hypnotics, antimuscarinics, dopamine agonists and warfarin. Conversely, decreased tissue sensitivity may occur on ageing (e.g. to isoprenaline or propranolol).

16.4 How do the increasing numbers of older people affect pharmacy?

As part of the UK's National Service Framework for older people, the Department of Health has highlighted the important role that pharmacists can play in the care of the elderly both in the community and in hospital.

As people get older their use of medicines tends to increase. Four in five people over 75 take at least one prescribed medicine, with 36% taking four or more medicines. Older people are also significant users of over-the-counter medicines. This creates a challenge to ensure that medicines are prescribed appropriately and used effectively, taking into consideration how the ageing process affects the body's ability to handle medicines (*see* Section 16.3), the existence of multiple diseases and the complicated medication regimens that are sometimes required.

There is a growing weight of evidence that adverse reactions to medicines are a significant cause of morbidity and hospital admissions. Moreover, while in hospital, 6–17% of older in-patients experience adverse drug reactions. Other problems in older people (as well as in others) include failure to prescribe medicines (e.g. antithrombotic treatment to prevent stroke, antidepressants) for patients who would benefit, failure to use medication as intended, changes in medication after discharge from hospital, which can create confusion for the patient, and sometimes duplication and/or omission in treatments. Dosage instructions on medicine labels are sometimes inadequate (e.g. 'Take as directed' or 'Take as required'), such that neither the patient nor the carer has access to the appropriate dosage information. Repeat prescribing can often be inefficient in that patients have to order different items at separate times, and may unintentionally receive the same medication at separate times, leading to wastage. Some older people may have difficulty in getting to the surgery to collect their prescription or to have it dispensed. Collection and delivery services for prescriptions have been successful in circumventing such difficulties, but many older people and their carers require further help and advice with their medicines.

Commonly reported symptoms in older people

In the pharmacy, the conditions most commonly reported by older people are arthritis and related conditions, followed closely by difficulty in walking and unsteadiness, forgetfulness and poor vision. In addition, falls are a common problem. Older people will often also describe deafness, back pain, breathlessness on slight exertion, swollen feet and indigestion. However, patients are frequently unable to describe their symptoms because of restricted knowledge and vocabulary. Older people have been shown to be especially poor at describing detail and depth of symptoms, and pharmacists must therefore be patient and often penetrating in their questioning. (For further discussion on all aspects of responding to symptoms *see* Section 18.3.) Moreover, older people often have a tendency to think that their symptoms are due entirely to old age and that there is little that can be done to help so they fail to mention them.

Pharmaceutical care in older patients

Prescribing and taking medicines is easy. But prescribing and taking medicines well is more difficult. Pharmaceutical care, which is a patient-centred approach that aims to care for all a patient's medicine-related needs, focuses on helping to ensure that medicines are both prescribed and used well. This may involve pharmacists in various activities such as prescribing support to doctors, medication review with both patients and carers, monitoring and review of repeat prescribing.

Prescribing support

Many pharmacists now provide prescribing advice and support to general medical practitioners and primary care organisations (primary care groups and trusts). Some advice may involve a reduction in prescribing, for example where a certain medicine is not required either because it has doubtful efficacy or because it is not indicated in that particular patient, while other advice might involve increased prescribing, such as appropriate use of antidepressants and antithrombotic therapy to prevent stroke and myocardial infaction. The BNF states that in older people, particular care is needed in the prescribing of diuretics, antihypertensives, digoxin, psychotropics, hypnotics, anti-Parkinson medication and non-steroidal anti-inflammatory drugs (NSAIDs).

Medication review

Because of the tendency for older people to use more medicines than younger people, medication review and monitoring of treatment is particularly important in this age group. While time sometimes does not allow for complete evaluation of all older people's medication as frequently as would be ideal, it is useful to target those older people who may be at particular risk of medicine-related problems, such as failure of therapy, compliance issues, drug interactions, adverse reactions and so on. These include older people prescribed four or more medicines, those in care homes, those who have suffered medication-related problems in the past or who have suffered recent adverse changes in their health status (e.g. dizziness, confusion).

Older patients recently discharged from hospital are also worthy of special consideration, in that patients or GPs may restart medication unintentionally that was stopped in hospital, or patients may run out of medication that was started in hospital and fail to continue with it as intended. Such discrepancies can be reduced dramatically by improved communication between hospital and community pharmacists, (e.g. ensuring that the community pharmacist receives a copy of the discharge prescription).

Monitoring of treatment

Older people should be monitored to ensure that medicines are producing the intended effects, are not creating any adverse effects and remain appropriate for the individual in the prescribed dosage. It is also important to check whether the patient has any problems taking the medicine and if so what can be done to help. In older people, difficulties in taking medication are exacerbated by impaired mental ability, inability to open containers and poor eyesight.

A further complication is the tendency to hoard medicines. Many pharmacists will have experience of vast quantities of medicines returned by relatives of recently deceased older patients, and this is also reflected in campaigns to encourage the return of unused and unwanted medicines.

Memory aids have been developed to improve compliance, together with supplementary written instructions. While these aids do not provide containers of BP standards, their use may be of benefit to some patients.

Repeat prescribing

Many pharmacists are involved in review of repeat prescriptions, and this is an intervention that can improve the quality of prescribing and patient care. Important issues to consider in reviewing repeat prescriptions include appropriate synchronisation of quantities and duration of therapies, given that some medicines are taken when required and in others quantities used are imprecise (e.g. creams and ointments). Under- and over-ordering of regular medication also needs to be identified and mechanisms to flag up the need for medication review and laboratory testing (e.g. urea and electrolytes, liver function tests) should be in place.

Self-medication

While polypharmacy in prescribed medicines has been recognised as a problem in the care of older people, concurrent self-medication with non-prescription medicines is an acknowledged factor that can aggravate management. Pharmacists should be alert to requests for non-prescription medicines, especially if a prescription has just been dispensed.

Falls

Falls are a major cause of disability and mortality among older people and in the UK, each year, nearly half a million older people have to go to hospital following a fall. Pharmacists can play an important role in reducing the risk of falls in older people by providing information on how to prevent them and by conducting reviews of medication that may precipitate falls. Medicines that increase the risk of falls include those that cause hypotension, sedatives and hypnotics and drugs that cause dehydration (e.g. diuretics, laxatives). Pharmacists should also be aware of older people who take oral corticosteroids because these increase the risk of osteoporosis.

Care homes

Homes for the older people may be classed as residential homes or nursing homes, although the distinction between the two is blurring. In England and Wales, residential homes are not required to employ medical or nursing staff, and are registered and inspected by the Social Services Department of the Local Authority; nursing homes provide professional care by registered nurses and are registered and inspected by the Health Authority.

In care homes, medicines may be administered by care staff, but many patients are encouraged to take charge of their own medicines and administration wherever possible. All prescription-only medicines should be supplied on a named-patient basis, with full directions on each container.

It is important that pharmacists visit care homes to ensure that records are kept correctly, check and advise on the storage of medicines, and provide any further professional advice needed, particularly medication review where appropriate. Pharmacists should also take note of any non-prescription medicine stores in the residential home, confirming there are no potential interactions between prescription and non-prescription medicines.

16.5 Advice on lifestyle

A healthy lifestyle is as important for older people as for other age groups and pharmacists can help to encourage this in their older patients. Stopping smoking, regular exercise, moderation in alcohol consumption and healthy eating are issues which the pharmacist can discuss with older people.

Healthy eating

Current healthy eating guidelines which emphasise the importance of starchy, high-fibre carbohydrate, fruit and vegetables, together with moderation in fat, sugar and salt are in general as applicable to older people as to younger adults. However, these guidelines do need to be applied with common sense, particularly in older people who may be frail, chronically sick or losing weight. There is no need to deny a 92-year-old woman a couple of custard creams or a bar of chocolate with her afternoon tea.

Energy requirements tend to decline with age, but the need for protein, vitamins and minerals does not, emphasising the need for a diet which is nutrient-dense, i.e. rich in vitamins and minerals without being rich in calories. Fat restriction remains relevant in people up to the age of 75, but after that it will probably be too late to reverse the atherosclerotic effects of a high-fat diet and fat restriction will be less beneficial. Moreover, fat reduction is not appropriate in patients who are frail or losing weight, or who have a small appetite. This is because fat is energy-dense and therefore an easy way to boost calorie intake.

Other nutrients which may require particular emphasis in older people include iron, since anaemia is a common feature in this age group, calcium, because it may help to slow down the rate of bone loss, and the B group vitamins, particularly folic acid and vitamin B_{12}. Older people often have reduced absorptive capacity for vitamin B_{12}, and marginal intakes may result in deficiency.

Vitamin D also needs to be considered because it controls calcium absorption. Dietary sources are few and far between (e.g. oily fish, eggs, margarine) and sunlight exposure, which is a significant source of vitamin D, is often limited in older people. A vitamin D supplement (10 μg daily) is therefore a wise precaution.

Malnutrition

Pharmacists should be aware of the risks of malnutrition in older people. This is an increasing problem in the UK, and figures show that at least 40% of older people admitted to hospital are malnourished. Malnutrition has profound effects on health, including reduced immune response and muscle strength, predisposition to hypothermia, impaired wound healing and recovery from illness, apathy, depression and self-neglect and increased length of hospital stay. Pharmacists are well placed to identify older people who may be at risk of malnutrition. Such people include those who live alone, those who have recently been bereaved, those who are housebound, suffer from memory loss, confusion, depression or are in poor general health, or have chronic illness.

Measurement of Body Mass Index (weight (kg)/height $(m)^2$) is a useful indicator of nutritional status, and a BMI of less than 20 is a cause for concern. Weight loss over three to six months is an acute risk factor for malnutrition and a loss of more than 10% of body weight over this time period is considered to be clinically significant. Where it is not possible to establish weight and height, the risk of malnutrition can be assessed by taking into account any history of reduced food intake, loss of appetite or dysphagia, whether clothes or jewellery have become loose fitting and any psychological and physical disturbances likely to have contributed to weight loss.

Advice should focus in the first instance on food. The energy content of the diet should be increased by encouraging consumption of tasty attractive food of high calorie content during and between meals. Organising assistance with shopping, cooking and eating may also be required. The use of nutritional supplements (e.g. sip feeds) can be a useful way of boosting energy intake in older people, but should only be used if it is genuinely not possible to meet nutritional requirements from food.

17

Communication, counselling and concordance

17.1 Introduction

The role of the pharmacist, especially in the community, has always involved communication. Most pharmacists, principally through experience, have become adept at adjusting their verbal comments to the appropriate level necessary for effective understanding by the other party.

Hospital pharmacists, especially, have established an active role as communicators, not only to medical personnel, nursing staff and patients, but also to other healthcare professionals working in, or from, the hospital environment. This extended communicator role has been further facilitated by the appointment in many health districts of community service pharmacists.

The importance of communication in pharmacists' roles was in the past taken for granted. There was, little, if any, attempt to include instruction in undergraduate pharmacy courses, leaving it to the pre-registration training period. The Nuffield Report (1986), which made several recommendations about communication skills and counselling services, has been a major influence and encouraged and confirmed some of the changes already being carried out in pharmaceutical education at that time and subsequently. The need for modern therapeutic agents to be used correctly and safely to minimise the risk of adverse effects is of crucial importance. Greater demands than ever before are being placed on the prescriber and pharmacist to communicate with, and counsel where necessary, all patients to improve adherence to their medication regime. Those particularly at risk may have reading or language difficulties, or be mentally confused or may not use English as their first language.

Although all human beings start to communicate from birth, some acquire greater expertise than others, reflecting the conscious effort required to achieve effective communication. The fundamental requirement in effective communication is that the information received is the same as that sent, and is understood in the way intended by the sender. From this statement it can be seen that communication consists of three components:

- a sender
- a message
- a receiver.

When applied to communication between pharmacist and patient, pharmacist and prescriber, or prescriber and patient, the sender and receiver are individuals while the message may usually be conveyed orally, or in writing as a prescription, a label, or a leaflet. Undoubtedly, increasing use will be made in future of the various electronic means now available.

Remarkable changes have occurred over the past four decades in the way in which medicines are presented. No longer are patients supplied solely with mixtures to be taken a spoonful at a time or lotions to be applied to the skin. Instead, they are treated with one or more of the sophisticated products of pharmaceutical research and development, ranging from modified-release tablets and capsules, through metered-dose inhalation aerosols, to percutaneously absorbed drugs impregnated in self-adhesive skin patches. The continued development of communication skills by the pharmacist is necessary for counselling in order to maximize the correct and effective use of medicines achievable through the understanding and concordance of the patient.

The dictionary definition of the word 'counsel' is consultation or advice, but the verb may also mean 'to warn', and the noun 'counselling', of American origin, means 'a service consisting of giving advice on miscellaneous problems to citizens and others'. In spite of the breadth of meaning of the term, it can more specifically be seen as part of the interaction which can usefully occur between pharmacist and patient. It also includes the potential for contributing to the most suitable choice of medication and resolving problems of administration or the use of medication. Throughout this discussion, the term 'patient' will be used to include either a member of the public who presents a prescription, or one who requests advice about a non-prescription medicine.

Just as the acquisition of effective communication skills requires effort, so too does the development of the ability to be an effective counsellor. Probably the most important and for some, difficult, attribute is a willingness to listen as well as to talk.

The third term included in the title of this chapter is concordance, which requires some explanation. The term 'compliance' in medicine was very widely used until relatively recently to describe the extent to which patients took or used their medication in accordance with the advice given. Compliance is now recognised as being somewhat paternalistic, when it reflects the dictionary definition: as 'agreement, consent, or yielding to the wishes of another'. 'Adherence', meaning 'to stick to' has meanwhile gained considerable acceptance, especially by social scientists, as a more neutral and relevant term. The rather belated recognition that patients must be properly involved with their therapy and treatment in partnership with the prescriber, and pharmacist where appropriate, has encouraged the use of the term 'concordance'. In this context, the term focuses on 'agreement', in order to achieve the optimum treatment, compatible with what the patient wishes and can manage. Thus an individual's behaviour, beliefs and associated dietary or lifestyle constraints may be involved and need to be included. Social changes that can affect the ways in which humans interact may result in the need to change the ways in which we communicate. The achievement of concordance between patient and health professional will involve the identification of beliefs about illness, about treatment and about medicines and their importance or otherwise. As a consequence, by achieving concordance, adherence and appropriate compliance to medication regimes, the result should be an improvement in health outcomes, to the primary benefit of the individual patient.

It is through effective communication and counselling by pharmacists that patients in turn can make an invaluable contribution to the correct and optimally safe use of prescribed medicines, medicines purchased from the pharmacy, or those supplied by the pharmacist in response to symptoms described.

The association of the three terms communication, counselling and concordance represents factors which may significantly contribute to enhancing patient care and to the greater fulfilment of the pharmacist's professional role.

17.2 Communication

Communication is a complex process which, to be effective, depends greatly on the continuing transmission and feedback oscillating between sender and receiver. There are also important non-verbal reactions which must be in sympathy with the verbal messages if the latter are to be correctly understood prior to any response.

Barriers to effective communication

Some common barriers to effective communication can be readily identified and are listed in Table 17.1. This short summary attempts to highlight the major problems which practising pharmacists may encounter and, by inference, how communication may be maximised for the patient's benefit and the more effective use of pharmacists' time.

It is the need to be able to adapt and respond to the individual patient's mood that makes the use of learning aids (e.g. a pre-recorded videocassette explaining how to use suppositories, or viewing a relevant internet screen) a less than ideal substitute for personal communication.

Recognising and overcoming barriers

Communication invariably prompts questions from one or both participants. Pharmacists must be sure to ask the right questions while avoiding the threat of appearing to interrogate. Patients must not feel inhibited to ask what they may feel are naive questions.

Table 17.1 Common barriers to effective communication

The message	The message is too faint or inaudible The language used is not understood The vocabulary is too sophisticated to be understood The accent is unfamiliar
The environment	Background noise or distraction Lack of privacy
Attitude	Human characteristics such as impatience Sender or receiver conveying the impression that 'they haven't time'

The message

Pharmacists must ensure that they do not give the impression that they are sorry for the patient or, that by using lay terminology and speaking in short sentences, they appear to be talking down to the patient.

The environment

The environment must be conducive to the communication process. If the pharmacist is literally speaking down to a patient from a raised platform, this may appear threatening and create difficulties, particularly for the elderly, to either hear or to respond. Many pharmacies built with raised dispensaries to make them more conspicuous, and which helped the pharmacist to literally oversee the pharmacy, have been refitted at floor level.

Physical barriers (e.g. a pharmacy counter or prescription reception point) may militate against relaxed conversation. If the pharmacist moves around the end of the counter, the patient may feel more at ease and in less of an interview-type situation. The trend for many more pharmacies to be refitted with counselling areas or rooms is to be applauded. Privacy is often crucial to counselling and the effective conveying and receiving of information. An anxious parent receiving basic dosage information about an antibiotic mixture prescribed for their young child may well be unhearing, because of the real or perceived invasion of privacy by other patients awaiting their prescriptions and who appear to be crowded around. Only later may the parent wonder whether confirmation was given as to whether the mixture should be given before or after food! Where advice relates to more sensitive forms of treatment, privacy, or the lack of it, may be even more critical. The opportunities for the development of pharmaceutical care and medicines management, as well as the recognition of the pharmacists' contribution to patient healthcare can only be enhanced by the improvement of counselling facilities.

For most people there is an optimum distance to be kept between communicators. Standing close to strangers may appear threatening and invasive, and is normally reserved for family and close friends. The optimum acceptable distance apart also varies with age group, culture and gender.

Attitude

It is obviously essential that the pharmacist possesses a sound and adequate knowledge of the patient's medication and an awareness of the most useful information sources to which the pharmacist may refer. The patient will therefore be reassured by the pharmacist's confidence and manner.

Perhaps surprisingly, only a small part of the impact of any message communicated is attributable to the verbal content. Emotion, tone of voice, gestures and body language are equally powerful influences.

The patient must perceive that the pharmacist has time; that he or she is genuine and wishes to establish an empathy with, and for, the patient; and that he or she is sympathetic and can encourage the patient to have trust and confidence. Once established, the patient's interaction and participation is the best foundation for concordance.

The manner of expression may be dramatically influenced by anger, joy, despair or weariness. The pharmacist must be sensitive to mood and be aware of the need to listen carefully to the patient before responding in a calm, resilient, non-aggressive and supportive manner. The need to gain the patient's confidence is paramount. In body language, the way in which the participants use their eyes in face-to-face communication may be crucial (although there may be significant differences between ethnic groups in the way in which eye contact is used). If either party fails to make eye contact, it can be extremely disconcerting to the other person and may easily convey disinterest. However, if one person stares hard and unwaveringly at the other, the effect may be equally disquieting and even threatening.

Eye contact conveys that the speaker has, even if only momentarily, the attention of the listener. In effective communication the skill is to regularly reaffirm attention by eye contact of varying duration, sensitive to avoiding either any threat, or any loss of attention by turning the head and eyes away to a distracting extent, especially if it were to be to look at the next patient or customer.

The timing of eye contact may also act as a means of emphasis and a vital feedback mechanism capable of registering the listener's reaction to what has been heard. Communication with patients who are blind or partially sighted may benefit from contact (e.g. touching the arm) as a substitute for eye contact.

The movement of head, arms and legs may all contribute to, or distract from, communication. The angle of the head may convey enquiry or, if tilted back, superiority or a haughty or aggressive attitude. A nod or a series of nods can confirm undivided attention and agreement on the part of the listener, although nods which appear too repetitive may be distracting.

Folded arms may convey, or at least exaggerate, a defensive reaction (i.e. a holding-at-arms-length type of response). However, facial expression in most people is very explicit, and in meaningful communication is a powerful indicator and feedback mechanism, showing emotions like happiness, anger, agreement, disagreement, interest and boredom. A fixed permanent smile may convey insincerity, whilst an encouraging smile confirms a willingness to start or advance a dialogue.

It is also most important to avoid any distracting tics (e.g. repetitively touching part of the head or face with a finger, the repetitive furrowing of the brow, or playing with spectacles).

Communication technique may be effectively studied and improved by role-play exercises, preferably aided by video filming and playback in order to objectively assess and appraise.

Communication with prescribers

The principles of communication are no different when the pharmacist telephones a prescriber with a prescription query than when explaining the dosage directions for a dispensed medicine to a patient. In both, it is necessary to avoid language which appears to threaten. No pharmacist would, when querying an unusually high dose, normally state that an overdose had been prescribed. Instead, having first identified him/herself and supplied the patient's name and address, the pharmacist should seek clarification whether or not the prescriber intended a dose in excess of that recommended in the BNF or by the manufacturer. These independent, authoritative sources, quoted objectively from one professional to another, are much more likely to elicit a constructive response. This is no subservient strategy. In the highly unlikely event of the prescriber being unable or unwilling to adjust the dose appropriately, or providing an adequate explanation for an unusually high dose (which should preferably be initialled and endorsed by the prescriber), the pharmacist should professionally consider whether the patient would be put at risk. In such circumstances, it may be wise to seek a second opinion (e.g. from the Royal Pharmaceutical Society, the National Pharmaceutical Association, or another pharmacist) before proceeding. Sensitivity to adjust the particular communication strategy to fit the situation is what is required.

In citing this 'traditional' example, it is relevant to note that significant numbers of the population are potentially identifiable today as either slow (about 7%) or fast metabolisers (about 20%). The testing of saliva samples with accessible equipment is likely to be soon available and will enable the identification of those who could be atypically affected by 'standard' dosages of certain drugs. The potential cause of adverse drug reactions or drug interactions relates to the cytochrome P450 (CYP) drug oxidation mechanism and is attributable to several main P450 cytochromes including CYP2D6. Certain drugs may either inhibit or induce particular CYP enzymes. Possible toxicity could result from enzyme inhibition or conversely clinical efficacy may be prejudiced following enzyme induction. Once this information is available, it should be possible to adjust the dosage of certain drugs to the specific needs of an individual. Such information could incur a new dimension to the form of the communication between prescriber and pharmacist exemplified in detail but not in principle.

It is worth noting that interprofessional communication and understanding is immeasurably enhanced when the pharmacist personally knows the prescriber. Attendance at local professional meetings may provide an excellent opportunity for social interaction which in turn can enhance mutual trust and confidence.

Table 17.2 Summary of influences on effective communication

- Create a suitable atmosphere for the patient or customer to be receptive including the absence of distracting noise, a sense of privacy, and the minimum of physical barriers
- Be prepared to listen carefully and patiently
- Ask logical questions where necessary in a systematic manner
- Ensure that the information conveyed is correct, relevant, and reliably up-to-date
- Facilitate communication by recognising the influence of non-verbal communication factors (e.g. body language, facial expression, gestures, head movement and posture)
- Avoid distracting tics
- Be sensitive to and keep to an acceptable distance apart
- Ensure that the language and vocabulary, including any technical terms used, are right for the receiver
- Be aware that the quality of the communication depends more on interaction than on duration. Be ready to respond to non-verbal clues
- Maintain empathy

A summary of influences on effective communication and the characteristics of successful communication is given in Tables 17.2 and 17.3.

Enhancing communication skills

The use of communication skills in counselling by the pharmacist has wide-ranging application, from the supply of dispensed medicines to healthcare advice and health promotion. However, it is most important to recognise that the label, verbal instruction or counselling and a leaflet are not and never can be alternatives but they are all complementary to each other and essential for optimising the patient's understanding and motivation to adhere to a medication treatment programme.

Labelling

The labelling of medicines is concerned with the communication of information. The pharmacist

Table 17.3 The characteristics of successful communication

- The purpose of communication is not just to deliver a message but to effect a change in the recipient through dialogue, in respect of his knowledge, attitude, and eventually behaviour
- The value of communication is to be judged not on its purpose or content, but on its effect on the recipient
- Good communication is difficult
- Communication must be matched to the knowledge, social background, interest, purposes and needs of the recipient
- Communication is effected not only by words, which must have the same meaning for giver and receiver, but also by attitudes, expressions and gestures
- If communication is to change behaviour, the required change in the recipient must be seen by him or her to have more advantages than drawbacks. The patient should feel empowered to cooperate in deciding upon the best medication strategy for him/herself
- To make sure that communication has succeeded, information about its effect (feedback), both immediate and subsequent, is needed
- Communication demands effort, thought, time and often money

should preferably check with the patient to ensure that the directions for use are properly understood, and reinforced where necessary by the opportunity for verbal interactive response. Where essential additional information cannot be included on a label, it may be supplied in the form of a leaflet.

In the UK, additional cautionary advice has been incorporated into a range of 'Cautionary and Advisory Labels for Dispensed Medicines', included as an appendix in the BNF and linked to correspond to code numbers in the preparation entries. The recommendations for their use reflect the need for patients to be given more precise information about their medicines. It also stresses the importance of counselling by pharmacists, reinforcing the care that should be taken during treatment (e.g. about the avoidance of alcohol, the risks of drowsiness especially related to driving, or the need to take the medicine with water, not milk).

The wording of additional labels has been carefully chosen, attempting to provide the information concisely but intelligibly. However, even with their use, it is vital that the pharmacist counsels the patient to confirm the information given on the label and that it is understood. The BNF notes that 'counselling needs to be related to the age, experience, background and understanding of the individual patient'.

Occasionally, it may be preferable to counsel the patient rather than provide a cautionary label (e.g. about the risk of the medicine staining either clothes or the skin). The BNF includes additional recommended counselling advice for some products.

Much work has been done, and ingenuity used, to support verbal communication and medicine labels (e.g. Braille labels for blind patients reproducing simple directions like 'one to be taken three times a day' on semi-rigid plastic strips). This is not a small problem as there are nearly one million people registered blind or partially sighted in the UK. Furthermore, about 45% of the UK population require optical appliances to assist vision and the numbers are increasing. Legibility is not solely dependent on print size, but it is the most influential contributor to legibility. A minimum of 6 point type is generally recommended, with preferably a minimum of 12 point type for any warnings. Colour selection and layout must also be considered. The Royal National Institute for the Blind (RNIB) would like to see a minimum type size of 14 point used where possible, and the production of large-print documents, perhaps using bold or semi-bold 16–22 point type with a single-colour background and good spacing.

The greater availability of more potent medications today requires the issues of legibility and understanding to be vigorously addressed. Pharmacists have a responsibility to make sure that patients who are not able to read labels are provided with some alternative. This could simply take the form of identifying in large letters the medicine as, for example, 'Heart Tablets', and/or ensuring that carers are adequately informed. The use of large print can appear to be the most obvious solution but may make attachment to a small original pack of a medicine impractical. If the label is detached, other problems may be created. Counselling is crucial in order to best resolve any difficulties.

Leaflets

Leaflets play an important part in the communication of information that is too detailed to include on the medicine label. The physical dimensions of many medicine containers are insufficient to allow the necessary information to be affixed to the surface in a print size that can be easily read. The advantage of leaflets derives from fewer constraints on space compared with labels, increasing the ease of readability and illustration potential. They are also more permanent than the spoken word and can be referred to at a later date by the patient. On 1 January 1994, Directive 92/27/EEC on labelling and leaflets came into force, which included the requirements for the format and content of patient information leaflets to be supplied with each medicine. Many medicines are now available in manufacturers' original packs complete with patient information leaflets or 'patient package inserts' (PPIs). The content of these leaflets, which are subject to official approval, is based on the Summary of Product Characteristics (SPC) which is replacing the Data Sheet. The leaflets are written in a form that is understandable to patients collectively and not for the individual. Unfortunately this inevitably means that extensive lists of contraindications and side-effects are included, many of which are likely to be irrelevant to the individual patient but must be included. The overall impact of such a leaflet if fully read and understood, may be a negative rather than a positive influence on adherence to a dosage regime. It is much to be preferred if the pharmacist takes time with a patient, opens the pack in the pharmacy, extracts the leaflet and goes through the PPI with the patient.

In Australasia pharmacy computer-generated leaflets, which have also been tried in UK, have the advantage of being personalized and made more relevant to the individual. This can be of considerable help in achieving concordance. Simple leaflets devised to help patients in the use of particular types of pharmaceutical preparations (e.g. eye ointments or nasal drops) have proved beneficial. It has been found that directions are best limited to five or six key points if possible and can be considerably helped by simple line drawings, such as confirming that the head is best tilted back when using an inhaler. This may seem a simple point, but was omitted from most first-generation inhaler PPIs.

Many leaflets include illustrations (pictograms), which may be especially helpful and easier for the poorly sighted and those with literacy or language difficulties to comprehend. One of the more successful and least ambiguous pictograms included in some PPIs involves the use of a clock face to indicate the most appropriate times for medication to be administered. The main disadvantages of leaflets, however, are that they may become detached from the product to which they apply and, unlike verbal advice, they are not interactive. When neatly packaged inside a secondary pack, the leaflet may not even be noticed by a patient, which is all the more reason for a pharmacist to initiate a dialogue while the patient is still present in the pharmacy. Web-based versions of some PPIs are now available on the Electronic Medicines Compendium (www.emc.vhn.net) and could be of increasing usefulness as a resource in facilitating the information offered by a pharmacist.

Leaflets containing detailed specific information on the use of more sophisticated products such as pressure inhalers, especially if required to be used with an inhaler device, are usually very well produced, often with colour printing, and frequently include step-by-step illustrations to aid comprehension. However, some of these leaflets may be too detailed to be meaningful without careful supportive explanation by pharmacists. This is especially important when such a product is issued to an elderly patient and particularly so, if for the first time. It is very important for pharmacists to have studied such leaflets before giving them out, enabling them to go through the salient points with confidence (Figure 17.1).

A number of investigations have studied the requirements for format, wording and range of leaflets. Reference must be made to several specialist treatment cards and booklets that have been developed over a number of years through the cooperation of various bodies including the

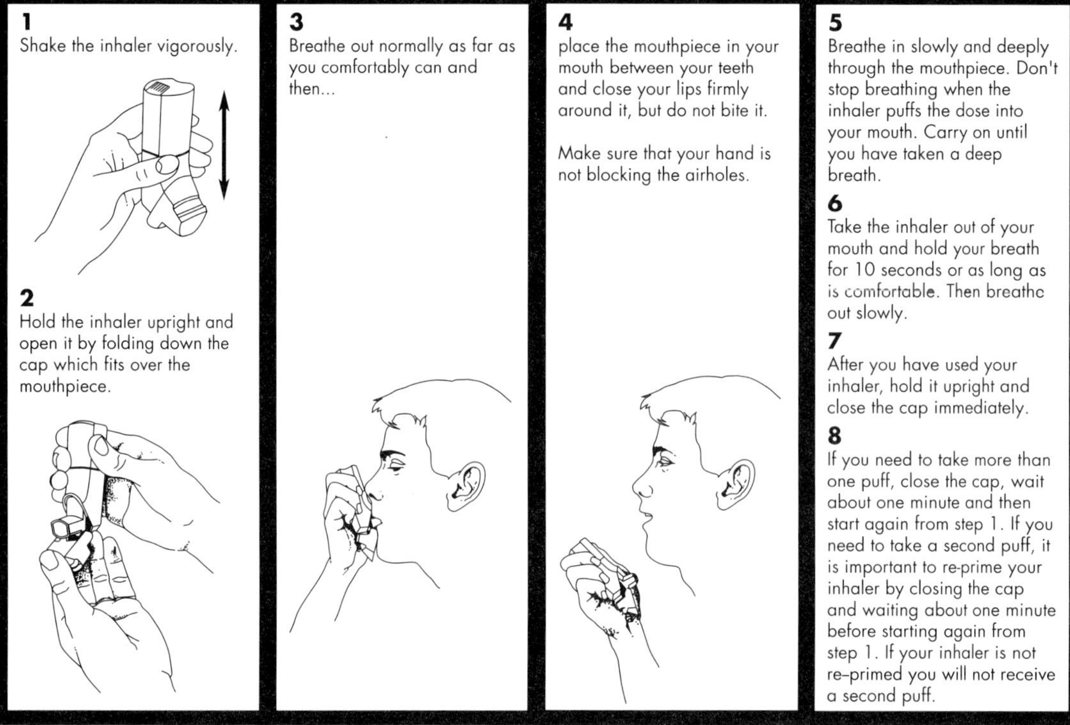

Figure 17.1 Use of a Salamol pressure inhaler.

Royal Pharmaceutical Society, the British Medical Association and the Department of Health. The purpose of these cards and booklets is primarily to warn patients undergoing certain treatments how to avoid some possible adverse consequences and side-effects, thereby aiding adherence to their therapy. Examples include the Lithium Treatment Card (obtainable from the National Pharmaceutical Association) shown in Figure 17.2; the Steroid Treatment Card (obtainable from the Department of Health and illustrated in the BNF) shown in Figure 17.3; and the Anticoagulant Treatment Booklet (obtainable from Health Authorities). These cards and booklets, in addition to PPIs, should be issued and the contents explained by pharmacists to those patients receiving relevant medication, especially on the first occasion.

The language of labels and leaflets

Pharmacy, like any other discipline has developed its own technical jargon terms. These may well be understood and taken for granted within a year of starting a pharmacy degree programme but may have little or no meaning to other people. The distinction between terms such as 'lotion' and 'liniment' or between 'suppository' and 'pessary' are not obvious in the absence of instruction, experience or a dictionary (preferably for technical terms). It is part of a pharmacist's professional responsibility to be satisfied that any such terminology is properly understood. Attention must be given when printing labels, counselling patients or designing leaflets to ensure that sentences are short and technical terms are avoided. Phrases like 'one drop to be instilled into the conjunctival sac' are better replaced by 'put one drop in each eye'. Some words and phrases are more easily substituted than others. 'Thinly' may be considered to be more widely understood than 'sparingly', where the latter word is used in relation to the application of topical corticosteroids. It is not, however, easy to find an entirely satisfactory word for 'discard' when giving advice about the

THINKING ABOUT STARTING A FAMILY?

Because Lithium can effect the unborn baby do NOT become pregnant without first talking to your doctor. If you are pregnant tell your doctor now.

KEEP YOUR TABLETS IN A SAFE PLACE WELL OUT OF THE REACH OF CHILDREN.

Produced by the National Pharmaceutical Association in collaboration with the Royal Pharmaceutical Society

PLEASE RECORD YOUR BLOOD LEVEL OF LITHIUM

DATE TAKEN	BLOOD LEVEL	DAILY DOSE

LITHIUM TREATMENT CARD

CARRY THIS CARD WITH YOU AT ALL TIMES. SHOW IT TO ANY DOCTOR OF NURSE WHO TREATS YOU AND ANY PHARMACIST YOU BUY MEDICINES FROM

NAME ....

PREPARATION OF LITHIUM ....

Should a different proprietary product be prescribed, the card must be suitably endorsed.

HOW SHOULD I TAKE THE TABLETS?

Swallow each tablet whole or broken in half, with water. Do NOT chew or crush it. Try to take the dose at the same time each day.

WHAT SHOULD I DO IF I MISS A DOSE?

Do NOT double your next dose. If you find you have missed a few doses, start taking your usual dose on the day you remember and tell your doctor.

WHY MUST I HAVE A BLOOD TEST?

This is to check the amount of lithium in your blood. It is very important to have the correct amount because too much can be dangerous. Take the blood test ABOUT 12 HOURS AFTER the last dose of lithium. It's also required to check your thyroid function is satisfactory.

CAN I DRINK ALCOHOL?

It is safe to drink SMALL quantities though it can make car driving more hazardous.

CAN I TAKE ANY OTHER MEDICINES WITH LITHIUM?

Some medicines can change the amount of lithium in the blood. These include diuretic (water) tablets, some pain killers and some indigestion mixtures. So check with your doctor or pharmacist before taking other medicines.

Please note: It is safe to take aspirin and paracetamol but not ibuprofen.

WHAT ELSE ALTERS THE LITHIUM LEVEL?

The level can be altered by the amount of fluids you drink, changes in the amount of salt in your food, sweating more than usual (in hot weather, fever or infection), severe vomiting, severe diarrhoea and a low salt diet. Check with your doctor if any of these things happen.

SIGNS OF A HIGH LITHIUM LEVEL

Vomiting, blurred vision, severe diarrhoea, unusual drowsiness, muscle weakness and feeling very giddy may mean that your level of lithium is too high. Stop taking the tablets and talk to your doctor IMMEDIATELY.

DOES LITHIUM HAVE SIDE EFFECTS?

Some slight effects (such as sickness, shaking, indigestion, thirst) may occur at first but they usually wear off if blood tests are normal. Discuss this with your doctor. Some patients may gain weight but this can be prevented with a sensible diet.

HOW LONG WILL I HAVE TO TAKE LITHIUM?

Lithium is a way of preventing illness so you may have to take it for many years. Never stop taking the tablets without asking your doctor.

Figure 17.2 Lithium treatment card.

disposal of a medicine that has expired. 'Do not use after . . .' is negative and does little to discourage hoarding while 'Throw away. . .' may be seen as an unfortunate choice of words. Familiar and understood as the legally required phrase 'For external use only' may be to pharmacists and doctors, it seems strange and possibly offputting to some patients when included on a mouthwash or gargle label.

It is no less important today than it was when typewritten and machine-produced labels were first required on all dispensed medicines from 1 January 1984 that the type used should be adequate, readable, and not too faint because the computer labeller needs a replacement ink-jet cartridge. Attention to such detail cannot be under estimated. Leaflets should also be designed to avoid these problems.

For those who do not speak, write or read English there are additional difficulties. In many cases, patients may be accompanied to their doctor's surgery, and later to the pharmacy, by a family member who does understand English. Sometimes, however, it is a very young member of the family who has to act as interpreter and the quality of translation due to a child's inexperience

INSTRUCTIONS

1 DO NOT STOP taking the steroid drug except on medical advice. Always have a supply in reserve.

2 In case of feverish illness, accident, operation (emergency or otherwise), diarrhoea or vomiting the steroid treatment MUST be continued. Your doctor may wish you to have a LARGER DOSE or an INJECTION at such times.

3 If the tablets cause indigestion consult your doctor AT ONCE.

4 Always carry this card while receiving steroid treatment and show it to your doctor, dentist, nurse or midwife whom you may consult.

5 After your treatment has finished you must still tell any new doctor, dentist, nurse or midwife that you have had steroid treatment.

I am a patient on

STEROID

TREATMENT

which must not be stopped abruptly

and in the case of intercurrent illness may have to be increased

Full details are available from the hospital or general practitioners shown overleaf

WZO 098

	Name and Address	Tel No.
Patient		
General Practitioner		
Hospital		
Consultant or Specialist		

Treatment was commenced on ....

Drug	Date	Dose

Have you had Chicken-Pox?

If you have not had chicken-pox before, it is important that you avoid contact with others who may have chicken-pox or shingles whilst you are taking this medicine, and for three months after stopping it. If you think that you may have been exposed to chicken-pox or shingles during this time **seek urgent medical advice**.

Figure 17.3 Steroid treatment card.

may be less than satisfactory. Some studies have shown that elderly immigrants unable to speak any English are frequently also illiterate in their own language. In such cases the otherwise excellent multilingual leaflets produced by some pharmaceutical companies and health authorities are of limited value. The pharmacist must take responsibility to check that any directions are properly understood and be able to come up with some alternative means of effective communication, however basic that may appear to be. One example is the use of impromptu pictograms drawn to ensure that the patient is clear about his or her medicine and its regime.

It must be re-emphasised, however, that the content of a leaflet or warning card is only likely to be of effect if it is drawn to the attention of the patient by the pharmacist. It has been reported recently that of the 80% who were aware of a PPI, only 40% had read some of it and only 21% had read all of it. It is to be hoped that increased awareness of the existence of PPIs, together with proactive counselling by pharmacists will dramatically correct an unsatisfactory situation.

There is now available on the internet an initiative set up by the Royal Pharmaceutical Society addressing some of the issues identified and discussed in this chapter and section. It is accessed on www.concordance.org.

17.3 Counselling

This term has been increasingly used to describe the sympathetic interaction between pharmacists and patients, which may go beyond conveyance of straightforward information about the medicine and how and when to use it.

Much greater attention is now paid to counselling and training for counselling by all healthcare professions. This is especially so in the context of the greater awareness of, and attention given to, holistic health, which is concerned with the integrated health and well-being of the person as a whole. While there are many forms of counselling, it is generally a way of relating to a person in need of guidance, using understanding, sympathy and sincerity. Most counsellors are eclectic, drawing from different types of counselling such as 'behavioural', which is concerned with modifying behaviour from the unacceptable to the acceptable, and 'humanistic', which is more concerned with personal growth and human potential. It is important to enable patients to feel empowered and in control of their medication regime. The reason for the medication, the desired therapeutic outcome, a balanced consideration of any potential side-effects and the dosage details all require to be understood in order to progress to concordance.

For the pharmacist, often conscious of how time-consuming successful counselling may be, it is important to recognise that to establish an initial pharmacist–patient relationship requires sufficient emphasis upon patient watching and listening.

Counselling may be described succinctly as helping people to help themselves. The importance of listening to and understanding the patient cannot be over-emphasised. Simple facts clearly expressed are fundamental to successful counselling.

With the advent of original pack dispensing, the pharmacist should ideally have the opportunity to devote more time to communication and counselling, which needs to be recognised as a professional priority.

Pharmacists should not only advise prescribers and patients about medicines, but also:

- monitor and report adverse drug reactions;
- consult with prescribers about prescribing and dispensing procedures;
- advise members of the public about non-prescription medicines; and
- continue to expand the primary healthcare role of giving advice to patients in response to symptoms.

Pharmacists may also contribute to health promotion, take part in diagnostic screening procedures and provide domiciliary pharmaceutical services. Counselling is the cornerstone of all these facets of the pharmacists' role which may be comprehensively embraced by the dynamic concepts of 'patient-oriented pharmaceutical healthcare' and 'medicines management'.

Pharmacists keep and maintain prescription-based patient medication records (PMRs) primarily for patients who regularly visit the same pharmacy and subject to the RPSGB Code of Ethics and Standards. Records are of particular benefit for those with chronic conditions on long-term medication and for the care of the elderly, especially for the detection of adverse reactions and drug interactions and the confirmation of dosage regimes. PMRs are not only of considerable benefit to patients but are a most useful resource for pharmacists in ensuring the highest standard of pharmaceutical care. The current limitation is that many PMRs cannot be reliably complete because not all of a patient's prescriptions have necessarily been dispensed at the same pharmacy. A flexible system of patient registration with a pharmacy of the patient's choice, in a manner analogous to NHS registration with a GP and a dentist, could make the efficacious and safer use of medication much more assured. PMRs could also include details of over-the-counter medicines where beneficial to the records and pharmacists' ability to monitor a patient's adherence to medication regimes would be further facilitated. The opportunity to be alerted to any potential problem at an early stage could be enormously helpful to a patient at risk.

One method of record-keeping used in France and trialled in the UK involves an electronic 'smart-card'. The prescriber records the patient's medication on the card, and this is retained by the patient. Subsequently, the patient may elect to show it to the pharmacist when he hands in a prescription or purchases a non-prescription medicine. The pharmacist may then check and update the card as appropriate, providing an invaluable aid to the more effective use of medicines. Problems arise, however, when 'smart cards' are forgotten, lost or stolen.

The lack of access by pharmacists to patient medical records, on the grounds of confidentiality, means that pharmacists are usually not aware or certain of the prescriber's diagnosis or reason for treatment. A further complication arises in the number of possible indications attributable to many medicines. If questioned by a patient, a pharmacist may need to respond with tact and care, and avoid giving the patient any cause for alarm. Patients may describe the prescriber's diagnosis, in which case pharmacists should make a calculated decision as to what information can responsibly be given. It may, however, be necessary to suggest that patients discuss those aspects of their treatment more fully with the prescriber, particularly where patients are uncertain of the basis of treatment. When a patient normally only uses the services of one pharmacy, there is an increased likelihood of the prescriber being willing to share some of the medical record relevant information confidentially with the pharmacist. The opportunity for closer professional cooperation between prescriber and pharmacist, both in dialogue with the patient, can contribute in a major way to the level and value of concordance by the patient and the quality of healthcare.

In addition, the opportunity may be provided to give further advice on how and when the medicine should be taken or used.

Most patients are only able to recall about a third of what they have been told, and it is recommended that, when counselling, the more important points should be stated at the beginning and repeated at the end of the interview. Among factors that have been found to decrease effective interaction between patients and prescribers, and which may equally handicap counselling by pharmacists, are the following:

- Patients are too fearful or nervous to ask questions.
- Patients are unwilling to ask questions for fear of appearing ignorant.
- Patients are confused by medical terminology or jargon.
- Patients do not appreciate the importance of the information conveyed.
- Prescribers or pharmacists devote insufficient time to explain instructions adequately.
- The consultation is inappropriately terminated (e.g. by prescribers writing a prescription, or pharmacists placing the medicine in a bag and handing it out with little or no explanation).

Pharmacists have the opportunity and responsibility to ensure that patients understand all relevant information relating to the prescribed treatment. Pharmacists should use, as appropriate, suitable verbal, written or audiovisual communication techniques (*see* Section 17.2) to inform, educate or reinforce the knowledge of patients about their medicines. Patients so enabled should then be in an informed position to recognise and agree to a medication regime appropriate to their needs.

Factors influencing effective patient counselling

Environment

Space, furnishing, privacy and noise can be significant influences on effective counselling. Many community pharmacies in the UK lack an adequate separate counselling area or room as previously noted. Some pharmacies have installed counselling booths which provide a measure of discreet confidentiality while still enabling the pharmacist to be available if required, to supervise pharmacy medicine sales. In the absence of a specifically designated area, a greater impression of privacy may be conveyed around a quiet end of a medicine counter or prescription reception point. Even subdued lighting at one end of a counter has been found to convey a measure of privacy. The dispensary is an inappropriate area for counselling purposes and could incur potential security risks. Pharmacists in pharmacies with established counselling facilities engender and experience a heightened awareness by the public of the profession's contribution to primary healthcare and they are more readily identified as members of the primary healthcare team.

Personal factors

To most people, a clean, well-fitting white laboratory coat or uniform, or smart business-like clothing, conveys a professional image which helps to put the patient at ease and conveys confidence. Although fewer community pharmacists wear white lab coats, it is still important that pharmacists should be distinguished from dispensing technicians and assistants. Name badges which include the word 'Pharmacist' and the green cross symbol for pharmacy are helpful.

Pharmacists' behaviour, as with any other professional, can also contribute to the ease and effectiveness of communication and counselling. An awareness of the non-verbal aspects of communication (*see* Section 17.2) is very important. Waiting patients and customers will instinctively observe pharmacists and staff and start to form a perception of the level of trust and confidence which they can expect in the pharmacy personnel.

Time

The major limiting factor determining how much patient counselling actually happens in pharmacy practice is time. This may be unfortunate but applies to many similar professional situations which also involve counselling. The structure of UK community pharmacy (consisting mostly of single-pharmacist pharmacies), the informal access and erratic workload often make it difficult for pharmacists to devote sufficient time to counselling.

In the last 10 years, NHS prescriptions dispensed annually in each pharmacy in Great Britain have increased in number by about 50% to nearly 50 000. In order to devote adequate time to counselling, dispensing should be performed by trained technicians under supervision, or a second pharmacist should be available, but in reality the erratic workload may make this difficult to implement.

17.4 Concordance and the limit of concordance

Concordance is a relatively new approach to the prescribing and taking of medicines. It has gradually evolved as a consequence of the recognition that patients should be actively engaged in determining their own approach, understanding and implementation of appropriate therapy for their condition, in partnership and in mutual agreement with relevant healthcare professionals. Concordance is defined or described in the November 2000 web base www.concordance.org as: 'an agreement reached after negotiation between a patient and a healthcare professional that respects the beliefs and wishes of the patient in determining whether, when and how medicines are to be taken. Although reciprocal, this agreement is an alliance in which the healthcare professionals recognise the primacy of the patient's decisions about taking the recommended medications.'

Some patients may decline to share the responsibility which forms part of an agreement, as is inherent in the term concordance. Adherence or compliance may then more accurately describe the position. While attitudes, especially among healthcare professionals may be changing, much variation exists and is reflected in many studies and journal papers.

It was only in the mid-1960s that compliance rates were studied in medical practice among groups of patients with various diseases (e.g. depression, acute infections, various chronic diseases) and in pregnancy. Since that time, many papers have been published, reporting and reviewing many facets of compliance or adherence and non-compliance. The term compliance is used in this section when reference is made to its use in other published sources.

Compliance in keeping appointments for disease screening initiated by healthcare professionals is often below 50%, but it rises markedly where children are involved. When an appointment is initiated by the patient for treatment, compliance again improves, representing a shift towards the concept of concordance.

Patients on short-term medication have tended to show greater compliance than those on long-term therapy, as might be expected. It is also apparent that the motivation for compliance is greater for the treatment of disease rather than its prevention. Many other factors may affect compliance (e.g. the age and intelligence of the patient, and whether any significant improvement may be noted by the patient as a result of continued treatment).

Patient perceptions of concordance

Research has not identified any one specific cause for non-compliance, nor does it seem possible to identify a special type of patient who lacks compliance. The active participation of patients in their treatment may be influenced by factors which limit or promote compliance, which may also be identified as moving towards the concept of concordance.

Factors contributing to a lack of concordance

(*see also* Table 17.4)

Among inhibiting factors are:

- anxiety
- lack of appropriate dosage aids
- length of illness
- personal characteristics (e.g. lack of independence, or despair)
- poverty
- social and cultural factors (e.g. illness as an excuse, or fatalism)
- social isolation
- wrong information.

These factors are essentially the same as those which contributed to poor compliance and often reflect the absence of engagement with one or more health professionals, loneliness and

Table 17.4 Factors contributing to a lack of concordance (formerly considered as poor compliance)

- The patient does not take the prescription to the pharmacy or collect the dispensed medicine
- The directions for use are not understood (e.g. due to inadequacy of directions, reading difficulty, language difficulty, or complexity of instructions)
- The purpose of the medicine, and the reasons for taking it, are not understood. This may be due to omission by the prescriber or pharmacist, or a lack of comprehension
- Physical difficulties (e.g. in opening the container or handling small tablets)
- Problems associated with administration of the drug (e.g. retention of a suppository, unpleasant taste, or difficulty in swallowing)
- The patient considers there is no improvement in his or her condition after dosage
- Real and imagined side-effects
- Inconvenience of dosage regimen (e.g. difficulty in arranging administration in the working day)
- The patient is unwilling to enter into a dialogue with a healthcare professional in order to consider his or her own beliefs and wishes in the context of prescribed medication

isolation. The need is for those who can help to resolve the situation to recognise that it is necessary to treat the whole person. This is of particular importance when counselling patients suffering from severe depression or other affective disorders, when it is crucial to gain their confidence first. Such patients may have a low attention span, be forgetful of advice given about their medication and be dismissive of their treatment. It can be an extremely time-demanding situation, which adds to the difficulties in many busy pharmacies.

The key factor in promoting patients' participation in their treatment is motivation. The way in which patients perceive their motivation for living and their resultant lifestyle are most important influences. The acceptance of being ill, handicapped or disabled, former experience of illness, and attitude are characteristics which may encourage patients to take part actively in their treatment, especially when promoted by the concept of concordance.

In practical terms, pharmacists may find that non-adherence is directly related to, or affected by, one or more of the following factors.

Difficulty in keeping to dosage regimen in daily living

Some formulations may not be as easily administered at work as a tablet or a cream. Many patients find it easier to remember to take medicines at meal times than an hour beforehand. If remembered later, the patient may be inhibited from taking the missed dose unless the situation has been anticipated in discussion with the pharmacist.

A common example is the administration of antacid preparations. These may need to be administered during the working day, and it may be easier for patients to carry tablets to work rather than a large mixture bottle.

The act of swallowing solid oral dosage forms may also pose problems for some patients. Pharmacists may be made aware of this difficulty during counselling, whereas patients may be reluctant to discuss this seemingly 'minor' point with the prescriber. A brief telephone call from the pharmacist to the prescriber may help to overcome this problem.

Treatment regimen too complex and not properly understood

What action might pharmacists take in the situation described in Figure 17.4? Pharmacists can design a chart to help the patient to understand the regimen. If the patient is not living alone, it may be possible to recruit a member of the family to help with the dosage schedule. Different types of container for different tablets or capsules may also be helpful.

In the case described, it would be most sensible to refer to the prescriber and discuss how critical the reducing dose steps are likely to be. Some clinicians consider it satisfactory to reduce the dose of prednisolone by 5 mg every 5–7 days down to 5 mg daily, which should then be reduced slowly. This results in a much simpler reducing dosage schedule. The importance of active communication between pharmacists and prescribers, and pharmacists and patients should be obvious. Concordance is of crucial importance in such situations.

A patient is presented with two containers of prednisolone tablets, bottle A containing 5 mg prednisolone tablets and bottle B containing 1 mg prednisolone tablets.

> On days 1 to 5, take TWO tablets from bottle A morning and night, then from days 6 to 10, take TWO tablets in the morning and ONE at night from bottle A, then from days 11 to 15, take TWO in the morning from bottle A. Do not take any tablets from bottle B on days 1 to 5, then on day 6 take FOUR at night with tablet from bottle A, then on day 7 take THREE at night from bottle B, TWO at night on day 8 from bottle B, ONE at night on day 9, and no tablets from bottle B on day 10. On day 11 start again with FOUR tablets from bottle B, THREE tablets from bottle B on day 12, TWO tablets from bottle B on day 13, ONE tablet from bottle B on day 14 and no tablet from bottle B on day 15.

Thus on days 1 to 5, a total of 20 mg prednisolone is to be taken, 19 mg total on day 6, 18 mg total on day 7, 17 mg on day 8, 16 mg on day 9, 15 mg on day 10, 14 mg on day 11, 13 mg on day 12, 12 mg on day 13, 11 mg on day 14, and 10 mg on day 15.

Figure 17.4 Prednisolone reducing dosage.

Another common contributor to non-compliance or non-adherence is polypharmacy. It has been frequently shown that patients receiving three or more drugs at the same time tend to have compliance or adherence problems.

Lack of confidence in prescriber or medication

Whatever the personal views of the pharmacist, it is imperative that the patient's confidence is maintained in both the medication and the prescriber. This may have the additional merit of improving the prescriber/pharmacist relationship which should be for the patient's ultimate benefit.

Influence of conflicting information derived from other sources

The patient may well pick up incorrect or conflicting information about their medication or condition being treated from the popular press or from family and friends.

It is a source of on-going concern that from time to time changes in the availability of medicines may be announced in the national press or the media before healthcare professionals are formally notified. Equally, patients may read an article in the press, see or hear a programme on TV or the radio about the possible harmful effects of medicines they are taking, and, not surprisingly, become reluctant to take them. In this situation, pharmacists should endeavour to discuss the benefits and risks of treatment, and try to convince patients that, where appropriate and to the best of their knowledge, such claims should not cause them undue concern. It should also be stressed that it may be harmful to stop treatment abruptly. Professional judgement will determine whether patients require further reassurance from their prescribers.

Child-resistant containers

Child-resistant closures and containers (British Standard 5321:1975) have been required for tablet and capsule formulations of aspirin and paracetamol since 1975 and certain liquid products since 1987 supplied without a prescription. Their original voluntary use became a requirement of professional practice in January 1989 for all dispensed medicines. However, patients who experience difficulty in the use of child-resistant containers may be supplied alternatives, but such patients should be counselled about the extra care needed in storage of such medicines. Users with potential problems (e.g. the elderly and patients with mild or moderate arthritis) benefit from counselling by pharmacists. Providing the technique in using child-resistant containers is demonstrated, and patients are convinced of their ability to use the closures by carrying out the procedure themselves, a significant majority subsequently experience few difficulties. It should be accepted that further counselling may be necessary to persuade some patients that such containers are desirable and have contributed significantly to decreased child mortality figures due to accidental poisoning. Young children visiting elderly grandparents or relatives can be particularly at risk.

The pharmacist's contribution to concordance

It is generally considered that patient education is the most important variable affecting compliance, adherence and concordance. Information provided to patients concerning their medicine must be understood. Faulty comprehension has been reported to contribute to many medication problems. If the medicine has been prescribed, information provided by pharmacists must reinforce and complement the prescriber's directions and that provided in the PPI.

As the involvement of pharmacists in the primary healthcare team is increasingly recognised, the importance of communication with patients cannot be overemphasized and sufficient time must be made available for this. The correct information at the appropriate level is the most important constructive influence to effect concordance that pharmacists can make. Information that pharmacists should consider important for patients includes:

- action to be taken in the event of a missed dose
- action to be taken in the event of suspected or confirmed pregnancy

- aim of the treatment
- arrangement of further supplies
- discarding of unused medicine beyond a specific expiry date
- dosage or amount to be used
- duration of treatment
- excipients which may potentially produce adverse effects
- expected side-effects which may be reduced by appropriate action by the patient (e.g. reduction of gastric irritation caused by some non-steroidal anti-inflammatory drugs by administration after food). A basic recognition of risk to benefit can be helpful and reassuring
- frequency and correct times of administration or use (administrative schedule)
- intended use and expected action, and advice in the event of no apparent effect
- maximum dose in 24 hours; in future adjustment may be necessary if a patient is identifiable as a slow or fast metaboliser
- medicines, food or activities the patient has to avoid during treatment
- method of use
- pharmaceutical form of the medicine and its identity
- side-effects to be referred to the prescriber
- storage of medication.

The aim of treatment is particularly relevant if pharmacists are responding to symptoms described by a patient, but should be considered with caution in regard to prescribed medicines as this is a professional matter between prescribers and patients. Patient confidentiality, as well as the patient's confidence in the prescriber, must be respected. Pharmacists must be selective with the range of the information conveyed. It would usually be inappropriate to counsel or advise patients on all the headings listed, as these can cover information as diverse as that in a product data sheet or Summary of Product Characteristics. Furthermore, these sources of information, as required by law, often tend to give most emphasis to the undesirable aspects of the drug in question, which can be offputting to the lay reader. The attention, understanding and memory of most patients would soon be overstretched, unfounded anxieties might be aroused, and the time required would be considerable and impractical.

What is essential is for pharmacists to ensure that patients possess sufficient information for the effective and safe use of medicines. Pharmacists who are able to develop a rapport with patients who regularly visit their pharmacy, and who can establish confidence in the minds of patients in a familiar and unthreatening environment, have the opportunity to contribute increasingly to patients' confidence in their medication. Patients are then in a position to feel comfortable in reaching a decision about taking their recommended medication.

Ways to improve adherence and promote concordance

(A list of tips that may be useful for patients is given in Table 17.5.)

Daily dose reminders

The design of special treatment packs, calendar packs and medication dose compartment aids, suitably labelled, have all been aimed at stimulating patient adherence through a better understanding of their treatment.

For difficult cases of non-adherence often aggravated by depression or forgetfulness,

Table 17.5 In the spirit of concordance: What can help me to remember to take my medication?

- Take it at the same time daily where appropriate
- Take it at other daily event times, such as cleaning teeth
- Put a sticker or reminder note on the refrigerator or other location
- Obtain a suitable medication dose compartment aid from my pharmacist and set a regular refill time, maybe with the pharmacist's guidance
- Get a member of my family or a friend to help remind me
- Get my pharmacist to boldly identify which medicine is which
- Make sure I understand what my medication is for and how soon I can expect results
- Make the commitment to go back to see my GP and pharmacist should I have a problem or feel that I am not making progress

especially in the elderly, pharmacists may find it helpful to introduce patients to one of the special medicine packaging devices. These compliance aids vary considerably in sophistication, design and cost.

Most daily dose reminders consist of a tray divided into compartments, which may be labelled with times during the day or days of the week. There may also be space for inclusion of a patient's individual label, and one device incorporates Braille markings to assist the blind and partially sighted.

Guidelines are laid down by the Royal Pharmaceutical Society for the use of daily dose reminders. Medicines should not be dispensed directly into these compliance aids unless the statutory labelling requirements can be fulfilled. If patients request that pharmacists load the daily dose reminder, this should be done using the dispensed medicine which carries the legally required label. An example of a widely used daily dose reminder is illustrated in Figure 17.5.

A number of other devices may be more useful. If an elderly infirm patient is visited regularly by a community nurse, the patient's medication can be prepared on a labelled tray, which may include liquid medicines already measured out in dispensing cups. Such cups, complete with lids, are made in different colours and capacities and are available from several sources.

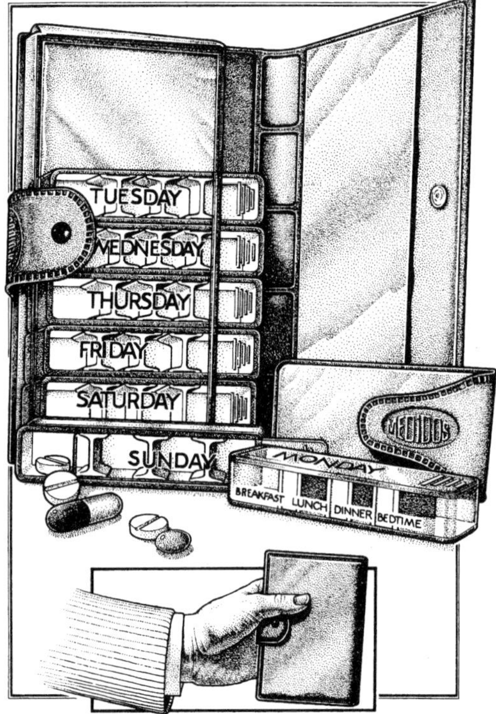

Figure 17.5 An example of a daily dose reminder.

However, such adherence aids are only available for limited distribution in special cases; in other cases, patients must purchase them.

A note of caution is appropriate, for although compliance aids are widely used with considerable benefit to many, their contribution to improved adherence is not universal. In many cases pharmacists cease to have either limited or any contact with the patients involved, especially with regard to repeat prescription items. Patients can become increasingly distanced from the identity and purpose of their medication, which can militate against adherence. The opportunity to benefit from supportive advice from a pharmacist is likely to be diminished and the pharmacist is not then in a position to reliably assess a patient's changing situation or needs. While medication dose compartment aids (MDC aids) can be beneficial, for many patients they should not be used as a compromise solution to more complex medication problems. Such problems are often associated with disadvantaged groups of patients such as the confused elderly or those suffering from depression on multiple medication and maybe living alone.

Family support

Where it is possible to invoke the support of other members of a patient's family who can give encouragement, improve understanding and, if necessary, supervise the taking or using of the medicine, adherence will invariably improve, at least in the short term. Such involvement is most helpful and should be considered essential where MDC aids (e.g. those described above) require regular refilling. It is in such circumstances that MDC aids are of value and the reservations identified above are offset.

Information

The information contained in the section describing pharmacists' contribution to achieving concordance (*see above*) is a comprehensive list of the range of advice that pharmacists could provide for patients. In reality, however, the oral information conveyed may be considerably more succinct, and may be summarised by the following points:

- How and when to take/use the medicine
- How much to take/use
- How long to keep taking/using the medicine
- What to do in the event of a missed dose
- What to do if something goes wrong
- Whether it is safe to drive
- Whether it is safe to take a small quantity of alcoholic drink.

17.5 Discussion

Pharmacists have the opportunity to play an exceptionally important role in ensuring that patients obtain the maximum benefit from the use of prescribed medicines. It should not be considered acceptable that patients be given their medicines with no input from pharmacists regarding use, the potential benefits and the action to be taken in the event of problems.

Communication plays a vital role in pharmacists' activities. Pharmacists must watch and listen carefully, paying particular attention to non-verbal signs (e.g. facial expression, posture and body movements). They must be able to convey sympathy and yet confidence, confirming and enhancing patients' attitude towards their treatment. This may be especially difficult if patients appear unreceptive. It should always be remembered that prescriptions are most likely to be presented by individuals who are unwell, or by someone who is concerned about a close relative or friend. If pharmacists can convey understanding, while at the same time maintaining professionalism, the attitude of patients can be correspondingly uplifted.

The type and range of information required for effective patient counselling is continually expanding and pharmacists must be aware of the sources that can provide useful information. Medicinal product entries in the BNF frequently include a 'counselling' prompt which may relate, for example to 'crushing a tablet before administration or it may be chewed', or it may be a more complex matter. The BNF appendix 9: 'Cautionary and advisory labels for dispensed medicines', cross references those products where counselling is advised with a capital 'C'. The BNF is also gradually incorporating evidence-based medicine information into its advice where this is currently available.

Conversely, the use of recommended cautionary and advisory labels may be deemed inappropriate by prescribers in certain circumstances. In such cases, prescribers may endorse the prescription NCL (no cautionary labels), and specify any alternative wording that is required.

In some instances, it is recommended that more than one cautionary label should be appended to a medicine. On occasions, however, pharmacists may use their professional knowledge and discretion to omit one or more of the labels. In this event, adequate counselling to compensate for the decision to delete an advisory label is required.

In addition to written aids to counselling, the organised use and availability of videotapes may provide a useful adjunct. Patients may watch a demonstration of the technique which should be used in administration of a drug (e.g. the use of a pressure inhaler), and the pharmacist should be available to answer any questions. Whatever audio-visual aids are used, however, it is important that pharmacists consider them an accessory to adequate patient counselling, not a substitute.

In 2000, the prescription net ingredient cost of NHS dispensed medicines in Great Britain was almost £5.6 billion, an increase in real terms of 35% in five years. The degree of non-compliance or non-adherence has been and is notoriously difficult to assess accurately, but figures of up to 30% have been suggested. It has been reported recently that 50–60% of patients prescribed inhalers have 'compliance problems'. Notwithstanding the vast waste of resources which these estimates represent, it also indicates that up to one-third of all medicines may not be used satisfactorily. Clearly, there is considerable scope for improving adherence, and pharmacists must play a vital role in the education of patients to achieve this. Equally, the increasing proportion of elderly people in the population, and their increasing dependence on medicines (*see* Chapter 16) suggests that problems in adherence may get worse rather than better. Many patients are bewildered by the complexity of dosage schedules, and pharmacists must fulfil their professional responsibilities by devoting time and effort to improving understanding and developing the positive partnership concept of concordance rather than relying on adherence.

Pharmacists should be alert to any indicators of poor compliance or adherence. Patients on long-term continuous therapy (e.g. beta-adrenoceptor blocking drugs, non-steroidal anti-inflammatory drugs or cardiac glycosides) may obtain repeat prescriptions from their surgery at regular intervals. Any indication by patients that they have sufficient tablets left not to require the full quantity on the prescription should prompt pharmacists to examine whether adherence has been satisfactory. This must obviously be approached sensitively, without appearing to criticise, and discreet questioning may highlight problems with side-effects or adverse reactions that may require supportive discussion and warrant referral.

At present it is not practically or economically feasible for community pharmacists to monitor adherence by the detection methods available for some drugs (e.g. penicillin, theophylline, digoxin or phenytoin) in urine, blood or saliva. Hospital pharmacists may be able to co-ordinate such analyses with procedures used for therapeutic drug monitoring. However, the range of drugs for which analysis may be easily carried out, and indeed the number of drugs for which monitoring would be cost-effective, is small. A far greater improvement in patient adherence can be achieved by effective communication and counselling which provides the foundation for effective concordance.

18

Minor illness and responding to symptoms

18.1 Introduction

People's ability and willingness to cope with minor ailments without consulting a doctor is of vital importance and is a significant area in which pharmacists can contribute to healthcare. The primary healthcare system would be totally unable to cope with the extra demand if all episodes of minor illness were referred to a doctor. More importantly, the public's willingness to deal with most problems themselves confirms their desire to take responsibility for their own health and can encourage a more sensible attitude to lifestyle to promote good health.

Perceptions of health

A patient's decision to seek medical advice is commonly based on a knowledge of health and health-related topics (e.g. obtained through experience or the media), perceptions of good health, and the advice given by others (e.g. relatives, friends and members of the primary healthcare team). It is essential that the information on which decisions are based is sound and factual. Pharmacists can play an important role in correcting misconceptions about ill-health and its treatment and they are viewed by the public as highly trained and easily accessible healthcare professionals.

Many minor illnesses do not require any medical treatment. Reassurance or suggestions about lifestyle modifications (e.g. smoking, diet or alcohol use) may be adequate. However, some conditions can benefit from the use of non-prescription medicines and patients may ask for these directly or purchase them after recommendation by the pharmacist.

Factors influencing the decision not to consult a doctor

The decision to seek medical advice, to self-medicate, or to do nothing when symptoms occur is complex. Only a small proportion of symptoms are reported to a doctor and many people do nothing at all to treat minor symptoms. Factors which determine whether a doctor is consulted include the severity of the symptom and the anxiety it may be causing, the desire to appease members of the family, and a need for sickness certification. Medical consultation is more commonly sought on behalf of the very young, by the elderly, women between 15 and 44 years of age, widows and widowers, and families with several children.

The greater proportion of minor illness for which medical advice is not sought has been called the 'iceberg' of illness. The reasons why people do not seek medical advice include the belief that their symptom cannot be altered through the use of drugs and must be accepted as part of their physical make-up, or concern that the symptom is too trivial to warrant the attention of the doctor (despite the anxiety the symptom may be causing the sufferer). Some patients may have experienced unpleasant side-effects through the former use of prescription medicines and be reluctant to take an unfamiliar drug. Some people may even prefer to take a non-prescription medicine that has been previously used with success, even if the reported symptoms are different. Other factors may include the relative inaccessibility of the doctor's surgery, the time spent in getting to the surgery and waiting for the consultation, and the potential loss in earnings of the visit.

18.2 Minor illness and its management

There is no agreed definition of what constitutes a minor illness, although the following criteria can be used as a framework. The condition should be:

- of limited duration
- self-limiting
- something which is perceived as non-threatening.

The range of minor illness changes with age. Many of the problems of the elderly are considered in Chapter 16 and of children in Chapter 15. Common minor illnesses in adults and their treatment are described in detail in Section 18.3.

Pharmacists' contribution to the treatment of minor illness

The reluctance of patients to seek a doctor's advice for the treatment of many episodes of minor illness and the ready accessibility of the community pharmacy highlights the important contribution which pharmacists make to maintaining health. Pharmacists can advise the public on many healthcare matters.

Some medicines which are considered appropriate for treatment of minor illness are legally classified in the UK as pharmacy [P] medicines, i.e. they must be sold under the direct supervision of the pharmacist. Pharmacists can therefore influence the public's choice of medicines and can ensure that such medicines are appropriately used. Equally importantly, pharmacists can use their considerable background knowledge on health and related subjects to positively influence aspects of the public's lifestyle (health promotion).

One way of increasing the potential contribution of pharmacists' response to symptoms is to increase the range of medicines that are available for recommendation. This can be achieved in the UK by changing drugs from prescription-only medicine [POM] status to pharmacy medicine [P] status (POM to P).

Table 18.1 Minor illnesses for which non-prescription medicines are available

Acne	Eczema	Pain
Allergic rhinitis	Eye infections and inflammation	Pruritus
Allergy	Fever	Psoriasis
Arthralgia	Fungal infections	Rashes
Athlete's foot	Haemorrhoids	Scabies
Birth marks	Halitosis	Sickness
Bruises and sprains	Hay fever	Sore throat
Chilblains and cramp	Headache	Sunburn
Cold sore and chapped lips	Head lice	Tear deficiency
Conjunctivitis	Heartburn	Teething and toothache
Constipation	Indigestion	Tinea
Corns and calluses	Infant colic	Thrush
Coughs and colds	Insect stings and bites	Tiredness
Cradle cap	Irritable bowel syndrome	Travel sickness
Cystitis	Lice (head, body, pubic)	Verrucas
Dandruff	Minor cuts and grazes	Warts
Diarrhoea	Mouth ulcers	Worm infections
Ear wax	Nappy rash	
Earache	Nasal congestion	

The range of products which can be recommended for minor illness

There is a tremendous variety of non-prescription medicines which the public can purchase for minor illness. The average number of non-prescription medicines held in the home (reportedly more than 7 in the UK and as high as 17 in the USA) suggests that patients may resort to these rather than visit the pharmacy on each occasion that symptoms are experienced. Medicines are often purchased for future expected symptoms, and this makes it difficult to be confident that the patient will make the best use of the advice given by the pharmacist.

The indications for the range of non-prescription medicines available are listed in Table 18.1.

Problems associated with the use of non-prescription medicines

Many members of the public are unaware that the misuse of non-prescription medicines has as great a potential for harm as misuse of prescription-only medicines. The purchaser may presume that, because the medicine is freely available and the pharmacist has been involved in its supply, there can be no problems associated with its use. In essence this is true, but only if the product is used for the purpose for which it was intended and at the correct dose and dosage interval. Consumers may ignore the contraindications and other detailed information on the package and administer drugs to inappropriate groups (e.g. young children and the elderly). Even if all adequate safety and precautionary measures are taken, non-prescription medicines can still provoke adverse reactions, interact with prescribed or other non-prescription medicines, and interfere with biochemical tests. More importantly the patient may delay seeking medical advice or overdose deliberately or accidentally.

In self-treatment, people have to assess their own symptoms and their diagnosis may be incorrect. The role of pharmacists in helping patients to come to the correct decision about their symptoms is crucial. Patients may overlook potentially more serious but less debilitating symptoms in preference to those which are more familiar. They may make a subconscious decision to ignore a symptom or its seriousness, and not seek professional advice because they cannot afford socially or financially to admit to its presence. In addition, in opting for self-medication patients assume that the symptom is self-limiting.

Patients who have previously used non-prescription medicines may visit their doctor but fail to inform him or her of the treatment they have already used or are still using. Many doctors do not ask their patients what, if any, non-prescription medicines they are taking.

Adverse reactions can occur with almost all non-prescription medicines, but some of the most common derive from the use of salicylates, paracetamol, iron preparations and antihistamines. Acute overdosing with non-prescription medicines forms a significant proportion of poisoning cases. A large proportion of the deaths from poisoning in adults are due to aspirin and paracetamol. Although it is acknowledged that these drugs are frequently supplied on prescription, their ready availability for purchase emphasises the public's responsibility to ensure their safe use and storage.

The inadequate storage of drugs in the home provides a potentially hazardous environment, especially for young children. Although there is a similar hazard with prescription medicines, a considerably larger number of non-prescription than prescription medicines are stored at home. The patient's perception that non-prescription medicines are less harmful than those that have been obtained from the doctor may lead to less care in their storage.

Educating the public about non-prescription medicines

Pharmacists can be an invaluable source of information on the safe and appropriate use of non-prescription medicines. However they are by no means the sole source of information on medicines that can be bought or prescribed by doctors.

Consumer magazines (and in particular those targeted at women and mothers), television and radio, home-doctor books and the internet are popular sources of advice. Self-care and healthcare books abound in non-specialist bookshops, and contain detailed reference to drugs that can be bought and prescribed.

Summary

Responding to symptoms plays an important part in healthcare. Most general-sales-list medicines and, by definition, all pharmacy medicines are sold through community pharmacies. Pharmacists have developed a counselling and advisory role in the treatment of minor illness. Some members of the public may know exactly which non-prescription medicine they want and input from pharmacists may be unwanted or indeed, on occasions, unwelcome. Despite this, pharmacists have a legal responsibility to supervise all sales of pharmacy medicines, and a professional responsibility to help consumers choose the most appropriate medicine for their symptoms. Conversely, other members of the public can be reassured and extremely grateful for a positive caring attitude from the pharmacist who clearly wishes to help, who devotes time to find out about their condition, and recommends the most appropriate treatment. Not only does the public benefit from the development of this role, but the pharmacist gains confidence and satisfaction in a professional and personal capacity.

18.3 Responding to symptoms

Introduction

The AIM of responding to symptoms is:

- A – Assessment
- I – Interpretation
- M – Management

Members of the public seeking advice from pharmacists about symptoms and self-medication usually fall into one of three categories. Some patients may have already made their own diagnosis from their symptoms, and will seek advice on treatment only. Others may describe a symptom, or group of symptoms, which require interpretation and a recommendation of a course of action or treatment. Thirdly, patients may request a specific category of medicine (e.g. an analgesic) but require advice on item selection.

By observing and interviewing patients, pharmacists must confirm a patient's self-diagnosis, interpret any symptoms described, and select the most appropriate regimen.

It must be remembered that a pharmacist's ability to respond to a patient's symptoms is limited because pharmacists cannot effectively examine patients. However, the following guidelines will prompt pharmacists to ask relevant questions in order to obtain a patient history to enable them to distinguish major illnesses from minor ailments.

Assessment and interpretation

For an account of effective communication between pharmacists and patients, *see* Section 17.2.

- Establish who the patient is.
  - Do not assume it is the person presenting the symptom.
- Evaluate appearance, demeanour, and manner. Does the patient appear ill?
  - Remember to act sympathetically towards those who are either unwell themselves, or who may be worried about a sick relative or friend.
- Establish a profile of the patient's symptoms by considering the following questions:
  - What is the primary symptom?
  - What is the present location of the symptom (e.g. where is the pain)?
  - What is the nature and severity of the symptom (e.g. is it a sharp or dull pain, or a dry or productive cough)?
  - Are there any accompanying symptoms?
  - Have any of these factors changed since their appearance (e.g. have the symptoms worsened, or has the pain moved or radiated elsewhere)?
  - Did the symptom appear gradually or suddenly? How long has it been present?
  - Can the presence of one symptom be linked to an associated event (e.g. alcohol consumption, emotional disturbances, diet, menstruation, injury, use of cosmetics or time of day)?
  - Does anything make the symptom worse or better (e.g. movement, posture or food)?
  - Is this an isolated occurrence of the symptom, or is it recurrent?
  - Have any family or friends complained of similar symptoms?
- Establish a treatment history.
  - Has the doctor been consulted for this symptom? If so, was treatment given?
  - Has self-medication already been tried? If so, what was the outcome?
  - Are any other drugs (prescribed or purchased from a pharmacy) being taken for an unrelated condition?
- Establish, by observation or questioning, the existence of any risk factors.
  - How old is the patient?
  - Is the patient pregnant?
  - Does the patient suffer from any chronic conditions (e.g. diabetes mellitus)?
  - Does the patient have any known drug allergies (e.g. to aspirin or lanolin)?

Management

Certain questions are particularly pertinent when considering specific symptoms, and these have been highlighted as Key Questions at the beginning of each of the following sections. The Key Questions are not, however, intended to be the only questions that might be asked, as all the above factors should always be considered when interviewing patients about their symptoms.

The answers obtained from interviewing the patient should indicate one of the following courses of action:

- Make a tentative diagnosis and give advice regarding the treatment. Pharmacists should take the opportunity to suggest the best course of action if the symptoms persist after a few days treatment (e.g. medical referral or return to the pharmacy).
- Refer the patient to a doctor either immediately if considered urgent, or by making an appointment for a consultation.
- Suggest no medicinal treatment, but counsel the patient (e.g. on diet). Often reassurance alone is an effective measure.

18.3.1 COUGHS AND COLDS

Introduction

Upper respiratory-tract infection may be caused by bacterial or, more commonly, viral invasion, resulting in the common cold. Although the symptoms of a cough and head cold may present separately, they often occur together.

Key questions 18.3.1

- When did the cough start?
- Was the cough preceded by symptoms of the common cold (e.g. sore throat, sneezing, nasal congestion)?
- Is the cough productive or dry?
- Is the cough painful?
- Does the patient have a fever?
- Has there been a change in character of a persistent cough?
- What is the appearance of the sputum?
- Is the cough worse at night?

Assessment and interpretation

Nature and severity

Patients with a head cold may complain of nasal congestion or nasal discharge (rhinorrhoea). The colour of nasal secretions is not normally a helpful sign, except when other symptoms (e.g. headache or facial tenderness and aching over and under the eyes) suggest sinusitis. In such instances, if the mucus is green or brown and symptoms have persisted for one week without improvement, then referral should be made so that the doctor may assess the condition.

The type of cough should be ascertained. Coughs broadly fall into one of three categories. First, a dry tickle felt in the throat may produce an irritating cough with no sputum. Secondly, a cough may be described as chesty, and sputum is produced. The third type is a chesty cough which does not produce sputum, and may represent congestion in the bronchi.

Onset and duration

The onset of most respiratory-tract infections is sudden, and the commonly described appearance of a sore throat, sneezing and rhinorrhoea herald the well-known syndrome of the common cold.

A cough which follows such symptoms will often arise because of irritation by a postnasal drip (mucus stimulating cough receptors in the pharynx) or clearing of the throat.

A cough at night may be related to the presence of an allergen. However, the presence of night-time cough is not helpful in differentiating the cause, except in children where it may be a sign of asthma.

In an otherwise healthy person, the duration of symptoms is an important factor which will determine whether non-prescription medicines may be recommended by pharmacists or referral is appropriate. Symptoms of the common cold generally last about one week, but may persist for two or three weeks. A cough that has not improved over two or three weeks should be referred for assessment to exclude any chronic condition, and this time period should be shorter if symptoms are causing distress or becoming more severe.

Long-standing recurrent cough (e.g. since childhood) may indicate a chronic lung disorder (e.g. bronchiectasis), and the decision whether to refer will be based on the patient's past experience and the severity of the current symptoms.

Smokers, who normally disregard their cough, may suffer from chronic bronchitis which can occasionally flare up into an acute attack. The decision to refer again rests on the severity of symptoms, but with this type of patient some professional advice about the damage caused by cigarette smoke may be warranted.

Accompanying symptoms

If there is sputum, its nature may be helpful in deciding management. Clear white sputum is of little clinical significance, but copious, white, frothy sputum may be coughed up by chronic bronchitic patients and smokers. Brown or green sputum suggests the presence of a chest infection but patients should generally only be considered for referral if they feel ill. The presence of blood-stained sputum requires referral. After a severe fit of coughing, it might be normal to pass one or two specks of blood in the sputum, but persistent blood specks or more obvious loss of blood requires referral as serious (but rare) problems (e.g. carcinoma, tuberculosis and pulmonary embolism) must be excluded.

A noticeably raised temperature is uncommon in adults suffering from the common cold. It may accompany more severe infections. If patients complain of night sweats and of feeling ill, or having a cough which has lasted for more than one week without improvement, referral is necessary to exclude serious conditions (e.g. tuberculosis).

General malaise, headache and myalgia are common accompaniments to viral illnesses (e.g. influenza). Providing no other symptom is present that would suggest the need for medical referral, the patient should be reassured that the illness will begin to resolve in a few days.

A sore throat is a frequent early symptom of the common cold, which usually resolves spontaneously. Referral is not necessary providing it is not painful or causing difficulty with swallowing (*see* Sore throat, Section 18.3.2).

Infected sinuses may cause sinus pain and headache. Sinus pain is usually characterised by a painful face, and tenderness to pressure below the eyes on the cheek bones and on the bony ridge above the eyes. Nasal mucus may be discoloured, indicating infection. Patients often complain of a long history of sinusitis, and a decision whether to refer will often depend on the benefit derived from previous treatment.

Patients may complain of persistent catarrh which exists for several days or weeks after other symptoms of a cold have disappeared. Providing they are otherwise well, symptomatic treatment is sufficient until the condition resolves.

Patients with rhinorrhoea or nasal congestion accompanied by itchy red eyes may be suffering from an allergy or infection. Allergy may represent a perennial rhinitis which may exist most of the year due to constant allergenic stimuli in the patient's environment (e.g. house-dust mite). More commonly, symptoms occur between April and August and are caused by seasonal allergies (e.g. hay fever). Under most circumstances, there are many symptomatic remedies which can be recommended before referral is necessary.

Wheezing represents an element of bronchoconstriction which, although more commonly associated by the layman with asthma, is not an uncommon component of other airways diseases (e.g. bronchitis and bronchiectasis). Wheezing in a child should be referred to the doctor. In adults, referral depends on the severity and whether patients are short of breath.

Patients who are short of breath, but have not normally been so in the past, require referral to exclude more serious conditions and to obtain early treatment. It should be remembered that patients with cardiac problems (e.g. heart failure) may also report this symptom, especially at night.

Severe pain on coughing or on inspiration requires referral to exclude conditions such as pleurisy and pulmonary embolism.

Patients with chronic chest symptoms should be questioned about weight loss. Severe weight loss may accompany serious conditions such as lung cancer and tuberculosis. It should always be enquired after in smokers and chronic bronchitics.

Causative and modifying factors

It may be possible to relate the onset of symptoms to a particular causative factor (e.g. an allergen in hay fever or previous exposure to cold or wet or other infected individuals with the common cold).

Drugs may precipitate respiratory problems. Aspirin and other non-steroidal anti-inflammatory drugs may provoke an asthmatic attack in about 5% of asthmatic patients. Beta-adrenoceptor blocking drugs may also cause bronchoconstriction in asthmatics. A small proportion of patients undergoing treatment with angiotensin-converting enzyme (ACE) inhibitors may develop a persistent, usually dry cough which disappears only when the treatment is withdrawn.

Some patients receiving antihypertensive therapy may develop nasal congestion.

Possible causes of cough are summarised in Part C.

Risk factors

Many risk factors (e.g. heart failure or smoking) may predispose patients to various pulmonary disorders.

In otherwise healthy people, age is the predominant risk factor for respiratory infections at both extremes of life. The elderly, especially the frail, the malnourished, and those who cannot keep warm are susceptible to chest infections. Such infections may make elderly patients take to their beds where they may develop pneumonia. Infections may also result in confusion and a fall, perhaps causing fractured bones and leading to several weeks in hospital. The elderly and other susceptible groups such as those with diabetes, asthma, chronic lung disease and heart failure should be encouraged to avail themselves of influenza vaccinations in the winter. If they become infected with the common cold virus, they need to take special care. If they feel ill, they should be advised to visit or call the doctor, who will assess their situation and decide on suitable treatment.

At the other end of the age spectrum, young children, especially those under nine months of age, require special attention. Infants who cannot feed because of nasal congestion, or who refuse to eat because they feel ill, require referral either to the doctor or health visitor. Any vomiting, breathing difficulties, noisy breathing or earache require referral. Similarly, those developing symptoms of a cold after immunisation should be referred. A night-time cough which persists needs assessment by a doctor, to exclude the presence of asthma.

Generally, children who are ill do not eat and it is this marker which will often give a clue as to whether it is necessary to refer.

Management

Non-drug treatment

Steam inhalations have been traditionally used to relieve nasal congestion. They are harmless and the addition of oils such as menthol may add a powerful placebo effect. There is no clear evidence from clinical trials to support their effectiveness.

Steam inhalations or an increased fluid intake may hydrate the inflamed pharyngeal mucosa and provide alleviation of dry coughs. Their use is also ideally suited for the treatment of productive coughs. Anecdotally, steam inhalations, or sitting in a bathroom with the hot water taps running, have been found to be helpful, possibly by hydrating the upper respiratory tree and encouraging loosening of viscid sputum and secretion from mucous glands.

Drug treatment

The management of coughs and colds with no underlying pathology is symptomatic and, despite the belief or expectations of many visitors to the pharmacy, there is no consistently good clinical evidence that any medication will curtail the natural progression of the infection. However, symptom relief is important since people with coughs and colds may otherwise take time off work. Although many clinical authorities dismiss cough medicines as placebos, the general public regard them with the greatest esteem. They are, at the very least, powerful placebos and some may be considered to have some pharmacological efficacy (*see below*).

Zinc is postulated to combine with the coat of the rhinovirus and prevent it entering cells and reproducing and has therefore been trialled as a 'cold cure'.

The evidence is unclear, but there are some claims that zinc lozenges, if taken within the first day of onset of a cold may reduce the duration and severity of symptoms. Similar claims have been made for megadoses of vitamin C.

Rhinorrhoea and nasal congestion may be alleviated by sympathomimetic agents. These vasoconstrictors shrink the inflamed tissues and reduce the activity of mucous glands in the nasal mucosa. They are available as systemic (BNF 3.10) or topical nasal (BNF 12.2.2) decongestants.

Oral products for the relief of coughs and colds are often combinations of a sympathomimetic agent, an antihistamine (to dry up secretions and to suppress any cough) and an analgesic with antipyretic properties. Sympathomimetic agents are contraindicated in diabetic patients as they stimulate beta-receptors and can counteract the effects of hypoglycaemic agents. They are also contraindicated in hypertension, hyperthyroidism and angina. In such cases, if a decongestant is deemed absolutely necessary, a topical formulation may be preferable, as local vasoconstriction should reduce its absorption from the nasal mucosa. Sympathomimetic agents should also be avoided in patients taking monoamine oxidase inhibitors and other antidepressant drugs.

Patients with glaucoma should not be given preparations containing antihistamines because of their intrinsic anticholinergic properties. These preparations may also cause a dry mouth, constipation, interference with accommodation and sedation.

If an antihistamine alone is recommended (e.g. in allergic rhinitis), it may be logical to select a non-sedating agent such as loratadine or cetirizine.

The use of topical decongestant sprays and drops for periods longer than one to two weeks may cause harmful effects and result in a rebound congestion (rhinitis medicamentosa).

Some patients with hay fever will benefit from topical steroids such as beclometasone in the form of a nasal spray, but continual regular use during the season is essential.

Patients who are feverish, have aching limbs and muscles, headache, or general malaise may benefit from using a simple analgesic with antipyretic properties (e.g. paracetamol). A streaming rhinorrhoea results in appreciable fluid loss and requires plenty of drinks to replace that loss.

Mild sore throats, though self-limiting, are traditionally temporarily relieved by sucking antibacterial pastilles or lozenges. Lozenges containing flurbiprofen may provide an anti-inflammatory effect, but should be avoided in asthmatic patients.

Cough suppressants have traditionally been used for dry, irritating, tickly coughs, but evidence to support their efficacy is largely anecdotal. Sufferers of coughs will expect something to alleviate their symptoms because the cough may keep them awake at night or irritate others who live or work within close proximity.

Codeine, dextromethorphan or pholcodine are found in many proprietary cough products. Codeine may be abused and the use of pholcodine, which has similar cough suppressant activity, is preferred.

Antihistamines are also cough sedatives and may be used alone or combined with opioids. They may, however, cause drowsiness and, if this is the case, are best used at night.

Demulcents (e.g. glycerol, honey and syrup) have been traditionally used to soothe the throat and tickly coughs.

For chesty, but non-productive coughs, a bronchodilator may encourage a clear airway and aid removal of sputum from the respiratory tree. Many products contain ephedrine and pseudoephedrine in combination with suppressants or expectorants. Contraindications to these sympathomimetic drugs are listed under nasal congestion (*see above*).

Productive coughs should be encouraged, not suppressed, to allow removal of sputum containing cell debris or irritating substances from the respiratory tract. There are many expectorant drugs used in non-prescription cough products (e.g. ammonium salts, guaiphenesin, ipecacuanha, squill and citric acid, *see* BNF 3.9.2.) but good clinical trial evidence in support of their efficacy is generally lacking.

18.3.2 SORE THROAT

Introduction

A sore throat is a common early accompaniment to the common cold and as such is unremarkable and self-imiting. However, certain causes of sore throats have potentially serious consequences and these should be enquired for where appropriate. (For a description of the relevant anatomy, *see* Section 12.4.)

Key questions 18.3.2

- Is swallowing affected?
- Is breathing impaired?
- Does the patient have persistent hoarseness or loss of voice?
- Are the tonsils red or swollen with white spots visible?
- Is the patient taking any prescribed drugs which are known to cause a sore throat?
- Has the sore throat persisted for more than one week without improvement?

Assessment and interpretation

Location and nature

The patient may complain of a dry irritating feeling at the back of the throat or oropharynx, and this is a common accompaniment to the common cold. If the throat is painful and the pain persists for more than two days, whether or not accompanied by symptoms of the common cold, it is possible that a bacterial infection, usually streptococcal, is the cause.

Examination in a well-lit area and asking the patient to say 'Ah' with the mouth open as wide as possible may reveal a red inflamed throat, and tonsils if present. White pus-filled spots on the tonsils will confirm tonsillitis and require referral for assessment and treatment. White spots elsewhere in the mouth (e.g. on the tongue and on the buccal mucosa) are likely to be due to candidiasis. However, aphthous ulcers, which are white patches on the mucosa, are more likely to be painful, especially when eating. Another disorder, lichen planus, may present with a white, lace-like pattern on the buccal mucosa, which may resemble candidiasis.

A sore throat causing a hoarse voice is likely to be due to laryngitis caused by bacterial infection. However, hoarseness in the presence of other symptoms may have different causes. Persistent hoarseness requires referral, as the possibility of sinister pathology (e.g. carcinoma of the respiratory tract) exists in a small number of cases.

Difficulty in swallowing may be a complication of a sore throat or may be due to obstruction from another source, and needs investigation to eliminate sinister causes.

Accompanying symptoms

If the sore throat is mild and symptoms of the common cold develop within 48 hours, the sore throat will normally resolve spontaneously within a short period.

Pain and general malaise may accompany a sore throat. If the throat is painful and there are large tender lymph nodes in the neck, a bacterial infection, possibly of the tonsils is likely. In such a case, referral for assessment of the value of antibacterial treatment is necessary. Alternatively, in young adults, the possibility of glandular fever should be borne in mind. Although a rash is associated with glandular fever, it may be late in appearing, and is often brought on by a course of amoxicillin. If the patient feels ill apart from symptoms of a cold, referral is advisable. Fever, night sweats or persistent aching muscles or joints accompanying a painful throat also demand referral.

Because of its proximity via the Eustachian tube, the ear often becomes infected from the throat. Ear pain is a sign of spread of infection and requires referral.

A rash accompanying a sore throat suggests a systemic disease (e.g. glandular fever, meningitis or one of the childhood infectious diseases). Cases should always be referred for a medical opinion, unless pharmacists are aware of local outbreaks of measles, mumps or chickenpox.

Awareness of a lump in the throat is a rare symptom, causing patients to complain of not being able to swallow or breathe normally. This may represent a quinsy-like illness and is characterised by ulceration of the tonsils in which inflammation interferes with the aperture of the trachea. If the patient cannot swallow normally or complains of an awareness of a lump in the throat, referral should be made.

Marked mouth ulceration is a painful condition. If patients have a history of ulceration, the decision to refer is based on the severity and the experience of the outcome of previous attacks. However, mouth ulceration which spreads to the outside of the lips and is accompanied by malaise or fever requires urgent referral to exclude serious disorders, especially when patients are taking immunosuppressant drugs (e.g. corticosteroids or cytotoxic agents), drugs capable of causing bone-marrow suppression (e.g. antiepileptics, carbimazole or tricyclic antidepressants), or drugs causing the Stevens–Johnson syndrome (e.g. co-trimoxazole, some antiepileptic drugs).

Causative and modifying factors

The most common cause of a sore throat is a bacterial or viral infection, although acid reflux and environmental influences (e.g. smoke or vapours) may also be implicated. Treatment with antibacterials can suppress the normal flora of the buccal cavity and allow an overgrowth of candida. Similarly, corticosteroid inhalations can cause a local immunosuppressive effect, resulting in candidiasis. Diabetics are particularly prone to recurrent infections, including oral thrush or candidiasis.

A summary of the possible causes of a sore throat is given under Throat discomfort, Part C.

Management

Non-drug treatment

Apart from medication, patients should avoid smoky or dusty atmospheres and reduce or stop smoking.

Drug treatment

Although it is difficult to distinguish between viral and bacterial throat infections, a rule of thumb may be applied that involvement of the tonsils or the ears should be referred for assessment of treatment with antibacterials. Patients with heart-valve disease should be referred to prevent secondary spread of streptococci to the endocardium. Other throat infections will usually be viral, for which antibacterial agents are of no use.

Infection presumed to be viral should be treated with a high fluid intake. If patients find swallowing painful, a light fluid diet should be taken. Lozenges may offer symptomatic relief. Their use is probably nothing more than placebo, but the flow of saliva which is stimulated by sucking may have a soothing effect. Flurbiprofen lozenges may provide some relief by an anti-inflammatory effect. Alternatively, gargling with two or three soluble aspirin tablets may provide adequate local relief of pain and inflammation. If pain spreads to the ears, non-opioid analgesics may be recommended as an interim measure until a doctor is seen.

18.3.3 HEADACHE

Introduction

Headache is possibly the most common symptom for which the lay public seek self-medication. It can usually be attributed to minor conditions (e.g. muscle tension), psychogenic causes or dilatation of cranial blood vessels. Rarely, serious causes (e.g. inflammation of the meninges, or tumours) are identified.

Key questions 18.3.3

- Where is the headache located (e.g. back, front)
- How severe is it?
- Did it come on suddenly for no apparent reason or is there an obvious cause (e.g. injury)?
- How long has it lasted?
- Are there any other symptoms?
- Does anything aggravate its severity?

Assessment and interpretation

Location

Frontal headache is most likely to be idiopathic or due to sinusitis, nasal congestion or migraine.

Pain in the back of the head (occipital headache) is frequently due to tension, stress or anxiety (referred to as psychogenic headache), especially if the pain radiates over the top or sides of the head. The patient will often describe a feeling of a tight band around or over the head. This type of headache is one of the most commonly reported. Tension may also be caused by neck injury or muscle spasm in the neck, back or shoulder. More serious causes include space-occupying lesions (e.g. tumours) and subarachnoid haemorrhage. Both of these conditions may also produce headache which is either felt in other parts or radiates to them.

Pain originating on one side of the forehead and face (unilateral headache) frequently accompanies sinusitis, whilst the unilateral pain of classical migraine can originate in any area of the head. Unilateral pain of both conditions can become bilateral.

Herpes zoster virus infections of the nerves running over the top of the scalp and into the eye can cause shingles on one side of the face. A severe lancing pain may be felt before the characteristic rash is apparent.

Cluster headaches are a type of migraine headache, which may affect one side of the head or face.

Trigeminal neuralgia involves the cranial facial nerve. The slightest touch or pressure on this area of the face can provoke an extreme pain often described as sharp or lancing.

Pain felt in the eye should be referred as it raises the possibility of serious problems such as glaucoma or trauma. Pain felt behind or around the eye can occur in sinusitis, migraine, or shingles.

Nature and severity

An extremely intense, often occipital headache which comes on very suddenly without warning and feels like a blow to the head, requires medical referral as it may indicate an emergency such as subarachnoid haemorrhage. If an equally intense pain has developed much more gradually, referral may be necessary to exclude the possibility of subdural haematoma. This possibility should be suspected following head injury, however trivial. Patients should be questioned about the occurrence of any possible trauma or incident.

Throbbing headache may be due to vascular changes (e.g. migraine or haemorrhage), or can accompany pyrexia of influenza or other viral infections.

Dull continuous headache may be due to tension, neck trauma or a tumour.

Onset and duration

An early morning headache, which usually abates during the day, can be caused by space-occupying lesions. A clear-cut diagnosis is not possible, however, because benign idiopathic and tension headaches may also be present from the moment patients awaken.

Patients known to be hypertensive should be made aware that persistent severe early morning headache may be associated with uncontrolled hypertension. Referral should be recommended, especially if nausea, vomiting, nose bleeds or bleeding from any other part of the body (e.g. haematuria) is noted. The nasal congestion of sinusitis is often worsened by lying down. Early morning headache is often associated with this condition.

An intense pain lasting more than 48 hours which disrupts normal lifestyle requires referral.

Stress and tension headaches, and sinusitis, produce a continuous dull pain over several days. Migraine varies in duration from a few hours to more than a day, but rarely lasts more than two days. Cluster headaches last for 1–2 hours (usually at night-time), often recurring at the same time for weeks or months.

Brief pain, or a consistent pattern of pain which has existed for several years, is unlikely to have a serious cause. However, changes in its nature, reflected by increasing severity or duration, require medical attention.

Accompanying symptoms

Symptoms accompanying headache can be useful in evaluating the cause of some types of headache.

General malaise, aching and fever may be indicative of a viral infection (e.g. the common cold, influenza). A less frequently encountered cause is meningitis. More specific diagnosis is possible if additional symptoms are present, and include a rash (e.g. mumps or meningitis) or nasal congestion (e.g. sinusitis or common cold).

Meningitis should also be suspected if the patient complains of fever, together with neck stiffness, extreme pain on both up-and-down and side-to-side movement of the head, nausea or vomiting, or rash. Restriction of movement in a horizontal plane can occur in muscle spasm caused by cervical spondylosis, torticollis or subarachnoid haemorrhage.

Headaches accompanied by nausea or vomiting may be characteristic of minor conditions (e.g. migraine) or serious illness (e.g. space-occupying lesions, haemorrhage, meningitis and glaucoma).

Disturbed vision may accompany various forms of headache. Blurred vision can accompany classical migraine, while restricted field of vision and haloes around artificial lights may occur in glaucoma. By comparison, common migraine does not affect normal visual fields.

Emotional disturbances (e.g. tiredness and an inability to fall asleep) may accompany headache caused by depressive disorders, tension and anxiety. Early morning awakening, poor appetite, and an inability to cope with worry are other indicators of emotional disturbances.

Patients reporting signs of central nervous system involvement in headache (e.g. drowsiness and irritability, numbness, paraesthesia and unilateral muscle weakness) should be referred immediately. Serious possible pathology suggested by these symptoms include stroke, subarachnoid or subdural haemorrhage, or a tumour. The gradual development and intermittent appearance of slurred speech and personality changes with headache may indicate space-occupying lesions.

A cyclical pattern of headache immediately before or during menstruation suggests hormonal imbalance.

Causative and modifying factors

Pain on movement of the head or neck may indicate a neck injury or inflamed meninges. Bending down will exacerbate the headache of space-occupying lesions, sinusitis, and other causes. Sudden movements produced by coughing and sneezing will worsen the headache of space-occupying lesions. Exercise may also precipitate migraine. Conversely, migraine and many other types of headache may be relieved by lying down, particularly in a darkened room.

Diet can play an important role in causing headache in individuals. Various foods and drinks (e.g. chocolate, coffee and alcohol) or hunger can precipitate migraine in some cases. Diabetic patients may also suffer headaches when their condition becomes unstable.

Bright daylight and artificial light may aggravate migraine and the headache of meningitis. Conversely, entering a darkened room may worsen the headache caused by glaucoma through pupillary dilatation.

It is important to be aware of a patient's treatment history. Patients should be asked about any current prescription or non-prescription medication and whether any link can be established between their symptoms and side effects of their medication.

Management

Non-drug treatment

Any obvious causative factors such as food, alcohol or eye strain should be excluded.

Once other possible causes, and the possibility of serious underlying pathology, have been excluded, long-term headaches may normally be attributed to stress and tension. Despite the absence of obvious physical causes, such patients should be treated sympathetically. Counselling in relaxation techniques (e.g. lying down, gentle exercise and massage) may be required to relieve the underlying cause. If the suggested measures show no improvement within, say, two weeks, patients could reasonably be referred if they are anxious, or their lifestyle is being disrupted.

Drug treatment

Headaches are generally more responsive to treatment by analgesics if treatment is started promptly. This is particularly true for migraine headaches, in which an early loading dose of analgesic followed by regular maintenance doses throughout the attack, is desirable.

Different formulations of analgesics may be more appropriate for certain types of headache. Although soluble or effervescent formulations achieve peak plasma concentrations more rapidly than non-soluble forms, there is no convincing evidence to suggest soluble forms relieve pain more quickly or effectively. Nevertheless, the placebo effect of such medicines is significant. Topical analgesics may be helpful in muscle tension or stiffness of the neck following trauma, or in tension headaches. The plethora of balms and rubs available may act through a counter-irritant effect, by local absorption of the analgesic, or both. The beneficial effects of local massage should also not be overlooked.

The choice of analgesic is empirical. Whenever possible, however, single-agent preparations are preferred to combination products.

Headache caused by minor neck injury, or tissue inflammation associated with nasal congestion or sinusitis, should theoretically benefit from the use of aspirin or ibuprofen rather than paracetamol. There is also some evidence to support the preferred use of ibuprofen in dental pain.

Aspirin and ibuprofen are contraindicated in several instances. Aspirin should not be recommended to children under 15 years of age because of its implication in Reye's syndrome. Aspirin and ibuprofen are also contraindicated in the presence of a history of heartburn, indigestion and peptic ulceration. Anyone with known hypersensitivity to aspirin should not be given ibuprofen.

Asthmatic patients may develop hypersensitivity to aspirin and other non-steroidal anti-inflammatory analgesics. Patients prescribed oral anticoagulant therapy should also not be given aspirin. Most patients will be aware of such interactions, but it is wise to ask all patients if they are taking other medication.

Aspirin may cause problems in the latter stages of pregnancy and paracetamol is a safer alternative. No teratogenic effects have been noted with ibuprofen use during pregnancy, but it should be avoided during pregnancy if possible.

Paracetamol may be used in children and in other patients in whom aspirin is contraindicated.

Codeine is only available in a non-prescription tablet form as a combination product with aspirin or paracetamol. If taken regularly for prolonged periods, constipation may result.

The addition of caffeine as an enhancer in combination analgesic formulations is probably of little real clinical benefit.

Feverfew has been used with variable success in the prophylaxis of migraine.

18.3.4 INDIGESTION

Introduction

Indigestion (dyspepsia) is a term commonly used to describe epigastric discomfort, heartburn or both, that may occur after eating or drinking. Patients will often use the term to describe a variety of non-specific gastrointestinal symptoms. It is important that pharmacists can evaluate the presenting symptoms in order to exclude any serious pathology before recommending remedial action. This section will deal with two descriptions of symptoms commonly presented to pharmacists by the public – heartburn and indigestion. Other abdominal conditions are described under abdominal pain (*see below*).

Heartburn is a symptom caused by reflux of acid from the stomach into the oesophagus causing oesophagitis, commonly felt as a burning sensation in the chest behind the sternum. Indigestion is a vague lay term which will be conveniently defined here as upper abdominal discomfort (i.e. epigastric symptoms) related to food or drink.

Key questions 18.3.4

- Can the patient pinpoint exactly where the discomfort is?
- Is there pain and if so has it spread?
- Do the symptoms occur after eating or drinking?
- Has the patient ingested anything which may have caused the symptoms?
- Is it relieved by antacids or food?
- Does anything aggravate it (e.g. bending down)?

Assessment and interpretation

Onset and duration

If this is the first episode of indigestion, it may be treated symptomatically with OTC medicines except where the patient is over 45 years of age. New occurrences should be regarded with caution particularly because carcinoma of the stomach, though a relatively rare condition, is more likely to be seen in this age group. It would be wise therefore to refer patients in this category for their doctors to follow them up.

If similar attacks of indigestion or heartburn have occurred before, they may be treated with OTC medicines (antacids or H_2-receptor antagonists) for up to seven days. If no improvement is felt, patients should be referred to the doctor for assessment. Attacks that are worse than in the past or are accompanied by new symptoms also require referral for assessment.

Symptoms of indigestion that are worse at night may be caused by duodenal lesions (e.g. duodenal ulcer), which are thought to be sometimes exacerbated by night-time secretion of gastric acid into the duodenum.

Accompanying symptoms

A bloated feeling or a sensation of fullness is common in patients with indigestion. Although such symptoms may transiently disappear along with indigestion after treatment with antacids, they may return and in such cases referral for further evaluation is required.

A loss of appetite often occurs in patients with abdominal symptoms, especially in peptic ulceration, which may lead to a loss in weight. Significant weight changes require referral as they indicate sinister pathology, which must be excluded at an early stage.

Vomiting or constipation, or both, in the presence of indigestion demands immediate referral because it may indicate obstruction in the gastrointestinal tract.

Similarly difficulty in swallowing or regurgitation of food after meals indicates possible obstruction in the oesophagus and requires medical assessment.

A patient with indigestion complaining of tiredness may have gastrointestinal blood loss in the vomit or stool. This may lead to anaemia and requires referral.

Causative and modifying factors

Drugs (e.g. non-steroidal anti-inflammatory drugs including aspirin, steroids, digoxin and iron) may cause indigestion.

Common dietary causative factors to enquire after include overindulgence in food or drink, rushed meals, and unusual or spicy foods. Indigestion may be relieved by eating small meals as food can act as a barrier between gastric acid and the mucosa. Alternatively, food may stimulate acid production and consequently aggravate the condition. This relationship with food merely reassures the patient that the origin of discomfort is in the gastrointestinal tract. Small amounts of food eaten frequently will usually offer the best relief of symptoms. If treatment with antacids or acid suppressants and dietary adjustment do not relieve the indigestion, then referral should be made to investigate for the presence of peptic ulceration. Coffee, tea, alcohol and smoking are likely to exacerbate indigestion and heartburn.

Bending over or lying down may aggravate acid reflux, leading to heartburn. Symptoms may be aggravated by obesity or hiatus hernia, again especially on bending down.

A summary of the possible causes of indigestion is given in Part C.

Isolated or recurrent factors

Recurrent symptoms of indigestion or heartburn require medical investigation, despite patients' assertions that the condition is normal for them. Nevertheless, many cases will show negative pathology.

If the patient has had indigestion in recent weeks and the symptoms are worse on this occasion, or other symptoms are present regardless of whether they respond to OTC medication, a referral should be advised.

In the second and third trimesters of pregnancy, the growing fetus and uterus may press against the bowel and stomach. This may cause indigestion, especially heartburn, which is aggravated on stooping or lying down. Oral iron preparations are a common cause of gastrointestinal upset in pregnant women.

Various chronic illnesses can also cause indigestion. Patients with heart failure may suffer gastrointestinal symptoms (e.g. indigestion, anorexia, and nausea) due to congestion and stasis of blood in the abdominal organs. Diabetic patients may have similar symptoms and require referral to check the control of their plasma glucose concentration.

Management

Non-drug treatment

If there is an obvious benign cause of an acute attack of indigestion, reassurance may initially be sufficient. Counselling on the avoidance of stress, smoking and coffee, and on the importance of small, regular, non-spicy meals and weight reduction, where appropriate, is important if the effects of drug therapy are not to be negated.

Simple measures such as sleeping with extra pillows can provide relief from night-time heartburn.

Drug treatment

Antacids and H_2-receptor antagonists are the primary, and often very effective, non-prescription treatments for indigestion and heartburn. Where reflux oesophagitis or heartburn is the problem, antacid products containing alginates are useful to help suppress the movement of acid through the oesophageal sphincter.

Antacids containing sodium bicarbonate (e.g. magnesium trisilicate mixture) should be avoided in patients with heart failure or with renal dysfunction because of the risk of sodium overload. The fact that magnesium salts are osmotic laxatives and aluminium salts can be constipating may influence the choice of antacid for individual patients.

Aluminium salts are thought to bind and inactivate pepsin which, in association with gastric acid, may be a major cause of gastric mucosal breakdown.

Antacids containing calcium carbonate may cause rebound indigestion by the direct stimulant effect of calcium on gastrin production, leading to increased secretion of gastric juice. A choice of an antacid containing a single magnesium or aluminium salt is recommended, depending on bowel habits. Antacids are best taken one hour after meals, at which time gastric emptying is slowed and contact time with the gastric contents is maximised.

Many proprietary antacids contain mixtures of magnesium and aluminium salts. The rationale for such mixtures may be to counteract the effects on the bowel habit of the individual agents, although otherwise these mixtures offer no advantages over single agents. Dimethicone, which may reduce flatulence by lowering the surface tension of bubbles of gas in the gastric fluid, is also present in many products.

In pregnancy, reassurance is often all that is required. However, a simple antacid (e.g. Milk of Magnesia) may be useful and is safe after the first trimester. Antacids interact with iron in the gastrointestinal tract, and this type of reaction may be reduced by arranging the dosage times so that the two are not taken within two hours of each other.

H_2-receptor antagonists (cimetidine, ranitidine and famotidine) are licensed as OTC medicines in the UK for the short-term treatment of dyspepsia and heartburn. They are extremely effective, as evidence from many clinical trials has shown. They can be taken either once or twice a day and are also useful in relieving night-time symptoms. It is important that patients who obtain relief from OTC H_2-receptor antagonists in the short term are cautioned not to use them continuously in the long term and to see their doctor for evaluation of their symptoms.

18.3.5 ABDOMINAL PAIN

Introduction

In this section abdominal pain refers to pain principally felt below the rib cage, but also includes pain felt in the chest as a result of pathology associated with the oesophagus (*see* Heartburn *above*).

Key questions 18.3.5

- Where exactly is the pain?
- Has the patient had a gastrointestinal illness before?
- When did the pain start?
- Is it an intermittent or a constant pain?
- Has the pain spread from its starting point?
- Is there anything that helps to reduce the pain?
- Has the patient vomited?
- Has there been a change in bowel habit?
- Has there been blood in the vomit or stool?
- Is there pain on passing urine?
- Is there abdominal tenderness?

Assessment and interpretation

Location

Pain in the midline sections of the abdomen, i.e. epigastric, central and suprapubic areas (*see* Figure 1.1), is usually indicative of an intestinal or gastric cause. The pain of peptic ulceration is typically epigastric, central, or both. In duodenal ulceration, the pain may also be felt slightly to the right. The pain of appendicitis begins in the central area but quickly radiates to the right iliac fossa. Pain in the right upper abdomen, just beneath the lower ribs, may be caused by spasm in the bile duct. However, this pain can sometimes be felt in the epigastrium.

The pain of irritable bowel syndrome is usually low down and typically occurs in the left iliac fossa, but may spread centrally or to the right iliac fossa.

Diverticular disease similarly causes pain in the right or left iliac fossae.

Sometimes gastrointestinal pain may be felt as a vague and generalised pain over most of the abdomen, as in gastroenteritis.

Reflux oesophagitis (*see* Heartburn *above*) may cause a burning pain in the epigastrium which may spread into the chest beneath the sternum.

Renal pain is felt in the loin area at the side or to the back of the abdomen. Infection or renal calculi affecting the ureters may cause pain radiating down from the loin to the iliac fossa on the affected side (ureteric or renal colic), and eventually the suprapubic area will be affected if the obstruction or infection affects the bladder and urethra.

Nature and severity

Pain in any hollow organ with a smooth muscular coat is usually colicky, reflecting the spasms of the circular smooth muscle in the wall of the organ. Colic is a spasmodic pain that is griping, reaches a peak, and then eases before returning. This type of pain may reflect involvement of the stomach, large and small bowel, the ureters, urethra and the bile ducts as well as the reproductive organs (e.g. the uterus and Fallopian tubes). Sometimes abdominal pain is less severe and specific, presenting as a dull ache (as in irritable bowel syndrome).

The pain of peptic ulceration is often described by patients as a gnawing pain and this is a typical description of ulceration. However, the pain may also be of the burning or boring type.

If patients describe the pain as the worst they have ever felt or as unbearable, and it has been present as a continuous severe pain for more than one hour, then immediate referral to a surgery or a hospital is necessary. Such symptoms are described as an acute abdomen, and in such cases, patients will be in obvious need of an urgent medical opinion. Possible causes of an acute abdomen include peritonitis, appendicitis, intestinal obstruction, biliary colic, bleeding or perforated peptic ulceration, renal colic, pancreatitis, strangulated hernia, occlusion of arteries in the abdomen and gynaecological conditions.

Onset and duration

If the pain is described as moderate, mild or occurring episodically with alternating periods of well-being, it is advisable to recommend medical referral after seven days. However, if patients have had similar bouts in the past, referral should be made earlier as this would suggest recurrence of an unresolved complaint with underlying pathology that requires investigation.

Persistent abdominal pain reported by patients over 45 years of age who have never suffered from dyspepsia before requires referral to exclude peptic ulceration and carcinoma of the stomach. The latter, though relatively rare, occurs more frequently in this older age group.

Accompanying symptoms

Details of the radiation of pain are useful diagnostic features. The pain of appendicitis commences centrally and, after a few hours, spreads to the right iliac fossa, and requires immediate referral. Patients who complain of pain in the abdomen radiating to the tip of the shoulder are probably experiencing referred pain from the diaphragm, and should be reassured that this is normal. Pain in the upper abdomen, especially the right hypochondrium, which is referred to the back or shoulder blades is suggestive of biliary colic, and in acute episodes will be severe enough to warrant referral.

Pain originating from kidney disorders and renal colic initially presents with loin pain and may radiate to the back or spread downwards to the iliac fossa and suprapubic area, and in males into the scrotum. It may also cause aching in the thighs.

Pain of ovarian and uterine disorders may also radiate to the thighs.

Pain can radiate from the stomach and spread into the chest as a result of acid reflux into the oesophagus. This may be caused by hiatus hernia, peptic or oesophageal ulceration, or milder forms of dyspepsia. If chest pain is severe, pharmacists should always refer patients immediately, unless patients can describe previous similar episodes and have no other signs of angina or myocardial infarction.

Recent weight loss over at least two to three weeks requires referral for investigation. It may represent the consequence of loss of appetite in someone with an abdominal complaint, but carcinoma of the stomach or large bowel, although relatively rare, requires exclusion in patients who are over 45 years of age.

Distension of the abdomen, described as a bloated feeling or sensation of fullness, may be caused by peptic ulceration. If it is persistent and accompanied by pain, referral is advised.

Vomiting, constipation, or both, in the presence of abdominal pain requires investigation to exclude the possibility of obstruction. Vomiting may also be a reflex action caused by intense pain. Difficulty in swallowing also requires referral.

The presence of blood in vomit or in the stools may be caused by a perforated ulcer or damaged inflamed areas in the gastrointestinal tract, and requires immediate referral. Blood may appear as a characteristic red colour or may be black ('coffee-ground' vomitus) in either vomit or stool.

Colicky pain accompanied by diarrhoea may be suggestive of gastroenteritis. Cases contracted in this country will normally resolve spontaneously, but if patients have recently returned from abroad, referral is advisable to exclude serious pathogens. Other possible diagnoses are ulcerative colitis, irritable bowel syndrome and diverticular disease.

Complications of cardiovascular disease can cause abdominal pain. Abdominal pain with chronic back pain and occasionally fainting may be indicative of an aortic aneurysm in the abdomen, which may be fatal if it ruptures. Older patients with a history of myocardial infarction or atrial fibrillation may develop mesenteric ischaemia due to embolism. This produces severe pain and can lead to necrosis of the intestinal wall.

Causative and modifying factors

The pain of peptic inflammation or ulceration may usually be related to food intake. It may be relieved or aggravated by food, as food can both buffer the effects of acid and stimulate acid production. Response to treatment with antacids or H_2-receptor antagonists suggests that the pain is more likely caused by a lesion in the gastrointestinal tract rather than urinary, genital or other abdominal organs.

Substances which stimulate gastric acid secretion (e.g. coffee, tea, alcohol, spicy foods or smoking) aggravate the pain of peptic ulceration or inflammation of the gastrointestinal tract.

Any upper abdominal pain which is aggravated by exercise or the cold, particularly if it radiates to the chest, requires referral to exclude angina. If the pain is severe and persists for an hour or more, immediate referral is required to exclude myocardial infarction.

Drugs can also provoke abdominal pain. Non-steroidal anti-inflammatory drugs may cause abdominal pain due to gastric or duodenal ulceration. Opioid drugs have a tendency to cause constipation, which may produce intestinal obstruction in some patients and result in abdominal pain. Some drugs can cause oesophageal ulceration (e.g. potassium chloride and tetracyclines).

Risk factors

The age of the patient should be considered in assessing the symptom. A child complaining of abdominal pain for more than a few hours should be referred for a medical opinion. If the child does not appear ill, pharmacists can advise the parent to take the child to see the doctor the next day, as this allows time to judge whether the condition is self-limiting.

Children may be judged to be ill, and therefore require immediate referral, if they show any of the following features:

- agitation
- behaviour significantly different from normal
- unconsolable crying, due to pain
- distress
- drowsiness
- fever
- pallor
- unable to keep still because of the pain
- vomiting.

Possible causes of continual crying in babies are gastroenteritis and obstruction. In gastroenteritis, the presenting symptoms may include pain, vomiting and diarrhoea. Obstruction may be caused by pyloric stenosis, in which forceful projectile vomiting occurs. It may also be due to an intestinal obstruction, producing vomiting with or without constipation, and the baby will rapidly decline towards shock. Each of these conditions requires urgent referral.

Management

Management of abdominal pain depends on the cause. If a patient does not require medical referral, symptomatic remedies may be helpful. Antacids (BNF 1.1, H_2-receptor antagonists (BNF 1.3.1) and laxatives (BNF 1.6) may be tried in appropriate cases. Pain may be relieved by paracetamol or a mixture of codeine and paracetamol, although codeine may be constipating. Aspirin and ibuprofen should be avoided in disorders of the gastrointestinal tract because of their tendency to irritate the gastric mucosa.

Spasmolytic drugs such as loperamide, dicycloverine and alverine are useful for the management of gastrointestinal colic and diarrhoea. Colic in babies is difficult to alleviate, especially since effective spasmolytics such as dicycloverine have age restrictions for their licensed use.

Patients with diarrhoea, and especially children, require adequate hydration (*see* Section 18.3.7).

18.3.6 NAUSEA AND VOMITING

Introduction

Nausea is a sensation of sickness accompanied by a loathing of food and often increased salivation.

Vomiting is the forceful ejection of the stomach contents caused by the diaphragm and abdominal wall being drawn in to press on the stomach.

Some patients may confuse vomiting with waterbrash, which is an effortless regurgitation of fluid into the mouth often accompanied by heartburn. Heartburn may be a normal event. However, it may accompany indigestion, particularly after meals or on lying down.

Key questions 18.3.6

- Has the patient eaten anything which may have caused the symptoms?
- Is the patient taking, or has been prescribed, any medicines?
- Does the patient experience any other symptoms at the same time?

Assessment and interpretation

Nature and severity

Projectile vomiting may be caused by pyloric stenosis, especially in babies, and also in adults with a history of peptic ulceration (usually duodenal) with a more recent onset of vomiting. Projectile vomiting demands a medical referral.

Vomit which is particularly sour smelling also requires referral as it indicates possible obstruction (e.g. pyloric stenosis).

Blood-stained vomit (haematemesis) should be regarded as unusual and requires referral. Blood may appear fresh and bright red, or dark with a clotted appearance. If the blood originates in the stomach, it will have been degraded by gastric acid, producing a dark-coloured vomit with an appearance like coffee grounds ('coffee-ground' vomitus).

Onset and duration

Vomiting which has occurred frequently during a period of more than 24–48 hours and is not improving requires referral. Similarly a deterioration in nausea or increased incidence of vomiting over a longer period of time requires investigation.

Vomiting which is preceded by nausea, even of short duration, usually indicates a gastrointestinal cause and is the most common presentation. However, sudden vomiting without nausea is characteristic of a central cause (e.g. a cerebral tumour or injury), and although much rarer, it should be borne in mind (*see also* Accompanying symptoms *below*).

Accompanying symptoms

Episodic or chronic vomiting accompanied by weight loss requires referral for investigation of the cause.

Abdominal pain may cause reflex vomiting as in liver disease, appendicitis, biliary colic, renal colic, hernias and genital disorders. Sometimes paroxysmal coughing can lead to vomiting. Other disorders that may lead to vomiting include Ménière's disease and acute pain in extra-abdominal body systems (e.g. in glaucoma).

Diarrhoea accompanying vomiting suggests gastroenteritis as the most likely cause, usually due to ingestion of some dietary insult or to infection. Recent travellers to hot countries should be referred to eliminate dysentery and food poisoning.

Central nervous system disorders (e.g. space-occupying lesions, meningitis, head injury and subdural haemorrhage) may result in vomiting, dizziness, drowsiness, loss of balance, and personality changes. Migraine attacks frequently terminate with nausea and vomiting. The presence of headache and any other symptoms of the aura of migraine should be ascertained.

A history of nausea or vomiting related to anxiety or an emotional disturbance requires appropriate treatment of the underlying psychological component. Reassurance may be all that is required but, in more severe cases, a medical referral is advised.

Some other psychiatric disorders may present with vomiting (e.g. anorexia nervosa and bulimia). These commonly occur in teenage girls and the history, although generally of long duration, is usually very difficult to elicit from the patient herself, although it may be reported by friends and relatives.

Causative and modifying factors

If the cause can be elicited, the decision of whether to refer or not becomes easier.

Common dietary causes are hot or spicy foods, overindulgence in food or alcohol, and sensitivity to certain foods (e.g. sea foods and pork). Such cases will usually begin to resolve spontaneously within 24 hours.

Many drugs can cause nausea and vomiting (e.g. non-steroidal anti-inflammatory drugs, colchicine, digoxin in toxic doses, iron, levodopa, theophylline, oestrogens, and cytotoxic drugs).

Motion is a common cause of nausea and vomiting and, in severe cases, may persist for a day or two after the journey.

Infection may cause vomiting, especially otitis media in children and the early stages of various viral illnesses (e.g. measles). Conditions affecting the abdomen may result in reflex vomiting (*see* Accompanying symptoms *above*).

Heart failure, particularly right-sided heart failure, may result in congestion of the abdominal organs with blood, giving a sensation of nausea and sometimes vomiting.

Episodes of vomiting, which may sometimes be severe, in patients with diabetes require immediate referral to exclude loss of control of the diabetes. Alternatively, any new symptoms of increased frequency of urination, thirst, weight loss or persistent fungal infections (e.g. in the skin and in women particularly in the perivulval area) should be treated with suspicion and diabetes excluded by immediate referral.

Chronic alcoholic patients may suffer from early morning vomiting.

Two types of vomiting may occur in pregnancy. The familiar syndrome of morning sickness comprises regular bouts of short-lived nausea, vomiting, or both, during the first few weeks of pregnancy. It may occur at any time of the day. It usually resolves spontaneously around the third month of pregnancy. Drugs should not be recommended, but reassurance, frequent small meals, rest, and bed rest in the mornings are sensible recommendations.

A more severe form of vomiting which may occur in early pregnancy is hyperemesis gravidarum. It may lead to dehydration and shock and requires medical referral.

Risk factors

Vomiting in children is usually self-remitting but certain points should be remembered. Many babies regurgitate their milk after a meal (posseting) and mothers should be reassured that this is normal. However, in cases of projectile vomiting (even though the baby may be alert and apparently normal) and in babies who appear distressed, irritable, or very drowsy, referral is required as soon as possible. Children over two years of age require referral if they have vomited for more than 24 hours.

Management

If the cause of vomiting has been identified or is suspected, the underlying disorder should be attended to as a priority.

Non-drug treatment

As in any self-remitting gastrointestinal disorder, vomiting should be treated by resting the stomach. Patients should be dissuaded from drinking milk or eating heavy or fatty meals for 24 hours, as these will exacerbate the situation. Sips of bland drinks, ideally water, should be taken regularly to prevent dehydration, although this is unlikely to occur in the cases of short duration commonly reported to pharmacies. Food should be avoided until the patient feels hungry, at which time items such as bread, toast or plain biscuits should be given. If tolerated, intake may be increased carefully until a normal diet is resumed.

Drug treatment

There are few oral drugs available to treat vomiting attacks. Both antihistamines and antimuscarinic drugs may be useful to prevent attacks, especially of motion sickness. Antihistamines such as cinnarizine, diphenhydramine and promethazine (BNF 4.6) which also possess anticholinergic properties, may be useful, but should be used with caution in patients with glaucoma, prostatitis, constipation and those who drive.

Babies and young children should be given oral rehydration fluids (BNF 9.2.1) that replace glucose, sodium and potassium lost during vomiting. Glucose enhances the absorption of electrolytes across the inflamed mucosa. The use of proprietary rehydration fluids in children should be encouraged in preference to home-made remedies which may result in inappropriate loads of sodium and potassium.

18.3.7 DIARRHOEA

Introduction

Diarrhoea is normally a self-limiting condition in which bowel frequency is increased and stool solidity is decreased. Patients in the UK usually recover within a few days with or without the aid of dietary measures or medication.

An awareness of the usual pattern of bowel frequency and motion consistency is essential in assessing the symptom and its severity. The age of patients also influences the urgency with which remedial action or referral should be undertaken. Babies and very old patients are particularly susceptible to the effects of dehydration caused by diarrhoea, but only when the diarrhoea lasts more than a few days and they appear very ill. See tables 18.2 and 18.3 for common causes of diarrhoea.

Key questions 18.3.7

- How old is the patient?
- Has there been a change in frequency *and* consistency of bowel motions? (i.e. is it really diarrhoea?)
- How long has the diarrhoea been present?
- Has the patient eaten or taken anything which might have caused the condition?
- Does the patient have a raised temperature?
- Has the patient recently returned from abroad?
- Is there blood in the stools?
- Has there been recent significant weight loss for no apparent reason?

Table 18.2 Common causes of acute diarrhoea

Infections
viral
bacterial (e.g. salmonella, campylobacter, *Escherichia coli*)
Food poisoning
Drugs (e.g. antibiotics)
Overindulgence in alcohol or spicy foods

Table 18.3 Causes of chronic diarrhoea

Infections (e.g. *Giardia*)
Diverticulitis
Bowel carcinoma
Inflammatory bowel diease (e.g. Crohn's disease, ulcerative colitis)
Drugs
Irritable bowel syndrome

Assessment and interpretation

Onset and duration

The frequency and urgency of emptying the bowels will indicate the severity of the problem.

Usually, if several bowel movements have occurred in the previous 24 hours, urgent medical referral will not be necessary, providing no other symptoms give cause for concern. Some patients will report looser motions than normal without a change in frequency. In this case, the urgency of the situation is minimal, but it should be reviewed after one or two days.

If diarrhoea has persisted in an adult for more than two to three days, and there is no sign of even slight improvement, it is wise to consider referral to the doctor. The presence of the accompanying symptoms described below will determine the necessity for referral.

Recurrence should be referred, since this is abnormal. Possible diagnoses to be considered are inflammatory bowel disease (such as ulcerative colitis or Crohn's disease) or irritable bowel syndrome. Typically, patients with inflammatory bowel disease will visit the toilet 10–20 times daily.

Accompanying symptoms

If diarrhoea is accompanied by blood in the stool, referral is essential since this could be a sign of a serious underlying condition (e.g. inflammatory bowel disease, dysentery, fissures or tears of the bowel mucosa, or colorectal cancer). The failure to report blood loss may not always indicate its absence, as it may be difficult for some patients to identify.

The appearance of mucus in the stool suggests that the integrity of the intestinal mucosa has been compromised, and usually requires referral. Small amounts may not be of any clinical significance but merely a sign of mucosal inflammation.

Diarrhoea accompanied by either severe abdominal pain that is persistent, or mild pain that has lasted for more than 48 hours, warrants urgent medical referral. Conversely, short-lasting episodes of colicky pain, relieved by evacuation of the bowel, are common and usually self-limiting, and do not normally warrant immediate action.

A long history of alternating periods of constipation and diarrhoea with colicky abdominal pain, or a continuous dull ache in adolescents and young adults, is suggestive of irritable bowel syndrome. In elderly patients, a history of either alternating or simultaneous diarrhoea and constipation may be an indication of spurious diarrhoea. Such symptoms are usually caused by impacted faeces producing partial obstruction of the bowel, in addition to liquid faeces that may squeeze past the obstruction, causing diarrhoea. Referral is recommended to permit investigation and treatment of the primary obstruction.

Patients with diarrhoea accompanied by vomiting over a period longer than 48 hours may require medical referral to exclude the possibility of gastroenteritis or rarer bacterial infections.

Any significant weight loss over a period of time before the current episode of illness in the absence of dieting requires referral. It may simply represent a loss of appetite through illness, but more serious pathology may exist (e.g. malabsorption or carcinoma) and any weight loss with diarrhoea should be medically investigated.

Causative and modifying factors

Changes to the diet may affect bowel movements. Overindulgence in alcohol or foods with high-fibre content (e.g. fruit and vegetables) may cause diarrhoea. Likewise unaccustomed intake of spicy or unusual foods may irritate the bowel and stimulate peristalsis. Food poisoning may be suspected if other people who have eaten the same food are similarly affected.

If there is a recent history of continental travel, gastroenteritis of viral or bacterial origin should be considered a possibility. If the symptoms last for 48 hours or more, medical referral is necessary. Patients returning from the Middle East or South East Asia, or Africa should be referred to exclude rarer causes such as dysentery, cholera and typhoid fever.

Diarrhoea may be caused by drug administration (e.g. laxatives, antibacterials, antacids containing magnesium, and specific agents such as iron, misoprostol, orlistat and high doses of metformin).

Patients who are known to have diabetes or thyrotoxicosis may suffer diarrhoea, which if persistent may require referral to check the control of their primary disease.

Babies

Babies may suffer diarrhoea, most commonly as a result of viral infections and teething but also due to poor sterilisation technique of feeding bottles or excessive intake of sugar. Diarrhoea which is not improving after 24 hours in a baby under six months should be considered for referral to the doctor or health visitor. With older babies a period of 48 hours without improvement is more appropriate.

Irritable bowel syndrome (IBS)

Patients who have been diagnosed with IBS by their doctor will often request OTC medicines and advice from the pharmacist. The cause of the condition is unclear and may be triggered by diet or lifestyle changes, stress or infection.

Management

Non-drug treatment
If the diarrhoea does not represent any serious pathology, it will resolve within a few days without treatment. However, a regular intake of fluids should be ensured, particularly in young children, to replace excessive losses in the faeces. Patients should be advised to sip plenty of fluids throughout the day.

Drug treatment
Oral rehydration salts (BNF 9.2.1) may be recommended for babies or elderly patients. Glucose, present in these solutions, acts as a carrier for the transport of sodium and water from the intestine into the blood.

Attempts to reduce diarrhoea may in some cases be counter-productive as it is an important means of flushing out toxins and irritants from the intestine. However, patients will request symptomatic relief for social reasons and personal convenience. Non-prescription medicines available (BNF 1.4.2) contain either opiates (e.g. morphine or codeine) or loperamide, and act by reducing the contractibility of the colon. Mebeverine and alverine are useful spasmolytic drugs in the treatment of irritable bowel syndrome. Dicyclomine is effective, but unlike the above spasmolytics, has anticholinergic effects. There is little evidence that adsorbent agents such as kaolin and chalk (BNF 1.4.1) give any reduction in diarrhoea, but their placebo effect may be considerable.

Management of IBS depends on the predominant symptoms – spasmolytics are effective in suppressing the abdominal pain and loperamide and codeine have been shown to be effective antidiarrhoeal drugs.

For bouts of constipation in IBS, fibre has been advocated for many years, but many patients cannot tolerate wheat bran which can cause pain and bloating.

18.3.8 CONSTIPATION

Introduction

The normal frequency of bowel movement in the population varies from about three times per day to once every three days. This wide variation makes definition of constipation difficult, but it may be defined as a diminished stool frequency from normal for that person, associated with the forced passage of a hard stool. As with the assessment of diarrhoea it is the change in bowel frequency that determines the severity of the condition. Table 18.4 lists some common causes of constipation.

Table 18.4 Common causes of constipation

Change in diet
Lack of exercise
Dehydration caused by reduced fluid intake or diuretics
Pregnancy
Haemorrhoids
Diverticular disease
Irritable bowel syndrome
Bowel obstruction (e.g. strictures, adhesions after surgery, inflammation, carcinoma)
Drugs

Key questions 18.3.8

- How often does the patient normally go to the toilet?
- How long has the patient been constipated?
- Can the symptoms be linked to any external factors?
- Is there blood in the stool?
- Does the patient have alternating diarrhoea and constipation?

Assessment and interpretation

Onset and duration

Uncomplicated constipation will resolve spontaneously within a few days. Constipation may be linked to lifestyle or dietary changes. If constipation does not improve after about four days of OTC treatment, then referral should be considered.

Nature and severity

If the condition is of recent origin, and is causing minor concern rather than significant discomfort, symptomatic relief may be suggested. Recurrent bouts of constipation should be referred, as any underlying pathology may still be present.

Accompanying symptoms

Blood passed through the rectum may appear mixed in the faeces or as leakage coating the stool. Its appearance warrants referral to the doctor. Recurrent constipation may result in the development of haemorrhoids, caused presumably by straining at stool. Subsequent constipation and straining may cause these rectal varices to tear or burst, producing blood which coats the stool or stains underwear. Less commonly, blood will arise from other bowel disorders (e.g. anal fissures, obstructions including tumours, and inflammatory bowel disease).

Any acute distension of the abdomen should be referred for medical examination.

The presence of severe pain warrants immediate referral. Mild or moderate pain of more than 48 hours duration requires prompt medical investigation.

For a discussion of constipation accompanied by, or alternating with, diarrhoea, *see* Diarrhoea, Section 18.3.7.

Patients who are constipated and are vomiting require referral to eliminate the possibility of an obstruction.

A recent history of weight loss should be referred to exclude serious causes.

Causative and modifying factors

A diet lacking in fibre will invariably result in constipation, particularly if patients lead a sedentary lifestyle. A reduced fluid intake will produce a similar effect since the colon will absorb the maximum volume of water possible in an attempt to conserve fluid.

A lack of physical activity (e.g. in immobile or bedridden patients) will be especially liable to cause constipation.

In the elderly, prescribed diuretics can cause constipation, when patients are not drinking adequate quantities of fluids. Other drugs which may cause constipation include iron; antacids containing aluminium, calcium or bismuth salts; opioids (e.g. in antidiarrhoeal medicines, cough suppressants and analgesics); antimuscarinic drugs and drugs with antimuscarinic activity (e.g. antiemetics, antihistamines, antipsychotics, tricyclic antidepressants and anti-parkinsonism agents).

Progesterone secreted in the latter stages of pregnancy has a spasmolytic action on most types of smooth muscle. The colon therefore becomes atonic, causing stasis of the faeces. This is a natural physiological consequence of pregnancy, and patients should be appropriately advised and reassured.

Constipation may also be caused by reduced patient mobility, faddish diets and prescription of iron supplements in the second and third trimesters.

Management

Non-drug treatment

Whenever possible, drug use in the treatment of constipation should be avoided.

In mild constipation, dietary adjustment and an increased fluid intake may be sufficient. Fruit, vegetables, wholemeal bread, brown rice and potatoes form the basis of a healthy non-constipating diet, together with avoidance of refined products (e.g. white bread and white sugar).

Adjustments to lifestyle to ensure adequate exercise and that the urge to defecate is not ignored, may be necessary. In particular, children should be taught to be regular and unhurried in their toilet habits.

Drug treatment

If laxatives are considered necessary, their use should be restricted to short courses of up to four days only, in the first instance. Referral should be advised if the condition has not resolved within one week.

Bulk-forming drugs (BNF 1.6.1) are recommended for simple constipation in the absence of impaction. When mixed with liquids, they swell in the colon, inducing peristalsis. Their action develops over several days, and so they are ineffective when a rapid effect is required. Care should be taken, particularly in the elderly, that sufficient fluid is taken with these products to prevent the risk of oesophageal obstruction.

Stimulant laxatives such as senna and bisacodyl (BNF 1.6.2) irritate the bowel mucosa, or stimulate the nerve plexus of smooth muscle, both of which increase bowel motility. They exert an effect within 6–12 hours. Short-term use only is recommended as prolonged usage can cause griping pain, diarrhoea and vomiting. Tolerance and bowel atony may develop.

Faecal softeners (BNF 1.6.3) are surfactant drugs. They increase the wetting efficiency of water, facilitating the mixing of fats and water to soften the faecal mass. Some agents are useful for patients with haemorrhoids and fissures where the passage of a hard stool is painful.

Liquid paraffin may cause lipoid pneumonia, especially in the elderly and should not be recommended.

Osmotic laxatives (BNF 1.6.4) such as magnesium salts are rapidly effective evacuants suitable only for short-term use. Their presence in the bowel leads to water retention due to an osmotic effect. This causes mechanical stimulation of the bowel and increased peristalsis.

Lactulose has a longer onset of action.

18.3.9 DYSURIA, FREQUENCY AND URGENCY

Introduction

A syndrome of painful, frequent and urgent urination (dysuria, frequency and urgency) occurs in lower urinary-tract infection, although bacteriuria cannot be proved in many instances. The condition is more common in women than men, and patients will often self-diagnose the symptoms as cystitis. However, the involvement of other parts of the urinary tract should always be borne in mind (e.g. the urethra causing urethritis, and the kidneys causing pyelonephritis).

Key questions 18.3.9

- Is the patient male or female?
- How long has the patient had the symptoms?
- How old is the patient?
- Is there any itching or discharge?
- Does the urine appear normal?
- Did the symptoms begin slowly, over a period of time, or abruptly?
- Does the patient notice having to get up during the night to pass urine more frequently than before?

Assessment and interpretation

The higher incidence of symptoms in females is thought to be due to the close proximity of the anus to the short urethra. This increases the likelihood of bacterial transmission to the bladder and urethra, which may result in cystitis and urethritis respectively.

When symptoms persist in men, the patient should be referred to exclude the possibility of prostatitis (particularly in older men), renal calculi, or other sources of inflammation and obstruction.

Nature and severity

Many patients report symptoms without severe pain or general malaise. Some, particularly men, may complain of hesitancy or a weak flow of urine during micturition. If these are present together with frequency or chronic dribbling, the patient should be referred.

Onset and duration

Dysuria, frequency and urgency usually present suddenly. Accompanying symptoms (e.g. mild back pain or abdominal pain, possibly due to renal involvement) may develop insidiously some time before the urinary symptoms.

Accompanying symptoms

The presence of any accompanying symptoms usually requires medical referral.

Localised symptoms in women include urethral itching and a pricking or stabbing pain, which further suggest the presence of an infection. In men, pruritus and soreness due to inflammation of the tip of the penis, often involving the foreskin, may occur without any symptoms of cystitis. The most likely diagnosis is balanitis caused by bacterial or fungal infection, or contact with soaps, disinfectants and other irritants. The presence of any penile discharge requires urgent referral either to the doctor or a specialist genito-urinary clinic at a local hospital.

Vomiting may occur either as a result of severe colicky pain in the ureters or urethra, or from infection. Fever and rigors also indicate the presence of infection.

Blood in the urine is not necessarily a serious sign as it may simply be due to inflamed tissue being sloughed off the urinary tract. The underlying pathology, however, may be serious (e.g. infection, bladder lesions, bladder and renal calculi, and kidney damage).

Vaginal symptoms (e.g. pruritus, discharge or stinging when urine makes contact with an inflamed vaginal labia) indicate involvement of the genital tract.

Lower urinary-tract pain may radiate to the loins or back. Equally, back pain or colicky pain in the loins may radiate to the groin and thigh, and in men to the testicles. Such symptoms indicate spasm of the urinary tract due to infection, obstruction (e.g. renal calculi) or other lesions.

Thirst and excessive fluid intake can also accompany dysuria, frequency and urgency. Fluid intake in excess of the normal 1–3 litres per day will cause frequency of micturition. If the patient is excessively thirsty as well as drinking large volumes, the possibility of diabetes should be considered.

Causative and modifying factors

Diuretics increase frequency of micturition. While most patients will realise their cause and effect relationship, their use should be enquired after.

Drinks (e.g. tea, coffee or alcohol) also have a diuretic effect, and can precipitate nocturnal frequency. They should therefore be avoided in the evening in susceptible individuals.

Irritants (e.g. bubble baths, nylon underwear and tights, vaginal deodorants, or even over-zealous use of strongly perfumed soaps) may cause perineal and urethral symptoms similar to those produced by cystitis.

The incidence of frequency and urgency may increase at the menopause, and may be followed by the development of postmenopausal urinary incontinence. Women reporting recurrent or prolonged episodes of frequency and urgency between 45 and 55 years of age should be referred for assessment.

Pregnancy is a common cause. Increased pressure on the bladder from the growing uterus is a normal consequence of pregnancy. Unless the resultant frequency is accompanied by pain or fever, the patient should require reassurance only.

Sexual intercourse can precede initiation or worsening of symptoms in women, probably as a consequence of infection arising from damage to the perineal mucosa.

Possible causes of painful, frequent and urgent urination are summarised under Urination abnormalities in Part C.

It should be ascertained whether the symptoms are similar to a previous acute episode, or whether they are persistent. If they represent a chronic problem, the patient should be referred, particularly if treatment previously initiated by the doctor has been unsuccessful.

Management

For symptoms without any complications, symptomatic treatment may be suggested for up to 48 hours. If no improvement is obvious by this time, referral should be recommended

Non-drug treatment

Patients should be advised to drink large volumes of fluid to dilute the bacteria in the bladder, and they should avoid delays in emptying the bladder.

Drug treatment

Symptomatic relief can usually be obtained by rendering the urine alkaline. Citric acid and its salts (e.g. potassium citrate and sodium citrate) are effective in this respect. However, care must be taken in the elderly, and patients with renal or heart disease, to prevent hyperkalaemia or hypernatraemia. Sodium bicarbonate powder may also be taken to alkalinise the urine, but similar precautions are required.

Pain or stinging on micturition may be relieved by paracetamol.

18.3.10 PERIANAL AND PERIVULVAL PRURITUS

Introduction

Itching of the skin around the anus (pruritus ani) and vulva (pruritus vulvae) may be a source of embarrassment to patients, many of whom will request advertised products rather than seek advice about its cause or the most appropriate form of treatment. Tactful and discrete questioning may therefore be required.

The conditions most commonly associated with pruritus ani are haemorrhoids in adults and threadworm infections, particularly (though not exclusively) in children. Pruritus vulvae commonly accompanies cystitis (*see* Section 18.3.9) and vaginal infections.

Key questions 18.3.10

Pruritus ani

- Is the patient a child or adult?
- If an adult, has the patient experienced these symptoms before?
- Is there any blood or mucus associated with the stools?

Pruritus vulvae

- Has the patient had the symptoms in the past?
- Can the patient identify the precise location of the discomfort? (The site of pruritus may be difficult to differentiate cystitis and vaginitis in women.)
- Is there a discharge?
- What is the appearance of the discharge?
- What is the patient's age?

Assessment and interpretation

Nature and severity

The mild itching associated with haemorrhoids often worsens within two to three days. In children, threadworm infection may be accompanied by severe or even painful itching at night. Pruritus vulvae frequently arises through the irritant effect of vaginal discharge on the vulva, which may be severe enough to disturb sleep. Similarly, cystitis may result in a burning sensation around the vulva.

Onset and duration

Pruritus caused by threadworm infection appears suddenly and, within 48 hours, may become excruciating at night-time due to severe excoriation of the anal region. Other forms of pruritus may develop insidiously.

Accompanying symptoms

Blood in the stool is an important symptom. Fresh blood coating the stool commonly derives from the rectum or anus, and usually indicates haemorrhoids or anal fissure. Blood mixed in the stool will have a higher origin in the gastrointestinal tract and could suggest more serious conditions such as ulcerative colitis, peptic ulceration or carcinoma. These all require referral. Blood spots on toilet paper following defecation may indicate haemorrhoids which may respond to symptomatic OTC treatment or resolve spontaneously, without the need for referral.

Perineal rash, sometimes spreading to the groin, may indicate candidal or tinea infection.

Threadworm infection can cause abdominal pain in children, as well as irritability and tiredness caused by lack of sleep. In addition, the presence of white threadworms on the buttocks at night-time may be detected, caused by the migration of females worms to the anus from the intestinal mucosa to lay their eggs.

Blisters, sores and rashes in the genital region are possible symptoms of sexually transmitted disease (STD) including bacterial and viral (herpes) infection. Such symptoms arising a few days after sexual intercourse with an infected partner require referral to a specialist genitourinary medicine (GUM) clinic at the local hospital for investigation and appropriate treatment. Susceptible individuals will be young adults, single persons, those returning from holiday or work abroad and those who have been treated previously for STD.

Recurrent attacks of pruritus may be associated with diabetes. The highly vascularised anal and vulval regions are vulnerable to bacterial and fungal infection, especially in the presence of high plasma glucose concentrations. Recurrent pruritus in known diabetic patients suggests poor disease control. If diabetes has not been diagnosed, enquiries should be made about the presence of associated symptoms (e.g. polyuria, nocturia, thirst and weight loss).

Perineal inflammation, and in particular pruritus vulvae, may produce painful urination. Equally the presence of a urinary-tract infection may produce pruritus.

Internal genital infections may produce a vaginal discharge which irritates the perineum. The discharge produced in candidiasis (vaginal thrush) is usually creamy white (described as a 'cottage cheese' appearance) and odourless.

A foul-smelling yellowish-green discharge results from trichomoniasis and bacterial infection produces either a greyish-white or clear discharge which may be odourless or have a fishy smell. Such symptoms require referral for appropriate antibacterial treatment.

Causative factors

Poor hygiene can be a factor in pruritus ani. It is a common misconception that haemorrhoids themselves produce pruritus. However, pruritus ani is most commonly due to faecal contamination, which itself can arise from haemorrhoids. Similarly, anal fissures produce extreme pain on defecation, impairing toilet hygiene. Excessive perspiration and poor ventilation of the skin due to folds of flesh (intertrigo) as occurs in obesity, are contributory factors which encourage infection of the skin by fungi or bacteria. Perfumed soaps, bath additives, toiletries and even sensitisers in topical medication used to treat the symptoms (such as local anaesthetics) may aggravate the pruritus.

Constipation may give rise to excessive straining at stool which will aggravate pruritus and the severity of haemorrhoids.

Broad-spectrum antibacterials (especially tetracyclines) are a frequent cause of candidiasis.

Inappropriate or tight clothing (e.g. close-fitting underwear and nylon tights) may also exacerbate perianal and perivulval pruritus.

A summary of the possible causes of pruritus ani and pruritus vulvae is given under Itch, Part C.

Risk factors

Pregnancy is a common risk factor. Vulval engorgement of pregnancy can produce perineal pruritus. Other common accompaniments to pregnancy may also contribute to its occurrence (e.g. constipation, dysuria and urinary-tract infection).

Management

If identified, the underlying cause of pruritus should be eliminated.

Non-drug treatment

One of the most important aspects of treatment is the attention to hygiene. Daily washing of the perineum will remove both faeces and perspiration; overfrequent washing, however, should be avoided. It is preferable to use soft washing materials rather than coarse flannels. Build-up of moisture may be reduced by the application of non-perfumed talcum powder. Loose underwear, preferably cotton rather than nylon, should be recommended.

Threadworm Non-drug hygienic measures, in addition to medication, may facilitate eradication of threadworm infection. After anthelmintic treatment has been started, a shower or bath should be taken each morning to remove the eggs. Hands should be washed thoroughly after going to the toilet and before meals, and fingernails kept trim and clean. Underwear and night clothes should be washed daily for two to three days following the initial anthelminthic dose. Bedding should be changed on the same day. Each member of the household should be given a separate towel which should be washed daily for two to three days. Bedrooms should be thoroughly dusted or cleaned following dosage to prevent re-infection from eggs shed on skin scales.

Drug treatment

Threadworm Oral, single-dose forms of piperazine and mebendazole are available as OTC medicines to treat threadworm infection. All family members should be treated for maximal effect, and a second dose, at least in the symptomatic members of the household, should be given after 14 days to kill any worms which have hatched since the time of the first dose. Any pruritus which persists after the first dose may be relieved with the application of crotamiton cream, but the patient should be reassured that the itching will subside in a few days.

Haemorrhoids A multitude of wipes, ointments and suppositories exist for the relief of symptoms. Care, however, should be taken in their use, as some medications such as benzocaine may sensitise the skin and aggravate the condition. They should not be used continuously for more than two or three days. Suppositories or ointment containing hydrocortisone can be used for a few days and will alleviate mild symptoms in most patients. Failure to do so requires referral to the doctor for appraisal of the situation.

Candidiasis (thrush) The medical treatment of vulvovaginal candidiasis has been well established over many years with imidazole antifungal agents and these are now available over the counter. OTC treatment of vaginal candidiasis with imidazole antifungal agents should only be started if the condition has been diagnosed on a previous occasion by a doctor and the woman recognises the symptoms to be the same as before. On the other hand, patients who have had more than two recurrences in the past six months as well as women over 65 years should be referred and not offered treatment at this stage. The pharmacist should explain that the doctor needs to investigate whether there is any predisposing cause for the frequent re-infections which can be modified.

Choice of treatment is between a single dose oral preparation such as fluconazole or a topical cream or pessary containing clotrimazole, econazole or miconazole. Although the creams are a useful adjunct in alleviating the symptoms in the vulval area, the infection is best treated with either an oral dose or insertion of a pessary high in the vagina where the infecting organism lies.

Men who suffer penile candidiasis (balanitis), perhaps as a result of infection from their female partners can be treated with a single dose of oral fluconazole.

Since the imidazoles are inhibitors of the hepatic metabolism of some other drugs, caution should be exercised in those taking warfarin (INR should be checked within a few days, if possible), antihistamines, drugs with arrhythmogenic potential such as terfenadine and astemizole, and ciclosporin (serum levels of ciclosporin may increase).

18.3.11 MUSCULOSKELETAL DISORDERS

Introduction

Disorders of the skeleton and muscles result in symptoms which most commonly present to pharmacists as pain in the back or limbs. Such disorders may be of multifactorial origin, but those which pharmacists commonly see will usually be due to wear, strain, injury or inappropriate and excessive movement of joints. These and other associated problems are described below.

Key questions 18.3.11

- Where is the pain?
- When did the pain start?
- Is there any stiffness, tenderness, swelling, numbness or tingling?
- Is the pain worse at certain times or aggravated by any activity?
- Is there any obvious deformity or abnormality in shape?
- Has the pain changed in nature or location?

Assessment and interpretation

Location, nature, and severity

The principal causes of a stiff or painful neck are likely to be due to injury or strain, torticollis (spasm of the muscles on one side of the neck), arthritis and more rarely cervical spondylosis or meningitis. These conditions can usually be differentiated by further history taking.

Pain or stiffness in the shoulder may be caused by injury to the joint or muscles (e.g. following overuse or excessive movement during exercise or sport). Stiffness in the shoulders and an inability to raise the arms may be caused by rheumatoid conditions in the older patient or by a frozen shoulder.

Pain at the elbow may be caused by strenuous overactivity of the muscles and their tendons which insert into the humerus at the elbow joint. Such pain is often due to sport or heavy manual work. It can cause golfer's elbow, which is characterised by pain on the inner side of the joint, and tennis elbow, which is more common and causes discomfort on the outer edge of the joint.

Gout predominantly affects men and may characteristically involve the metatarsophalangeal joint of the great toe, which becomes extremely painful and tender. Other joints may be similarly affected.

Apart from trauma, the two conditions most likely to present with pain in the forearm are tenosynovitis and carpal tunnel syndrome. The pain of tenosynovitis usually traces a line down the flexor surface of the forearm, wrist, thumb, and sometimes palm. The fingers become stiff and remain curled, and stretching causes pain. Sometimes numbness and tingling in the fingers is felt. Crackling or grating noises on movement may be heard or felt, especially in the wrist.

Carpal tunnel syndrome, caused by pressure on a nerve in the wrist, may present with symptoms similar to tenosynovitis. It is characterised by pain in the forearm, and numbness and tingling in the thumb and three fingers, the little finger rarely being affected. It is more common in women than men.

Rheumatoid arthritis commonly affects the wrist and finger joints, causing pain, swelling, and stiffness. Whereas osteoarthritis classically affects the distal and proximal interphalangeal joints, metacarpophalangeal joints and the wrists, rheumatoid arthritis in adults rarely affects the distal interphalangeal joints.

A fracture of the wrist commonly occurs after a fall on an outstretched hand. There is pain and tenderness and the hand cannot be moved.

Pain in the upper back or thoracic spine is unusual. The ribs attach to the 12 thoracic vertebrae, and strains or tears of the muscles of the chest or upper back may cause pain on breathing after coughing, or lifting heavy weights.

Pain from internal organs may penetrate to the upper back (e.g. biliary colic). Shingles may present as a unilateral superficial pain in the back and chest.

The lower back, comprising the lumbar and sacral regions of the spine, is more commonly associated with back pain than is the upper back. Low back pain is often termed lumbago, but this is a very general term and gives no indication of the cause.

Ankylosing spondylitis can cause pain anywhere in the spine, but most often occurs in the neck and lumbar regions. Similarly, osteoarthritis affects the lumbar region. The most common cause of acute lumbar pain is a prolapsed intervertebral disc (slipped disc). This causes severe pain, particularly after a major strain, injury or fall. Sometimes the muscles or ligaments surrounding the lumbar vertebrae may be torn or strained without significant prolapse of the disc, giving rise to milder symptoms.

Chronic back pain may indicate conditions such as osteitis deformans, osteoporosis (particularly in postmenopausal women), and rarely a tumour, or aortic aneurysm.

Any back pain that fails to resolve needs a medical assessment. Often the cause will not be sinister but merely poor posture or failure of an acute back injury to heal. Nevertheless, other causes require exclusion by the doctor.

Vascular disorders may present symptoms in the lower limbs. A common disorder that pharmacists encounter is chilblains, which may occur in the feet as a burning sensation. Other sites affected include the hands, earlobes and nose.

A painful calf that is swollen, hot, red and tender suggests the possibility of deep vein thrombosis. It may be particularly suspected in women taking combined oral contraceptives, those who have experienced previous episodes, and those with cardiovascular disease. It may also be seen in patients who have been bedridden for some time or undertaken long journeys (in a sitting position) and, in all cases, requires immediate referral.

Blue painful feet, which may accompany similar symptoms in the fingers, can be caused by Raynaud's syndrome and this is precipitated by cold, emotional disturbances or non-selective beta-adrenoceptor blocking drugs.

Pain in the calf or foot may be due to cramp, especially at night and in pregnancy. Pain in the back of the thigh and lower leg, arising suddenly especially during physical exercise, may be caused by an Achilles tendon or hamstring injury.

Rheumatoid arthritis and osteoarthritis may affect the knees and feet, causing pain, swelling, stiffness and difficulty in walking. Pain over the knee joint may also arise as a result of bursitis (housemaid's knee). A swelling behind the knee is likely to be caused by leakage from an inflamed knee joint into the space at the back of the knee (Baker's cyst).

Pain or stiffness in the legs accompanied by difficulty in movement or weight bearing should always be referred to exclude fractures and other causes.

Ankle sprains are the most common soft tissue injury, often caused by excessive movement on the joint. The ligament which covers the outer side of the ankle joint attaches the outer bone of the lower leg to the heel and foot. When the ankle is 'twisted' during activity, an inversion injury occurs to this lateral ligament and the familiar swelling and pain of the ankle and foot will occur.

Varicose veins are painful and unsightly and are usually easily recognisable, but any oedematous swelling or redness requires referral. Swollen legs, particularly involving the ankles and feet, may be symptomatic of heart failure and require referral.

Pain along the sole of the foot and heel bone may be a consequence of torn tendons causing plantar fasciitis, often arising through trauma or running.

Bunions occur predominantly in the elderly through deformed joints in the great toe caused by osteoarthritis. In the presence of ill-fitting shoes, this causes a painful toe and bony protrusion on the inside of the foot at the base of the great toe.

Accompanying symptoms

General malaise can accompany musculoskeletal symptoms. Inflammation or trauma may occur in various parts of the body. This is because some rheumatoid disorders are systemic diseases, and some bone disorders cause symptoms unrelated to the initial site of pain (e.g. weight loss or muscle wasting may occur in rheumatoid arthritis or polymyalgia rheumatica). Fever, fatigue, skin rashes and general malaise may also be seen and should be referred for investigation, as anaemia is a common accompaniment of chronic diseases (e.g. rheumatoid arthritis). Headache with back pain or muscle weakness require referral since they may accompany osteitis deformans or the arteritis of polymyalgia in older patients.

Paraesthesia (a tingling or 'pins and needles' sensation) may commonly indicate a trapped nerve and can occur in patients with inflamed joints. Symptoms in the fingers, hands or arms may occur in spondylitis, torn muscles or strained ligaments around the cervical and upper thoracic spinal vertebrae. Pain and stiffness spreading from a frozen shoulder may reach the back, chest and arms. Care must be taken to differentiate these symptoms from those which might occur after myocardial infarction, where typically pain in the chest radiates to the neck, jaw, and sometimes to the arms, often in the form of paraesthesia. It should be remembered that myocardial infarction does not always present with a classical chest pain. Symptoms of sudden onset in the jaw, neck and arms accompanied by a feeling of being unwell or distressed should be referred immediately for a medical opinion, especially if a history of cardiac problems is reported.

A rare cause of tingling sensations in the extremities is a form of focal epilepsy, and persistent or recurring bouts of symptoms require referral.

The most common spread of symptoms in a musculoskeletal disorder is sciatica, which follows a prolapsed intervertebral lumbar disc. Pain and paraesthesia may spread from the lower back to the buttock, thigh, calf or foot. A tear of a back muscle rarely radiates pain below the knee. Any back pain accompanied by bowel or bladder symptoms could indicate that there is pressure on sacral nerve roots and a referral is necessary in such cases.

Pain, either chronic back pain or abdominal pain, requires referral. In older patients the cause may be serious (e.g. an aortic aneurysm), although such cases will be rarely seen in the pharmacy. Chronic back pain, especially in the presence of fatigue, anaemia, infection and weight loss should always be referred to exclude sinister pathology (e.g. myeloma).

Renal colic may be felt as pain in the lower back at the level of the kidneys, which often spreads to the loins, groin and testes. Dysmenorrhoea causes lumbar pain that may radiate to the thighs and is experienced around and during the time of menstruation.

Causative and modifying factors

Movement and extremes of temperature can affect many musculoskeletal symptoms. Most are worsened by movement of the affected tissues, and serious injury (e.g. a fractured bone) results in immobility as a protective mechanism. Tennis and golfer's elbow are made worse by gripping, and by turning the forearm; tenosynovitis is worsened by stretching the forearm, wrist or hand. Walking precipitates the painful symptoms of a deep vein thrombosis or of intermittent claudication, whilst cramp is likely to occur at rest or lying down. Back pain caused by a prolapsed disc is made worse by movement and even by apparently unrelated activity (e.g. coughing or sneezing).

Vascular disorders (e.g. Raynaud's syndrome or chilblains) are exacerbated by exposure of the affected extremities to low temperatures. Arthritic symptoms appear to be exacerbated by cold and wet conditions.

A wide variety of additional factors can influence symptoms. Many symptoms are worse at different times of the day. Rheumatoid arthritis produces a characteristic stiffness, and osteoarthritic joints are especially painful in the morning. The pain of tenosynovitis and of frozen shoulder is worse at night.

Varicose veins are most painful and troublesome during menstruation. Some disorders are more common in certain age groups and in one sex. Tenosynovitis, carpal tunnel syndrome, Raynaud's syndrome and polymyalgia rheumatica are more common in women than men. The age of the patient may be helpful in identifying some disorders. Osteoporosis and osteitis deformans rarely occur before 40 years of age and polymyalgia is more common over 50 years of age. Rheumatoid arthritis, however, may occur at any age.

Vascular problems (e.g. cold extremities and Raynaud's syndrome) may be precipitated by beta-adrenoceptor blocking drugs.

Back pain due to a strain or prolapsed disc has traditionally been treated by rest for several days (*see* Non-drug treatment *below*). If this is unhelpful, referral is recommended. If the primary disorder is in other organs (e.g. urinary tract, gastrointestinal tract, aorta or reproductive organs), rest will not be helpful.

Risk factors

Age is an important risk factor, and elderly patients presenting with musculoskeletal complaints should generally be referred. Many symptoms may be attributable to chronic inflammatory disease or may be the trigger for such disease processes to take a hold. Some of the causes of inflammatory conditions may be serious and warrant investigation. Many accompanying factors, which sometimes remain clinically silent for a long period (e.g. the anaemia of chronic disease), are potentially serious and will often only be revealed upon medical investigation.

Management

Non-drug treatment

Treatment of an acute soft tissue injury such as a sports injury requires rest, ice, compression and elevation of the affected limb or joint. This procedure, commonly referred to by the acronym 'RICE', aims to reduce inflammation and bleeding or bruising. The symptomatic management of painful and inflammatory conditions should involve up to 72 hours with ice packs at regular intervals. When systemic symptoms or other accompanying factors suggest a more serious disorder or trauma a medical referral is necessary. Similarly symptoms which persist for more than a few days without improvement require a medical evaluation. Although medical therapy cannot always alleviate painful conditions, the patient should be advised to see a doctor to confirm the absence of any chronic systemic disease.

Acute localised inflammatory disease may be alleviated by local application of ice packs. Resting the affected part of the body is essential and is only effective if the rest is complete. For severe back pain caused by a prolapsed disc, the bed or mattress should be firm. Nowadays, patients are encouraged to mobilise as soon as possible with the aid of analgesics and ice packs to reduce acutely inflamed tissues.

A simple back muscle strain may show improvement in a matter of days, but a prolapsed disc can take up to six weeks to completely resolve. The latter condition, or one not resolving in a few days, therefore requires medical supervision.

In those who have recovered from a musculoskeletal disorder or who are prone to relapse, the importance of preventive measures (e.g. weight reduction if appropriate, gentle exercise, swimming and good posture) should be emphasised. Posture may be improved by remembering to keep the back straight, to support it when sitting, and to bend the knees when lifting.

Drug treatment

Non-opioid analgesics (e.g. aspirin or ibuprofen) will be helpful because of their anti-inflammatory properties. Care should be taken to establish that there are no contraindications to these drugs (e.g. a history of gastrointestinal symptoms, allergy or asthma). Combination analgesic products such as mixtures of aspirin and codeine or paracetamol and codeine may be beneficial. Topical preparations such as those inducing a sensation of warmth (e.g. 'heat balms', liniments) have traditionally been used, but should be reserved for background aches and pains and not acute flare ups. Topical NSAIDs can provide symptomatic relief in some individuals with muscular aches, sprains and strains, although the evidence for their efficacy in chronic conditions appears to be unclear.

18.3.12 SKIN CONDITIONS

Introduction

Skin lesions are often difficult to diagnose because of the wide variability in appearance, location, and severity of signs and symptoms. Although there is an important visual aspect to examination of skin disorders, questioning patients is as important as with other illnesses and minor symptoms. Nevertheless, those with skin complaints in which the skin surface is intact (i.e. there is no break in the skin surface and no ulceration) will rarely be in a life-threatening situation, providing there are no accompanying systemic symptoms. Thus self-medication for a short time will usually be appropriate.

Key questions 18.3.12

- What is the nature and distribution of the lesion?
- When did it appear?
- Is the patient aware of having been in contact with an infected person?
- What food has the patient recently eaten?
- What medicines, if any, is the patient taking?
- What chemicals or household cleaners has the patient been using?
- Has the patient been in contact with any animals?

Assessment and interpretation

Nature of the lesion

(A diagrammatic representation of common skin lesions is illustrated in Figure 13.1.) A rash may be defined as a raised or flat patch of skin, of a colour which is different from the normal surrounding skin. This definition covers the majority of skin lesions, but the more popular lay description is of an area of redness. An erythematous rash may be seen in the various types of eczema, urticaria, psoriasis, tinea infections, photosensitivity, sunburn, cellulitis, rosacea, acne and lichen planus.

Eczematous rashes will often produce scales and appear erythematous. In time they become dry and the scales become more obvious. A greasy or shiny rash with scaling may indicate seborrhoeic dermatitis. In young babies this scaling can be profuse on the scalp and face, producing areas of adherent white to yellow scales, called cradle cap. Extensive scaling also typifies psoriasis, in which thick, silvery white, scaly plaques may totally or partially overlie a pink or red lesion.

Small blisters containing clear fluid are termed vesicles, whereas larger versions are referred to as bullae. If the fluid is purulent, the blisters are described as pustules.

Pustular lesions are typically seen on the face in acne, impetigo, and herpes simplex virus infection; vesicles occur on the trunk and limbs in chickenpox and shingles, and on hands and feet in pompholyx and psoriasis. Bullae are seen in some drug rashes, sunburn and atopic dermatitis.

Characteristics of shape are important features of identification. Psoriatic lesions usually occur as patches with well defined edges, distinguishing them from the normal skin. Small, red, discrete patches may be seen in tinea infections and eczema, and in particular discoid or nummular eczema. (Nummular eczema derives its name from the latin word *nummus*, meaning a coin, which describes its red, round or oval appearance.) Tinea lesions have better delineated edges to the red patches, whereas eczematous patches blend into normal skin. Tinea lesions have redder margins compared to the centre of the lesion, giving the impression of spreading from the centre outwards.

Sometimes erythema may present as streaks or lines, especially on the arms or face. This is characteristic of contact dermatitis (e.g. caused by handling plants such as the primula, and hair dyes and other scalp preparations).

Confluent erythematous patches with irregular but well demarcated outlines can occur, especially on the trunk and limbs. They have white centres caused by oedema, and are characteristic of urticaria.

Pigmentation can occur. Eczematous spots may eventually change to a brown colour after a few weeks, especially after chronic scratching. Brown spots are also typical of a resolving lichen planus. Psoriatic lesions may present on close examination as brown spots on an erythematous background.

Changes in pigmentation (e.g. variability in the colour seen in a mole or an increase in its size) require referral for a medical opinion to exclude malignancy (e.g. melanoma). This is also true if bleeding, ulceration or pain occurs in a pigmented mole. However, melanoma may develop as a new lesion and not necessarily as an extension of a pre-existing mole.

An ulcer is a cavity or pit which most commonly occurs on the skin at sites of pressure sores on the sacrum, buttocks, legs and feet. In diabetic patients, ulceration may develop because of poor circulation in the lower leg, feet, and toes.

Neoplasms of the skin are usually raised lesions, but they may be described as ulcers by the lay public if they are inflamed. The most common benign tumour of the skin is the wart, which is a raised papular lesion usually of normal skin tone or greyish colour. Warts are self-limiting lesions (although facial and genital warts require medical referral) and most people will develop them at some time. Sometimes warts may appear pedunculated, resembling a cauliflower or bunch of grapes (mosaic warts).

The two most common skin cancers are the slow-growing basal cell carcinoma (rodent ulcer) and the faster growing squamous cell carcinoma. These are located on exposed areas.

Basal cell carcinoma may present initially as a small nodule with telangiectases over the surface (i.e. discrete dilated capillaries can be seen). The nodule may ulcerate or bleed, and its edges are usually raised or 'rolled' so that the lesion has the appearance of a volcano with the ulcer in the middle. Cystic forms may appear like raw warty lesions. It is sound policy to refer any chronic ulcerated or sinister looking lesions on sun-exposed areas. Sometimes, however, basal cell carcinoma presents as a flat slowly spreading area, and location and duration are the clues to diagnosis.

Squamous cell carcinoma may appear as a nodule or an ulcer and often the edges are rolled, as in basal cell carcinomas.

Location

The distribution of a rash or other skin lesions can be very helpful in determining the type of skin disorder. A useful guide is that if an imaginary vertical line is drawn down the body to split it in two, a symmetrical distribution of lesions on both sides generally points to an endogenous skin disorder (e.g. atopic eczema). Conversely, asymmetrical lesions indicate an exogenous type caused by contact or infection (e.g. contact dermatitis, tinea or cellulitis).

An area of erythema appearing on skin areas exposed to sunlight (e.g. face, neck and arms) suggests photosensitivity caused by applied or ingested chemicals, usually drugs (Table 18.5). This type of lesion will have a defined edge corresponding to the limits of coverage by clothing. It should be remembered that photosensitivity can occur at any time of year, not just summer.

If the palms of the hands are involved, photosensitivity can be excluded as these are not light-sensitive areas. Small lesions on sun-exposed areas which do not resolve require a medical opinion to exclude malignancy.

Conversely, a rash appearing on skin which has been, or is, covered by an article of clothing, jewellery or cosmetics should alert pharmacists to the possibility of a contact dermatitis.

Atopic eczema is characteristically located on the cheeks of babies and on the flexures of the neck, front of wrists and elbows, and behind the knees in young children. The distribution is usually symmetrical on each side of the body.

Table 18.5 Examples of photosensitising drugs

Oral	Amiodiarone
	Azapropazone and other non-steroidal anti-inflammatory drugs
	Bendrofluazide
	Chlorpromazine
	Ciprofloxacin
	Sulphonamides (especially co-trimoxazole)
	Tetracyclines
	Tricyclic antidepressants
Topical	Antihistamines
	Sunscreen agents
	Coal tar derivatives

Seborrhoeic dermatitis, seen more commonly in children than adults, may occur on the scalp, ears and eyebrows but may be more widespread on the axillae and groin, and in babies in the napkin area.

Psoriasis is commonly seen on the backs of the elbows, the front of the knees, the scalp, and anywhere on the trunk. It may also appear on the groins and axillae, but the face is rarely affected. The nails may be affected in psoriasis, giving a pitted appearance.

Acne vulgaris is a common problem in adolescents and young adults and may occur on the face, neck, upper back and shoulders. Rosacea occurs on the forehead and cheeks of older people.

Certain skin areas are invaded by ringworm. Tinea pedis attacks the spaces between the toes and the sole of the foot. This should be easily distinguishable from contact dermatitis caused by leather shoes or sandals, which has a wider distribution over the foot. The groin area may become infected with tinea (tinea cruris), producing an area of inflamed skin with a pronounced border. The napkin area of babies may become inflamed due to primary irritant dermatitis, usually caused by the formation of ammonia in the urine. The dermatitis may sometimes be contaminated (e.g. by *Candida*) in the area where the skin folds in the legs become erythematous. In a simple napkin rash these areas are normally spared.

Isolated, red, small discrete, round lesions of 1 or 2 cm diameter on the trunk and limbs may represent tinea corporis, but a similar appearance can be seen in nummular eczema, contact dermatitis and small plaques of psoriasis.

Isolated, small, red spots commencing at the wrists or between the fingers and spreading to the arms and trunk may indicate scabies. Larger red lumps occurring anywhere on the limbs or trunk may be due to insect bites. The legs or arms are particularly affected after walking in grass or working in the garden in the summer. Bed bugs will cause lesions noted particularly on awaking.

An erythematous rash covering a large proportion of the body is likely to be an allergic reaction to ingested food or drugs, or in a child, an infectious disease (*see* Management of special cases *below*).

Other typically located lesions seen on the face are impetigo around the mouth (in children), herpes simplex virus infections (cold sore), varicella-zoster virus infections (on the scalp, around the eye, the trunk, usually unilaterally). Perianal lesions may be caused by tinea (although anal irritation may also be due to haemorrhoids or threadworm) and genital lesions may be caused by warts or lice.

Infections of the skin (e.g. cellulitis) may be seen as an erythematous patch usually about 5 cm wide. The patch may occur anywhere on the body but commonly appears on the face or limbs. A red area on the lower leg might also be caused by thrombophlebitis or deep vein thrombosis. Such lesions require early medical attention, especially if they are painful. An erythematous rash over the inside of the ankles and shins may be due to stasis eczema, caused by poor circulation, especially in patients with ankle oedema.

Onset, spread and duration

The initial lesion of most skin disorders usually occurs suddenly and this may allow its relationship to a possible allergen or irritant in eczema to be identified. Sometimes an infective event may herald a skin condition (e.g. a sore throat before guttate psoriasis or the upper respiratory symptoms seen before the common infectious diseases of children, *see* Management of special cases *below*).

Scabies presents, initially, with a few isolated, itching, red spots on the back of the hands, wrist or forearm before spreading to other parts of the limbs and trunk, but not the face and scalp.

In babies, a rash in the napkin area may be a simple contact dermatitis, but if it spreads to the rest of the trunk it may indicate seborrhoeic dermatitis.

The duration of a skin lesion may be the determinant of whether to recommend treatment or refer the patient to a doctor. Any rash which has not resolved after one week and is causing symptomatic distress should be referred. Similarly individual lesions that are slow growing or insidiously changing in shape or colour can represent malignancy (e.g. melanomas, or basal and squamous cell carcinomas) and should be referred.

Accompanying symptoms and family history

Any systemic symptoms (especially of malaise) experienced by patients with an undiagnosed skin lesion require referral to exclude serious pathology.

Patients with psoriasis may also have arthritis, as the two are sometimes seen together as part of a disease complex.

The symptom mostly associated with skin lesions is pruritus. This is not a very discriminating symptom. A rash which is painful requires referral and such a rash on the face, scalp, trunk or arm may suggest shingles.

Sometimes symptoms may develop in the skin without the appearance of a visible lesion (Table 18.6). Pain without a rash requires referral, but pruritus is common without a rash as, for example, on the scalp (head lice), the body (body lice), and more rarely in systemic disease (e.g. kidney or liver disease).

Bleeding from skin lesions is generally regarded as serious, especially if melanoma or other skin cancer is a possibility. Warts, however, often bleed with little consequence, usually as a result of the patient paring down the lesion with a file or blade.

An inquiry about any family history of the suspected disorder may help diagnosis of skin disorders. Patients with atopic eczema will often report a family history of atopy which manifests itself as a triad of conditions – hay fever, asthma and atopic eczema. They will often have at least one other of these conditions in addition to the eczema themselves. Patients with psoriasis often have relatives who suffer from the disorder too.

Table 18.6 Conditions causing generalised pruritus with no visible lesion

Diabetes mellitus
Dry skin (especially in the elderly)
Gallstones
Hodgkin's disease
Iron-deficiency anaemia
Kidney failure
Liver failure
Pregnancy
Thyroid disorders

Table 18.7 Common primary irritants and contact allergens causing contact dermatitis

A. Primary irritants	Acids Alkalis Antiseptic solutions Bleach Degreasing solvents Detergents Mineral oils Soaps Shampoos
B. Contact allergens	Adhesive plaster Cement Clothing Cosmetics Deodorants Elastic Glues and resins Hair colourants Jewellery Leather Ointments and creams containing lanolin, local anaesthetics, antihistamines, sulphonamides and preservatives Plants (e.g. primula and chrysanthemum) Rubber gloves Watch strap Wood resins

Causative and modifying factors

Because most skin lesions itch, patients will scratch, although the temporary relief afforded by this is outweighed by the harmful consequences of scratching. Deleterious effects can include exacerbation of erythema (as in urticaria), spread of infected lesions to other parts of the body (e.g. tinea, impetigo), infection through scratching with dirty nails or fingers (infective eczema), or delayed healing.

A variety of factors may exacerbate or relieve skin lesions and symptoms. Exposure to sunlight may initiate or exacerbate photosensitivity reactions (e.g. those due to drugs) and rosacea, while other conditions (e.g. acne vulgaris and psoriasis) will often improve on exposure to ultraviolet light. Acne tends to be worse in the winter months. Exposure to irritants or allergens will initiate or cause recurrences of contact dermatitis (Table 18.7), and several topical agents (e.g. coal tar, industrial cutting oils and cosmetics) or ingested drugs (e.g. corticosteroids and antiepileptics) may exacerbate acne. There is no convincing evidence that dietary constituents (e.g. fats, chocolate, nuts or coffee) cause or aggravate acne, although individual patients may be allegedly affected more than others.

Trauma to the skin may initiate or worsen psoriasis. Less obvious trauma may allow penetration by viruses or fungi. This is thought to occur particularly when the soles of the feet are wet and the skin becomes macerated.

Conversely a dry skin, which can result from a chronic skin disorder (e.g. eczema or ichthyosis), will aggravate the condition with which it presents, causing further itching, scratching and general worsening of the condition.

Drugs may cause erythematous skin eruptions. Patients sensitive to penicillin may develop anything from a mild localised rash to a florid erythema covering the whole body. Some drugs (e.g. aspirin) may cause urticaria.

Drug rashes usually develop soon after administration, but not exclusively so. Finally, it should be remembered that failure to find the cause of a rash is often a signal to claim it to be of nervous origin, particularly by patients. Indeed, stress is thought to aggravate psoriasis and endogenous eczemas.

Management

The general principles of the treatment of skin disorders follow the same rules of treatment of other disorders. If the condition has not resolved by the end of one week (or earlier if patients are feeling ill), referral should be considered.

Pruritus

Pruritus can be alleviated by cooling (e.g. with cold compresses), calamine lotion, by oral antihistamines, or topical hydrocortisone (if pruritus is caused by allergic contact or primary irritant dermatitis, or insect bites and stings). Dry skin which itches should be hydrated by regular long-term application of emulsifying ointment or aqueous cream or other emollient.

Eczema

If eczema is of exogenous origin, avoidance of, or protection from, the offending causative agent, if known, is the first line of treatment. Rubber gloves should be worn to prevent contact with detergents, and barrier creams used to protect hands from irritant oils or chemicals in the workplace. Factors which exacerbate eczema (e.g. exposure to cold winds, wool and man-made fibres) should also be avoided.

Hydrocortisone cream (1%) is effective in the treatment of mild irritant or allergic contact dermatitis as well as insect bites. Patients with flare-ups of more severe lesions of either atopic or contact eczema may be treated with the more potent clobetasone cream (0.05%) for one week. If there is no improvement after this time, referral is recommended.

Napkin rash requires frequent nappy changes to keep the skin dry and to prevent contact with irritant ammonia in the urine.

There are a number of proprietary creams available to treat napkin rash. It should be remembered that creams are used for treatment to allow evaporation of water from the skin, preventing further maceration and damage. Barrier silicone creams or zinc and castor oil cream are suitable as preventative measures as they form a barrier to irritants. On tender skin where a rash is already present, this type of product will only exacerbate the problem.

Dry eczematous patches due to contact dermatitis or atopy require hydration with emulsifying ointment, aqueous cream or a proprietary product, to prevent painful cracking of the skin surface. Perfumed soap often acts as an irritant and the use of emulsifying ointment as a soap replacement or as a soak added to the bath in eczematous conditions can be helpful.

Wet or weeping eczematous lesions are usually treated with potassium permanganate soaks or compresses for about 15 minutes three times each day.

Stasis eczema on the ankles and shins is best referred to elicit and treat the cause. Graduated compression hosiery, topical steroids or coal tar-impregnated bandages may be prescribed.

In babies and children, atopic eczema can be treated with emulsifying ointment, but recurrences require referral.

Infantile seborrhoeic dermatitis (cradle cap) may respond to shampoos containing cetrimide or to gentle rubbing with olive oil to soften the scales before washing the hair. More resistant cases may require keratolytic agents (e.g. 1% salicylic acid in aqueous cream). If the rash has spread to the trunk, referral is advisable to assess the value of a topical corticosteroid. In adults, seborrhoea of the scalp may be relieved by a shampoo containing ketoconazole. Severe or chronic cases may require referral.

Psoriasis

Psoriasis should be referred when lesions recur. They may require potent corticosteroid preparations, dithranol, and sometimes psoralens with ultraviolet light treatment (PUVA). Psoriasis of the scalp may be treated with coal tar lotions.

Infections and infestations

Candida and tinea infections may be treated topically with imidazole derivatives (e.g. clotrimazole, miconazole or econazole) as they are effective against both fungi and some staphylococci. In the presence of a moist environment, which encourages growth of microorganisms (e.g. in skin folds or between digits), the liberal use of talcum powder will also promote healing by drying the skin. When the feet (tinea pedis) or groin (tinea cruris) are involved, daily washing to promote hygiene is also recommended. Tinea corporis, tinea capitis and nail infections are more resistant to treatment and should be referred. If treatment is recommended, patients should be advised to continue for at least two weeks, to prevent relapses, even if resolution of the rash is rapid.

Impetigo is a staphyloccocal infection which should in all cases be referred to the doctor.

Warts are extremely difficult to cure. Success depends on the ability of the immune system to counter the virus rather than the use of non-prescription products. However, caustic solutions containing salicylic acid abound on the market. They dissolve the keratin layers on the epidermis and, together with abrasion using an emery board or pumice stone, allow a pleasing cosmetic appearance by paring the wart so that it is less prominent. Care must be taken that surrounding normal skin is not exposed to the keratolytic agent. A solution of formalin 4% has traditionally been prescribed for plantar warts. The affected part of the foot is soaked for 15 minutes each day in the solution.

Head lice (*Pediculosis capitis*) should only be treated when lice have been detected by wet combing. They are treated by the careful application of insecticide (either malathion or a pyrethroid such as permethrin or phenothrin) in an alcoholic or aqueous lotion to the scalp and the hair close to the scalp. The lotion should be allowed to dry and left in contact with the scalp overnight, then shampooed off the next day. The application should be repeated after one week so that any lice which hatch after the first application will be killed. Only if lice are detected after the second application, should another insecticide be considered and the process repeated. Failures after use of a second insecticide should be referred for consideration of a prescription for carbaryl.

Patients and parents should be educated that the scalp may continue to itch for up to two weeks after successful treatment. Treatment failure is thought in most cases to be due either to poor application technique, use of inadequate quantities of lotion, resistance of lice, failure to treat contact persons or failure to appreciate that itching persists even when the lice have been eradicated. Close contacts (i.e. friends and family) should only be treated if lice have been detected by wet combing.

Phenothrin, permethrin and malathion are equally effective. Clinical studies have shown that children treated with insecticidal lotion have twice the cure rate of those treated by wet combing alone. Alcoholic lotions should be avoided in patients with asthma, eczema or other skin conditions.

Lice on eyelashes should be treated by applying petroleum jelly which blocks the respiration of the lice.

Pubic lice should be treated as described for head lice.

Body lice (*Pediculosis corporis*) may be treated after bathing, with an aqueous malathion lotion applied to the whole body from the neck down. Bedding and clothes should be washed.

Oral antihistamines, crotamiton cream, or both may relieve the associated itch.

Scabies may also respond to a sufficient quantity of aqueous malathion lotion (0.5%) or 5% permethrin cream applied from neck to toe in adults. Young children, the elderly and alcoholics should also be treated above the neck, because of reduced immunity to the scabies mite. Special care should be taken to apply the insecticide to the fingernails, toenails, groin and behind the ears. Bathing beforehand is not necessary. The insecticide should be washed off 12 hours later. Patients should be warned that itching may persist after the mite has been cleared from the skin, and can be relieved by oral antihistamines. The application should be repeated one week later. Close physical contacts of the patient should also be treated.

Acne vulgaris

A wide range of products are available for the treatment of acne. Non-prescription products may be classed as keratolytics (e.g. benzoyl peroxide, potassium hydroxyquinoline sulfate and salicylic acid) and antibacterials, although some are claimed to have a combination of properties. The keratolytic agents break down the keratin plugs in the hair follicles and allow sebum to drain to the skin surface. They should be used cautiously, initially using the lowest concentration products and increasing as necessary. Patients should be warned that the face may become red and sore after the initial application of a keratolytic agent and that this may be alleviated by initially applying less frequently. Antibacterial agents (including benzoyl peroxide) allegedly act by reducing the population of *Propionibacterium acnes*, one of the bacteria that split the triglycerides of sebum into irritant fatty acids, which cause inflammation in the sebaceous ducts.

Patients should be warned that the treatment of acne vulgaris is prolonged and at times unrewarding. Difficult cases, especially those associated with emotional disturbances may benefit from a referral. It may be helpful in unresponsive cases to recommend alcohol-based cleansing lotions or surgical spirit as an adjunct for short periods to degrease the skin and give a temporary respite.

The effects of sunlight
Sunburn and photosensitivity reactions are more difficult to treat than to avoid. Patients should be educated about the effects of sunlight, with recommendations to use sunscreens with high protection factors, particularly for the fair skinned and those going on summer holidays to a hot climate. Despite the apparently healthy look of a suntan, over-exposure can be painful and in the long term damaging.

Management of special cases

Diabetes
Diabetic patients are susceptible to recurrent infections of the skin, especially with candida and tinea. They are also prone to ulceration arising from injuries to the skin of the foot, and to ischaemia in the feet. Foot ulcers may become serious before they are brought to the attention of healthcare personnel, because diabetes can cause a peripheral neuropathy and make many skin disorders painless.

Infectious diseases of childhood
Although the infectious diseases of childhood are dealt with in this separate section, it should be remembered that these disorders may also occur in adulthood in a minority of cases.

Measles is less common as vaccination (*see* Section 15.5), is now more widespread in infants. Similarly, triple vaccination with MMR vaccine in infants has reduced the incidence of rubella (*see* Section 15.5), although chickenpox and scarlet fever may still be seen. Since these diseases usually occur only once in a lifetime and often occur in epidemics, especially amongst schoolchildren and playgroups, it should be enquired whether the child has had the suspected illness before, if they have had any vaccinations, and whether any of the child's friends have had similar symptoms recently.

Distinguishing the type of rash is important. Measles is a flat blotchy rash, whereas that of rubella is less well defined with smaller erythematous marks. The rash of chickenpox consists of pustules surrounded by small reddened areas. The pustules eventually burst and dry to form crusts. Scarlet fever appears as a bright red flush of the face and as a gooseflesh appearance around the neck.

The location and spread of the rash is also diagnostic. The rash of measles begins usually on the face and neck, and spreads downwards to the trunk and limbs. Rubella also begins on the face or back of the neck and spreads down over the trunk, but it can be extremely variable and transitory in appearance. Chickenpox and scarlet fever do not spread in the same way as measles and rubella. Spots occur on the trunk and face in chickenpox and then increase in number, whereas the flush of scarlet fever is limited to the face and gooseflesh to the neck and upper half of the trunk. A summary of the onset and accompanying symptoms is given in Table 15.7.

Measles is a notifiable disease (i.e. doctors are obliged to notify the local authority of any incidence). Parents of children with suspected measles should be advised to telephone the surgery to relate their suspicions, and the doctor can decide whether the child should be brought to the surgery or warrants a home visit. Unless otitis media is suspected or the child appears otherwise unwell, symptomatic treatment only of the upper respiratory symptoms and of the rash (with calamine lotion or an oral antihistamine) is required.

Rubella rarely requires treatment, but advice about avoiding contact with pregnant or suspected pregnant women should be given.

Chickenpox causes intense pruritus, for which oral antihistamines and calamine lotion are useful. Scratching should be discouraged.

Since scarlet fever is caused by a streptococcal infection, referral is necessary so that treatment with an antibacterial can be instituted.

18.3.13 EYE DISORDERS

Introduction

Ocular symptoms most likely to be encountered in the pharmacy are red eye, styes, swollen painful lids and sore gritty eyes. Responding to

Key questions 18.3.13

- Is there disturbance of normal vision?
- Is the eye painful?
- Is pain present within the eye or is the irritation or discomfort on the surface of the eye or eyelid?
- Is the eye watering?
- Has there been any trauma to or around the eye?

such symptoms requires care to avoid confusing common symptoms of minor disorders with potentially more serious conditions. Whenever advice on eye problems is sought, all available information must be obtained from patients before recommending a course of action.

Symptoms are discussed according to involvement of either the eyeball or eyelids. (For information on the structure of the eye, *see* Section 11.2.)

Assessment and interpretation – eyeball

Primary symptoms and location

Redness and inflammation of the eye commonly indicates conjunctivitis of bacterial, environmental or allergic origin. Confirmation of inflammation may be observed by noting the increased redness of the conjunctiva when the lower lid is pulled down. The degree of redness may vary, being particularly marked in allergic conjunctivitis due to either pollen or cosmetics.

Similar symptoms may be caused by dry eye. More serious pathology (e.g. uveitis, including iritis, and glaucoma) may be suggested if the conjunctiva close to the pupil is more inflamed than the periphery, and in the presence of other symptoms (*see below*).

Accompanying symptoms

The presence or absence of accompanying symptoms is the most important indicator of any underlying pathology.

Superficial discomfort (e.g. a feeling of soreness or grittiness) is characteristic of conjunctivitis. However, the presence of pain, especially within the eye, indicates a much more serious condition (e.g. glaucoma or uveitis) and requires immediate referral to a doctor.

Sticky eyes in the morning, or the daytime accumulation of pus in the corner of the eye, suggests an infective conjunctivitis.

Disturbed vision is not a consequence of conjunctivitis as the inflammation does not affect the cornea. Pharmacists should therefore be alert to reports of visual disturbances, as these indicate more serious conditions. The appearance of haloes around lights, particularly when leaving a darkened room, suggests closed-angled glaucoma. Blurred vision, difficulty in focusing, double vision and tunnel vision may be caused by conditions such as a thrombosed artery, intraocular haemorrhage, retinal detachment, optic nerve damage and closed-angle glaucoma. Gradual loss of vision may be caused by chronic glaucoma, cataracts, and retinal or macular degeneration. Any such symptoms therefore require immediate referral.

If there is abnormal redness of the facial or peri-orbital skin, eye symptoms may be secondary to another focus of infection (e.g. cellulitis and herpes virus infection).

Hazy pupils can occur in certain eye disorders. In conjunctivitis, the pupils will be bright and normal. However, in uveitis and glaucoma, the iris and pupil may appear hazy or cloudy. Additional indications of uveitis include pupillary constriction due to a swollen iris, and a misshapen pupil caused by the adhesion of the iris to the lens.

In closed-angle glaucoma, the pupils appear partially dilated and do not respond to light. They may also be oval in shape. These effects are less pronounced in open-angle glaucoma.

Severe eye pain can produce nausea and vomiting. In this event, or in any associated change in visual acuity or appearance of the pupil, the patient should be referred immediately.

Subconjunctival haemorrhage, appearing as a red haemorrhagic spot in the white of the eye, can appear spontaneously following sneezing or as a result of trauma to the head or eye. In the latter case, the patient should be referred but otherwise the patient requires reassurance that this represents nothing more than a spontaneous, small superficial bleed which will resolve naturally within one or two weeks provided that there are no accompanying symptoms.

Assessment and interpretation – eyelids

Primary symptoms and location

Inflammation, either on the margin or under the eyelid, is the most common symptom. A stye is due to inflammation of a hair follicle at the base of an eyelash on the eyelid margin. Glandular inflammation of the eyelid margin is termed blepharitis. Small, hard lumps which usually appear under the upper eyelid indicate a chalazion or meibomian cyst ('internal stye').

Accompanying symptoms

A stye may cause superficial pain whereas a chalazion and blepharitis are associated with soreness.

Skin changes around the eye and eyelid can develop. Some eyelashes may be lost in blepharitis and there is frequently scaling and crusting of the lid margins. Seborrhoea of the face and scalp, together with dandruff, is commonly present.

Outward (ectropion) and inward (entropion) turning of the eyelid is often associated with eye irritation by the eyelashes.

Duration

Styes usually resolve spontaneously within a few days. Blepharitis and chalazion are chronic disorders which may subside temporarily, but frequently recur.

Risk factors for eye disorders

Age is an important risk factor. Many eye disorders (e.g. glaucoma, ectropion and entropion) have a high incidence in the elderly. In the very young, symptoms suggesting an eye infection in a baby under two months of age may have derived from the delivery, and be particularly serious if the mother had a sexually transmitted disease. All newborn babies with eye disorders should be referred.

Diabetes mellitus commonly causes reversible changes in lens shape or serious retinal pathology, especially if diabetic control is poor. All diabetic patients who complain of visual disturbances or eye infection should be referred for medical assessment.

Management

Non-drug treatment

Red inflamed eyes due to allergic conjunctivitis may be relieved by elimination of the allergen whenever possible. Styes will resolve spontaneously within two or three days, although healing can be facilitated by applying a clean piece of cotton wool or lint soaked in warm water, as a hot compress, for 15 minutes each day. This procedure should be repeated until the stye comes to a head. In blepharitis, the eyelid margins should be bathed in warm water or a dilute solution of a baby shampoo to assist descaling. The accompanying presence of dandruff should also be treated with a suitable shampoo. The use of a non-medicated moisturising base (e.g. emulsifying ointment or aqueous cream) will help prevent skin flaking and keep the eyelid margins soft and hydrated.

Despite its dramatic appearance, subconjunctival haemorrhage will heal spontaneously, in a similar way to a bruise under the skin, within two weeks and requires only reassurance.

Drug treatment

Infective conjunctivitis may be treated with non-prescription antibacterial agents. Two related compounds available as eye-drops (propamidine) and an eye ointment (dibromopropamidine) have been shown to be active against the common pathogens (e.g. streptococci, staphylococci and *Haemophilus*). For optimal effect, the eye drops can be instilled every 1–2 hours during the day (which is more frequent than recommended by the manufacturer's licence) and the eye ointment applied at night, to give sustained action. If the symptoms show no sign of improvement within 48 hours, the patient should be referred.

Allergic conjunctivitis may be treated with eye drops containing a vasoconstrictor (e.g. xylometazoline, naphazoline) either alone or in combination with an antihistamine (e.g. antazoline), or with cromoglicate eye drops. Patients should be advised that these preparations may cause transient stinging when applied to an inflamed eye.

18.3.14 EAR DISORDERS

Introduction

The ear is closely associated anatomically with the upper respiratory tract. Many symptoms and disorders in the ear may present as features that may be identified with disorders in the upper respiratory system.

Key questions 18.3.14

- Is there pain or discomfort?
- Is the patient's hearing affected?
- Is the patient feeling dizzy?
- Can the patient hear ringing or humming noises?
- Has there been any recent trauma or injury to the affected ear?
- Is any inflammation or an unusual lesion visible on the outer ear?

Assessment and interpretation

Nature and severity

The most serious disorder affecting the outer ear is a tumour. The outer ear is exposed to the sun and it may be the site for solar keratosis, which is the precursor of malignant epithelioma. Any recently noticed sore area, which does not resolve and is growing in size, should be referred. Basal cell carcinoma (rodent ulcer) may arise on the pinna, often on its upper edge, in the form of an ulcer with a raised border.

Trauma to the pinna may result in profuse bleeding because of its abundant blood supply. Similarly, contusions may produce large haematomas between the skin and cartilage, eventually producing fibrous scarring which may result in the deformed 'cauliflower ear'. Bleeding points should be compressed with a clean gauze pad and patients referred to a hospital. Contusions require surgical drainage.

The pinna and auditory canal may sometimes appear red and inflamed due to eczema or infection. Various substances may cause obstruction of the auditory canal (e.g. wax or foreign bodies, including insects).

Pain within the ear may be due to inflammatory causes in the outer ear. However, if no lesions are visible, then the source of the pain or ache is most likely to be inflammation in the middle ear caused by infection (i.e. otitis media). It may affect one or both ears.

Severe injury (e.g. a blow to the head or directly on the ear) may rupture the tympanic membrane and cause pain. Similarly, the eardrum may rupture when the pressure inside the middle ear is less than on the outside (e.g. due to aircraft making a descent or divers descending below 10 metres). The Eustachian tube, which normally equalises the pressure, becomes occluded.

Deafness may be due to congenital or occupational causes as well as wax, otosclerosis, secretory otitis media (glue ear) and old age.

Disorders of the inner ear may affect hearing and balance, causing vertigo or dizziness.

Onset and duration

The cause of sudden deafness may be obvious (e.g. following poking of the ear with a variety of instruments from matchsticks to pencils). Noise damage may also cause sudden hearing loss.

Sudden dizziness may be caused by a viral infection of the inner ear, whereas a more chronic progressive onset may be due to the ageing process or, less commonly, Ménière's disease.

Causative and modifying factors

Previous episodes of inflammation may indicate otitis externa. There are two causes, infective and reactive, although both may be present at any one time. Reactive otitis externa represents a chronic tendency to eczema. The auditory canal may be sore and pruritic. Scaling and red skin may be present. The infective form may be caused by bacteria, viruses, or fungi and is usually acute. It may be recognised by the presence of a discharge, together with soreness and irritation which, if untreated, may lead to painful ears.

Some patients may have an aural fistula (i.e. a congenital blind pit in front of the external canal) which is of no significance, except when it becomes infected.

An insect sting in the ear canal can produce oedema, causing occlusion of the canal. Immediate referral is necessary.

Deafness caused by wax in the auditory canal usually affects one ear, although eventually both ears may be involved if untreated.

Environmental factors can also precipitate ear disorders. Patients subject to excessive noise in their occupation or domestic environment may suffer noise damage and deafness. Transient deafness may accompany the other symptoms of otitis media.

Accompanying symptoms

Otitis media classically presents as earache which may be accompanied by symptoms of an upper respiratory-tract infection, and occurs commonly in children. The pain may be intense and throbbing, affecting one or both ears. There may be fever and tenderness around the ear. Inflammation of the middle ear may cause the drum to bulge out and possibly burst, which is painful. A discharge of pus and blood may be found in the auditory canal after perforation of the drum.

Glue ear also occurs in children and is similar to otitis media but produces a sticky effusion. It is a chronic form of otitis media.

Disorders of the inner ear are characterised by vertigo or dizziness, often with nausea and vomiting. Tinnitus may also be present. Repeated attacks are characteristic of Ménière's disease. Dizziness without deafness, accompanied by upper respiratory-tract infection, may be caused by viral infection of the inner ear. It should be remembered that elderly people often have dizzy spells unrelated to the ear, and such patients require referral.

Excessive wax may produce a feeling of numbness on the affected side of the face, and an uncomfortable feeling in the ear.

Risk factors

Occupations and sports can increase the risk of ear disorders. Swimmers should be especially careful to occlude the ear canal (e.g. by using ear plugs) if they are prone to otitis externa. This helps keep the ears clean and dry, excludes microorganisms, and prevents a warm, wet environment in which they would proliferate. High-speed water sports (e.g. water-skiing) may subject some people to ruptured eardrums due to barotrauma.

Workers in environments of excessive noise should be protected by the use of ear protectors.

Children are especially prone to ear disorders. They may be the victims of their own mischievous pastimes by lodging foreign bodies in their ear canals. Developmental changes (e.g. teething) may subject them to earache. The enlargement of the adenoids may cause obstruction of the Eustachian tube. Upper respiratory-tract infections in small children frequently cause earache and otitis media because of inflammation and blockage of the Eustachian tube, which is narrow in children.

Management

Ear wax is difficult to remove other than by syringing. However, softening the wax using cerumenolytic ear drops (BNF 12.1.3) is recommended, with drops instilled regularly for a few days before syringing. Olive oil and sodium bicarbonate ear drops are claimed to be effective, but there is little clinical evidence to support their use. If patients have a history of ear infections accompanied by perforation, or have a chronically discharging ear, then drops must not be instilled until a doctor has examined the eardrum to check for perforation.

The entry of flies and other insects into the auditory canal may cause great irritation and panic. Instillation of olive oil should kill the intruder and the ear should be syringed that day. If the insect has stung the ear, referral should be made as quickly as possible.

Otitis externa should be referred for antimicrobial treatment. However, pharmacists may advise patients that improved ear hygiene may be helpful and enhance antimicrobial therapy by leaving the canal clean and dry so that invading microorganisms cannot colonise it. Ear plugs should not be used during infection as they serve only to retain the exudate and provoke further infection.

Pain in the ears, especially in a child, indicating the likelihood of a middle ear infection should be considered for referral. However there is a substantial body of evidence which supports the view that the course of such infections is not altered by antibiotics and that symptoms will resolve spontaneously after a few days. Thus many general practitioners delay or avoid giving antibiotics routinely and pharmacists working closely with doctors can assist in educating the parents of young children and offer paracetamol to relieve the pain until the symptoms subside. If there has been pain for three days, then most doctors would consider prescribing a course of antibiotics. The presence of a discharge requires referral.

Any trauma to the outside of the ear, especially that resulting in bleeding, requires immediate referral for assessment.

18.4 Emergency hormonal contraception

Introduction

Emergency hormonal contraception (EHC) is used to prevent a pregnancy after unprotected intercourse or after a contraceptive method has failed. Recent figures show that Britain has the highest teenage birth-rate in Europe – twice that of Germany, three times that of France, and six times the Dutch rate, and one of the targets of the government's sexual health strategy is to reduce pregnancy rates in the under 18s by 50% by the year 2010.

EHC is available from a number of sources, including general practitioners, NHS walk-in centres, family planning clinics and sexual health clinics. It is also available from pharmacies through the traditional route on prescription as a prescription-only medicine (POM). However, since January 2001, an emergency contraceptive pill containing levonorgestrel (Levonelle) has been available from pharmacists without prescription under a patient group direction (PDG) or as a pharmacy only (P) medicine.

A patient group direction is 'a written direction, signed by a doctor or dentist, and by a pharmacist, relating to supply and administration only, of a prescription only medicine (POM) or P medicine to persons generally, subject to any specific exclusions set out in the Direction.' A PGD is therefore a written document which states the circumstances in which the medicine can be supplied. It lists those excluded from treatment, states when further advice should be sought from the doctor and includes details of any follow-up action and records needing to be kept. Under a PGD scheme EHC may be supplied to under 16s if the PGD specifies this, while the P medicine can only be supplied to women over 16. Moreover, EHC may be provided free under a PGD scheme, but the woman has to pay for it if she buys it as a P medicine. PGDs can be authorised by primary care trusts (and their equivalents in Scotland and Northern Ireland), NHS Trusts and other NHS bodies.

The Society's Code of Ethics allows pharmacists to follow their own conscience in the supply of EHC, while ensuring that patients have access to it. If pharmacists are unhappy about supplying EHC on moral or religious grounds, they should treat the matter sensitively and provide information on an alternative source of supply, which can be accessed within the required timeframe (i.e. within 72 hours of unprotected sex).

Types of emergency contraception

There are three methods of emergency contraception:

- Progestogen-only pills – Levonelle or Levonelle-2 (Levonelle-2 being the POM equivalent of Levonelle). Each pack contains two tablets of levonorgestrel 750 µg. The first tablet should be taken as soon as possible (and no later than 72 hours) after unprotected intercourse or contraceptive failure. The second tablet should be taken 12 hours (and no later than 16 hours) after the first tablet.
- The older combined progestogen and oestrogen pills (Schering PC4 – the Yuzpe method). The dose is two tablets followed by a second dose of two tablets 12 hours later.

Both types of pill work in a similar way, and depending on the point in the menstrual cycle the pill is taken, it either prevents or delays ovulation, prevents fertilisation or prevents implantation of the fertilised egg into the uterus. Clinical opinion is that EHC is not an abortifacient, and pharmacists should explain this.

- The copper IUD, which, provided it is fitted within five days of unprotected intercourse, works by preventing the implantation of the fertilised egg.

Dealing with requests for EHC

The Council of the Royal Pharmaceutical Society has approved five professional standards for the sale of EHC as a P medicine. These are mandatory requirements to be adopted by all pharmacists. In brief, they state that pharmacists should:

- deal with the request personally and decide whether to supply or refer
- provide all the necessary information to enable the woman to decide whether or not to use the product
- handle all requests sensitively with due regard to the customer's right to privacy
- supply the product to a person other than the woman concerned only in exceptional circumstances
- inform patients of the benefits of regular methods of contraception, disease prevention and sources of help.

Pharmacists need to obtain sufficient information from the client to assess whether EHC is needed. The essential issue is whether the woman has been placed at risk of pregnancy in the last 72 hours due to unprotected sex or contraceptive failure. EHC is not always needed, and it is important to check the following points.

- Is the woman presenting in person?
- Is she 16 or over? This is a requirement of the OTC licence, but is not for a POM supply and may or may not be for a PGD supply.
- Has she used any other form of emergency contraception during the current menstrual cycle? If appropriate, clients may be given more than one supply of EHC within a cycle, but they should be advised about possible cycle disruption and encouraged to use regular methods of contraception.
- Is she taking any other medication? Several drugs interact with levonorgestrel. Carbamazepine, griseofulvin, phenytoin, primidone, phenobarbitone, phenylbutazone, rifampicin, rifabutin and St John's wort may increase the rate of metabolism of levonorgestrel, reducing its blood levels and efficacy. Levonorgestrel may reduce the metabolism of ciclosporin and increase the risk of toxicity with this drug.
- Does she suffer from any condition that could compromise the absorption of EHC (e.g. vomiting, severe diarrhoea or Crohn's disease)?
- Does she suffer from hepatic dysfunction? The use of progestogen-only EHC is not recommended for such clients.
- Is she pregnant or likely to be pregnant? In other words, is the period late? If so, how late? Was the last period unusual in any way (e.g. lighter or shorter)? Has there been in any other unprotected sex in the cycle already?
- Has she experienced severe clinical problems (e.g. allergy) with progestogen-only products before?
- Did she have her last period normally (bearing in mind that menstrual cycles vary in length), without any differences (e.g. late or light)?

Pharmacists should give the following advice when EHC is supplied:

- The first tablet should be taken as soon as possible (and not later than 72 hours) after unprotected sex or contraceptive failure, and the second 12 hours (but not more than 16 hours) later.
- Some women feel sick after taking progestogen-only EHC. Actual vomiting, however, is very rare. If a woman is sick within 3 hours of taking the first tablet, she should take the second tablet straightaway and get a further supply. If she vomits within 3 hours of the second tablet, she must get another supply.
- EHC does not provide protection against pregnancy for the rest of the cycle. If a woman takes the contraceptive pill, she should continue to take it after taking EHC, but a barrier method should be used in addition until the next period.
- EHC can alter the timing of the next period, which may be either early or late, but usually occurs within three days of the expected time. If the next period is lighter, shorter or later than usual, the woman should be advised to see her GP or family planning clinic to get a pregnancy test.
- Women who are breastfeeding should be advised that levonorgestrel appears in the breast milk in too small an amount to harm the baby. However, mothers who are concerned can be advised to take the pill just after a breast feed, so minimising the secretion of levonorgestrel in the next feed.

18.5 Smoking cessation

Introduction

Smoking is the single greatest cause of preventable illness and premature death. In the UK, the number of deaths from tobacco is estimated to be in excess of 120 000 a year. The constituents of tobacco smoke include nicotine, carbon monoxide and more than 1000 polycyclic hydrocarbons. The consequences of smoking on disease and mortality are well documented and include not only cancer of the lung, but also cancers of the mouth, lip, throat, pancreas, bladder, kidney, liver, cervix and stomach. Smoking doubles or trebles the risk of myocardial infarction, and increases the risk of development of osteoporosis. During pregnancy, smoking increases the risk of spontaneous abortion, premature birth, congenital malformations, low birth weight babies and haemorrhage during pregnancy. Smoking irritates the upper airways and is linked to many disorders of the respiratory system in addition to cancer, particularly bronchitis and eventually, with persistent smoking, to chronic obstructive airways disease and emphysema.

Helping smokers to stop smoking and preventing smoking from being started represent enormous challenges, but pharmacists, with their ready accessibility to the public and the range of smoking cessation aids available without prescription are well placed to meet them.

Methods of stopping smoking

Stopping smoking is generally a matter of self-motivation and discipline and many smokers give up, once they are determined to do so without any special aids. However, various products are helpful for those who wish to give up but feel unable to do so unaided. Most of the licensed products now available over the counter are in the form of nicotine replacement therapy. However, bupropion is available on prescription (*see* BNF 4.10). Where possible, smokers should have access to a specialist smokers' clinic for behavioural support.

Nicotine replacement therapy

Nicotine replacement therapy (NRT) helps smokers to stop on account of the nicotine it contains, albeit at a lower level than is found in cigarettes, by reducing withdrawal symptoms and cravings. It is well absorbed through the buccal and sublingual mucosa, skin and lungs, routes which are employed in the various NRT products (i.e. chewing gum, sublingual tablets, lozenges, transdermal patches, inhalator, nasal spray). The choice of product depends on the number of cigarettes smoked each day and the time to the first cigarette of the day, with higher strengths recommended in people who smoke their first cigarette within 20 minutes of waking and who smoke more than 20 cigarettes each day. There is little difference in the efficacy between the various formulations, although a particular smoker may choose one product over another.

Nicotine chewing gum is available in two strengths – 2 mg and 4 mg. Heavier smokers (more than 20 cigarettes a day) and those who crave a cigarette within 20 minutes of waking up should be recommended to use the 4-mg product, while less heavy smokers should start with the 2-mg product and transfer to the higher strength product if they use more than 15 pieces a day. Correct chewing technique involves chewing the gum slowly until the taste becomes strong, then resting the gum between the cheek and gum until the taste fades. The process is then repeated until the gum has lost its flavour, which normally takes about 30 minutes. A piece of gum can be chewed whenever the urge to smoke is felt, and the same quantity of gum should be continued for about three months, after which the number of pieces chewed each day should be gradually reduced to zero.

Nicotine sublingual tablets and lozenges are another option, both of which can be used up to three months, then gradually reduced over a period of a further three months.

Nicotine patches are available in several strengths. The patch should be applied to a non-hairy area of the chest, upper arm or thigh. The recommended treatment period and length of time on each strength varies between brands, but in general the highest strength is used for between four and eight weeks, followed by stepwise reduction to the lower strengths over two to eight weeks before stopping altogether.

The inhaler consists of a cartridge impregnated with nicotine which is inserted into a holder. When inhaled through a plastic mouth piece, the cartridge releases the nicotine over a period of about 20 minutes. This device may be particularly useful for people who feel the need to continue with the hand-to-mouth activity of cigarette smoking. The inhalator can be used when the urge to smoke occurs, and normally between six and 12 cartridges will be used each day during the first eight weeks. In the following weeks the number of cartridges should be reduced by half then stopped after a further two weeks.

A nicotine nasal spray is also available. This can be used up to a maximum of one spray into each nostril twice an hour for 16 hours each day for eight weeks then reducing gradually over a total period of three months.

NRT products contain lower doses of nicotine than cigarettes and are less harmful than smoking. However, they are not licensed for use in pregnancy and breast feeding and should be used with caution in all individuals with cardiovascular disease, hyperthyroidism, diabetes mellitus, phaeochromocytoma, renal and hepatic impairment and in those with a history of peptic ulcer.

19

Diagnostic procedures

19.1 Introduction

Patients may be subjected to a variety of diagnostic procedures at different points in their journey of medical care, for example in hospital, at the doctor's surgery, in the workplace, sometimes at sports centres and increasingly in community pharmacies. When such tests are conducted in pharmacies, the pharmacist has an obvious role, but even when tests are conducted elsewhere, the pharmacist can be a useful source of information about the procedure and what it may mean for the patient.

Diagnostic procedures can be roughly classified according to two main types:

- Directly investigative procedures, which require the presence of the patient for the duration of the procedure. Such procedures vary in complexity from the routine and fairly simple, such as measurement of blood pressure, pulse, height and weight, through to X-rays and monitoring of heart function by electrocardiography to more sophisticated techniques such as magnetic resonance imaging (MRI), ultrasound and computed tomography scans.

- Tests on samples. These tests are performed on samples such as blood, urine and faeces, which are removed from the patient and tested in a laboratory.

Diagnostic tests are used in three main ways:

1. To confirm a diagnosis (e.g. bone densitometry in suspected osteoporosis, biopsy in suspected coeliac disease)
2. To assess the severity of a disease (e.g. magnetic resonance imaging for staging of a tumour or creatinine clearance to assess the level of renal impairment)
3. To monitor response to treatment (e.g. serum cholesterol following initiation of lipid-lowering therapy, blood pressure following body weight loss, reduction in salt intake and/or anti-hypertensive drug therapy).

Role of the pharmacist

Pharmacists have a variety of roles in relation to diagnostic testing. First, they are frequently asked questions by patients who have concerns or who want further information about the tests which they have been recommended to undergo. Patients who have never undergone such a procedure before may well have anxieties about what is involved, why the test is being conducted and what the results are likely to indicate. Pharmacists can do a great deal to allay such fears by giving clear, confident explanations about the procedure of concern, and most of the common procedures pharmacists are likely to be asked about are covered in Sections 19.2 and 19.3.

Secondly, pharmacists can use diagnostic tests in the context of overall medicines management. They can use the results of a test to advise prescribers on the choice of a drug and dosage, for example in heart failure or hypertension. When drugs are used in renal or hepatic failure, pharmacists can advise on parameters to monitor and changes in drug dosage where appropriate. Diagnostic tests can be used to detect and prevent adverse drug reactions (e.g. hypokalaemia with loop diuretics) and interactions (e.g. those involving oral anticoagulants) and to monitor a patient's response to drugs (e.g. oral anticoagulants, medicines for asthma).

Thirdly, pharmacists may also be directly involved in diagnostic testing, or point of care testing, themselves. The development of technology is increasingly allowing 'near-patient testing' and pharmacists may be involved, for example, in the measurement of blood cholesterol and lipids, blood glucose and glycated haemoglobin and testing for *Helicobacter pylori*, as well as pregnancy testing and measurement of blood pressure and body weight. Other point-of-care tests that can be carried out in a pharmacy include C-reactive protein for inflammatory conditions, streptococcus A for sore throat, microalbuminuria for diabetes mellitus and hypertension, blood testing for glandular fever, and food allergy testing.

Code of ethics

Pharmacists wishing to offer diagnostic testing in the pharmacy should be aware that the Royal Pharmaceutical Society's Code of Ethics has a section on diagnostic testing and health screening. This section includes requirements for competencies of staff involved in providing the service, a designated area (not in the dispensary) with suitable facilities for performing the test and providing counselling. An appropriate quality-assurance programme must be in place and the equipment must be properly maintained. The Code of Ethics also states that it is important to keep up to date with developments in the field and to make sure advice given to the patient is in line with current guidelines. Patients should be fully informed about the significance of the results in a manner they can understand and they must be referred to the GP when appropriate.

Interpretation of test results

Any pharmacist who has looked at patient case notes and medical records will know that patients can generate a huge amount of diagnostic and laboratory data. There are many types of laboratory reports due to the diversity in diagnostic techniques used. Reports may be expressed qualitatively, quantitatively or semi-quantitatively. Results from the various types of scans, such as computed tomography, magnetic resonance imaging and ultrasound, and endoscopic procedures are largely qualitative. They will describe the appearance of the tissue under investigation and will explain the clinical significance of any abnormalities in the tissue. Haematology and biochemistry results are generally expressed quantitatively, i.e. as a set of numbers, while microbiological results tend to be semi-quantitative in that the report will identify which microorganisms have been detected, with their sensitivities described semi-quantitatively.

Normal and reference values

In the interpretation of test results it is important to distinguish between the use of the terms 'normal' and 'reference'. Indeed, the term normal should not be used at all in relation to results expressed quantitatively. Such results will be provided by the laboratory in the context of a reference range which is quoted alongside the patient's test result to aid interpretation. The term reference is used in preference to normal because there is no clear-cut distinction between normal and abnormal concentrations of any constituent in blood or urine. Using the term normal implies that any concentration outside the stated range is abnormal and unhealthy, while any concentration inside is normal and therefore healthy.

However, the reference range typically represents the mean result ±2 standard deviations observed in a large population of apparently healthy individuals (*see* Figure 19.1). In other words, it covers 95% of the 'normal' population,

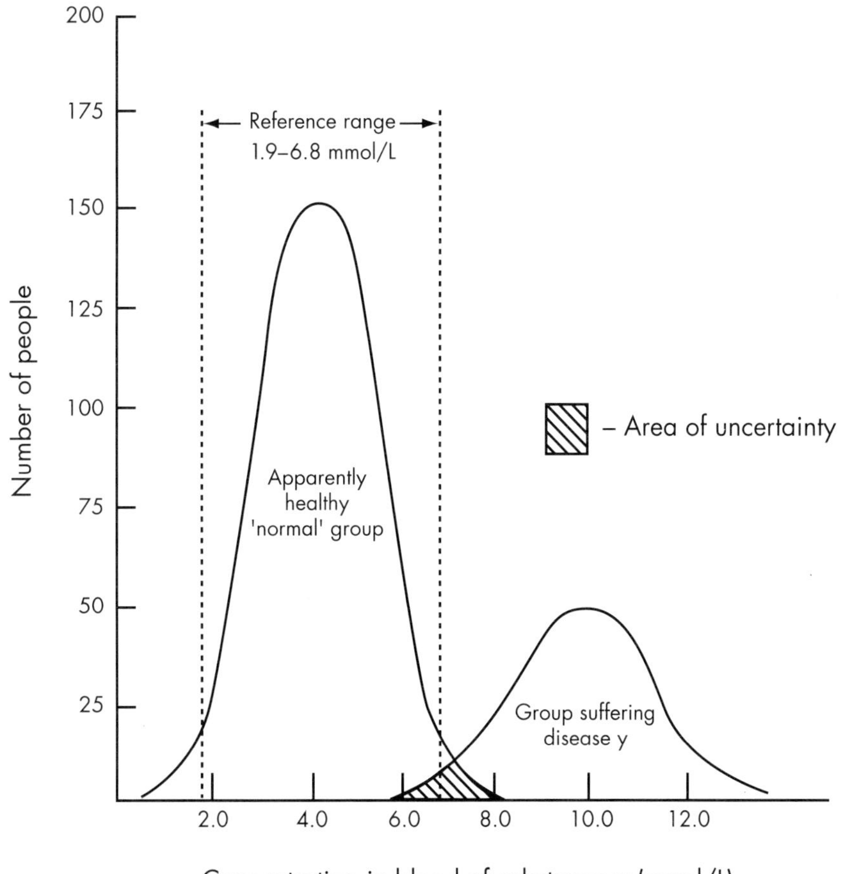

Figure 19.1 The overlap in reference range and values occurring in disease.

which means that 5% of healthy individuals will fall outside that range. So, because the reference range excludes 5% of healthy people, the term normal is inappropriate.

In the sections that follow, reference ranges are quoted for all quantitative tests. However, it is important to be aware that reference values vary from one laboratory to another and it is always advisable to refer to the reference values of the laboratory where the sample has been tested. With some tests, such as serum sodium and potassium, or red and white blood cell counts, differences between laboratories will be negligible; others, such as enzyme assays, may vary considerably.

Factors that affect test results

A variety of factors can influence test results, and these should always be considered before the patient is assumed to have a disease. Test results which fall outside the reference range can be caused by disease, and this is why diagnostic tests are used to screen for disease, confirm a clinical diagnosis or monitor a disease process. However, test results can also be affected by other factors such as:

- *Drugs.* Some drugs may affect blood concentrations directly, while others may interfere with the analytical procedure.
- *Age of the patient.* For example, white cell count is higher at birth than in adulthood and blood urea concentration increases with age.
- *Sex of the patient.* Blood hormone levels differ between men and women. Red cell counts and haemoglobin concentrations may be lower in women than in men.
- *Pregnancy.* Thyroid function tests, for example, can be altered during pregnancy.
- *Time of day* the sample was collected. Several blood constituents fluctuate throughout the day, and several tests require that a sample be taken at a specific time.
- *Diet.* The concentration of some blood constituents varies depending on whether the patient is fasting or not.
- *Ethnicity.*
- *Recent exercise.*
- *Posture* when the sample was taken (i.e. recumbent or sitting upright).

19.2 Directly investigative procedures

Thirty-three commonly used investigative procedures are described in this section. Pharmacists will not be directly involved in performing many of these, but may be questioned by patients about them. Each of the following procedures is described under three main headings: a definition, an explanation of what the procedure involves and findings (i.e. what the procedure may show).

Amniocentesis

Definition

Amniocentesis is a prenatal diagnostic technique that involves using a needle to withdraw fluid for analysis from the amniotic cavity.

Explanation of procedure

During the procedure, the fetus is monitored by ultrasound scanning. The fetal heart beat, the position of the placenta and location of amniotic fluid are all noted. Guided by ultrasound, a needle is inserted through the patient's abdominal and uterine walls into the amniotic cavity. Fluid is withdrawn for analysis and the needle is removed.

Amniocentesis is performed for a variety of reasons. It is important in assessing chromosomal and genetic aberrations (e.g. haemophilia), hereditary metabolic disorders, (e.g. cystic fibrosis), anatomic abnormalities (e.g. neural tube closure defects – spina bifida), fetal maturity status, sex of the fetus, fetal status affected by rhesus isoimmunization and fetal distress.

It may be performed at different times into the pregnancy depending on the reason for the test. If chromosomal or genetic aberrations are suspected, it is best performed between 14 and 16 weeks. If performed to find out fetal maturity status, then it should be after the 35th week of pregnancy.

Amniocentesis poses small risk for the patient and fetus.

Findings

Findings vary depending on the reason for the test.

Angiography

Definition

Angiography is a technique used to aid visualization of the arteries on X-rays. It involves injection of a contrast medium through a catheter into the area of clinical concern.

Explanation of procedure

The catheter is inserted percutaneously into an artery in the arm or groin. Before insertion of the catheter, a topical anaesthetic is applied to the area, then, guided by fluoroscopy (X-ray images) a short, thin wire with a rounded tip is carefully inserted into the artery using a needle. The needle is then removed and a vascular sheath inserted round the wire which is also removed. The catheter may then be inserted along the guide wire. When the catheter is correctly positioned, the wire is removed and contrast medium inserted through the catheter. Finally, the blood vessels are checked on a series of rapidly recording X-rays or on a screen.

Angiography is performed for evaluation of the arteries in the area of clinical interest for abnormalities such as aneurysm, atherosclerosis, embolism, fistula, haemorrhage, neoplasm, arteriovenous shunting, stenosis, thrombosis and vasculitis.

Nowadays angiography is used less commonly, having been replaced to some extent by procedures with less discomfort to the patient (e.g. computed tomography, magnetic resonance imaging (MRI) and ultrasound).

There is a small risk of the catheter damaging the blood vessels, and a small minority of patients are allergic to the contrast medium. Patients suffering from severe hepatic, renal or cardiovascular disease may be at greater risk.

Findings

The visualized arteries should be smooth with no evidence of vessel wall irregularity, aneurysm, occlusion or extravasation.

Arthroscopy

Definition

Arthroscopy is a technique used to evaluate a joint, including the cartilage, ligaments, menisci and connecting bursa. It involves the use of an athroscope inserted into the joint.

Explanation of procedure

A local anaesthetic is instilled at the appropriate site, and a small-gauge needle inserted into the joint space. Any fluid in the joint space is aspirated and sent for the appropriate biochemical or bacteriological analysis. Contrast medium is then inserted into the space with the aid of an arthroscope.

Arthroscopy is used for the evaluation of any damage to the cartilage, ligaments and bony structures composing the joint or soft tissue masses in the joint. It is used to identify the reasons for pain and swelling in joints and can also be used for surgery such as repair of cartilage.

Findings

The surfaces of the cartilage and menisci should be smooth without evidence of erosion or disintegration, and there should be no fluid in the joint space.

Audiometry

Definition

Audiometry is used to assess hearing sensitivity using an audiometer to generate electrically a set of pure tones.

Explanation of procedure

The patient is presented with a series of pure tones over a range of frequencies and instructed to signal the audiologist each time a tone is perceived. The auditory threshold (i.e. the minimal intensity of sound required for audibility) is determined for each frequency. The threshold hearing level is plotted against the frequency for each pure tone and the audiogram is inspected to quantify the degree of hearing loss. In addition, it may sometimes indicate the cause of the hearing loss.

Audiometry is used for three main reasons: first to evaluate hearing loss, secondly as periodic screening during prolonged ototoxic drug therapy, and thirdly in some cases of tinnitus. It is regarded as an initial screening test for hearing dysfunction.

Findings
Normal values for auditory thresholds have been defined and a 'normal' audiogram plotted. This is compared with the audiogram obtained from the patient. The test is highly dependent on patient reliability and cooperation.

Barium meal/enema

Definition
A barium meal is an imaging technique that involves radiographic and fluoroscopic evaluation of the oesophagus, stomach and duodenum while the patient is drinking a barium solution. A barium enema is used to study the bowel using a similar technique.

Explanation of procedure
The patient will be advised not to eat for a period of time before the procedure (e.g. after midnight if the test is to be performed in the morning) and some radiologists may recommend a mild laxative subsequent to the procedure, particularly in older, constipated patients. The patient is asked to drink the solution (or is given an enema) and spot films are obtained while the solution is moving through the gastrointestinal tract.

These procedures are used to evaluate the gastrointestinal tract for the presence of neoplasms, ulcers, hiatus hernia, diverticula, gastro-oesophageal reflux and inflammatory bowel disease.

Findings
Findings vary depending on the reason for the test.

Bone densitometry scans

Definition
A bone densitometry scan is an imaging test to measure the density of the bone, usually in the lumbar region and hips. The gold standard technique is dual energy X-ray absorptiometry (DEXA), which involves passage of a narrow beam X-ray through the bone to be measured.

Explanation of procedure
The patient should remove all metal (e.g. metal zips, metal buttons) in the path of the X-ray. The X-ray is collected at a detector, the X-ray energy changed to electrical energy then sent to a computer for analysis and display. The amount of calcium in the bone is then calculated. The procedure is performed in hospital, although portable scanners, which can be used in GPs' surgeries to check the bone mineral density of the heel bone, are growing in popularity.

Bone densitometry is used in patients considered to be at risk of osteoporosis, and hence of fracture, although its value in predicting risk of fracture is controversial. Such patients include oestrogen-deficient women with a family history or other risk factors for osteoporosis, those with primary hyperparathyroidism and those on long-term glucocorticoid therapy.

Findings
The World Health Organization has developed standards for bone density based on T scores (standard deviation units below peak bone mass minus bone mass in young healthy individuals of 20–40 years). Normal = T score > –1; osteopenia = T score –1 to –2.5; osteoporosis = T score < –2.5.

Bronchoscopy

Definition
Bronchoscopy is a telescopic examination of the upper airway, vocal chords, trachea and bronchi, which involves the use of a bronchoscope introduced into the trachea.

Explanation of procedure
The procedure may be done with or without general anaesthesia depending on the type of bronchoscope. If a flexible bronchoscope is used, the patient is premedicated with a benzodiazepine or narcotic and the nasopharynx anaesthetized with lidocaine gel or spray. The tip of the bronchoscope is lubricated with lidocaine gel and introduced nasally or orally with the patient in the sitting or supine position. Lidocaine solution is injected through the bronchoscope to anaesthetise the vocal cords, trachea and bronchi and when adequate anaesthesia has been achieved, a

visual inspection of the airways is made. If a rigid bronchoscope is used, the procedure is conducted under general anaesthesia.

Bronchoscopy is used in the diagnosis and staging of bronchial carcinoma, the assessment of recurrent pneumonia and a range of other lung conditions. Indications for rigid and flexible bronchoscopy overlap to some extent, although rigid bronchoscopy tends to be used largely for therapy (e.g. control of haemoptysis, foreign body removal, laser therapy) rather than diagnosis.

Possible complications include painful mouth and throat and occasionally bleeding.

Findings
The examination should reveal normal mucosa and no lesions.

Cholangiography

Definition
Cholangiography is a radiological technique, which involves injection of a contrast medium to enable visibility of the biliary system.

Explanation of procedure
This procedure may be performed after cholecystectomy before closure of the abdominal incision. A contrast agent is injected into an indwelling T-tube and the bile ducts assessed by X-ray. In this instance, cholangiography is used to evaluate the patency of the biliary system and any filling defects in the bile ducts.

Alternatively, the procedure is used in the absence of surgery to determine the cause and location of any biliary obstruction, such as gallstones, inflammatory stricture, pancreatitis, pancreatic carcinoma, gall bladder carcinoma and cholangiocarcinoma. In this case, a needle is inserted into the liver until a bile duct is found. Contrast medium is then injected and X-ray films obtained.

Any complications are usually secondary to haemorrhage or sepsis.

Findings
The bile duct should be smooth, without evidence of filling defects, dilatation, bile duct narrowing or extravasation.

Colonoscopy

Definition
A colonoscopy is a telescopic examination of the colon, ileo-caecal valve and portions of the terminal ileum by means of a fibreoptic or video endoscope.

Explanation of procedure
On the day before the examination, the patient will be given a laxative or bowel cleansing solution to ensure that the bowel is empty. Nothing to eat or drink is allowed for 6 hours before the procedure. Premedication is routinely given before the examination to decrease the comfort of bowel stretching and produce mild sedation. The patient is then placed on his or her side and the lubricated endoscope inserted into the rectum and advanced through the various portions of the lower gastrointestinal tract. Significant anatomical landmarks are identified and mucosal surfaces examined for ulceration, haemorrhage, neoplasms, polyps, etc. Minor surgical operations may also be performed at the same time.

Colonoscopy is used to investigate unexplained gastrointestinal symptoms, unexplained rectal bleeding, abnormality in a barium enema, the severity of inflammatory bowel disease, diverticular disease, colitis and endometriosis. Therapeutic indications include polypectomy, tumour resection and foreign body removal.

Possible complications include perforation and haemorrhage, but the risk is small.

Findings
Findings vary depending on the reason for the test, but the report following the examination will comment on any mucosal abnormalities.

Colposcopy

Definition
A colposcopy is a telescopic examination of the epithelium and underlying blood vessels of the cervix and surrounding anogenital area. It involves the use of a colposcope, which is a magnifying instrument with a powerful light source that provides three-dimensional images.

Explanation of procedure

The patient is placed on her back and a vaginal speculum is inserted gently to expose as much of the cervix and vagina as possible. The colposcope is then inserted and positioned to optimise visibility of the cervix and vagina. After inspection of the cervix and vagina, acetic acid is applied to the cervix to assist in the differentiation of normal squamous epithelium from dysplastic epithelium; it achieves this by coagulating the nuclear and cystoplasmic proteins of the squamous epithelium, turning it opaque and white. The speculum is then removed and the perianal region examined in a similar manner.

Colposcopy is used to aid diagnosis of patients with abnormal cervical cytology or evaluation of an observed cervical, vaginal or perianal lesion.

Findings

Findings vary depending on the reason for the test.

Computed tomography (CT)

Definition

A computerised tomogram (CT) is a radiographic technique using specialised X-rays to show internal organs in great detail.

Explanation of procedure

The procedure is performed using a CT scanner (Figure 19.2), which is a specialised type of X-ray machine sending out several beams simultaneously from different angles. After the beams have passed through the tissue being investigated, their strength is measured. Beams that have passed through dense tissue (e.g. bone) will be weaker than beams that have passed through less dense tissue (e.g. lung). The relative density of the tissues investigated is measured by computer and displayed as a two-dimensional image on a monitor. Some CT scanners can reconstruct the information from two-dimensional computer images to produce three-dimensional images.

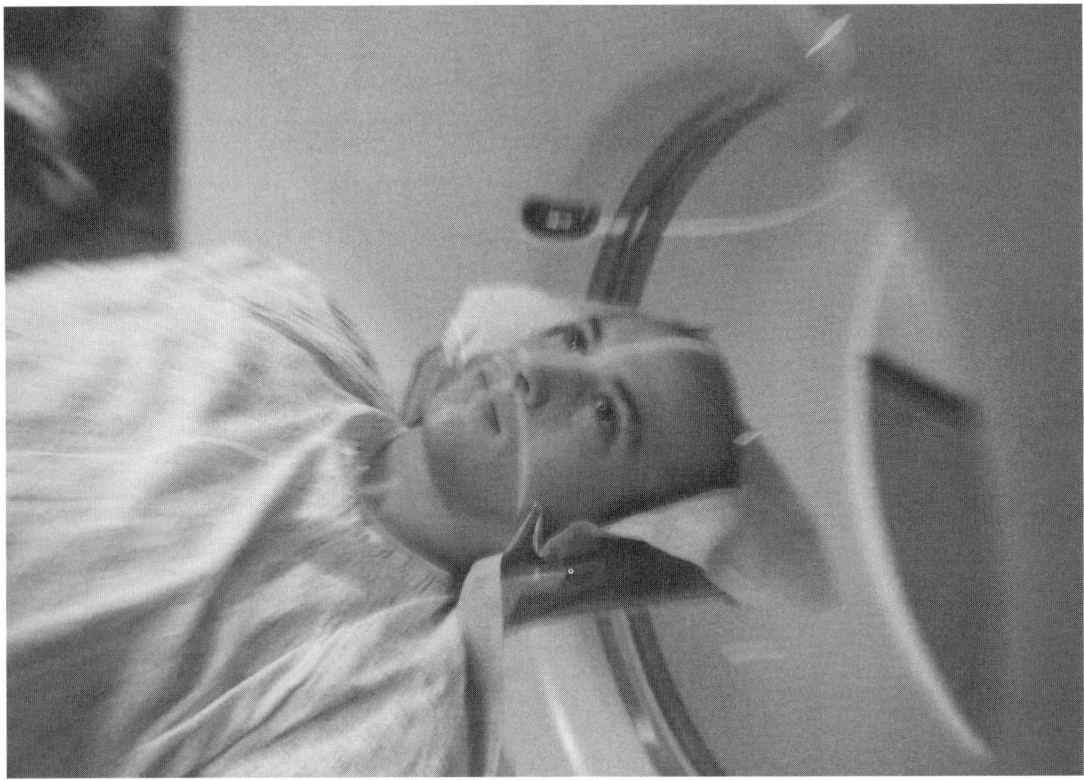

Figure 19.2 Patient undergoing a CT scan. (Reproduced with permission of Michael Donne/Science Photo Library.)

During the procedure the patient lies on a bed with the body part under examination placed in the round tunnel or opening of the scanner. The bed moves slowly backwards and forwards to allow the scanner to take pictures of the appropriate parts of the body.

Originally designed for scanning the brain, CT scanners are used to examine virtually any part of the body. The procedure is used to investigate aneurysms, brain damage, tumours and abscesses throughout the body, internal injuries such as torn kidney, spleen or liver and bone injury. It can also be used to guide biopsies, staging known tumours and planning radiotherapy.

Although there should be no complications, far more X-rays are involved in a CT scan than in an ordinary X-ray examination, so CT scans are not recommended without good medical reason. Some patients may experience an allergic reaction to the contrast medium injected into the veins.

Findings
Findings vary depending on the reason for the test.

Cystoscopy

Definition
A cystoscopy is a telescopic examination of the anterior and posterior urethra, bladder neck and bladder. It involves the use of a cystoscope.

Explanation of procedure
Before the procedure, topical anaesthesia is applied to the urethra and the cystoscope inserted into the urethra. The cystoscope is continually advanced with careful inspection of the urethra and the entire bladder surface. An attached camera allows a view of the bladder to be projected on to a television monitor.

Cystoscopes can be either flexible or rigid. Flexible cystoscopes are more comfortable for the patient, allow for ease of inspection by deflection of the instrument tip and the examination can be conducted with the patient in the supine position. Rigid cystoscopes have the advantage of better optics, easier orientation inside the bladder and a wider range of instruments can be used, making it easier to take biopsies or cauterise bladder tumours.

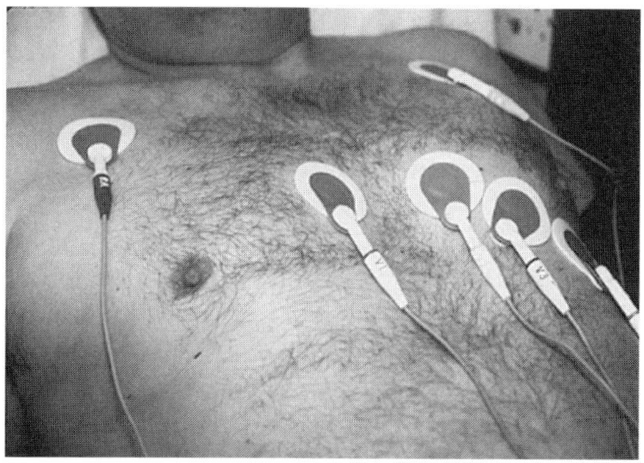

Figure 19.3 Electrocardiography. (Reproduced with permission of Antonia Reeve/Science Photo Library.)

The procedure is used for the diagnosis of lower urinary tract disease, especially the evaluation of microscopic and gross haematuria. Additional indications include voiding symptoms which can be caused by neurological, inflammatory, neoplastic or congenital abnormalities.

In general, cystoscopy is considered to be a low-risk procedure. Microscopic bleeding is common but self-limiting, while urethral and bladder perforation is rare.

Findings
Findings vary depending on the reason for the test.

Electrocardiography

Definition
An electrocardiogram (ECG) is a diagnostic procedure that measures the electrical activity of the heart.

Explanation of the procedure
To obtain an ECG, up to 12 self-adhesive electrodes are attached to locations on the arms, legs and chest (Figure 19.3). Areas where the electrodes are to be located are prepared, then the electrodes are placed. Appropriate recording of the 12 leads is achieved by automatic pens on moving paper, then the electrodes are removed.

The ECG is widely used in patients with known or suspected heart disease. In those without known heart disease, the ECG is used as a screening test for occult coronary artery disease, cardiac arrhythmias, ventricular hypertrophy and cardiomyopathy. It is invaluable for the investigation of patients with acute chest pain and can be used to assess whether the patient has had a heart attack. It can also be used to monitor the effects of drug therapy for cardiovascular disease and can provide useful insight into metabolic abnormalities such as hypercalcaemia, hypocalcaemia, hyperkalaemia and hypokalaemia.

ECG is considered a safe procedure.

Findings
Interpretation of an ECG is quite complex and requires thorough training.

Electroencephalography

Definition
An electroencephalogram (EEG) is a diagnostic procedure that records the electrical activity of the brain using scalp electrodes.

Explanation of procedure
The principle of the procedure is based on the fact that neurons within the cerebral cortex generate low-amplitude electrical signals. Electrodes placed over the cortex are able to detect these signals. From 8 to 20 electrodes are placed in a pattern designated by convention, and the underlying activity of the brain is recorded. The brain rhythms are then amplified, filtered and transmitted to a polygraph and recorded as wave forms by automatic pens on moving paper.

EEG is used to evaluate patients with suspected seizure disorder, to assess coma and other impairments in mental status and in the diagnosis of certain infections of the central nervous system (e.g. Alzheimer's disease). It is also used to evaluate sleep disorders, for monitoring of cerebral activity intra-operatively, and to evaluate cerebrovascular disease and head injury.

EEG is considered a safe procedure.

Findings
Interpretation of an EEG is quite complex and requires thorough training.

Endoscopy

Definition
An endoscopy involves visual examination of hollow organs of the body (e.g. stomach, lungs) using a fibreoptic endoscope. An endoscope can also be used to take a biopsy.

Explanation of procedure
The instrument is gently placed into the area of interest and the examination takes place. Depending on the area being examined, a local anaesthetic may be given.

This procedure is used to examine the surfaces of hollow organs to detect the presence of tumours and other lesions.

Findings
Findings vary depending on the reason for the test.

Exercise tolerance test

Definition
The exercise tolerance test is a diagnostic test for various cardiovascular and respiratory parameters involving the patient walking on a treadmill.

Explanation of procedure
Baseline 12-lead electrocardiograms are recorded in the supine and standing positions. During testing the patient wears a nose clip and breathes out through a valve that separates expired air from room air. An appropriate exercise protocol is selected based on clinical assessment and the patient's expected exercise ability.

Blood pressure, 12-lead ECGs, heart rate, ST segments, arrhythmias, symptoms and subjective patient responses are monitored during the exercise programme. The test is stopped when the patient reaches maximal exercise capacity, significant ischaemic changes are recorded, significant rhythm disturbances are observed, haemodynamic status is compromised or the patient asks to stop the test. During the test, measurements of expired air are obtained, including oxygen tension, carbon dioxide tension and air flow, as well as respiratory rate and tidal volume. Total body oxygen consumption and carbon dioxide production are calculated.

After the test the patient is monitored until haemodynamically stable and blood pressure and pulse return to near baseline level.

The test is used to determine the presence and severity of exercise induced myocardial ischaemia and to evaluate the potential for rhythm disturbances and haemodynamic disturbances with activity. It is also useful for evaluating the effect of any medical therapy and for prescribing exercise and activity. The patient's exercise tolerance and oxygen and carbon dioxide consumption can be assessed.

Findings

Findings vary depending on the reasons for the test.

Gastroscopy

Definition

Gastroscopy is a telescopic examination of the inside of the oesophagus, stomach and duodenum. It involves the use of a thin fibreoptic instrument.

Explanation of procedure

The back of the throat is sprayed with a local anaesthetic (e.g. xylocaine), the instrument is gently placed in the mouth and the patient asked to swallow it. Sometimes premedication is used, but the procedure may be carried out without sedation. In addition, a biopsy may be taken for microscopic examination. This procedure has reduced the use of barium meals, of which relatively few are performed nowadays.

Gastroscopy is used to examine the mucous membrane of the upper gastrointestinal tract to check for the presence of tumours, ulcers or other abnormalities.

Findings

Findings vary depending on the reason for the test.

Glucose tolerance test

Definition

The glucose tolerance test is a 2-hour (occasionally a 3-hour) blood and urine test for glucose. It involves consumption of a glucose-containing drink.

Explanation of procedure

Patients should continue with their normal diet (including habitual carbohydrate intake) for at least three days prior to the test, but they are usually asked to fast from about 10 pm on the evening before. The glucose drink can be a carbohydrate drink (e.g. Maxijul), 75 g glucose dissolved in water and flavoured with sugar-free squash or citric acid, or 395 mL Lucozade. A blood sample is taken before the drink is consumed, then at 1 hour and 2 hours after taking the drink. Urine is also collected before and 1 hour after the test.

Glucose tolerance tests are occasionally used to diagnose diabetes mellitus. However, diabetes is more usually diagnosed from measurement of fasting blood glucose. Glucose tolerance tests may also be used to investigate an impaired fasting glycaemia, which may have been identified from a fasting blood glucose test.

A modified glucose tolerance test which involves taking a fasting specimen then a second specimen 2 hours after a meal, or preferably after a 75 g glucose load is, however, a useful screening tool for diabetes.

Findings

The World Health Organization (1998) has set the following criteria and cut-off points.

Plasma glucose:

Fasting <5.5 mmol/L and 2 hour <7.8 mmol/L (diabetes mellitus unlikely)

Fasting <7.0 mmol/L and 2 hour 7.8–11.1 mmol/L (impaired glucose tolerance).

Fasting 6.1–7.0 mmol/L (impaired fasting glycaemia)

Fasting ≥7.0 mmol/L and 2 hour ≥11.1 mmol/L (diabetes mellitus)

Blood glucose:

Fasting <4.9 mmol/L and 2 hour <6.7 mmol/L (diabetes mellitus unlikely)

Fasting <6.0 mmol/L and 2 hour 6.7–10.0 mmol/L (impaired glucose tolerance)

Fasting 5.3–6.1 mmol/L (impaired fasting glycaemia)

Fasting ≥6.1 mmol/L and 2 hour ≥10.0 mmol/L (diabetes mellitus).

Helicobacter pylori test

Definition

This is a test for the presence of *Helicobacter pylori*, which is implicated in peptic ulcer and its eradication can lead to healing of ulcers. However, *H. pylori* testing does not detect which patients have *H. pylori*-related disease.

Explanation of procedure

H. pylori can be detected from biopsy specimens at endoscopy, most commonly with a rapid and reliable biopsy urease test.

The gold standard non-invasive *H. pylori* test is a carbon urea breath test in which the patient is required to swallow a radiolabelled carbon isotope. This is exhaled as radiolabelled carbon dioxide, and the test can be performed in hospital or in general practice surgeries.

In addition, blood tests can be used to detect *H. pylori* antibodies. Both laboratory-based and near-patient blood tests are available, but concerns have been raised about the accuracy of these tests, particularly the near-patient test. Breath tests are more accurate, with higher sensitivity and specificity than either laboratory-based or near-patient serological tests.

Stool antigen tests are also available. These appear to have a high level of accuracy, but they are not widely used.

Intravenous pyelography

Definition

Intravenous pyelography is a radiographic procedure for the evaluation of the morphology and function of the urinary tract. It involves the intravenous administration of a contrast material.

Explanation of procedure

Patients are encouraged to take nothing by mouth after midnight the night before the examination. The contrast material is administered intravenously and is concentrated and excreted by the kidneys. Appropriate radiographs are exposed during the concentration and excretion of the contrast medium.

The procedure is used to investigate abnormalities involving the urinary tract.

Complications are rare, but some patients may suffer reactions to the contrast medium.

Findings

Findings vary depending on the reason for the test.

Laparoscopy

Definition

Laparoscopy is a telescopic procedure for viewing the anterior intra-abdominal structures by means of a laparoscope.

Explanation of procedure

A laparoscopy is generally performed under general anaesthetic. A needle is inserted into the peritoneal cavity, followed by insufflation of carbon dioxide to create a space for the surgeon to view or operate. The laparoscope is introduced through a small cut made in the abdomen.

There are various indications for laparoscopy, including ascites of unknown aetiology, liver disease of unknown aetiology, suspected peritoneal cancer, cancer staging in malignancies such as ovarian cancer or Hodgkin's disease. It may also be used to investigate chronic abdominal or pelvic pain, such as endometriosis, appendicitis, ovarian cysts, and in cases of primary or secondary amenorrhoea and suspected ectopic pregnancy.

Laparoscopy can also be used operatively for procedures such as tubal ligation, treatment of endometriosis with laser, lysis of cysts caused by ovarian diseases or other pelvic disease. Most sterilisations are now performed through a laparoscope.

This procedure is considered safe, with serious complications being estimated to affect between one and two per 1000 patients. Risks include accidental injury or perforation of the bowel, liver, spleen, ovary and gall bladder. Minor complications include bleeding or bruising especially at the site of the skin incision.

Findings

Findings vary depending on the reason for the test.

Lumbar puncture

Definition
Lumbar puncture involves the collection of cerebrospinal fluid (CSF) for chemical, microbiological and cellular analysis.

Explanation of procedure
A spinal needle is passed into the intravertebral space, generally between the fourth and fifth lumbar vertebrae and the CSF is allowed to drain into sterile collection tubes. The CSF is examined visually (normally it is clear) and the spinal fluid pressure measured. Routine tests performed on the CSF include cell counts, protein and glucose. The procedure is generally performed under local anaesthesia with the patient in either the seated or the prone position.

Lumbar puncture is used in suspected cases of encephalitis, meningitis, subarachnoid haemorrhage, multiple sclerosis and malignancies of the central nervous system such as lymphoma or leukaemia. It is also used in lymphoma staging.

The procedure is relatively safe and complications are rare. Headache is the most frequent complication. Low backache may also occur and infection may develop if there has been insufficient attention to sterile technique during the procedure.

Findings
Interpretation of CSF findings is complex and should always be made in conjunction with the clinical presentation. Findings vary depending on the reason for the test. For example in bacterial meningitis, the classic findings include raised white blood cells, predominance of polymorphonuclear leucocytes and decreased glucose.

> *Normal ranges:*
> Lymphocyte cells: $<5\ mm^3$
> Red blood cells or white blood cells: $<1 \times 10^6/L$
> Protein: 0.1–0.5 g/L
> Glucose: 2.1–4.5 mmol/L
> Culture: no growth
> CSF pressure: 70–200 mmH_2O

Magnetic resonance imaging

Definition
Magnetic resonance imaging (MRI) is a diagnostic technique which relies on radio frequency or radio signals induced within the patient by a magnetic field to obtain images. Unlike most conventional radiological procedures, MRI does not utilise ionizing radiation.

Explanation of procedure
The patient lies inside a large cylinder-shaped magnet and radio waves 10 000–30 000 times stronger than the magnetic field of the earth are passed through the body. The magnet then induces radio signals from the patient's body, and the signals are picked up by a scanner and computer.

Prior to the scan the patient will be asked to remove all metallic objects from their person, including loose change, belts, hair pins, earrings and so on. Dentures should also be removed. Patients should inform medical staff if they have a pacemaker or any surgical clips, but orthopaedic metalwork such as artificial joints are not usually a problem. Credit cards and other bank cards should not be taken into the scanner because the magnetic field can permanently erase information carried on them.

An MRI scan gives clear, detailed pictures of almost all tissues in the body, including those surrounded by bone. MRI is better able to distinguish between normal and abnormal tissue than computed tomography (CT) and unlike CT, which can only scan tissues horizontally, MRI can take pictures from almost every angle.

The procedure can be used to identify and stage tumours in any part of the body, and is also a useful diagnostic tool for detection of abnormal tissue in patients with multiple sclerosis. The method can also be used to detect bleeding or ischaemia in the brain and to examine the spine, joints, heart, liver, pancreas, spleen and kidneys.

There are no known risks associated with an MRI scan. Patients have to lie still in a cylinder while the scan is being performed, and claustrophobia may be experienced by some people.

Findings

Findings vary depending on the reason for the test.

Mammography

Definition

A mammogram is a type of breast X-ray used to examine the breasts.

Explanation of procedure

The patient is asked to undress to the waist and stand in front of the X-ray machine. Each breast is compressed in turn between two perspex plates, and two images of each breast are taken using a brief X-ray pulse. Some patients find the experience painful, but for the majority there is no more than minor discomfort.

A mammogram is indicated in the evaluation of any newly appearing breast lump considered suspicious for tumour. However, because of the high incidence of breast cancer among the female population, screening mammography is also recommended in the asymptomatic patient. In the UK, this means having a mammogram every three years between the ages of 50 and 64 years. In the US, the American Cancer Society recommends a mammogram every one to two years in women aged 40–49, and those aged 50 years or older are recommended to have a mammogram on an annual basis.

However, young women who are considered to be at high risk of developing breast cancer because of their family history or in whom a biopsy has shown an abnormality are offered screening at an earlier age in both the UK and the USA.

Findings

A mammogram will detect abnormalities in breast tissue, but does not necessarily show whether those abnormalities are benign or malignant. Further investigations such as ultrasound or fine needle aspiration cytology may be required.

One in 20 women who have a mammogram will be recalled for assessment. This can be either because there is a technical problem with the first mammogram or because there is a need for further investigation. However, women should be reassured that being recalled does not mean they have breast cancer. Of those recalled after the first mammogram, about one in 10 will have cancer.

Myelography

Definition

Myelography involves collection of spinal fluid for laboratory analysis and viewing of the cervical, thoracic and/or lumbar spinal cord by injection of contrast material.

Explanation of the procedure

The procedure is performed under local anaesthesia, and using fluoroscopy, an appropriate entry site is selected over the lumbar spine, or occasionally over the upper cervical spine. A spinal needle is guided fluoroscopically to the thecal sac and spinal fluid may be withdrawn for laboratory analysis (e.g. cell count, protein, immunoglobulins, cytology). Contrast material is then injected into the subarachnoid space of the spinal canal and films of the lumbar, thoracic and/or cervical spine are obtained.

Patients taking medication which lowers the seizure threshold (e.g. antipsychotics) should stop these medicines 24–48 hours before the procedure.

Myelography is used to identify abnormalities of the spinal cord, including those due to trauma, malignancy or compression of spinal nerve roots. It is usually performed in patients unable to undergo MRI or in those with MRI findings that are equivocal.

Findings

There should be no evidence of displacement of the spinal cord or the nerve roots. There should be no evidence of any compression or any filling defect in the thecal sac.

Paracentesis

Definition

Paracentesis is a procedure for diagnostic and/or therapeutic purposes in patients with ascites. It involves sampling ascites fluid from the peritoneal space.

Explanation of procedure
The procedure involves withdrawal of ascites fluid (usually 50–100 mL, more in cases of suspected malignancy or infection) with a needle and syringe. The fluid is routinely analysed for cell count, bacteriology, cytology, albumin and protein.

Paracentesis is indicated in patients with ascites of recent onset, ascites of unknown aetiology and those with suspected ascites fluid infections.

The risk of complications from paracentesis is controversial in that some of the literature emphasises the possible complications while others conclude that it is a relatively safe procedure. Complications include needle perforation of the liver or spleen, intraperitoneal haemorrhage from laceration of an umbilical vein or infection of ascites fluid by non-sterile technique.

Findings
Findings vary depending on the reason for the test.

Patch tests

Definition
A patch test is an objective method of demonstrating allergic contact dermatitis. It involves application of multiple test materials to the skin surface.

Explanation of procedure
Patch testing is performed on an area of the skin where there is no dermatitis, and the site chosen is usually the upper back. The skin is premarked in vertical rows using a fluorescent pen and a small amount of allergen is applied to an aluminium disc, which is then fixed to the skin with non-allergenic tape. The standard selection of allergens used is known as the European Standard Battery, which consists of the commonest allergens. Additional allergen batteries are available for specific occupations (e.g. hairdressers, printers) and the patient's personal cosmetics may also be tested.

The patches are left in place for 48 hours then removed by the patient. Heavy exercise is not permitted during this period to avoid excessive perspiration. Skin response is recorded at 1, 24 and 48 hours after patch removal. Additional readings may be taken after that. The patient will be asked to refrain from washing the area until the last reading is taken.

The patch test is used to confirm the diagnosis of suspected allergic contact dermatitis and to determine the responsible allergen where many allergens are suspected.

Findings
Results will vary depending on whether the patient is allergic to any of the test substances. Spurious results (false negatives and false positives) may occur and represent a major clinical challenge.

Pleural biopsy

Definition
Pleural biopsy involves biopsy of the pleura using a needle passed through the intercostal space.

Explanation of procedure
Pleural biopsy is performed under local anaesthesia. The appropriate intercostal space is located and the needle advanced between the ribs and into the pleural space. The needle is blunt tipped and wide bored with a special device to grip and cut the pleura. Pleural fluid may be withdrawn and several pleural samples are collected. The needle is then removed. Pleural specimens are sent for bacterial culture.

The procedure is used for suspected malignant pleural effusion, pleural effusion of unknown aetiology and suspected tuberculous pleural effusions.

The procedure is not without risk and the most common complication includes pneumothorax. Other complications include haemothorax, lung perforation, local infection at the needle entrance site and local pain.

Findings
Findings vary depending on the reason for the test.

Positron emission tomography

Definition

Positron emission tomography (PET) is a medical imaging technique that provides functional information about particular tissues or organs. It involves the use of radio-isotopes.

Explanation of procedure

Patients are asked to fast for about 4–6 hours before the procedure. A radioactive tracer is injected into the bloodstream about 1 hour before the study is undertaken. The tracer emits positrons which interact with electrons in body tissue to release gamma radiation. This is received by a circular array of detectors surrounding the patient then subsequently reconstructed into a computerised image.

PET scans are used in the diagnosis of brain tumours and stroke, and in the investigation of epilepsy, schizophrenia, manic–depressive disorder, Alzheimer's disease and other mental illnesses. They are also used to investigate ischaemic heart disease and to study brain functions such as speech, reading, memory and reading.

This procedure is low risk. As with most other imaging techniques, the patient receives a small dose of radiation.

Findings

Findings vary depending on the reason for the test.

Sigmoidoscopy

Definition

A sigmoidoscopy is a telescopic examination of the rectum, sigmoid colon and proximal portions of the colon by means of a flexible fibreoptic endoscope.

Explanation of procedure

On the day before the examination, the patient will be given a laxative or bowel cleansing solution to ensure that the bowel is empty. Premedication is not normally necessary. The patient is then placed on his or her side and digital rectal examination is performed first. Then the lubricated sigmoidoscope is gently inserted into the rectum and advanced through the various portions of the lower gastrointestinal tract. Insufflation of the bowel is necessary but only to a minimal extent compared with that required for colonoscopy. Significant anatomical landmarks are identified and mucosal surfaces examined for ulceration, haemorrhage, neoplasms, polyps, etc. Minor surgical operations may also be performed at the same time.

Sigmoidoscopy is used to investigate unexplained rectal bleeding, the severity of inflammatory bowel disease, sigmoid diverticulitis, colitis and screening for colorectal cancer.

Possible complications include perforation and haemorrhage, but the risk is small.

Findings

Findings vary depending on the reason for the test, but the report following the examination will comment on any mucosal abnormalities.

Ultrasound

Definition

Ultrasound scans are images of internal organs created from sound waves directed into the body then reflected back to a scanner.

Explanation of the procedure

A gel is applied to the skin over the area of interest and a handheld transducer is swept across the area to image the appropriate organs (Figure 19.4). The scanner can also be used through natural orifices of the body such as the vagina. Sound waves are used for the imaging and no radiation exposure is present. Images are recorded on X-ray film.

Ultrasound scanning is used to diagnose conditions in many areas of the body such as the abdomen, heart, liver and kidneys. It is commonly used in the detection of malignancies and the staging of tumours. Ultrasound is also used in pregnancy to assess the growth and development of the fetus.

This procedure is low risk and there is no evidence that ultrasound scans harm the unborn child.

Findings

Findings vary depending on the reason for the test.

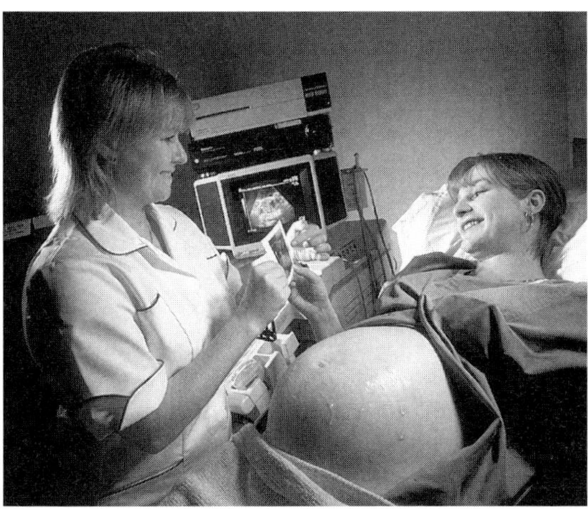

Figure 19.4 Ultrasound. (Reproduced with permission of Deep Light Productions/Science Photo Library.)

Vaginal smear

Definition
A vaginal smear involves taking a scraping of cells from the cervix.

Explanation of procedure
A speculum, made of either metal or plastic, is passed into the vagina. The two halves of the speculum are opened to hold the vaginal walls apart and the device is placed so that the doctor or nurse can see the cervix. There are many devices for taking the smear itself, including wooden ones and small brushes.

The purpose of a cervical smear is to detect cells which are pre-cancerous or cancerous. In the UK it is currently recommended to have a smear every three years.

Findings
Findings depend on the reason for the test.

X-ray examinations

Definition
X-rays are a form of electromagnetic radiation, which have high energy and short wavelength and are able to pass through tissue.

Explanation of procedure
The patient stands between the X-ray machine and a screen used for obtaining the image. The X-rays are converted into light, and the denser tissues (e.g. bones) which block more of the rays than less dense tissues (e.g. the lung) appear whiter.

An X-ray image can be extremely informative and can be used, for example, to detect fractures or a shadow on the lung. X-rays (radiotherapy) are also used in the treatment of some forms of cancer.

Nowadays, with the very small doses of radiation used, the risk after appropriately supervised X-ray examination is extremely small. However, radiation can cause damage to the fetus and the use of X-rays during pregnancy is avoided or kept to a minimum.

Findings
Findings depend on the reason for the test.

19.3 Tests on samples

Blood tests

Blood tests (Table 19.1) are a very useful diagnostic tool and can be performed on all the various constituents of blood (*see* Section 9.4). The most commonly requested blood test is the full blood count (FBC), which includes a count of the three cellular elements: erythrocytes (red cells), leucocytes (white cells) and thrombocytes (platelets).

Red cell tests

Tests relating to red cells are used primarily to diagnose anaemia and to investigate the possible causes of the anaemia. These include:

- The red blood cell (RBC) count is the number of red cells in the blood. This is decreased in anaemia (*see* Section 9.1.2) and raised in polycythaemia (*see* Section 9.1.1) or in cases of dehydration due to any cause.

Table 19.1 Haematology. Typical adult reference intervals

Test or cell	Reference range
Red cell count (RCC)	
Men	$4.5–6.5 \times 10^{12}$/L
Women	$3.9–5.6 \times 10^{12}$/L
Reticulocyte count (0.8–2.0% of RCC)	$25–100 \times 10^{9}$/L
Haemoglobin	
Men	13.5–17.5 g/dL
Women	11.5–15.5 g/dL
Packed cell volume (PCV) or haematocrit	
Men	0.4–0.54
Women	0.37–0.49
Mean cell volume (MCV)	80–100 fL
Mean cell haemoglobin (MCH)	27–32 pg
Mean cell haemoglobin concentration (MCHC)	30–36 g/dL
White cell count (WCC)	$4.0–11.0 \times 10^{9}$/L
Neutrophils (40–75% WCC)	$2.5–7.5 \times 10^{9}$/L
Lymphocytes (20–40% WCC)	$1.5–4.9 \times 10^{9}$/L
Monocytes (2–10% WCC)	$0.2–0.8 \times 10^{9}$/L
Eosinophils (1–5% WCC)	$0.04–0.44 \times 10^{9}$/L
Basophils (<1% WCC)	$0.01–0.10 \times 10^{9}$/L
Platelet count	$150–400 \times 10^{9}$/L
Erythrocyte sedimentation rate (ESR)	<10 mm/h
Prothrombin time (factors I, II, VII, X)	10–14 seconds
Activated partial thromboplastin time (VIII, IX, XI, XII)	35–45 seconds
Thrombin time	14–16 seconds

- Haemoglobin is the concentration of the protein haemoglobin in the blood. Concentrations are reduced in anaemia and raised in polycythaemia, hypoxia, renal conditions where excess erythropoietin is produced, or dehydration due to any cause. In addition, smoking may raise haemoglobin (due to increased carboxyhaemoglobin).
- Packed cell volume (PCV or haematocrit) is the percentage of the total blood volume occupied by red cells. PCV can be used as a screen for anaemia and to indicate the degree of fluid loss in dehydration. A drop in PCV can also indicate internal haemorrhage before other symptoms of internal bleeding become apparent. PCV is raised in polycythaemia and in chronic hypoxia associated with pulmonary disease and congenital heart disease.
- Mean cell volume (MCV) is a measure of the average (mean) volume of red cells. Raised MCV suggests vitamin B_{12} or folate deficiency, myxoedema, alcoholism or liver disease, haemolysis, aplasia or marrow filtration. Reduced MCV suggests chronic blood loss, iron deficiency anaemia, thalassaemia, sideroblastic anaemia or anaemia of chronic disease.
- Mean cell haemoglobin concentration (MCHC) is a measure of the average (mean) concentration of haemoglobin in red cells. Reduced MCHC suggests iron deficiency, or chronic blood loss.

The MCV and the MCHC, together with the microscopic examination of red cells, help in identifying causes of anaemia. Thus, according to these two indices anaemias can be classified into three types:

1 Normocytic (normal MCV), normochromic (normal MCHC) anaemia. Anaemias in this group include those which result from haemorrhage, leukaemia or chronic renal failure, and also the haemolytic anaemias (*see* Section 9.1.2) and aplastic anaemia (*see* Section 9.1.2). Most cases of anaemia associated with chronic disease fall into this category.
2 Microcytic (low MCV), hypochromic (low MCHC) anaemia. Iron deficiency anaemia and thalassaemia fall into this group.
3 Macrocytic (raised MCV) anaemia. This type of anaemia is caused by deficiency of vitamin B_{12} and folate, which leads to abnormal red cell production. MCV may be raised in patients who are not anaemic, and the main causes of this are alcohol abuse and cirrhosis of the liver.

Erythrocyte sedimentation rate (ESR)

This is defined as the length of clear fluid at the top of a tube (a narrow-bore tube specifically used to measure ESR) left for 1 hour when blood is left to stand at room temperature.

ESR is a non-specific test and is raised in many different types of illness, including those involving inflammation, injury and malignancy. However, in most of these conditions, it is quite possible that ESR will be normal. In clinical practice ESR is used as supportive evidence of inflammation in conditions such as rheumatoid arthritis, Crohn's disease and ulcerative colitis. It may also be used to monitor the effectiveness of therapy in those suffering chronic infection (e.g. tuberculosis and subacute bacterial endocarditis). Many patients with cancers of all types have a raised ESR and the test has no place in the diagnosis of cancer, with the exception of multiple myeloma where raised ESR is found so consistently that it is one of the diagnostic criteria for the condition. In addition, ESR is raised in Hodgkin's disease, in which the test is used not for diagnostic purposes but for monitoring progress of the disease and effectiveness of therapy.

White blood cell tests

An increase in the leucocyte count (leucocytosis) occurs most commonly as a result of infection, inflammation or any major tissue damage. A large increase occurs in leukaemia. A reduction in white cell count (leucopenia) is much less common than an increase. Unlike leucocytosis, which may be benign, occurring as an appropriate response to infection or inflammation, leucopenia is never appropriate.

Abnormal white cell counts are the result of an increase or decrease in one or more of the five types of white cell:

- *Neutrophils*. An increased neutrophil count (neutrophilia) is a feature of most acute bacterial infections, acute inflammatory conditions (e.g. rheumatoid arthritis), pregnancy, surgery, burns, myocardial infarction and solid tumours (e.g. lung cancer). A low neutrophil count (neutropenia) is a feature of some viral infections (e.g. mumps, influenza, HIV, viral hepatitis), aplastic anaemia, acute leukaemia and some advanced cancers (particularly those tumours which have spread to the bone).
- *Eosinophils*. A raised eosinophil count (eosinophilia) may be caused by allergic conditions (e.g. hay fever, allergic asthma, eczema, food allergy), allergic drug reactions and parasitic worm infections.
- *Basophils*. Abnormal counts of these cells are fairly rare, but basophil numbers are raised in chronic myeloid leukaemia.
- *Lymphocytes*. An increased lymphocyte count (lymphocytosis) is a feature of glandular fever. Lymphocytosis may also occur in the early stages of HIV infection, viral hepatitis, mumps, rubella, chickenpox, tuberculosis and whooping cough. Causes of reduced lymphocyte count include acquired immune deficiency syndrome (AIDS), systemic lupus erythmatosus (SLE), influenza, burns and surgery.
- *Monocytes*. An increased monocyte count (monocytosis) may occur in tuberculosis, subacute bacterial endocarditis and other chronic bacterial infections.

Platelet count

A reduced platelet count (thrombocytopenia) is a feature of immune thrombocytopenic purpura (ITP). It may also be caused by drugs, such as some antibiotics (e.g. penicillin, sulphonamides), some diuretics (e.g. frusemide, acetazolamide) and some anti-inflammatories.

A severe increase in platelet count may occur in malignant disorders of the bone marrow characterised by abnormal proliferation of myeloid stem cells (e.g. chronic myeloid leukaemia, polycythaemia vera, essential thrombocytopenia). A mild to moderate increase is more common and may be seen in severe infectious illness (e.g. septicaemia), chronic inflammatory conditions (e.g. rheumatoid arthritis), as well as after haemorrhage, surgery or other severe trauma.

Blood coagulation tests

Blood coagulation tests measure the ability of the blood to form fibrin in the blood clotting cascade (*see* Section 9.4). In essence they measure the time taken for a sample of patient's blood plasma to form a fibrin clot in a test tube after addition of a reagent that initiates the clotting cascade. In addition to the international normalised ratio (INR *see below*), there are three main coagulation tests:

- *Prothrombin time (PT).* This is one of the tests used to monitor oral anticoagulants. Commercially produced thromboplastin (factor III) is added to the plasma and the time taken in seconds for the plasma to clot is measured. The test is sensitive to reduced levels of factors V, VII and X, prothrombin and fibrinogen, and deficiency of one of more of these factors will result in an abnormally long time for a fibrin clot to form (i.e. PT will be increased).
- *Activated partial thromboplastin time (APPT).* Also known as kaolin cephalin clotting time (KCCT), this test is a measure of the intrinsic clotting cascade. An abnormally prolonged clotting time indicates a deficiency of one or more of the factors required by the intrinsic pathway (e.g. factors VIII, IX, XI and XII). This test is used for monitoring intravenous heparin.
- *Thrombin time (TT).* In this test thrombin is added to the patient's plasma. This is a test specifically for the final stages of the common pathway converting fibrinogen to fibrin. An abnormally long thrombin time indicates deficiency of factor I (fibrinogen).

International normalised ratio (INR)

This is a blood test measuring prothrombin time reported as the international normalised ratio (INR). INR is the ratio of the patient's prothrombin time to the mean normal prothrombin time, exponentially equalised by the international sensitivity index (ISI) of the reagent/instrument combination.

$$\text{Patient's INR} = \frac{\text{Patient's prothrombin time (seconds)}}{\text{Mean normal prothrombin time (seconds)}}$$

Reported INR results are therefore independent of the reagents and methods used.

INR is used for assessing patients stabilised on long-term oral anticoagulant therapy. Initially, the INR may be checked daily or on alternate days after commencing therapy. After hospital discharge INR estimation is generally performed every week for four to six weeks, and thereafter measurement can be extended to every 12 weeks if control and compliance are satisfactory. Changes in the patient's medical condition (e.g. drug therapy, heart disease, thyroid status) may alter anticoagulant control and require more frequent monitoring.

For patients not on anticoagulant therapy, the INR equals 1. INR values in properly anticoagulated patients will range between 2.0 and 3.5, depending on the condition being managed. Full details and target INRs currently recommended by the British Society for Haematology can be found in the BNF (2.8.2).

Urine tests

Urine tests (*see* Table 19.2) can provide information about a wide range of diseases. Urine can be examined visually or tested by dipstick methods, which can be used to show abnormalities such as sugar, protein or blood. Pregnancy is also detected using a urine test. In addition, if more detailed information is required, urine can be sent for laboratory analysis, which may include microbiological examination.

Table 19.2 Urine. Typical adult reference ranges

Test	Reference range (per 24 hours)
5-Hydroxyindole acetic acid	<31 μmol
17-Oxosteroids	
Men	17–76 μmol
Women	10–52 μmol
17-Oxygenic steroids	
Men	17–70 μmol
Women	10–63 μmol
Cortisol (free)	
Men	<270 nmol
Women	<260 nmol
Creatine	<380 mol
Creatinine	
Men	9.7–23.0 mmol
Women	9.0–11.7 mmol
Homovanillic acid (HVA)	<42 μmol
Potassium	35–80 mmol
Protein	<150 mg
Sodium	120–220 mmol
Urate	0.5–5.9 mmol
Urea	209–475 mmol
Vanillylmandelic acid (VMA)	<36 μmol

Visual examination

Normal urine is a clear, straw-coloured or yellow fluid, and a simple visual examination of a specimen can sometimes provide evidence of an infection. As in other bacterial infections, urinary-tract infection is associated with recruitment of the white blood cells, and white blood cells are removed from the site of infection in the form of pus. Pus causes urine to become cloudy. However, cloudy urine does not always mean the presence of a urinary-tract infection (UTI) and clear urine does not always mean absence of an infection.

Dipstick tests

There are various dipstick tests which can be used to test urine for glucose, protein, blood and bacteria.

- *Glucose*. Glycosuria (sugar in the urine) can be caused by diabetes mellitus, pregnancy, sepsis or renal tubular damage.
- *Protein*. Proteinuria (protein in the urine) can be caused by urinary-tract infection (UTI), diabetes mellitus, glomerulonephritis, nephrosis, pyrexia and pregnancy.
- *Blood*. Haematuria (blood in the urine) can be caused by renal conditions such as glomerulonephritis, interstitial nephritis, carcinoma and vasculitis (e.g. endocarditis, systemic lupus erythematosus or other connective tissue diseases). It can also be caused by infection (e.g. cystitis, prostatitis and urethritis), bladder catheterisation, calculi and after administration of cyclophosphamide.
- *Bacteria*. Assuming that the urine has been collected appropriately (i.e. it is not contaminated with the mixture of bacteria normally present in the lower third of the urethra or ano-genital area), bacteria in the urine indicates a UTI. The dipstick method for detection of urinary bacteria is based on the fact that all common bacteria causing UTI convert nitrate present in urine to nitrite. Thus, an increase in urinary nitrite concentration indicates bacterial infection. In addition, the enzyme leucocyte esterase indicates the presence of white cells and detection of this enzyme in urine provides further evidence of infection. The dipstick consists of two pads, one for detection of nitrite, the other for detection of the enzyme, and following immersion of the dipstick in freshly voided urine, the two pads are examined for a colour change, indicating the presence of bacteria, white cells or both. Although very convenient, these dipstick methods are limited by the number of false positives and positive tests should always be submitted for urine culture to confirm the presence of bacteria. A negative dipstick result, however, is strong evidence that the patient is not suffering from a UTI.

Twenty-four-hour urine tests

Twenty-four-hour urine collections are used to measure a number of metabolites such as calcium, creatinine, nitrogen, oxosteroids, potassium, sodium, urea and urate. The accuracy of such measurements depends mainly on the accuracy of the urine collection. Errors may occur due to misunderstandings on the part of the patients or lack of clarity of explanation on the part of the doctor or nurse as to exactly what is required.

The procedure involves collecting urine over a 24-hour period. For a 24-hour urine collection required, say, between 9 am on Tuesday and 9 am on Wednesday, the patient will be asked to empty the bladder completely at 9 am on Tuesday morning and discard this specimen. Urine already in the bladder at the time of the start of the test must not be included in the collection. All urine passed until 9 am on Wednesday will be collected. Then at 9 am on Wednesday the bladder should be emptied completely and this specimen added to the collection. The urine sample must be analysed within 1 hour of collection.

Midstream specimen of urine (MSU)

This procedure is used to obtain a specimen of urine uncontaminated by bacteria surrounding the urethra. These bacteria can be the same as those causing a urinary-tract infection and can therefore result in a false positive test. Collected midstream, the urine can be analysed for the presence of infection in the kidneys and bladder.

Collection of the specimen involves cleaning the skin around the urethra to avoid contamination of the urine specimen with bacteria that can make the collected specimen inaccurate or unusable. The patient then urinates, stops urination, then urinates again into a collection container. The aim is to collect a midstream specimen.

Microscopical examination

A tiny drop of urine is placed under a microscope and examined mainly for the presence of red and white blood cells. Urine normally contains a few red and white blood cells but a significant increase in red blood cells is indicative of haematuria (*see above*) and a significant increase in white cell numbers is evidence of infection. The only reliable method of confirming the presence or absence of bacteria in the urine and identifying the species is to culture the urine.

Stool tests

Stool specimens may be examined for a number of reasons, including the presence of gastrointestinal infective organisms, such as those causing food poisoning (*Salmonella* species, *Staphylococcus aureus, Bacillus cereus, Clostridium perfringens, Clostridium botulinum*), shigella, cholera and giardia. Stools may also be tested for occult blood, urobilinogen and fat.

Faecal occult blood

The faecal occult blood test may be a useful screening tool for colorectal cancers and polyps. Although safe and inexpensive it is limited by the fact that it will only detect larger polyps and cancers. In addition, colorectal cancers bleed intermittently so the test is relatively insensitive and many false negatives occur. Moreover, other non-malignant lesions can bleed, causing a positive result so the test is therefore non-specific. In addition, oral iron preparations can cause false positive reactions and aspirin can cause gastrointestinal bleeding unrelated to gut pathology.

Screening of asymptomatic people over 45 years shows that 2% of people test positive. Of these, one in 10 will have carcinoma and one in three an adenoma.

Faecal urobilinogen

Urobilinogen is produced in the small intestine by the action of the intestinal bacteria on bile and it is the compound which gives the stool its brown colour. Increased faecal urobilinogen levels are found where there is increased haemolysis of red blood cells. Decreased levels suggest obstructive biliary disease.

Faecal fat

The test for faecal fat is used to help diagnose the malabsorption syndrome. Stool specimens are collected to see if fat is being digested. If there is steatorrhoea or excess fat in the stools, stools will be frothy, foul smelling and greasy. Fat will not be digested if the patient has pancreatic disease with a deficiency of lipase, biliary obstruction or some other intestinal malabsorption condition.

Table 19.3 Liver function tests. Typical adult reference ranges

Test	Reference range
Albumin	35–55 g/L (S)
Bilirubin	
Total	3–20 μmol/L (S)
Conjugated	0–14 μmol/L (S)
Alanine aminotransferase (ALT)	0–45 iu/L
Aspartate amintransferase (AST)	0–50 iu/L
Gamma-glutamyltransferase (GGT)	
Men	0–70 iu/L
Women	0–40 iu/L
Alkaline phosphatase (AP)	90–300 iu/L

Liver function tests

Liver function tests (LFTs, *see* Table 19.3) are a group of biochemical measurements that are useful in identifying patients who are suffering from disease of the liver or biliary tract. Parameters measured to investigate liver function include:

- Albumin
- Bilirubin
- Alanine aminotransferase (ALT) and aspartate aminotransferase (AST)
- Gamma-glutamyltransferase (GGT)
- Alkaline phosphatase (AP).

None of these tests is specific for liver or biliary disease, in that other diseases not involving the liver might cause one of more of these tests to be abnormal. In addition, even in cases of liver disease, one or more of the tests might be normal. However, it is extremely unlikely that all tests would show normal results in a patient with liver or biliary disease. Together, therefore, the combination of tests is more useful than a single test on its own.

Albumin

Albumin is synthesised from amino acids in the liver and is the single most abundant protein in plasma, accounting for around 60% of plasma protein. Since albumin is made in the liver, it might be expected that levels would always be low in patients with liver disease. However, this is not always the case because albumin has a long half-life and plasma concentrations change slowly. Thus, while albumin levels are low in chronic liver disease (e.g. cirrhosis), levels may remain normal in cases of acute liver disease (e.g. infective hepatitis).

Albumin levels may also be reduced in conditions other than liver disease (e.g. malnutrition, diseases associated with malabsorption such as Crohn's disease, chronic renal failure, nephrotic syndrome, severe burns and post-operatively). The patient's state of hydration may also affect albumin concentration; dehydration raises concentration and overhydration lowers it.

Bilirubin

Bilirubin is a breakdown product of haemoglobin. In the blood it is bound almost exclusively to albumin and is taken up by the liver cells where it is conjugated and excreted in the bile. The concentration of bilirubin in serum therefore reflects the balance between the amount produced by destruction of red blood cells and that removed by the liver. There are three main reasons for raised bilirubin levels in adults:

- Diseases associated with damage to the hepatocytes (e.g. acute or chronic hepatitis, cirrhosis, primary liver cancer, liver metastases). This leads to a reduced capacity to conjugate bilirubin for excretion into the bile.
- Diseases causing restriction of bile flow and consequent reduction in bilirubin excretion (e.g. cholestasis, gallstones obstructing the bile duct, carcinoma of the pancreas).
- Diseases causing increased red blood cell destruction and consequent increased production of bilirubin (e.g. haemolytic anaemias).

In healthy individuals, almost all of the serum bilirubin is in the unconjugated form. As bilirubin levels rise above 35 $\mu mol\ L^{-1}$, the patient becomes visibly jaundiced, and in severe jaundice bilirubin levels can rise as high as 500 $\mu mol\ L^{-1}$ or even higher. In jaundice, determination of the ratio of conjugated to unconjugated bilirubin can give some indication of the cause of the jaundice. If the proportion of conjugated bilirubin is high, this suggests obstruction, while if the proportions are about equal, hepatocellular damage is likely.

Alanine aminotransferase (ALT) and aspartate aminotransferase (AST)

Alanine aminotransferase (ALT), previously known as serum glutamic pyruvic transaminase (SGPT), is present in high concentrations in the liver. It is also found in heart and skeletal muscle, but in much lower concentrations. Aspartate aminotransferase (AST) is more widely distributed than ALT and is present in liver, heart, kidney, skeletal muscle and red blood cells. These enzymes are released from damaged cells, both in the liver and at other sites. AST is raised in shock, while there is little elevation of ALT unless liver disease is present. ALT is therefore more specific for liver disease and AST is not included in the LFT profile in all laboratories.

Raised levels of these enzymes are found in any form of liver disease, with particularly high levels in acute liver damage (e.g. viral hepatitis) and more modestly raised levels in chronic liver disease (e.g. cirrhosis) and obstructive jaundice.

Gamma-glutamyltransferase (GGT)

Gamma-glutamyltransferase (GGT) is present in high concentrations in the liver, kidney, prostate and pancreas. Levels of the enzyme are raised in all types of liver and biliary tract disease (e.g. acute and chronic hepatitis, cirrhosis, obstructive jaundice) and also in carcinoma of the pancreas. The test can be used to identify those with liver or biliary disease but is not useful in establishing the cause.

However, measurement of GGT is useful in patients at risk of liver disease due to alcoholism. This is because GGT, unlike the other liver enzymes, is raised by alcohol consumption even if there is no liver damage. Levels return to normal on cessation of drinking, but if high levels of GGT persist, it is likely that some liver damage has been sustained or that the patient is actually still drinking. Measurement of GGT is therefore useful in the management of patients with alcoholic liver disease.

Alkaline phosphatase (AP)

Alkaline phosphatase (AP) is widely distributed in the body and is produced by the liver, bone and the gut. Levels of the enzyme are raised in diseases of the liver and biliary tract, with the highest levels found in obstructive jaundice. AP is usually raised in cirrhosis and liver cancers, but levels may be normal or only slightly raised in acute hepatitis. In addition, increased levels are found in some diseases of the bone (e.g. Paget's disease, osteomalacia and bone tumours).

Blood gases

The test for blood gases includes the measurement of oxygen (pO_2) and carbon dioxide (pCO_2) in the blood and also the pH of the blood together with other parameters of acid–base balance, such as the concentration of bicarbonate (HCO_3^-) (*see* Table 19.4). It is used mainly for monitoring of critically ill patients, in whom blood gas measurements may sometimes be required every few hours. Acid–base disturbances can be classified as either acidosis or alkalosis (*see* Section 9.3.3).

Table 19.4 Blood gases. Typical adult reference ranges

Test	Reference range
pH	7.35–7.40
pCO_2	4.5–6.0 kPa (35–45 mmHg)
pO_2	10.6–13.3 kPa (80–100 mmHg)
Bicarbonate	22–28 mmol/L
Base/excess deficit	−3 to +3 mmol/L

Urea and electrolytes (U&Es)

Measurement of serum or plasma urea, creatinine and various electrolytes (e.g. sodium, chloride, potassium, calcium, magnesium and phosphate) is one of the groups of tests most commonly carried out (*see* Table 19.5). Together with clinical

Table 19.5 Urea and electrolytes. Typical adult reference ranges

Test	Reference range
Urea	2.5–6.5 mmol/L (S)
Creatinine	
Men	50–100 μmol/L (S)
Women	50–80 μmol/L (S)
Mild renal impairment	150–300 μmol/L (S)
Moderate renal impairment	300–700 μmol/L (S)
Severe renal impairment	>700 μmol/L (S)
Creatinine clearance	70–130 mL/min
Bicarbonate	22–28 mmol/L (S)
Calcium	
Total	2.10–2.65 mmol/L (S)
Ionized	1.0–1.25 mmol/L (S)
Chloride	95–105 mmol/L (S)
Copper	16–31 μmol/L (S)
Magnesium	0.7–1.2 mmol/L (S)
Potassium	3.5–5.0 mmol/L (S)
Phosphate	0.8–1.45 mmol/L (S)
Sodium	135–145 mmol/L (S)
Zinc	8–23 μmol/L (S)

(S) = serum concentration.

assessment, they are used to monitor patients with fluid and electrolyte disturbances (*see* Section 9.3.3).

Concentrations of both blood urea and creatinine give an indication of kidney function. Urea is a waste product of amino acid metabolism and creatinine of muscle metabolism. Both are eliminated in the urine, and if the ability of the kidneys to excrete them is compromised, they accumulate in the blood, leading to a rise in serum concentration of both. However, no increase in concentration of either occurs until around 50% of renal function is lost, so they are poor indicators of renal disease. Serum urea may also be raised in congestive heart failure, while serum creatinine is likely to be normal.

Creatinine clearance, which is a direct measure of glomerular filtration rate (GFR) is a more sensitive and specific measure of early renal disease than either serum urea or creatinine. It measures the volume of plasma which is cleared of creatinine during passage through the kidneys in one minute. The greater the clearance the more effective are the kidneys at clearing creatinine from the blood and excreting it in the urine. A reduction in creatinine clearance indicates renal damage.

Cardiac enzymes

Measurement of the amount of cardiac enzymes in blood (*see* Table 19.6) is used to identify those patients who have suffered a myocardial infarction. The three enzymes most commonly measured for this purpose are:

- Creatine kinase (CK)
- Lactate dehydrogenase (LD)
- Aspartate aminotransferase (AST).

Table 19.6 Cardiac enzymes. Typical adult reference ranges

Test	Reference range
Creatine kinase (CK)	
Men	24–195 iu/L
Women	24–170 iu/L
Lactate dehydrogenase (LD)	100–500 iu/L
Aspartate aminotransferase (AST)	5–50 iu/L

Creatinine kinase

Creatinine kinase (CK) is an enzyme that catalyses the transfer of phosphate from creatinine phosphate to adenosine diphosphate. It is present mainly in cardiac muscle, skeletal muscle and brain and raised plasma levels of CK are indicative of damage to these tissues. Three isoenzymes exist CK(MM), CK(BB) and CK(MB). When CK is measured in plasma, it is the sum of all three isoenzymes that is measured but the isoenzymes can also be measured separately. Most of the CK(MB) is found in cardiac muscle so this is a more specific measure for cardiac muscle cell damage than CK. CK(MB) is the most sensitive enzymatic indicator of MI in routine use. Following a myocardial infarction there is a characteristic increase in CK(MB) activity between 4 and 6 hours post-MI, followed by a rise in CK from around 8 hours. Levels peak between 20 and 30 hours and return to normal after two to four days.

Lactate dehydrogenase (LD)

This enzyme catalyses the dehydrogenation of lactic acid to produce pyruvate. LD is widely distributed throughout body tissues, but especially in liver, heart muscle and skeletal muscle. Five isoenzymes exist and LD1 is the predominant form in the heart muscle while the liver and skeletal muscle contain primarily LD4 and LD5. Unlike the other LD isoenzymes, LD1 can utilise hydroxybutyrate as a substrate as well as lactate, and an alternative name for LD1 is hydroxybutyrate dehydrogenase (HBDH). In most laboratories, total LD is measured, but in some the more specific isoenzyme for cardiac muscle (LD1) is measured. LD and HBDH rise at around 10–12 hours after an infarct, peak after two to three days, after which they decline over seven days or more.

Aspartate aminotransferase (AST)

Aspartate aminotransferase (AST) catalyses the transfer of an amino group from the amino acid aspartic acid to ketoglutamic acid. AST is widely distributed throughout the tissues, but particularly in heart muscle, skeletal muscle and liver. AST rises at around 8 hours after an infarct, peaks after one to two days and returns to normal after 6–10 days.

Thyroid function tests

Thyroid function tests (*see* Table 19.7) include the measurement of the concentration of thyroid hormones in the blood and such tests contribute to the diagnosis and monitoring of thyroid disorders. The profile of tests used for testing of thyroid function varies between laboratories, but usually includes the following:

- *Total thyroxine (T4).* This includes measurement of free (biologically active) thyroxine and protein-bound (biologically inactive) thyroxine in serum. Sometimes, free thyroxine (FT4) is measured separately.

Table 19.7 Thyroid function tests. Typical serum adult reference ranges

Test	Reference range
Thyroid-stimulating hormone (TSH)	0.5–5.5 miu/L
Thyroxine	
T4	60–135 nmol/L
Free	9.4–25 pmol/L
Tri-iodothyronine	
T3	1.1–2.8 nmol/L
Free	3.0–8.6 pmol/L

- *Total triiodothyronine (T3).* This includes measurement of free (biologically active) triiodothyronine and protein-bound (biologically inactive) triiodothyronine in serum. Sometimes, free triiodothyronine is measured separately.
- *Thyroid-stimulating hormone (TSH).* This measures the serum concentration of the pituitary hormone TSH.

Abnormal thyroid function tests are found in patients with hyperthyroidism and hypothyroidism (*see* Section 6.2). The results which would be expected in hyperthyroidism are:

- Increase in serum T4, FT4 and T3 concentrations, although occasionally T4 and FT4 are normal while only T3 is raised.
- Reduction in serum TSH concentration. In severe disease concentrations may be undetectable.

The results which would be expected in hypothyroidism are:

- Reduction in serum T4 and FT4 concentrations (although both may be at the low end of normal in the early stages of the disease).
- Increase in serum TSH.

Blood lipids

This test includes measurement of cholesterol (including the individual fractions) and triglyceride (*see* Table 19.8). It is used to help assess an individual's risk of coronary heart disease or to

Table 19.8 Serum lipids. Typical adult target ranges

Test	Target range
Cholesterol	<6.5 mmol/L; desirable <5.2 mmol/L
LDL	<3.35–4.0 mmol/L (abnormal >5 mmol/L)
HDL	
Men	Ideally >0.9 mmol/L
Women	Ideally >1.2 mmol/L
Triglycerides	<2.3 mmol/L

monitor the effectiveness of diet and/or drug therapy aimed at reducing blood lipids.

Three measurements are usually made in the laboratory. These are:

- the concentration of total cholesterol, i.e. cholesterol contained in low-density lipoprotein (LDL), high-density lipoprotein (HDL) and very-low-density lipoprotein (VLDL)
- the concentration of HDL cholesterol
- the concentration of triglycerides, i.e. the triglycerides contained in VLDL, LDL and HDL.

Initial samples need not be taken in the fasting state. This is because fasting does not affect the total cholesterol concentration, although it does influence the triglyceride level. A fasting lipid profile (including breakdown into LDL, HDL and triglycerides) is required only if total cholesterol (non-fasting) is raised.

Patients who should have their lipid levels measured include those with:

- existing CHD, peripheral vascular disease or cerebrovascular disease
- a first-degree relative with CHD before the age of 55 years in men or 65 years in women.
- a family history of raised cholesterol or triglyceride levels
- other risk factors for CHD, such as diabetes mellitus, hypertension, obesity or smoking.

Unlike other blood tests, the concept of a reference range is inappropriate for cholesterol testing. This is because a large proportion of apparently healthy individuals have cholesterol levels which are associated with an increased risk of CHD. In other words, normal levels of cholesterol in a population are sometimes unhealthy. Thus, the concept of target, rather than reference, ranges is used to interpret cholesterol results.

Microscopy

Microscopy is used to examine tissue samples removed from a patient to aid in the diagnosis of disease. Many disease processes such as malignancy, infection and inflammation, are characterised by specific changes in the tissues which are visible under the microscope and microscopy is probably most widely used in the diagnosis and staging of malignant tumours. It is also used in the diagnosis of non-malignant disease of the gastrointestinal tract, liver, lungs and kidney, in disorders of the skin and connective tissue, and more recently it has been used in the diagnosis of tissue rejection among patients who have received transplanted organs.

Individual cells, rather than tissue samples, can be removed for microscopy, and this is less invasive than recovery of tissues. Typically cells are scraped from the surface of organs such as the cervix, the stomach, duodenum and lungs. Cells can also be recovered by fine needle aspiration from the pleural and peritoneal cavities or from solid tumours (e.g. in the breast).

Microscopy is also used to examine samples such as blood, urine, sputum, faeces and cerebrospinal fluid and swabs taken from sites where infection is suspected, to identify pathogenic microorganisms. This helps in the diagnosis of disease caused by infective agents. Bacteria can often be identified by examining such specimens under the microscope, but more precise identification can only be achieved after culture (growth of organisms on nutrient-rich media).

Miscellaneous tests

Reference values for a variety of tests not included in the text of this chapter can be found in Table 19.9. Conversion factors from traditional to SI units can be found in Table 19.10.

Table 19.9 Miscellaneous tests. Typical adult reference ranges

Test	Reference range
Acid phosphatase	0.5–11 units/L
Aldosterone	70–350 pg/mL (S)
Amylase	70–300 iu/L (S)
Ferritin	
Men	24–300 μg/L (S)
Women	15–300 μg/L (S)
Folate (red cell)	150–700 μg/L
Globulins (total)	16–37 g/L (S)
Gamma globulins	
IgA	1.5–2.5 g/L (S)
IgC	8–18 g/L (S)
IgM	0.4–2.9 g/L (S)
Glucose (fasting)	3.3–6.7 mmol/L
HbA1c (glycated haemoglobin)	
Normal	<6.5%
Acceptable	6.5–7.5%
High risk	>7.5%
Elderly	<11% is acceptable
Iron	10–30 μmol/L (S)
Lead (RBC)	0.5–1.7 μmol/L
Osmolality	282–295 mOsm/kg
Total iron binding capacity (TIBC)	40–75 μmol/L (S)
Transferrin	1.7–3.4 g/dL (S)
Uric acid	0.15–0.47 mmol/L (S)
Vitamin B_{12}	150–1000 ng/L (S)
Sex hormones	
Follicle stimulating hormone (FSH)	
Follicular phase	2.5–9.7 iu/L (S)
Mid-cycle	up to 7.6–19.0 iu/L (S)
Luteal phase	0.9–5.8 iu/L (S)
Postmenopause	12–100 iu/L (S)
Luteinising hormone (LH)	
Follicular phase	0.8–9.0 μmol/L (S)
Mid-cycle	<65 μmol/L (S)
Luteal phase	0.7–14.5 μmol/L (S)
Oestradiol	
Follicular phase	40–170 pmol/L (P)
Mid-cycle	440–1400 pmol/L (P)
Luteal phase	180–1000 pmol/L (P)
Postmenopause	36–175 pmol/L (P)
Progesterone (7 days before onset of period)	
Normal ovulation	>30 nmol/L (P)
No ovulation	<15 nmol/L (P)
Postmenopause	0.1–1.0 nmol/L (P)
Prostate specific an tigen (PSA)	0–4 μg/L
Testosterone	
Men	10–35 nmol/L (S)
Women (premenopause)	0.3–2.8 nmol/L (S)
Women (postmenopause)	0.3–1.2 nmol/L (S)

(S) = serum; (P) = plasma.

Table 19.10 Conversion from traditional to SI units

Test	Unit	Conversion to SI unit
Acid phosphatase	0.56 KA	1 iu/L
Amylase		1 iu/L
Aspartate transaminase		iu/L
Blood gases		
pCO_2	mmHg × 0.133	1 kPa
pO_2	mmHg × 0.133	1 kPa
Serum albumin	10 × g/100 mL	1 g/L
Serum bicarbonate	1 mEq/L	1 mmol/L
Serum bilirubin	1 mg/100 mL × 17.1	1 mmol/L
Serum calcium	1 mg/100 mL × 0.25	1 mmol/L
Serum chloride	1 mEq/L	1 mmol/L
Serum creatinine	mg/100 mL × 88.4	1 mol/L
Serum globulin	g/100 mL × 10	g/L
Serum glucose	mg/100 mL × 0.555	mmol/L
Serum iron	mg/100 mL × 0.18	mol/L
Serum magnesium	mEq/L × 0.5	mmol/L
Serum phosphate	mg/100 mL × 0.32	mmol/L
Serum potassium	mEq/L	mmol/L
Serum sodium	mEq/L	mmol/L
Serum triglycerides	mg/100 mL × 0.011	mmol/L
Serum urate	mg/100 mL × 0.17	mmol/L
Total iron-binding capacity	mg/100 mL × 0.18	mmol/L
Urinary calcium	mg/24 h × 0.025	mmol/24 h
Urinary creatinine	mg/24 h × 0.0088	mmol/24 h
Urinary phosphate	mg/24 h × 0.032	mmol/24 h
Urinary urea	g/24 h × 0.032	mmol/24 h

From the *SK&F Clinical Pharmacy Handbook*, 2nd edition, 1989. Smith Kline & French Laboratories, Welwyn Garden City.

20

Professional and self-help organisations

20.1 Introduction

Pharmacists are often approached by patients for information about self-help groups, and it is important to be aware of the basis of their existence. The importance of the concept of self-help in preventing the available health services from being overwhelmed has been explained in Section 18.1. Many people, and in particular those suffering from chronic illness or those who have gone through a traumatic experience (e.g. the loss of a child through a 'cot death'), benefit from contact with others who have had similar experiences. This fact should not be taken as a failure on the part of professionals to be of any assistance, but should be recognised as an important means of helping individuals to overcome their health problems themselves.

Other important functions of self-help organisations include the provision of literature for patients (either paper versions or on the internet), which reinforces the advice given by medical and pharmacy staff. The publication of literature promotes self-reliance and self-determination, and, equally importantly, can help in raising funds for the group, many of which are run on a shoestring budget. Self-help organisations can act as a stimulus for government to introduce innovations in patient care, especially in 'less attractive' areas of healthcare (e.g. for the mentally handicapped).

This chapter provides background details and addresses of a wide range of health organisations located in the UK. It includes organisations of the pharmaceutical and medical professions, and organisations which have been established to provide help for patients suffering from particular conditions or in certain predicaments (e.g. disability). Although only British details have been provided, sister or comparable organisations with the same or similar titles frequently exist in other countries; readers in other countries should therefore seek local addresses.

For ease of use, the information has been divided in two sections. Section 20.2 lists the conditions with which particular organisations are associated; with some self-help groups, this is obvious from the title of the organisation, but others aim to help a broader range of patients with differing conditions. Section 20.3 provides a directory of organisations, with current details of addresses and telephone numbers. Only those self-help organisations that have been considered as non-ephemeral and based at a relatively fixed address have been included. Details of the organisations have been included in other dedicated directories, where many details have been constant in two or more editions. Although all addresses and telephone numbers have been checked immediately before going to press, certain minor changes are inevitable during the expected life of this book.

It must be stressed, however, that inclusion in this listing should not be taken as a statement of approval of that organisation by the RPSGB; equally, non-inclusion should not be interpreted as non-approval.

One final point is of particular importance. If self-help organisations are recommended to patients, remember that, in addition to giving details of the address and telephone number, it would be beneficial to ask patients to enclose a stamped addressed envelope when they write to the organisation, to help offset administrative costs.

20.2 Categories of organisations

Abortion
Birth Control Trust
British Pregnancy Advisory Service
Family Planning Association
Marie Stopes International
National Abortion Campaign
Pregnancy Advisory Service

Acne
Acne Support Group

Addison's disease
Addison's disease self-help group

Adoption and fostering
British Agencies for Adoption and Fostering
Post-adoption Centre

Adrenoleukodystrophy
Attia Research Trust into ALD

AIDS
AIDS Care Education and Training
Body Positive
Haemophilia Society
London Lighthouse
National AIDS helpline
Terrence Higgins Trust

Alcohol dependence
Accept Services
Al-Anon
Alcohol Concern
Alcoholics Anonymous
Alateen
Medical Council on Alcoholism
Scottish Council on Alcohol
Turning Point

Allergy
Action Against Allergy
Anaphylaxis Campaign
British Allergy Foundation
Food and Chemical Allergy Association
Medic-Alert Foundation
Migraine Trust
National Eczema Society

Alopecia
Hairline International

Alzheimer's disease
Alzheimer's Disease Society

Angina pectoris
British Heart Foundation
Family Heart Association
Chest Heart and Stroke Association
Coronary Prevention Group

Ankylosing spondylitis
Arthritis Care
National Ankylosing Spondylitis Society

Anxiety
First Steps to Freedom
Phobics Society

Arthritis and related conditions
Arthritis Care
Leonard Cheshire Foundation
National Ankylosing Spondylitis Society

Asthma
Action Against Allergy
British Lung Foundation
National Asthma Campaign

Ataxia
Ataxia
Friedreich's Ataxia Group

Autism
International Autistic Research Organisation
National Autistic Society

Back pain
Back Care

Bereavement
Age Concern England
Compassionate Friends
CRUSE
Foundation for the Study of Infant Deaths
Miscarriage Association
National Association of Widows

Blindness
Guide Dogs for the Blind Association
Royal National Institute for the Blind
National Deaf-Blind League
National Federation of the Blind
Partially Sighted Society
SENSE
Wales Council for the Blind

Bone disorders
Brittle Bone Society
National Osteporosis Society

Brain tumours
United Kingdom Brain Tumour Society

Breast cancer
Breast Cancer Care

Breast care
Breast Care Campaign

Breast feeding
La Leche League
National Childbirth Trust
Twins and Multiple Births Association

Bronchitis
Age Concern England
British Lung Foundation
Chest Heart and Stroke Association

Cancer
Breast Cancer Care
British Association of Cancer United Patients
British Colostomy Association
Cancer and Leukaemia in Childhood (CLIC)
Cancer Care Society
Cancer Research Campaign
Cancerlink
Colon Cancer Concern
CRUSE
Hospice Information Service
Leukaemia Research Fund
Macmillan Cancer Relief
Marie Curie Cancer Care
National Cancer Alliance
Ovacome
Prostate Cancer Charity
United Kingdom Brain Tumour Society
Womens Nationwide Cancer Control Campaign

Care in the community
BNA
National Association of Hospital and Community Friends

Cerebral palsy
SCOPE

Children and young people, care of
Action for Sick Children
Association for Brain Damaged Children and Young Adults
Association for Children with Heart Disorders
Association of Parents of Vaccine Damaged Children
Association for Spina Bifida and Hydrocephalus (ASBAH)
Attention Deficit Hyperactivity Disorder (AD/HD) Family Support Groups UK
Baby Life Support Systems (BLISS)
Barnardo's
British Agencies for Adoption and Fostering (BAAF)
British Institute for Brain Injured Children (BIBIC)
British Institute of Learning Disabilities
Child Accident Prevention Trust
Child Growth Foundation
ChildLine
Children's Liver Disease Foundation
Cleft Lip and Palate Association (CLAPA)
Contact a Family
Council for Disabled Children
FAB-UK
Foundation for the Study of Infant Deaths
Gingerbread
Glue Ear Society
Hyperactive Children's Support Group

Justice for all Vaccine Damaged Children
National Council for One Parent Families
National Organisation for Counselling Adoptees and Parents (NORCAP)
National Society for the Prevention of Cruelty to Children (NSPCC)
Restricted Growth Association
Scottish Down's Syndrome Association
Scottish Spina Bifida Association
Society for the Protection of Unborn Children

Cerebral palsy
Bobath Centre for Children with Cerebral Palsy
Leonard Cheshire Foundation

Cirrhosis
British Liver Trust

Cleft lip
Cleft Lip and Palate Association (CLAPA)

Coeliac disease
The Coeliac Society

Complementary therapy
British Herbal Medicine Association
British Holistic Medical Association
British Homoeopathic Association
Centre for the Study of Complementary Medicine
National Institute of Medical Herbalists
National Register of Hypnotherapists and Psychotherapists
Natural Medicines Society

Contraception and birth control
British Pregnancy Advisory Service
Brook Advisory Service
Family Planning Association
International Planned Parenthood Federation
ISSUE (National Fertility Association)
Marie Stopes International
Pregnancy Advisory Service

Cot death
Scottish Cot Death Trust

Creutzfeldt-Jakob disease (CJD)
CJD Support Network

Crime
National Association for the Care and Resettlement of Offenders (NACRO)
Victim Support

Crohn's disease
Crohn's in Childhood Research Association
National Association for Colitis and Crohn's Disease

Cross dressing
The Beaumont Society

Cushings disease
Association for Cushings Treatment and Help

Cystic fibrosis
Cystic Fibrosis Trust

Deafness and ear problems
Breakthrough
British Tinnitus Association
Council for the Advancement of Communication with Deaf People
Hearing Dogs for Deaf People
National Deaf Children's Society
National Deaf-Blind League
Royal National Institute for the Deaf
Scottish Association for the Deaf
SENSE
Wales Council for the Deaf

Deep vein thrombosis
British Vascular Foundation

Dental health
British Dental Health Foundation
British Fluoridation Society

Depression
Depression Alliance
Manic Depression Fellowship
SAD Association

Dermatitis herpetiformis
Coeliac Society

Diabetes mellitus
Diabetes UK
Medic-Alert Foundation

Digestive disorders
British Digestive Foundation

Disability, physical
Association of Disabled Professionals
British Limbless Ex-Servicemen's Association (BLESMA)
Centre for Accessible Environments
Council for Disabled Children
DIAL UK
Disability Alliance
Disability Information Trust
Disability Law Trust
Disability Sport England
Disability Wales
Disabled Drivers' Association
Disabled Living Foundation
Disfigurement Guidance Centre
Limbless Association Rehabilitation Centre
Leonard Cheshire Foundation
Queen Elizabeth Foundation for Disabled People
Royal Association for Disability and Rehabilitation (RADAR)
Values into Action

Down's syndrome
Down's Syndrome Association

Drug dependence and abuse
Alcoholics Anonymous
DrugScope
Families Anonymous
Narcotics Anonymous
Northern Ireland Community Addiction Service
Release
Re-Solv
Standing Conference on Drug Abuse
Terrence Higgins Trust
Turning Point

Dyslexia
British Dyslexia Association
Dyslexia Institute

Dystonia
Dystonia Society

Eating disorders
Eating Disorders Association

Eczema
National Eczema Society

Elderly, care of the
Action on elder abuse
Age Concern Cymru
Age Concern England
Age Concern Nothern Ireland
Age Concern Scotland
Alzheimer Scotland
Alzheimer's Disease Society
Alzheimer's Disease Society Northern Ireland
Counsel and Care
Help the Aged
National Federation of Retirement Pensions Associations
Nursing Home Fees Agency (NHFA)

Emphysema
Chest Heart and Stroke Association

Encephalitis
Encephalitis Support Group

Endometriosis
National Endometriosis Society

Enuresis
Enuresis Resource and Information Centre

Epilepsy
British Epilepsy Association
Epilepsy Association of Scotland
National Society for Epilepsy

Euthanasia
Human Rights Society

Eye care
British Retinitis Pigmentosa Society (BRPS)
Eye Care Information Service

Fabry disease
Fabry Disease Research Fund and Support Group

Family support
Family Welfare Association

Fragile X syndrome
Fragile X Society

Franconi's anaemia
FAB-UK

Gallstones
British Liver Trust

Gaucher's disease
Gaucher's Association

Glaucoma
International Glaucoma Association

Genetic disorders
Genetic Interest Group

Glycogen storage disease
Association for Glycogen Storage Disease

Gout
Arthritis Care

Guillain-Barré syndrome
Guillain-Barré Syndrome Support Group

Haemophilia
Haemophilia Society

Hay fever
British Allergy Foundation

Heart disease
Association for Children with Heart Disorders
British Heart Foundation
British Hypertension Society
Cardiomyopathy Association
Chest Heart and Stroke Association
Coronary Prevention Group
Family Heart Association
National Heart Forum
Northern Ireland Chest, Heart and Stroke Association

Herpes simplex virus infection
Herpes Viruses Association

Homelessness
Shelter

Huntington's disease
Huntington's Disease Association

Hydrocephalus
Association for Spina Bifida and Hydrocephalus

Hypertension
British Heart Foundation
British Hypertension Society
British Kidney Patient Association
Chest Heart and Stroke Association

Incontinence, urinary
Continence Foundation
Disabled Living Foundation

Infertility
British Pregnancy Advisory Service
Child
Family Planning Association
ISSUE (National Fertility Association)
Marie Stopes International

Ileostomy
IA (Ileostomy and Internal Pouch Support Group)

Impotence
Impotence Association

Incontinence
Continence Foundation

Irritable bowel syndrome
IBS Network

Kidney disease
British Kidney Patient Association
National Kidney Federation
The National Kidney Research Fund and Kidney Foundation

Laryngectomy
National Association of Laryngetomee Clubs

Leukaemia
Anthony Nolan Bone Marrow Trust
Leukaemia Care Society
Leukaemia Research Fund

Liver disease
British Liver Trust
Children's Liver Disease Foundation

Lupus
Lupus UK

Lymphoedema
Lymphoedema Support Network

Lymphoma
Lymphoma Association

Marfan syndrome
Marfan Association UK

Medical and other professional organisations (non-pharmacy)
British Acupuncture Council
British Chiropractic Association
British Dental Association
British Dietetic Association
British Medical Association
British Nutrition Foundation
British Red Cross Society
Consumers' Association
General Medical Council
National Consumer Council
Office of Fair Trading
Office of Health Economics
Royal Society of Health
St John Ambulance
Society of Chiropodists and Podiatrists

Medical accidents
Action for Victims of Medical Accidents

Meningitis
Meningitis Research Foundation
National Meningitis Trust

Menopause
Marie Stopes International

Mental health/illness
Age Concern England
Leonard Cheshire Foundation
MIND (The Mental Health Charity)
Scottish Association for Mental Health

Mental retardation/handicap
Down's Syndrome Association
Leonard Cheshire Foundation
MENCAP
National Autistic Society

Migraine
Action Against Allergy
Migraine Action Association
Migraine Trust

Motor neuron disease
Motor Neurone Disease Association
Scottish Motor Neurone Disease Assocation

Multiple sclerosis
Federation of Multiple Sclerosis Therapy Centres
Leonard Cheshire Foundation
Multiple Sclerosis Society

Muscular dystrophy
Muscular Dystrophy Group

Myalgic encephalomyelitis (ME)
Action for ME

Myasthenia gravis
Myasthenia Gravis Association

Myocardial infarction
British Heart Foundation
Coronary Prevention Group

Neurofibromatosis
The Neurofibromatosis Association (NFA)

Nutrition
Vegan Society
Vegetarian Society
Weight Watchers
Women's Nutritional Advisory Service

Obsessive compulsive disorder
Obsessive Action

Ovarian Cancer
Ovacome

Paget's disease
National Association for the Relief of Paget's Disease

Pain
Back Care
Pain Interest Group
Pain Relief Fund
Pain Society

Parkinsonism
Age Concern England
Leonard Cheshire Foundation
Parkinson's Disease Society

Pharmacy organisations
Association of the British Pharmaceutical Industry
Association of Pharmacy Technicians
British Pharmaceutical Students' Association
Centre for Pharmacy Postgraduate Education
Clinical Pharmacokinetics Society
College of Pharmacy Practice
Guild of Healthcare Pharmacists
Institute of Pharmacy Management International
National Association of Women Pharmacists
National Pharmaceutical Association
Northern Ireland Centre for Postgraduate Pharmaceutical Education and Training (NICPPET)
Pharmaceutical Services Negotiating Committee
Proprietary Articles Trade Association
Proprietary Association of Great Britain
Radiopharmacy Group
Rural Pharmacists Association
Scottish Centre for Post Qualification Pharmaceutical Education
Society of Apothecaries of London
United Kingdom Clinical Pharmacy Association
Welsh Centre for Postgraduate Pharmaceutical Education

Phenylketonuria
National Society for Phenylketonuria (NSPKU)

Phobias
Phobics Society

Poliomyelitis
Disabled Living Foundation

Post-traumatic stress disorder
Trauma Aftercare Trust

Prader-Willi syndrome
Prader-Willi Syndrome Association

Pregnancy and childbirth
Action on Pre-eclampsia
Ante-natal Results and Choices
Birth Control Trust
Birth Defects Foundation
British Pregnancy Advisory Service
Family Planning Association
National Childbirth Trust
Pre-eclampsia Society
Pregnancy Advisory Service
Stillbirth and Neonatal Death Society
Twins and Multiple Births Association

Premenstrual syndrome
National Association for Premenstrual Syndrome (NAPS)

Prostate
Prostate Association

Prostate Cancer
Prostate Cancer Charity

Psoriasis
Psoriasis Association
Psoriatic Athropathy Alliance

Raynaud's disease
Raynaud's & Scleroderma Association

Relationships
Relate

Reye's syndrome
National Reye's Syndrome Foundation of the UK

Sarcoidosis
British Lung Foundation

Schizophrenia
National Schizophrenia Fellowship (NSF)
National Schizophrenia Fellowship (Scotland)
Schizophrenia Association of Great Britain

Scleroderma
Raynaud's & Scleroderma Association

Scoliosis
Scoliosis Association

Seasonal Affective Disorder
SAD Association

Sexually transmitted diseases
Family Planning Association
Herpes Viruses Association

Sickle-cell anaemia
Brent Sickle Cell/Thalassaemia Centre
Sickle Cell Society

Sleep
British Snoring and Sleep Apnoea Association (BSSAA)

Sjögren's Syndrome
British Sjögren's Syndrome Association

Smoking
Action on Smoking and Health
QUIT

Sotos syndrome
Sotos Syndrome Group

Speech disorders
Action for Dysphasic Adults
Association for Stammerers
British Dyslexia Association
Chest Heart and Stroke Association
Motor Neurone Disease Association

Spinal cord injury
The Back-up Trust
Spinal Injuries Association

Spina bifida
Association for Spina Bifida and Hydrocephalus
Urostomy Association

Stoma therapy
British Colostomy Association
Ileostomy Association of Great Britain and Northern Ireland
Urostomy Association

Stroke
Action for Dysphasic Adults
British Heart Foundation
Stroke Association

Sturge Weber syndrome
Sturge Weber Foundation

Sudden infant death syndrome
Foundation for the Study of Infant Deaths

Systemic lupus erythematosus
Arthritis Care

Telangiectasia
Telangiectasia Self-Help Group

Thalassaemia
Brent Sickle Cell/Thalassaemia Centre
Sickle Cell Society
UK Thalassaemia Society

Thalidomide
Thalidomide Society

Tourette syndrome
Tourette Syndrome UK Association

Travel
MASTA

Ulcerative colitis
Ileostomy Association of Great Britain and Northern Ireland
National Association for Colitis and Crohn's Disease

Valvular heart disease
British Heart Foundation
Chest Heart and Stroke Foundation

Varicose veins
British Vascular Foundation

Vitiligo
Vitiligo Society

Williams syndrome
Williams Syndrome Foundation

Women
Positively Women
Wellbeing
Women's Health
Women's Nationwide Cancer Control Campaign
Women's Nutritional Advisory Service

20.3 Directory of organisations

A

ACTION AGAINST ALLERGY (AAA)
PO Box 278
Twickenham
Middlesex TW1 4QQ
Tel: 020 8892 2711
Fax: 020 8892 4950
Website: www.actionagainstallergy.co.uk

Action Against Allergy is a registered charity which aims to promote an understanding of clinical ecology, the causative role of foods and chemicals in chronic illness (e.g. migraine, asthma, catarrh, skin rashes and hypertension). It provides members with a personal information service, advice on where specialist help can be obtained, a postal book service, and arranges films and lectures. It also provides details to people of other sufferers in the same area so that local groups may be formed.

ACCEPT SERVICES
724 Fulham Road
London SW6 5SE
Helpline: 020 7371 7477
Tel: 020 7371 7455

Accept Services uses facilitators who help group members towards understanding the feelings and personal issues that have played a part in problems with alcohol.

ACNE SUPPORT GROUP
PO Box 230
Hayes
Middlesex UB4 0UT
Helpline: 020 8841 4747
Fax: 020 8845 5424
Website: www.stopspots.org

The Acne Support Group provides support for sufferers of acne.

ACTION FOR DYSPHASIC ADULTS (ADA)
Northcote House
1 Royal Street
London SE1 7LL
Helpline: 020 7261 9572
Tel: 020 7261 9572
Fax: 020 7928 9542

Action for Dysphasic Adults is a registered charity which provides information and advice to dysphasics and their carers, and aims to create greater awareness among professionals and the general public of the nature of the condition and needs of dysphasic adults. Long-term and, where possible, intensive rehabilitation for dysphasic adults is encouraged in association with speech therapy services.

ACTION FOR ME
PO Box 1302
Wells
Somerset BA5 2WE
Helpline: 0891 122976
Tel: 01749 670799
Fax: 01749 672561

Action for ME provides advice and support, such as welfare benefits information, therapy advice, lists of sympathetic doctors, factsheets, books and a journal, to sufferers of myalgic encephalomyelitis and their carers.

ACTION FOR SICK CHILDREN
300 Kingston Road
London
SW20 8LX
Helpline: 020 8542 4848
Fax: 020 8542 2424

Action for Sick Children is a national charity dedicated to improving the standards and quality of healthcare for children in hospital, at home and in the community.

ACTION FOR SICK CHILDREN (SCOTLAND)
15 Smith's Place
Edinburgh EH6 8NT
Helpline: 0131 553 6533
Tel: 0131 553 6553
Fax: 0131 553 6553

ACTION FOR VICTIMS OF MEDICAL ACCIDENTS
44 High Street
Croydon
Surrey CR0 1YB
Helpline: 020 8686 8333
Tel: 020 8686 8333
Fax: 020 8667 9065

Action for Victims of Medical Accidents aims to help people who have suffered as a result of medical treatment or the failure to give medical treatment. In addition, it aims to promote change in the attitudes of health carers towards victims and in procedures for ensuring accountability and obtaining redress.

ACTION ON ELDER ABUSE
Astral House
1268 London Road
London SW16 4ER
Helpline: 0808 808 8141
Tel: 020 8764 7648
Fax: 020 8679 4074
Website: www.elderabuse.org

Action on Elder Abuse aims to prevent abuse in older people by promoting changes in policy and practice, through raising awareness, providing education, promoting research and the provision of information. In addition, it offers a membership service, a national information service for all enquirers and a confidential helpline for anyone concerned about the abuse of an older person.

ACTION ON PRE-ECLAMPSIA (APEC)

31–33 College Road
Harrow
Middlesex HA1 1EJ
Helpline: 020 8427 4217
Tel: 020 8863 3271
Fax: 020 8424 0653
Email: info@apec.org.uk
Website: www.apec.org.uk

Action on Pre-eclampsia provides information for parents and health professionals about pre-eclampsia, supports sufferers and their families and promotes and publicises relevant research.

ACTION ON SMOKING AND HEALTH (ASH)

109 Gloucester Place
London W1H 4EJ
Tel: 020 7935 3519
Fax: 020 7935 3463
Website: www.ash.org.uk

ASH is a charity which aims to work with others to eliminate smoking by influencing policy and public opinion on tobacco use.

ADDISON'S DISEASE SELF-HELP GROUP

21 George Road
Guildford
Surrey GU1 4NP
Helpline: 01483 830673
Tel: 01483 830673
Fax: 01483 830673

Addison's Disease Self-help Group aims to put people with this disease in touch with each other.

AGE CONCERN ENGLAND

Astral House
1268 London Road
London SW16 4ER
Helpline: 0800 009966
Tel: 020 8765 7200
Fax: 020 9765 7211
Email: ace@ace.org.uk
Website: www.ace.org.uk

Age Concern England is the national centre for approximately 950 independent local Age Concern groups serving the needs of elderly people with help from over 120 000 volunteers. Age Concern England's governing body also includes representatives of 70 national organisations, and works closely with Age Concern Scotland, Wales, and Northern Ireland. Age Concern groups provide a wide range of services, including visiting, day care, clubs, and specialist services for physically and mentally frail elderly people. Age Concern England supports and advises groups through national field officers, and a variety of grant schemes.

Other work includes training, research, information, campaigning and publishing.

AGE CONCERN CYMRU

1 Cathedral Road
Cardiff CF1 9SD
Tel: 029 2037 1566
Fax: 029 2039 9562
Email: enquiries@accymru.org.uk
Website: www.accymru.org.uk

AGE CONCERN NORTHERN IRELAND

3 Lower Crescent
Belfast BT7 1NR
Tel: 028 9024 5729

AGE CONCERN SCOTLAND

113 Rose Street
Edinburgh EH2 3DT
Tel: 0131 220 3345
Fax: 0131 220 2779
Email: enquiries@acsinfo3.freeserve.co.uk

AIDS CARE EDUCATION AND TRAINING (ACET)

PO Box 3693
London SW15 2BQ
Helpline: 020 7511 0110
Tel: 020 8780 0400
Fax: 020 8780 0450
Email: acet@acetuk.org
Website: www.acetuk.org

ACET provides unconditional care for those with HIV/AIDS and practical education and training about HIV and its prevention. Worldwide, ACET works with international agencies to promote policies to reduce the spread of HIV and supports others who are responding to AIDS in their community.

AL-ANON FAMILY GROUPS

61 Great Dover Street
London SE1 4YF
Helpline: 020 7403 0888
Fax: 020 7378 9910
Email: alanonuk@aol.com
Website: www.hexnet.co.uk

Alcoholics Anonymous is a fellowship of men and women who share their experience, strength and hope with each other that they may solve their common problem and help others to recover from alcoholism. The only requirement for membership is a desire to stop drinking. There are no dues or fees for AA membership; it is self-supporting through its own contributions. AA is not allied with any sect, denomination, politics, organisation or institution; does not wish to engage in any controversy; and neither endorses nor opposes any causes. Its primary purpose is to help other alcoholics achieve sobriety.

AL-ANON INFORMATION CENTRE

Room 338
Baltic Chambers
50 Wellington Street
Glasgow G2 6HJ
Helpline: 0141 221 7356
Tel: 0141 221 7356

ALATEEN

61 Great Dover Street
London SE1 4YF
Tel: 020 7403 0888

Alateen is part of Al-Anon for teenagers with an alcoholic relative.

ALCOHOL CONCERN

Waterbridge House
32–36 Loman Street
London SE1 0EE
Helpline: 020 7928 7377
Tel: 020 7928 7377
Fax: 020 7928 4644

Alcohol Concern aims to reduce the costs of alcohol misuse and to develop the range and quality of services available to problem drinkers and their families. Activities include service development, policy, library, publications and a workplace advisory centre.

ALCOHOLICS ANONYMOUS

PO Box 1
Stonebow House
Stonebow
York
North Yorkshire Y01 7NJ
Helpline: 020 7833 0022
Tel: 01904 644026
Fax: 01904 629091
Website: www.alcoholics-anonymous.org.uk

A voluntary fellowship of men and women who are alcoholics and who help each other achieve and maintain sobriety through sharing experiences and giving mutual support.

ALZHEIMER'S DISEASE SOCIETY

Gordon House
10 Greencoat Place
London SW1P 1PH
Helpline: 0845 3000 336
Tel: 020 7306 0606
Fax: 020 7306 0808
Email: info@alzheimers.org.uk
Website: www.alzheimers.org.uk

The Alzheimer's Disease Society is a registered charity which supports professionals and relatives of those suffering from Alzheimer's disease. It also promotes, funds and disseminates information on research. Local branches organise relative support groups, day centres, sitting services, and resource and information centres. The Society also has central Caring and Research Funds.

ALZHEIMER'S DISEASE SOCIETY (NORTHERN IRELAND)

86 Aglantine Avenue
Belfast BT9 6EU
Helpline: 028 9066 4100
Tel: 028 9066 4100
Fax: 028 9066 4440

ALZHEIMER SCOTLAND (ACTION ON DEMENTIA)

22 Drumsheugh Gardens
Edinburgh EH3 7RN
Helpline: 0808 808 3000
Tel: 0131 243 1453
Fax: 0131 243 1450
Email: alzheimer@alzscot.org
Website: www.alzscot.org

ANAPHYLAXIS CAMPAIGN

PO Box 149
Fleet
Hampshire GU13 0FA
Tel: 01252 542029
Fax: 01252 377140
Website: anaphylaxis.org.uk

The Anaphylaxis Campaign aims to raise awareness of potentially fatal food allergies and provide information and guidance to sufferers.

ANTE-NATAL RESULTS AND CHOICES (ARC)

73 Charlotte Street
London W1T 4PN
Helpline: 020 7631 0285
Tel: 020 7631 0280
Fax: 020 7631 0280

ARC aims to help parents who discover their unborn baby may have an abnormality.

THE ANTHONY NOLAN BONE MARROW TRUST

The Royal Free Hospital
Pond Street
Hampstead
London NW3 2QG
Helpline: 020 7284 1234
Fax: 020 7284 8226

The Anthony Nolan Bone Marrow Trust provides unrelated bone-marrow donors for patients suffering from leukaemia and other allied bone-marrow disorders, regardless or race, colour or creed. In addition, it undertakes research into improving the outcome of bone-marrow transplantation.

ARTHRITIC ASSOCIATION

First Floor Suite
2 Hyde Gardens
Eastbourne
East Sussex BN21 4PN
Helpline: 020 7491 0233
Tel: 020 7491 0233
Fax: 01323 639793

The Arthritic Association helps people who are suffering or who have suffered from arthritis, or any similar illness, to regain freedom from pain. In addition, the association provides services or facilities to alleviate suffering and help recovery.

ARTHRITIS CARE

18 Stevenson Way
London NW1 2HD
Helpline: 0808 800 4050

Tel: 020 7380 6500
Fax: 020 7380 6505
Website: www. arthritiscare.org.uk

Arthritis Care is a registered charity and a national welfare organisation for sufferers from arthritic diseases. Membership of the charity is open to all sufferers, and all those interested in their welfare. It provides practical help for those with special needs, as well as information about facilities and aids available. There are over 370 local branches in the UK, a residential home for the severely disabled, specially adapted holiday centres and self-catering units.

ASSOCIATION FOR BRAIN DAMAGED CHILDREN AND YOUNG ADULTS (ABDC)

Clifton House
3 St Paul's Road
Coventry CV6 5DE
Helpline: 024 7666 5450
Tel: 024 7666 5450
Fax: 024 7666 5450

ABDC provides a residential home and respite care for children with learning difficulties. It strives to help each person to reach his or her own potential in a supportive or caring environment in partnership with their families and schools.

ASSOCIATION FOR CHILDREN WITH HEART DISORDERS

Killieard House
Killiecrankie
Pitlochry
Perthshire PH16 5LN
Helpline: 01796 473204
Tel: 01796 473204
Fax: 01796 473204

The Association for Children with Heart Disorders provides support in everyday care and welfare to parents and families of children with heart disorders. In addition, it raises money for research into congenital heart disorders and assists children's heart units improve facilities and maintain improvements in hospitals as new technology is developed. It provides weekend breaks for young adults and families.

ASSOCIATION FOR CUSHINGS TREATMENT AND HELP

54 Powney Road
Maidenhead
Berkshire SL6 6EQ
Helpline: 01628 670389
Tel: 01628 670389
Fax: 01628 415603
Email: cushingsacth@btinternet.com

The Association for Cushings Treatment and Help aims to support patients with Cushings syndrome. It acts as a resource for easing their experience during diagnosis, treatment and follow-up and helping them to achieve the best quality of life.

ASSOCIATION FOR GLYCOGEN STORAGE DISEASE (UK)

9 Lindop Road
Hale
Altrincham
Cheshire WA15 9DZ
Helpline: 0161 980 7303
Tel: 0161 980 7303
Fax: 0161 226 3813

The Association for Glycogen Storage Disease acts mainly as a family contact and support group for all persons affected by glycogen storage disease. In addition it encourages the provision of specialist centres for the diagnosis, treatment and monitoring of patients and to act as a focus for educational, scientific and charitable activities in relation to glycogen storage disease.

ASSOCIATION OF BREASTFEEDING MOTHERS

PO Box 207
Bridgwater
Somerset
TA6 7YT
Helpline: 020 7813 1481
Email: abm@clara.net
Website: http://home.clara.net/abm

The Association of Breastfeeding Mothers is a registered charity and aims to educate parents about the means and advantages of breastfeeding. This is achieved by local meetings countrywide, training counsellors and the encouragement of local support groups. Publications and seminars help to educate health professionals to advise mothers on breastfeeding, and on twins, insufficient milk and other topics. A books-by-post service is also operated.

ASSOCIATION OF DISABLED PROFESSIONALS

BCM ADP
London WC1N 3XX
Helpline: 01924 283253
Tel: 01924 270335
Fax: 01924 283253

The Association of Disabled Professionals aims to improve education, rehabilitation, training and employment opportunities available to disabled people. It encourages disabled people to develop their physical and mental capacities to the full, to find and retain employment suitable for their abilities and qualifications and to participate fully in everyday life of society.

ASSOCIATION OF THE BRITISH PHARMACEUTICAL INDUSTRY (ABPI)

12 Whitehall
London SW1A 2DY
Tel: 020 7930 3477
Website: www.abpi.org.uk

The Association of the British Pharmaceutical Industry is the trade association representing manufacturers of prescription medicines. The Association was formed in 1930 and now represents 152 companies which produce nearly 99% of medicines supplied to the NHS. The main functions of the Association are to maintain and improve the reputation of the industry and its contribution to the health and economic welfare of the nation; to assist contact between member companies and government departments, professional, scientific and trade organisations and other similar bodies; and to act as a channel of communication and to act on collective decisions made by its members.

ASSOCIATION OF PARENTS OF VACCINE DAMAGED CHILDREN

78 Campden Road
Shipston on Stour
Warwickshire CV36 4DH
Helpline: 01608 661595
Fax: 01608 663432

The Association of Parents of Vaccine Damaged Children campaigns for state compensation for vaccine damage.

ASSOCIATION OF PHARMACY TECHNICIANS UK

Lesley Morgan MBE
WCPPE
9 North Road
Cardiff CF10 3DY
Tel: 029 2087 4784
Website: www.aptuk-online.org

This association seeks to ensure and continually improve upon professional, educational and practice standards for registered pharmacy technicians and allied support staff in all healthcare and pharmaceutical organisations.

ASSOCIATION FOR SPINA BIFIDA AND HYDROCEPHALUS (ASBAH)

ASBAH House
42 Park Road
Peterborough PE1 2UQ
Tel: 01733 555988
Fax: 01733 555985
Website: www.asbah.org

The Association for Spina Bifida and Hydrocephalus is a welfare and research organisation which provides information, advisory and welfare services, and practical assistance in all aspects of life with spina bifida and hydrocephalus. It also supports and promotes research into the prevention, treatment and management of spina bifida and hydrocephalus. There is a regular magazine, LINK, and a group for young people, LIFT. A national organisation supports the work of approximately 80 local associations. Specialist field workers and counsellors are also provided.

ATAXIA

10 Winchester House
Kennington Park
Cranmer Road
London SW9 6EJ
Helpline: 020 7582 1444
Fax: 020 7582 9444

Ataxia provides information, advice and support to sufferers, their families and carers. It also raises money for research and offers a limited care services fund.

ATTENTION DEFICIT HYPERACTIVITY DISORDER (AD/HD) FAMILY SUPPORT GROUPS UK

1a High Marsh
Dilton Marsh
Westbury
Wiltshire BA13 4DL
Helpline: 01380 726710
Tel: 01373 826045
Fax: 01373 825158

The Attention Deficit Hyperactivity Disorder Family Support Groups UK aims to promote awareness, remove isolation, assist with educational and medical issues, social services, benefits and to link up families of sufferers. It also organises conferences, seminars and workshops.

ATTIA RESEARCH TRUST INTO ALD

36 Baker Street
London W1M 1DG
Helpine: 020 7580 5089
Fax: 020 7224 0681

The Attia Research Trust offers support to families with children with adrenoleukodystrophy (ALD), provides respite care, aims to raise public awareness of the condition and to encourage medical research into ALD.

B

BABY LIFE SUPPORT SYSTEMS (BLISS)

17–21 Emerald Street
London WC1N 3QL
Helpline: 0500 618140
Tel: 020 7820 9471
Fax: 020 7820 9567
Email: information@bliss.org.uk
Website: www.bliss.org.uk

The aim of BLISS is to give every baby born in the UK an equal chance. To achieve this, BLISS donates life-saving equipment to neonatal units, sponsors specialist nurse training and offers information and support for parents with infants needing specialist care at birth.

BACK CARE

16 Elmtree Road
Teddington
Middlesex TW11 8ST
Tel: 020 8977 5474
Fax: 020 8943 5318
Website: www.backpain.org

Back Care is a registered charity which supports research and education into the causes, prevention and treatment of back pain. It organises local branches, which are supported by a regional organisation, in which information on back pain is disseminated and exercise classes carried out.

THE BACK-UP TRUST

The Business Village
Broomhill Road
London SW18 4JQ
Helpline: 020 8875 1805
Fax: 020 8870 3619
Email: back-up@dialpipex.com

Back-up is a national charity whose aim is to encourage individuals with spinal cord injury to become re-integrated into the community and regain independence and motivation through sporting activities.

BARNARDO'S

Tanners Lane
Barkingside
Ilford
Essex IG6 1QG
Tel: 020 8550 8822
Fax: 020 8551 6870
Website: www.barnardos.org.uk

Barnardo's provide accommodation and support for young people who are leaving care, day care in deprived areas, special education for children with diabilities, youth training, adoption and fostering. It works with children and youngsters affected by poverty, HIV/AIDS, homelessness and abuse.

THE BEAUMONT SOCIETY

27 Old Gloucester Street
London WC1N 3XX
Helpline: 01582 412220
Website: www.beaumontsociety.org.uk

The Beaumont Society is a self-help organisation for people who cross-dress and their families.

BIRTH CONTROL TRUST

16 Mortimer Street
London W1N 7RJ
Tel: 020 7580 9360

The Birth Control Trust, together with its sister organisation the Birth Control Campaign, aims to advance medical and sociological research into contraception, sterilisation, and legal abortion. It operates from a national office in London, and produces leaflets and booklets, which may be obtained by post.

BIRTH DEFECTS FOUNDATION

Martindale
Cannock
Staffordshire WS11 2XN
Tel: 01543 4262777
Fax: 01543 468999
Email: help@birthdefects.co.uk
Website: www.birthdefects.co.uk

The Birth Defects Foundation aims to improve child health by the prevention and management of birth defects. It gives support and information to affected families.

BNA

The Colonnades
Beaconsfield Close
Hatfield
Herts AL10 8YD
Helpline: 0800 657575
Tel: 01707 263544
Fax: 01707 272250
Email: info@bna.co.uk
Website: www.bna.co.uk

BNA provides care in the community in hospitals, nursing homes, offices and factories. In addition, it offers affordable and flexible care to people in their own homes.

THE BOBATH CENTRE FOR CHILDREN WITH CEREBRAL PALSY

250 East End Road
East Finchley
London N2 8AU
Tel: 020 8444 3355
Fax: 020 8444 3399
Email@ info@bobathlondon.co.uk
Website: www.bobathlondon.co.uk

The Bobath Centre gives advice and support for children suffering from cerebral palsy. It also provides training for doctors and therapists.

BODY POSITIVE

51b Philbeach Gardens
London SW5 9EB
Helpline: 020 7373 9124
Fax: 020 7373 5237

Body Positive is a self-help group providing information and support to all people living with or affected by HIV/AIDS. Facilities available include helpline, drop-in centre, health/legal advice, complementary therapies, hospital visiting, information room, monthly newsletter and support groups.

BREAKTHROUGH TRUST

(Deaf-Hearing Integration)
Alan Geale House
The Close
Westhill Campus
Bristol Road
Selly Oak
Birmingham B29 6LN
Tel: 0121 472 6447
Fax: 0121 415 2323
Website: www.breakthrough-DHI.org.uk

Breakthrough is a trust whose aim is the integration of deaf and hearing people of all ages.

BREAST CANCER CARE

Kiln House
210 New Kings Road
London SW6 4NZ
Helpline: 0808 800 6000
Tel: 020 7384 2984

Fax: 020 7384 3387
Email: bcc@breastcancercare.org.uk
Website: www.breastcancercare.org.uk

Breast Cancer Care is the national organisation providing information and support to those affected by breast cancer.

BREAST CARE CAMPAIGN

Blythe Hall
100 Blythe Road
London W14 0HB
Tel: 020 7371 1510
Fax: 020 7371 4598
Website: www.breastcare.co.uk

Breast Care Campaign aims to promote information and education on non-malignant breast disorders.

BRENT SICKLE CELL/THALASSAEMIA CENTRE

122 High Street
Harlesden
London NW10 4SP
Tel: 020 8961 9005
Fax: 020 8453 0681

The Brent Sickle Cell/Thalassaemia Centre offers advice, information and support for people with sickle cell, thalassaemia and related conditions. In addition, it offers free screening and counselling services and aims to promote awareness of these conditions.

BRITISH ACUPUNCTURE COUNCIL

63 Jeddo Road
London W12 9HQ
Tel: 020 8735 0400
Fax: 020 8735 0404
Email: info@acupuncture.org.uk
Website: www.acupuncture.org.uk

The British Acupuncture Council aims to maintain common standards of education, discipline, ethics and codes of practice to ensure the health of the public at all times. In addition, it is committed to promoting research and promoting the role that acupuncture can play in public health.

BRITISH AGENCIES FOR ADOPTION AND FOSTERING (BAAF)

Skyline House
200 Union Street
London SE1 0LX
Tel: 020 7593 2000
Fax: 020 7593 2001
Email: mail@baaf.org.uk
Website: www.baaf.org.uk

The British Agencies for Adoption and Fostering is a registered charity and the professional association for all those concerned with adoption, fostering and social work with children and families. It aims to promote good standards of professional practice; to increase public understanding of the issues involved; and to bring children with special needs improved opportunities for family life. It provides training and consultancy, gives advice and information, and publishes books, leaflets and a journal.

BRITISH ALLERGY FOUNDATION

Deepdene House
30 Bellegrove Road
Welling, Kent DA16 3PY
Tel: 020 8303 8525
Fax: 020 8303 8792

The British Allergy Foundation aims to improve awareness of allergy, produce educational materials and raise money for research.

BRITISH ASSOCIATION OF CANCER UNITED PATIENTS (BACUP)

3 Bath Place
Rivington Street
London EC2A 3JR
Helpline: 0808 800 1234
Tel: 020 7696 9003
Fax: 020 7696 9002
Website: www.cancerbacup.org.uk

BACUP is a registered charity which was set up to provide information and support to cancer patients, their families and friends, health professionals and the general public. A team of experienced cancer nurses answer telephone and written enquiries on all aspects of cancer care. It has a comprehensive directory of both local and national resources (e.g. support groups, counselling services, home care services, insurance brokers and transport services). BACUP produces leaflets and booklets on the main types of cancer and on the emotional and practical problems of coping with the disease. Publications are sent free of charge to patients and their relatives. *BACUP News*, published three times a year, is sent regularly on request.

The Cancer Information Service is available Monday to Friday 10 am to 5.30 pm, extended to 7 pm Tuesdays and Thursdays.

BRITISH CHIROPRACTIC ASSOCIATION

Blagrave House
17 Blagrave Street
Reading
Berkshire RG1 1QB
Helpline: 0118 950 5950
Tel: 0118 975 7557
Fax: 0118 958 8946

The British Chiropractic Association promotes high standards of professional practice, conduct and training for chiropractors. In addition, it aims to improve awareness of chiropractic among the public and healthcare professionals as a safe and effective means of treatment for a variety of musculoskeletal complaints.

BRITISH COLOSTOMY ASSOCIATION

15 Station Road
Reading
Berkshire RG1 1LG
Helpline: 0800 328 4257
Fax: 0118 956 9095

The British Colostomy Association is a registered charity which exists to provide help, advice and reassurance to colostomy patients in the UK, and to represent their interests. Members of the group involved in patient care themselves have a colostomy. There is a national headquarters, with area officers throughout the UK and Eire. The group is also a member of the International Ostomy Association.

BRITISH DENTAL ASSOCIATION (BDA)

64 Wimpole Street
London W1M 8AL
Tel: 020 7935 0875
Website: www.bda-dentistry.org.uk

The British Dental Association is the professional body which represents dentists in a trade union and scientific role, and holds the initiative on all key issues which affect them. It aims to protect and promote the image of dentistry. Activities include an annual conference; national and local meetings of the different standing committees; and the publication of the *British Dental Journal* and *BDA News* which are circulated free to members. The BDA has 21 branches, and 120 sections, with regional offices in both Scotland and Northern Ireland.

BRITISH DENTAL HEALTH FOUNDATION

Eastlands Court
St Peter's Road
Rugby CV21 3QP
Tel: 01788 546365
Fax: 01788 541982
Website: www.dentalhealth.org.uk

The British Dental Health Foundation promotes the benefits of dental care to the general public and answers written requests on any aspects of dentistry.

THE BRITISH DIETETIC ASSOCIATION

5th Floor
Elizabeth House
22 Suffolk Street
Queensway
Birmingham
West Midlands B1 1LS
Tel: 0121 616 4900
Fax: 0121 616 4901
Email: info@bda.uk.com
Website: www.bda.uk.com

The British Dietetic Association is a registered charity which aims to advance the science and practice of dietetics through promotion of training and education of dieticians; spreading the knowledge and further understanding of dietetics; and to facilitate the exchange of information amongst members, other professionals, and the general public. Groups within the association with special interests include parenteral and enteral nutrition, renal disease, community nutrition, paediatric nutrition and the elderly. Pharmacists may obtain advice on the use of therapeutic dietary products from their local dietician.

BRITISH DIGESTIVE FOUNDATION

3 St Andrews Place
London NW1 4LB
Tel: 020 7486 0341
Fax: 020 7224 2012
Email: dds@digestivedisorders.org.uk
Website: www.digestivedisorders.org.uk

The British Digestive Foundation produces leaflets and supports research on common digestive disorders including indigestion, heartburn, peptic ulcer, irritable bowel syndrome, diarrhoea, travellers' diarrhoea, constipation, gall bladder disease, food poisoning and hepatitis.

BRITISH DYSLEXIA ASSOCIATION

98 London Road
Reading
Berks RG1 5AU
Helpline: 0118 966 8271
Tel: 0118 966 2677
Fax: 0118 935 1927
Website: www.bda-dyslexia.org.uk

The British Dyslexia Association is a registered charity committed to encouraging the early identification of children handicapped by specific learning difficulties. It offers a comprehensive counselling, information and referral service for dyslexic children and their parents, dyslexic adults and teachers. It organises courses, conferences, produces leaflets, and seeks to provide professional expertise to both parents and children. There are 68 local associations, and 57 corporate members (e.g. independent schools, and university and hospital departments).

BRITISH EPILEPSY ASSOCIATION

New Anstey House
Gateway Drive
Yeadon
Leeds LS19 7XY
Helpline: 0808 800 5050
Tel: 0113 210 8800
Fax: 0113 391 0300
Email: epilepsy@bea.org.uk
Website: www.epilepsy.org.uk

The British Epilepsy Association is a registered charity concerned with the interests of people with epilepsy, their families, and professionals working with them. It produces a comprehensive range of literature giving information and practical advice on coping with epilepsy and investigates, through the British Epilepsy Research Foundation, medical and social aspects of the condition. Services are provided by a headquarters and six regional offices.

BRITISH FLUORIDATION SOCIETY

4th Floor
University of Liverpool School of Dentistry
Liverpool L69 3BX
Helpline: 0151 706 5216
Tel: 0151 706 5216
Fax: 0151 706 5845

The British Fluoridation Society aims to improve dental health by ensuring the optimum fluoride content of drinking water.

BRITISH HEART FOUNDATION

14 Fitzhardinge Street
London W1H 4DH

Helpline: 0870 600 6566
Tel: 020 7487 7178
Fax: 020 7486 5820
Website: www.bhf.org.uk

The British Heart Foundation is a registered charity which supports research projects into cardiovascular disease; informs doctors throughout the country of advances in the field through the issue of a Factfile; and provides the public with proven risk factors related to heart diseases. It also strives to improve facilities for cardiac care by providing life-saving equipment for hospitals and ambulance services.

BRITISH HERBAL MEDICINE ASSOCIATION

Sun House
Church Street
Stroud
Gloucestershire GL5 1SL
Helpline: 014533 751389
Tel: 01453 751389
Fax: 01453 751402

The British Herbal Medicine Association aims to encourage the availability of herbal medicine, and to promote a wider knowledge and recognition of its value. It seeks to advance the science and practice of herbal medicine by modern techniques, and to promote high standards of quality and safety in herbal products. It also fosters research into phytotherapy. The Association publishes the *British Herbal Pharmacopoeia*.

BRITISH HOLISTIC MEDICAL ASSOCIATION

Rowland Thomas House
Royal Shrewsbury Hospital South
Shrewsbury SY3 8XF

The British Holistic Medical Association was set up by a group of doctors and medical students interested in the whole-person approach to healthcare. It publishes books, tapes and a journal, and has a nationwide network of local groups run by professional members for personal growth, education and support.

BRITISH HOMEOPATHIC ASSOCIATION

15 Clerkenwell Close
London
Helpline: 020 7566 7800
Website: www.trusthomeopathy.org

The British Homeopathic Association is a registered charity which works to widen the availability of homeopathy by doctors both within and outside the NHS. It acts as an advice centre, dealing with many enquiries annually. It holds first aid and self-help seminars for the general public, and special meetings to encourage pharmacists and veterinarians. It is a national organisation with a Council, of whom two members are pharmacists.

BRITISH HYPERTENSION SOCIETY

Blood Pressure Unit
St George's Hospital Medical School
Cranmer Terrace
London SW17 0RE
Tel: 020 8725 3412
Fax: 020 8725 2959
Email: bhsis@sghms.ac.uk
Website: www.hyp.ac.uk/bhsinfo

The British Hypertension Society provides information on self-help for people with high blood pressure and gives advice on prevention and treatment.

BRITISH INSTITUTE FOR BRAIN INJURED CHILDREN (BIBIC)

Knowle Hall
Knowle
Bridgwater
Somerset TA7 8PJ
Tel: 01278 684060
Fax: 01278 685573

BIBIC provides programmes of home stimulation therapy for children with brain injury as an alternative to accepting brain injury as untreatable. Treatment techniques are taught to the parents who thereafter carry them out at home. Assessment is conducted every four months to enable adjustments to be made to the treatment programme if necessary.

BRITISH INSTITUTE OF LEARNING DISABILITIES

Wolverhampton Road
Kidderminster DY1O 3PP
Tel: 01562 850251
Fax: 01562 851970
Website: www.bild.org.uk

Aims to improve the quality of life for people with learning difficulties.

BRITISH KIDNEY PATIENT ASSOCIATION

Bordon
Hampshire GU35 9JZ
Tel: 01420 472021
Fax: 01420 475831

The British Kidney Patient Association is a national registered charity concerned with the welfare of kidney patients (both dialysis and transplant patients), and the provision of kidney machines and holiday dialysis centres. It also aims to create a greater awareness of the needs for kidney donors, and the problems caused by their lack of availability.

BRITISH LIMBLESS EX-SERVICEMEN'S ASSOCIATION (BLESMA)

Franklin Moore House
185–187 High Road
Chadwell Heath
Essex RM6 6NA
Tel: 020 8590 1124
Fax: 020 8599 2932
Email: blesma@btconnect.com
Website: www.blesma.org

BLESMA aims to promote the welfare and well-being of serving and ex-service amputees and their widows and families. It provides grants, rehabilitation, residential and nursing homes.

BRITISH LIVER TRUST

Ransomes Europark
Ipswich IP3 9QG
Helpline: 0808 800 1000
Tel: 01473 276326
Fax: 01473 276327
Email: info@britishlivertrust.org.uk
Website: www.britishlivertrust.org.uk

The British Liver Trust is the support group for people with cirrhosis, hepatitis and other liver disorders. It offers information and advice to sufferers and their families and carers.

BRITISH LUNG FOUNDATION

78 Hatton Garden
London EC1N 8JR
Tel: 020 7831 5831
Fax: 020 7831 5832
Email@ blf-user@gpiag-asthma.org.uk
Website: www.lunguk.org.uk

The British Lung Foundation works to fund research into lung disease, to support people with lung conditions and to provide information on lung diseases and good lung health.

BRITISH MEDICAL ASSOCIATION (BMA)

BMA House
Tavistock Square
London WC1H 9JP
Tel: 020 7387 4499
Website: www.bma.org.uk

The British Medical Association was founded in 1832 to promote the medical and allied sciences, and to maintain the honour and interests of the medical profession. Five autonomous committees represent and negotiate on behalf of doctors in general practice, hospitals (consultant and junior staff), community medicine, and universities. Publications include the *British Medical Journal*, *BMA News Review*, scientific medical journals, abstracts of medicine and surgery, and special reports.

THE BRITISH NUTRITION FOUNDATION

High Holborn House
52–54 High Holborn
London WC1V 6RQ
Tel: 020 7404 6504
Email: postbox@nutrition.org.uk
Website: www.nutrition.org.uk

The British Nutrition Foundation is a charity, supported by contributions from its member companies, which aims to provide sound, impartial and objective information about food and nutrition. It aims to help individuals understand how they may best match their diet with their lifestyle, and sets out to achieve these aims through education, information, and research. Its resources are available to healthcare professionals, educators, the media, MPs and government departments, industry, and the public.

THE BRITISH PHARMACEUTICAL STUDENTS' ASSOCIATION (BPSA)

c/o 1 Lambeth High Street
London SE1 7JN
Tel: 020 7735 9141
Website: www.bpsa.org.uk

The British Pharmaceutical Students' Association is the only organisation to cater solely for the needs of pharmacy students, and especially pre-registration graduates. The organisation encourages and facilitates interchange of ideas and opinions between its members, and provides a platform for communication to other pharmaceutical organisations. The BPSA tries to achieve its aims by organising national and regional events to which both students and graduates are invited. Local conferences, sports matches and social events have been commonplace in past years.

BRITISH PREGNANCY ADVISORY SERVICE (BPAS)

Austy Manor
Wootton Wawen
Solihull
West Midlands B95 6BX
Helpline: 08457 304030
Tel: 01564 793225
Fax: 01564 794935
Website: www.bpas.org

The British Pregnancy Advisory Service is a registered charity providing education, research and a range of services, including counselling and treatment of problems connected with fertility and infertility. It carries out pregnancy tests, vasectomies, female sterilisation and sterilisation reversals at its five nursing homes.

BRITISH RED CROSS SOCIETY

9 Grosvenor Crescent
London SW1X 7EJ
Tel: 020 7235 5454
Fax: 020 7245 6315
Email: information@redcross.org.uk
Website: www.redcross.org.uk

The British Red Cross Society offers training in first aid and related skills to its members and the general public. Welfare duties are carried out for home-bound patients, and elderly and disabled people. It also raises funds and provides relief supplies internationally.

BRITISH RETINITIS PIGMENTOSA SOCIETY (BRPS)

PO Box 350
Buckingham MK18 5EL
Helpline: 01280 860363
Tel: 01280 860195
Fax: 01280 860195
Email: lynda@brps.demon.co.uk
Website: www.brps.demon.co.uk

BRPS provides a network for sufferers to meet fellow sufferers and works with others towards finding a cure for the disease.

BRITISH SJÖGREN'S SYNDROME ASSOCIATION

20 Kingston Way
Nailsea
Bristol BS19 2RA
Helpline: 01275 854215
Tel: 01275 854215
http://ourworld.compuserve.com/homepages/bssassociation

The British Sjögren's Syndrome Association aims to help patients and their families and carers understand and cope with the disease and aims to improve awareness of patients' problems among health professionals.

BRITISH SNORING AND SLEEP APNOEA ASSOCIATION (BSSAA)

How Lane
Chipstead
Surrey CR5 3LT
Helpline: 01249 557997
Tel: 01249 701010
Fax: 01737 248744

BSSAA provides advice and information, advises on and provides prevention devices and gives help and support to people with snoring and sleep apnoea.

BRITISH SOCIETY FOR MUSIC THERAPY

25 Rosslyn Avenue
East Barnet
Hertfordshire EN4 8DH
Tel: 020 8368 8879

The British Society for Music Therapy promotes music therapy through meetings, conferences, publications and videos.

BRITISH STAMMERING ASSOCIATION

15 Old Ford Road
London E2 9PJ
Helpline: 0845 603 2001
Tel: 020 8983 1003
Fax: 020 8983 3591
Email: mail@stammering.org
Website: www.stammering.org

The British Stammering Association helps people who stammer to communicate more effectively and it also produces literature for people who stammer.

BRITISH TINNITUS ASSOCIATION

4th Floor
White Building
FitzAllen Square
Sheffield S1 2AZ
Helpline: 0800 0180527
Tel: 0114 279 6600
Fax: 0114 279 6222
Email: bta@tinnitus.org.uk
http://www.tinnitus.org.uk

The British Tinnitus Association provides advice, information and support for people with tinnitus and aims to promote awareness of the condition.

BRITISH VASCULAR FOUNDATION

Griffin House
West Street
Woking GU21 1EB
Tel: 01483 726511
Fax: 01483 726522
Email: bvf@care4free.net
Website: www.bvf.org.uk

The British Vascular Foundation promotes research and provides information on a number of vascular disorders such as varicose veins, deep vein thrombosis and aneurysms.

BRITTLE BONE SOCIETY

30 Guthrie Street
Dundee DD1 5BS
Helpline: 0800 0282459
Tel: 01382 204446
Fax: 01382 206771
Email: bbs@brittlebone.org
Website: www.brittlebone.org

The Brittle Bone Society aims to promote research into the causes and treatment of osteogenesis imperfecta and similar bone diseases characterised by excessive fragility of the bones. In addition, it provides advice and support for sufferers and their carers and families.

BROOK ADVISORY CENTRES

421 Highgate Studios
53–79 Highgate Road
London NW5 1TL
Helpline: 08000 185 023
Tel: 020 7284 6040
Fax: 020 7284 6050
Email: information@brookcentres.org.uk

Brook Centres offer young people free, confidential contraceptive advice and supplies as well as help with sexual and emotional difficulties.

C

CANCER AND LEUKAEMIA IN CHILDHOOD TRUST (CLIC)

Abbey Wood
Bristol BS34 7JU
Helpline: 0117 3112600
Fax: 0117 3112694

CLIC aims to help children suffering from cancer and leukaemia and their parents. The trust receives no government money and relies on voluntary donations to fund its services which include welfare grants, research and treatment.

CANCER CARE SOCIETY

11 The Corn Market
Romsey
Hampshire SO51 8GB
Tel: 01794 830300
Fax: 01794 518133
Email: info@cancercaresoc.demon.co.uk
Website: www.cancercaresoc.demon.co.uk

The Cancer Care Society provides information, counselling, support groups, complementary therapies, holiday accommodation and a wig-fitting service.

CANCER RESEARCH CAMPAIGN

10 Cambridge Terrace
London NW1 4JL
Helpline: 0800 226237
Tel: 020 7224 1333
Fax: 020 7487 4310
Email: crcinformation@crc.org.uk
Website: www.crc.org.uk

The Cancer Research Campaign is a registered charity aiming to defeat cancer. To achieve this, it supports research at centres throughout the UK, providing funds for projects on the recommendation of its Scientific and Education Committees. A field staff of 22 area appeals organisers provide the link between about 1000 voluntary local committees and the headquarters.

CANCERLINK

11–21 Northdown Street
London WC1X 9JN
Helpline: 0808 808 0000
Tel: 020 7833 2818
Fax: 020 7833 4963

Cancerlink provides emotional support and information for patients, their families, carers and friends, and health professionals on all aspects of cancer. It acts as a resource for over 500 cancer support and self-help groups throughout the UK.

CARDIOMYOPATHY ASSOCIATION

40 The Metro Centre
Tolpits Lane
Watford
Hertfordshire WD1 8SB
Tel: 01923 249977
Fax: 01923 249987
Email: cmassoc@aol.com
Website: www.cardiomyopathy.org

The Cardiomyopathy Association provides support and information to potential and diagnosed sufferers of cardiomyopathy.

CENTRE FOR ACCESSIBLE ENVIRONMENTS

Nutmeg House
60 Gainsford Street
London SE1 2NY
Tel: 020 7357 8182
Fax: 020 7357 8183
Email: info@cae.org.uk
Website: www.cae.org.uk

Centre for Accessible Environments is a registered charity which provides information, training and consultancy on the design and adaptation of buildings and spaces to ensure that they are accessible to everyone, including disabled and older people. It appraises architect's drawings for access criteria and provides in-house training and publishes design guides.

CENTRE FOR PHARMACY POSTGRADUATE EDUCATION (CPPE)

University of Manchester
School of Pharmacy and Pharmaceutical Sciences
Coupland III Building
University of Manchester
Oxford Road
Manchester M13 9PL
Tel: 0161 778 4000
Fax: 0161 778 4030
Website: www.pa.man.ac.uk

CPPE provides education and training for all pharmacists in England.

CENTRE FOR THE STUDY OF COMPLEMENTARY MEDICINE

51 Bedford Place
Southampton
Hants SO15 2TG
Tel: 023 8033 4752

The Centre for the Study of Complementary Medicine was set up by medically qualified practitioners who work at the centre and offer skills in a wide range of complementary medical techniques. Clinical services are offered in acupuncture, manipulative medicine, homeopathy and clinical ecology. The techniques are also taught, largely at postgraduate level, and research is also carried out.

CEREBRAL PALSY HELPLINE (SCOPE)

PO Box 833
Milton Keynes MK12 5NY
Helpline: 0808 800 3333
Tel: 01908 321047
Fax: 01908 321051
Email: cphelpline@scope.org.uk
Website: www.scope.org.uk

The Cerebral Palsy Helpline is the national information and support line for SCOPE. It offers support, advice and information on cerebral palsy and similar disabilities and provides information about SCOPE and its activities.

CHILD

Charter House
43 St Leonards Road
Bexhill on Sea
East Sussex TN40 1JA
Tel: 01424 732361
Fax: 01424 731858
Email: office@email2.child.org.uk
Website: www.child.org.uk

Child provides support and information to people suffering the effects of infertility and promotes public awareness and encourages mutual support.

CHILD ACCIDENT PREVENTION TRUST

4th Floor, Clerks Court
18–20 Farringdon Lane
London EC1R 3HA
Tel: 020 7608 3828
Fax: 020 7608 3674
Email: safe@capt.demon.co.uk

The Child Accident Prevention Trust works to reduce the number and severity of preventable childhood accidents in the UK, through information, research and national campaigns.

CHILD GROWTH FOUNDATION

2 Mayfield Avenue
Chiswick
London W4 1PW
Helpline: 020 8995 0257
Tel: 020 8995 0257
Fax: 020 8995 9075

The Child Growth Foundation cares for children whose growth is too great or too little. It acts as an umbrella organisation for the Growth Hormone Insufficiency Group, Turner Syndrome, IUGR/Russell Silver, Bone Dysplasia, SOTOS and Premature Sexual Maturation support groups for patients and parents. In addition, it funds research, organises educational programmes and markets measuring equipment.

CHILDLINE

2nd Floor, Royal Mail Building
Studd Street
London N1 0QW
Helpline: 0800 1111
Tel: 020 7239 1000
Fax: 020 7239 1001
Website: www.childline.org.uk

Childline is the free national helpline for children and young people in danger and distress. It provides a confidential telephone service for any child with any problems 24 hours a day and refers children in danger to appropriate helping agencies. Childline also brings to public attention issues affecting children's welfare and rights.

CHILDREN'S LIVER DISEASE FOUNDATION

36 Great Charles Street
Birmingham B3 3JY
Tel: 0121 212 3839
Fax: 0121 212 4300
Email: info@childliverdisease.org
Website: www.childliverdisease.org

The Children's Liver Disease Foundation offers support and promotes research into all aspects of paediatric liver disease. It provides new facilities and trained staff and helps to ensure emotional support for families of children with liver disease.

CLEFT LIP AND PALATE ASSOCIATION (CLAPA)

235–237 Finchley Road
London NW3 6LS
Tel: 020 7431 0033
Fax: 020 7431 8881
Email: clapa@cwcom.net
Website: www.clapa.cwc.net

CLAPA provides information and support to children and parents of children with cleft lip and/or cleft palate.

CLINICAL PHARMACOKINETICS SOCIETY

Department of Clinical Biochemistry
St Luke's Hospital
Warren Road
Guildford
Surrey
Tel: 01483 571122

The Clinical Pharmacokinetics Society aims to establish and develop pharmacy involvement in drug level monitoring and pharmacokinetic interpretation services. A wide range of objectives include the evaluation of therapeutic drug monitoring (TDM) services; education and training in TDM; and an extension of databases for the evaluation of population pharmacokinetic parameters.

COELIAC SOCIETY OF THE UNITED KINGDOM

PO Box 220
High Wycombe
Bucks HP11 2HY
Tel: 01494 437278
Fax: 01494 473349
Email: admin@coeliac.co.uk
Website: www.coeliac.co.uk

The Coeliac Society is a registered charity which exists to help those who have been medically diagnosed as having coeliac disease or dermatitis herpetiformis. It is a national organisation with 57 local groups. The Society publishes the *Coeliac Handbook*, a list of gluten-free manufactured products, and other aids for patients.

COLLEGE OF PHARMACY PRACTICE

University of Warwick Science Park
Barclays Venture Centre
Sir William Lyons Road
Coventry CV4 7EZ
Tel: 024 7669 2400
Fax: 024 7669 3069
Website: www.collpharm.org.uk

The College of Pharmacy Practice was established by the Council of the PSGB as a company, limited by guarantee, and with charitable status. The principle purposes of the College are to promote and maintain a high standard of practice to advance education and training in all pharmaceutical disciplines and at all levels; to establish standards of vocational training; to advance knowledge of the application of pharmacy in total healthcare; and to conduct, promote, and facilitate research into the practice of pharmacy, and to publish the results of those endeavours. All pharmacists registered in Great Britain are eligible to become student members and can take the College's two part Practitioner Membership Examination after being registered for three years and being a College member for one year.

COLON CANCER CONCERN

9 Rickett Street
London SW6 1RU
Tel: 020 7381 9711
Email: help@coloncancer.org.uk

This is a support group for people affected by colon cancer and their families and friends.

COMPASSIONATE FRIENDS (Bereaved parents support group)

53 North Street
Bristol BS3 1EN
Helpline: 0117 953 9639
Tel: 0117 966 5202
Fax: 0117 966 5202

Compassionate Friends is a nationwide organisation of bereaved parents which offers friendship and understanding to other bereaved parents, and also to bereaved siblings and grandparents after the death of a child from any cause.

CONSUMERS' ASSOCIATION

2 Marylebone Road
London NW1 4DX
Tel: 020 7830 6000

The Association for Consumer Research (ACRE) is a registered charity which undertakes research and comparative testing of goods and services. Its trading subsidiary, the Consumers' Association, publishes a range of *Which?* Magazines, and also *Self Health* and the *Drug and Therapeutics Bulletin*. The Research Institute for Consumer Affairs (RICA) is a sister organisation to ACRE which carries out projects aimed at helping elderly and disabled people.

CONTACT A FAMILY

170 Tottenham Court Road
London W1P 0HA
Tel: 020 7383 3555
Fax: 020 7383 0259
Email: info@cafamily.org.uk
Website: www.cafamily.org.uk

Contact a Family provides advice, information and support to families caring for children with any form of disability or special need.

CONTINENCE FOUNDATION (INCONTINENCE INFORMATION HELPLINE)

307 Hatton Square
16 Baldwins Gardens
London EC1N 7RJ
Helpline: 020 7831 9831
Fax: 020 7404 6876
Email: continence.foundation@dial.pipex.com
Website: www.continence-foundation.org.uk

The Continence Foundation Helpline aims to encourage people whose lives are affected by incontinence to discuss their problem in confidence with a trained person.

CORONARY PREVENTION GROUP

2 Taviton Street
London WC1H 0BT
Tel: 020 7927 2125
Fax: 020 7927 2127
Website: www.healthnet.org.uk

The Coronary Prevention Group is a registered charity devoted to the prevention of coronary heart disease. It provides information and practical advice on the major causes of the disease. The group is run by the country's leading experts on heart disease and deals with issues ranging from nutrition, farming, smoking and exercise to recovering from a heart attack. The group also publishes a range of information on the subjects.

COUNCIL FOR COMPLEMENTARY AND ALTERNATIVE MEDICINE (CCAM)

Tel: 020 8735 0632

The Council for Complementary and Alternative Medicine provides a forum for communication and cooperation between professional bodies representing acupuncture, chiropractic, homeopathy, medical herbalism, naturopathy and osteopathy. It also aims to promote and maintain the highest standards of training, qualification and treatment in these therapies, and to facilitate the dissemination of information about them. A register of CCAM member practitioners is held at the headquarters.

COUNCIL FOR DISABLED CHILDREN

8 Wakley Street
London EC1V 7QE
Helpline: 020 7843 6058
Tel: 020 7843 6061
Fax: 020 7278 9512

The Council for Disabled Children promotes collaborative work among organisations providing services and support for children with disabilities and special needs.

COUNCIL FOR MUSIC IN HOSPITALS

74 Queens Road
Horsham
Walton-on-Thames
Surrey KT12 5LW
Tel: 01932 252809
Fax: 01932 252966

The Council for Music in Hospitals provides concerts in England, Wales and Northern Ireland, given by professional musicians.

COUNCIL FOR THE ADVANCEMENT OF COMMUNICATION WITH DEAF PEOPLE

Durham University Science Park
Block 4
Stockton Road
Durham DH1 3UZ
Tel: 0191 383 1155
Fax: 0191 383 7914
Email: durham@cacdp.demon.co.uk
Website: www.cacdp.demon.co.uk

CACDP is the national examining body for communication skills between deaf and hearing people, including British sign language, lipreading, communication with deaf-blind people and deaf awareness. In addition, the council sells curricula for each of the examinations and produces sign language videos.

COUNSEL AND CARE

Twyman House
Lower Ground Floor
16 Bonny Street
London NW1 9PG
Helpline: 0845 300 7585
Tel: 020 7485 1550

Fax: 020 7267 6877
Email: advice@counselandcare.demon.co.uk

Counsel and Care provides information and advice for people over 60 on a wide range of issues such as welfare benefits, accommodation and residential and nursing care. In addition, it maintains a database of home care agencies from which it can advise individuals. It can also issue single payment grants for specified items.

CREUTZFELDT-JAKOB DISEASE (CJD) SUPPORT NETWORK

Birchwood
Heath Top
Ashley Heath
Market Drayton
Shropshire TF9 4QR
Tel: 01630 673 973
Fax: 01630 673 993
Email: cjdnet@alzheimers.org.uk
Website: www.alzheimers.org.uk/cjd/index.html

The CJD Support Network provides help and support for people with CJD, their carers and concerned professionals.

CROHN'S IN CHILDHOOD RESEARCH ASSOCIATION

Parkgate House
356 West Barnes Lane
Motspur Park
Surrey KT3 6NB
Tel: 020 8949 6209
Fax: 020 8942 2044

Crohn's in Childhood Research Association provides help and support to sufferers and their families. It also raises funds for research into Crohn's disease, ulcerative colitis and related conditions.

CRUSE, THE NATIONAL ORGANISATION FOR THE WIDOWED AND THEIR CHILDREN

126 Sheen Road
Richmond
Surrey TW1 1UR
Tel: 020 8940 4818
Fax: 020 8940 7638

CRUSE is a registered charity which offers help, advice and information on practical problems, and opportunities for social contacts, to all bereaved people. It also runs training courses in bereavement counselling, and a number of fact-sheets and other literature are available either through the national organisation or from its 130 branches in the UK.

CYSTIC FIBROSIS TRUST

11 London Road
Bromley
Kent BR1 1BY
Tel: 020 8464 7211
Fax: 020 8313 0472
Email: enquiries@cftrust.org.uk
Website: www.cftrust.org.uk

The Cystic Fibrosis Trust is a registered charity which finances research into a cure for cystic fibrosis and to improve current methods of treatment. Branches throughout the UK help and advise parents with the everyday problems of caring for children with cystic fibrosis. The Trust also aims to educate the public about the disease and to promote its earlier diagnosis in children.

DEPRESSION ALLIANCE

35 Westminster Bridge Road
London SE1 7JB
Tel: 020 7633 9929
Fax: 020 7633 0559
Email: hq@depressionalliance.org
Website: www.depressionalliance.org

Depression Alliance provides information and support to sufferers of depression and their carers and promotes research into the causes and management of depression and dissemination of such research.

DIABETES UK

10 Queen Anne Street
London W1M 0BD
Tel: 0207 323 1531
Website: www.diabetes.org.uk

Diabetes UK is a registered charity which was formed to provide advice and information for all diabetics and their families, to promote greater public understanding about diabetes, and to support research into the prevention, treatment, and cure of the disease and its complications. There are over 350 local groups and branches throughout the UK, which arrange regular meetings and social events. BDA also publishes a wide range of literature, provides videos and posters, and arranges educational activity weekends for diabetics and their families.

DIAL UK

Park Lodge
St Catherine's Hospital
Tickhill Road
Balby
Doncaster DN4 8QN
Tel: 01302 310123
Fax: 01302 310404
Email: dialuk@aol.com
Website: www.number.aol.com/dialuk

Dial UK is a disability helpline.

DISABILITY ALLIANCE

Universal House
88–94 Wentworth Street
London E1 7SA
Helpline: 020 7247 8763
Tel: 020 7247 8776
Fax: 020 7247 8765

Disability Alliance provides information for disabled people on their entitlements and aims to break the link between disability and poverty.

DISABILITY INFORMATION TRUST

Mary Marlborough Centre
Nuffield Orthopaedic Centre
Headington
Oxford OX3 7LD
Tel: 01865 227592
Fax: 01865 227596
Email: www.ditrust@btconnect.com
Website: www.home.btconnect.com/ditrust/home.htm

The Disability Information Trust publishes a series of reference books giving details of the range of equipment and aids available to help disabled people. These include specially manufactured equipment, everyday consumer goods and DIY ideas. Practical advice, and points to consider before purchase, are also given. All items are tested and assessed by disabled people either at home or in the hospital prior to their inclusion.

DISABILITY LAW SERVICE

39–45 Cavell Street
London E1 2BP
Helpline: 020 7791 3131
Tel: 020 7791 9800
Fax: 020 7791 9801

Disability Law Service gives free legal advice and representation to disabled people and their families and/or carers. It advises on benefits, community care, discrimination, education, employment, housing, wills, trusts and other matters affecting the lives of disabled people.

DISABILITY SPORT ENGLAND

13–27 Brunswick Place
London N1 6DX
Helpline: 020 7490 4919
Fax: 020 7490 4914
Email: infor@dse.org.com
Website: www.britsport.com

A national organisation that aims to provide, develop and co-ordinate opportunities in sport and recreation for people with disabilities.

DISABILITY WALES

Llys Ifor
Crescent Road
Caerphilly
Mid Glamorgan CF83 1XL
Tel: 029 2088 7325
Fax: 029 2088 8702
Email: info@dwac.demon.co.uk

The national organisation of disability association which aims to provide advice and information on disability issues in Wales.

DISABLED DRIVERS ASSOCIATION

National Headquarters
Ashwellthorpe
Norwich NR16 1EX
Tel: 01508 489449
Fax: 01508 488173
Email: ddahq@aol.com
Website: www.justmobility.co.uk/dda

The Disabled Drivers Association provides information for disabled drivers, obtains concessions with many ferry companies and campaigns through government and local bodies to advance the cause of disabled people.

DISABLED LIVING FOUNDATION (DLF)

380–384 Harrow Road
London W1 2HU
Tel: 020 7281 6111
Website: www.dlf.org.uk

The Disabled Living Foundation provides information on all non-medical aspects of living with a disability (including mental, physical and sensory, together with multiple handicaps and the infirmities of age). It provides a general information service on aids and equipment (including a subscription service for updated information and enquiry service), and advisory services on incontinence, visual handicap, clothing and music. There is a demonstration centre in which equipment may be viewed and tried out. The DLF also organises publications and seminars.

DISFIGUREMENT GUIDANCE CENTRE

PO Box 7
Cupar
Fife KY15 4PF
Tel: 01337 870281
Fax: 01337 870310

The Disfigurement Guidance Centre provides information (for a small fee) and targets different areas with the aim of meeting needs in the field of disfigurement.

DOWN'S SYNDROME ASSOCIATION

155 Mitcham Road
London SW17 9PG
Tel: 020 8682 4001
Website: www.dsa-uk.com

The Down's Syndrome Association is a registered charity which aims to create and develop the environment in which people with the condition may realise their full potential. It provides information about health, education, teenage problems and life after school. The Association promotes research into ways of improving life of people of all ages with Down's syndrome. The Association has a national administrative office and resource centre based in London, and a network of branches throughout the UK.

DRUGSCOPE

Waterbridge House
32–36 Loman Street
London SE1 0EE
Tel: 020 7928 1211
Fax: 020 7928 1771
Email: services@drugscope.org.uk
Website: www.drugscope.org.uk

DrugSCope is the UK's leading drugs charity and centre of expertise on drugs. It provides up-to-date drug information to professionals and the public, conducts research and develops policies on drugs and drug-related issues, promotes humane and effective ways of responding to drugs and drug use, encourages informed debate and provides a voice for over 800 member bodies.

THE DYSLEXIA INSTITUTE

133 Gresham Road
Staines
Middlesex TW18 2AJ
Tel: (0784) 59498/63851/63852
Website: www.dyslexia-inst.org.uk

The Dyslexia Institute aims to provide a teaching, teacher-training, assessment and advisory service for dyslexics and those working with them. It also hopes to increase general awareness of the difficulties encountered by dyslexics at school and at home. In order to ensure that more teachers nationally are informed and skilled in dealing with the problem, the Institute aims to increase the provision made for it at teacher-training level. It is a national organisation with assessment and teaching centres around the country.

DYSTONIA SOCIETY

46–47 Britton Street
London EC1M 5UJ
Helpline: 020 7490 5671
Tel: 020 7490 5671
Fax: 020 7490 5672
Website: dystonia.org.uk

The Dystonia Society supports individuals who have any form of dystonia and their families and carers, through the promotion of improved awareness, research and welfare.

E

EATING DISORDERS ASSOCIATION

Wensum House
103 Prince of Wales Road
Norwich
Norfolk NR1 1DW
Helpline: 01603 621414
Tel: 01603 619090
Fax: 01603 664915

The Eating Disorders Association provides support and information to people with eating disorders, their families, friends and carers. It promotes local groups, local help and a membership scheme.

ENABLE

6th Floor
7 Buchanan Street
Glasgow G1 3HL
Helpline: 0141 226 4541
Fax: 0141 204 4398
Email: enable@enable.org.uk

Enable is a voluntary association which represents the interests of people with learning disabilities. It was formed by parents in 1954 and has over 70 branches across Scotland and a membership of around 6000. It provides information and legal advice and support for families as well as holidays, jobs, training, day services and respite care. It also has 12 family-sized homes for people with profound and complex needs.

ENCEPHALITIS SUPPORT GROUP

44a Market Place
Malton
North Yorkshire YO17 7LW
Helpline: 01653 699599
Tel: 01653 699599
Fax: 01653 699599

The Encephalitis Support Group provides support to sufferers of encephalitis and their families and works to raise awareness of the condition and to raise funds for research.

ENURESIS RESOURCE AND INFORMATION CENTRE (ERIC)

34 Old School House
Britannia House
Kingswood
Bristol BS15 2DB
Tel: 0117 960 3060
Fax: 0117 960 0401
Email: info@eric.org.uk
Website: www.enuresis.org.uk

ERIC provides support and information to children, youngsters, parents and professionals on all aspects of wetting and soiling.

EPILEPSY ASSOCIATION OF SCOTLAND

48 Govan Road
Glasgow G51 1JL
Helpline: 0141 427 4911
Tel: 0141 427 4911
Fax: 0141 427 7414
Email: support@epilepsyscotland.org.uk
Website: www.epilepsyscotland.org.uk

The Epilepsy Association of Scotland promotes the welfare of people with epilepsy. It provides information, support, counselling service and social work. It is involved in field and community projects, as well as training a wide range of professional groups in understanding and managing epilepsy.

EYE CARE INFORMATION SERVICE

PO Box 131
Market Rasen
Lincolnshire LN8 5TS
Tel: 01673 857847
Fax: 01673 857696

The Eye Care Information Service supplies the public with information on general eye care. Advice may also be obtained by telephone. Any detailed questions are answered by an ophthalmic optician (optometrist).

F

FAB-UK

4 Pateley Road
Woodthorpe
Nottingham NG3 5QF
Helpline: 0115 926 9634

FAB-UK provides support and information for families of children with Fanconi's anaemia. It also undertakes fundraising to assist research into bone marrow transplants.

FABRY DISEASE RESEARCH FUND AND SUPPORT GROUP

10 Broadmeadow Road
Wyke Regis
Weymouth DT4 9BS
Helpline: 01305 774443
Tel: 01305 774443
Fax: 01305 774443
Email: fabry@wdi.co.uk

The Fabry Disease Research Fund and Support Group aims to promote awareness of Fabry disease and to raise money for research.

FAMILIES ANONYMOUS

Unit 37
The Doddington and Rollo Community Association
Charlotte Despard Avenue
London SW11 5JE
Helpline: 020 7498 4680
Tel: 020 7498 4680
Fax: 020 7498 1990
Website: www.famanon.org.uk

Families Anonymous provides support to families and friends of people who use and abuse drugs.

FAMILY HEART ASSOCIATION

7 North Road
Maidenhead, Berkshire SL6 1PE
Tel: 01628 628638
Fax: 01628 628698
Website: www.familyheart.org

The Family Heart Association provides information for people with inherited hyperlipidaemias or who are prone to premature angina or myocardial infarction for other reasons.

FAMILY PLANNING ASSOCIATION (FPA)

2–12 Pentonville Road
London N1 9FP
Helpline: 020 7837 4044
Tel: 020 7837 5432
Fax: 020 7837 3042
Website: fpa.org.uk

The Family Planning Association is a registered charity which provides information, advice, and education on birth control, fertility, reproductive health, sex education, sexuality and relationships. It aims to preserve and protect the good health, physical and mental, of individuals, couples, and families, and prevent the hardship and distress caused by unwanted conceptions.

FAMILY PLANNING ASSOCIATION SCOTLAND

Unit 10
Firhill Business Centre
74 Firhill Road
Glasgow G20 7BA
Helpline: 0141 576 5088
Tel: 0141 576 5088
Fax: 0141 576 5006

FAMILY PLANNING ASSOCIATION WALES

Ground Floor
Riverside House
31 Cathedral Road
Cardiff CF11 9HB
Tel: 029 2064 4034
Fax: 029 2064 4306
Email: fpa@cymru@compuserve.com

FAMILY WELFARE ASSOCIATION

501–505 Kingsland Road
London E8 4AU
Tel: 020 7254 6251
Fax: 020 7249 5443

Family Welfare Association provides practical, financial and social care to families.

FEDERATION OF MULTIPLE SCLEROSIS THERAPY CENTRES

Bradbury House
155 Barkers Lane
Bedford MK41 9RX
Tel: 01234 325781
Fax: 01234 365242
Email: info@ms-selfhelp.org
Website: www.ms-selfhelp.org

The Federation of Multiple Sclerosis Therapy Centres provides information, support and training for the MS therapy centres within the Federation.

FIRST STEPS TO FREEDOM

7 Avon Court
School Lane
Kenilworth
Warwickshire CV8 2GX
Helpline: 01926 851608
Tel: 01926 864473
Fax: 0870 164 0567
Email: info@firststeps.demon.co.uk
Website: www.firststeps.demon.co.uk

First Steps to Freedom is a helpline for sufferers and carers of people with anxiety, panic attacks, obsessional compulsive disorder, borderline personality disorder, phobias, anorexia, bulimia and tranquilliser withdrawal. It also provides telephone self-help groups, factsheets, booklets, audio tapes, videos and books.

FOOD AND CHEMICAL ALLERGY ASSOCIATION

27 Ferringham Lane
Ferring
West Sussex BN12 5NB
Tel: 01903 241178

The Food and Chemical Allergy Association provides advice on how to identify and overcome allergies.

FOUNDATION FOR THE STUDY OF INFANT DEATHS

Artillery House
11–19 Artillery Row
London SW1P 1RT

Helpline: 020 7233 2090
Tel: 020 7222 8001
Fax: 020 7222 8002

The Foundation for the Study of Infant Deaths is a registered charity which raises funds for research into the causes and prevention of cot death (sudden infant death syndrome). It gives personal support to bereaved families by letter, telephone and leaflets, and puts parents in touch with previously bereaved parents (Friends of the Foundation) who offer an individual befriending service. It also acts as a centre of information on cot death for parents and professionals, and for the exchange of knowledge within the UK and abroad.

FRAGILE X SOCIETY

53 Winchelsea Lane
Hastings
East Sussex TN35 4LG
Tel: 01424 813147

The Fragile X Society provides advice and information to sufferers of Fragile X syndrome and their families.

FRIEDREICH'S ATAXIA GROUP

The Stable
Wiggins Yard
Bridge Street
Goldalming
Surrey GU7 IHW
Tel: 01483 424006
Fax: 01483 417111

The Friedreich's Ataxia Group provides advice and information to sufferers of Friedreich's ataxia and their families.

G

GAUCHER'S ASSOCIATION

25 West Cottages
London NW6 1RJ
Helpline: 020 7433 1121
Tel: 020 7433 1121
Email: office@gaucher.net
Website: www.gaucher.org.uk

Gaucher's Association provides information about Gaucher's disease (an inherited enzyme-deficiency disorder) and encourages the availability of treatment.

GENERAL COUNCIL AND REGISTER OF OSTEOPATHS

176 Tower Bridge Road
London SE1 3LU
Tel: 0118 957 6585

The General Council and Register of Osteopaths exists to protect the public by insisting for its membership on a standard of excellence in osteopathic training, practice and behaviour. This is achieved by accrediting four-year full-time courses at certain educational establishments approved by Council, and by maintaining a strict Code of Ethics. Only graduates of accredited courses are entitled to membership of the Register and to use the abbreviation of MRO. Details of local registered osteopaths may be obtained by contacting the secretary at the above address.

GENERAL MEDICAL COUNCIL (GMC)

178–202 Great Portland Street
London W1N 6JE
Tel: 020 7580 7642
Fax: 020 7915 3641
Website: www.gmc-uk.org

The General Medical Council is the statutory body for the regulation of the medical profession. Its duties include the promotion of high standards and coordination of all stages of medical education; keeping and publishing a register of duly qualified doctors; providing advice for doctors on standards of professional conduct and on medical ethics; and taking action in cases of serious professional misconduct or where a doctor's fitness to practice appears to be seriously impaired by reason of a mental or physical condition. Its membership comprises representatives nominated by the Crown, appointed by the universities having medical faculties, and by the medical corporations, and elected directly by members of the profession.

GENETIC INTEREST GROUP

Unit 4d
Leroy House
436 Essex Road
London N1 3QP
Helpline: 020 7430 0090
Tel: 020 7704 3141
Fax: 020 7359 1447
Email: post@gig.org.uk
Website: www.gig.org.uk

The Genetic Interest Group is the national alliance for voluntary groups supporting families with genetic disorders. It works to raise awareness, to provide training for lay and professional people, to fight discrimination and to promote development of appropriate, high-quality services to people who need them.

GINGERBREAD

16–17 Clerkenwell Close
London EC1R 0AN
Helpline: 020 7336 8184
Tel: 020 7336 8183
Fax: 020 7336 8185
Email: office@gingerbread.org.uk
Website: www.gingerbread.org.uk

Gingerbread provides a support network for single parents and their children.

GLUE EAR SOCIETY

1 Annington Road
London N2 9NB

The Glue Ear Society is a contact group for parents of children with glue ear.

THE GUIDE DOGS FOR THE BLIND ASSOCIATION
Hillfields
Burghfield Common
Reading RG7 3YG
Helpline: 0118 9835555
Fax: 0118 9835433

The Guide Dogs for the Blind Association is a registered charity responsible for the breeding and training of guide dogs, and training blind people (and associated aftercare services) to work with them. The Association has approximately 420 branches throughout England, Scotland and Wales whose members operate on a voluntary basis.

GUILD OF HEALTHCARE PHARMACISTS
MSF
50 Southwark Street
London SE1 1UN
Tel: 020 7717 4000
Fax: 020 7717 4010
Website: www.ghp.org.uk

The Guild of Healthcare Pharmacists represents the interests of hospital pharmacists in professional matters and in negotiations on salaries and conditions of employment. The Guild merged with the Association of Scientific, Technical and Managerial Staff (ASTMS) in order to provide the professional negotiating skills needed within the Pharmaceutical Whitley Council where salaries and conditions of service are decided. Membership of the GHP is open to all practising hospital pharmacists. They participate in the work of the Guild through local groups, which conduct professional, business and social meetings throughout the year. Policies at national level on professional and non-professional matters are decided by a council of 24 members, who are elected by the membership.

GUILLAIN-BARRÉ SYNDROME SUPPORT GROUP OF THE UK
Lincolnshire County Council Offices
Eastgate
Sleaford
Lincolnshire NG34 7EB
Helpline: 0800 374803
Tel: 01529 304615
Fax: 01529 304615

The Guillain-Barré Syndrome Support Group provides support to patients, relatives and friends, if possible through personal visits by former patients. It supports research into the causes and treatment of the illness, educates and maintains awareness and encourages local and special interest groups.

H

HAEMOPHILIA SOCIETY
3rd Floor
Chesterfield House
385 Euston Road
London NW1 3AU
Helpline: 0800 0186068
Tel: 020 7380 0600
Fax: 020 7387 8220
Email: info@haemophilia.org.uk
Website: www.haemophilia.org.uk

The Haemophilia Society is a registered charity which represents the interests of people with haemophilia, and provides them, their families and healthcare professionals with help, advice and assistance as appropriate. The problems of HIV and AIDS are particularly important with respect to the safety of blood products. It is a national society, with a number of locally run groups.

HAIRLINE INTERNATIONAL
Lyons Court
1668 High Street
Knowle
West Midlands B93 0LY
Tel: 01564 775281
Fax: 01564 782270
Website: www.hairline.international.co.uk

Hairline International gives support and information to people suffering from alopecia and other types of hair loss. It provides newsletters, telephone service and meetings.

HALLEY STEWART LIBRARY
St Christopher's Hospice
51 Lawrie Park Road
Sydenham
London SE26 6DZ
Tel: 020 8778 9252

The Halley Stewart Library contains a small specialised collection of books and journal articles on all aspects of terminal care and bereavement, and lists of references on specific topics can be sent to enquirers. Books and reprints are also available through a mail order service.

HEADWAY
4 King Edward Court
King Edward Street
Nottingham NG1 1EW
Helpline: 0115 924 0800
Tel: 0115 924 0800
Fax: 0115 958 4446
Email: enquiries@headway.org.uk
Website: www.headway.org.uk

Headway aims to promote understanding of all aspects of head and brain injury and to provide information and support to people with head injury and their families and carers.

HEARING DOGS FOR DEAF PEOPLE
London Road
Lewknor
Oxfordshire OX9 5RY
Helpline: 01844 353898
Tel: 01844 353898
Fax: 01844 353099

Hearing Dogs for Deaf People trains dogs to be the ears of deaf people. Dogs are trained to respond to sound (e.g. doorbells, telephone) and lead the deaf person to the sound. The service is provided free of charge.

HELP THE AGED

207–221 Pentonville Road
London N1 9UZ
Tel: 020 7253 0253
Website: www.helptheaged.org.uk

Help the Aged is a registered charity which works to improve the quality of life of all elderly people in the UK and overseas, especially those who are frail, neglected and forgotten. It provides food and clothing, supports day centres and self-help projects. Through its publications, it advises on the welfare of elderly people, including safety, health, mobility and finance.

HERPES VIRUSES ASSOCIATION

41 North Road
London N7 9DP
Helpline: 020 7609 9061
Tel: 020 7607 9661
Website: www.herpes.org.uk

The Herpes Viruses Association provides advice and counselling for people affected by herpes viruses and gives accurate information on the virus to the public, media and health professionals.

HOSPICE INFORMATION SERVICE

St Christopher's Hospice
51/59 Lawrie Park Road
Sydenham
London SE26 6DZ
Tel: 020 7778 9252

The Hospice Information Service provides a resource and link for members of the public and healthcare professionals. A directory of Hospice Services in the UK and Eire is published annually. A list of overseas organisations is also available. A varied educational programme is offered by the teaching hospice, including courses for pharmacists.

HUMAN RIGHTS SOCIETY

Mariners Hard
Cley, Nr Holt
Norfolk NR25 7RX
Tel: 01263 740404
Fax: 01263 740404

The Human Rights Society opposes the legalisation of euthanasia because it sees no way that the law could provide the necessary safeguards.

HUNTINGTON'S DISEASE ASSOCIATION

108 Battersea High Street
London SW11 3HP
Tel: 020 7223 7000
Fax: 020 7223 9489
Website: www.hda.org.uk

The Huntington's Disease Association provides advice and support to patients suffering from Huntington's disease and their families and carers.

HYPERACTIVE CHILDREN'S SUPPORT GROUP

71 Whyke Lane
Chichester
West Sussex PO19 2LD
Tel: 01903 725182
Fax: 01903 734726
Website: www.hascg.org.uk

The Hyperactive Chhildren's Support Group is a contact and support group for parents of hyperactive children.

I

IA (THE ILEOSTOMY AND INTERNAL POUCH SUPPORT GROUP)

PO Box 123
Scunthorpe
DN15 9YW
Helpline: 0800 0184724
Fax: 01724 721601
Website: www.ileostomypouch.demon.co.uk

The Ileostomy and Internal Pouch Support Group formed the Ileostomy Association (IA). IA's aim is to support people who have an ileostomy and to help improve their quality of life. IA works closely with health professionals, manufacturers and others.

IMPOTENCE ASSOCIATION

PO Box 10296
London SW17 9WH
Tel: 020 8767 7791

The Impotence Association provides information on the management of male erectile dysfunction.

INSTITUTE FOR COMPLEMENTARY MEDICINE

PO Box 194
London SE16 1QZ
Helpline: 020 7237 5165
Tel: 020 7237 5175

The Institute for Complementary Medicine is a registered charity which aims to increase public awareness of natural therapies through education and research. It is concerned with the establishment of national standards of professional training for natural therapy practitioners, and can provide members of the public with information on practitioners, research documents and books. It also has begun a programme of research into the workings of complementary treatment. It runs special courses introducing natural therapies. Some of the therapies covered are acupuncture, osteopathy, chiropractic therapy, herbal medicine and homeopathy. A directory of registered practitioners is held by the Institute.

INSTITUTE OF PHARMACY MANAGEMENT INTERNATIONAL

c/o Nicholas Wood
The Seasons
Park Wood
Doddington
Brentwood
Essex CM15 0SN
Tel: 01277 823889
Email:enelwood@compsuserve.com
Website:
www.pharmweb.net/pwmirror/pw9/ipmi/index.html

The Institute of Pharmacy Management International initiates fundamental and practical research programmes and promotes up-to-date teaching of pharmaceutical administration relevant to all branches of the profession. A journal is published quarterly, and an annual conference permits members to present original work concerning pharmacy practice. The college of the Institute enables members to qualify for a diploma of the Institute through attendance of study modules during a residential course.

INTERNATIONAL AUTISTIC RESEARCH ORGANISATION

49 Orchard Avenue
Shirley
Croydon CR0 7NE
Helpline: 020 8777 0095
Tel: 020 8777 0095
Fax: 020 8776 2362
Email: iaro@lineone.net

The International Autistic Research Organisation provides information and seeks to raise awareness of research into autism.

INTERNATIONAL GLAUCOMA ASSOCIATION (IGA)

108c Warner Road
Camberwell
London SE5 9HQ
Helpline: 020 7737 3265
Tel: 020 7737 3265
Fax: 020 7346 5929
Email: info@iga.org.uk
Website: www.iga.org.uk/home.htm

The International Glaucoma Association is a registered charity which offers all those interested in preventing blindness from glaucoma a forum for the exchange of ideas, and aims to increase awareness of the problems of the disease. It sends out information booklets free on receipt of a large SAE. It also supports research into the causes and treatment of glaucoma from donations received.

INTERNATIONAL PLANNED PARENTHOOD FEDERATION

Regents College
Inner Circle
Regents Park
London NW1 4NS
Tel: 020 7486 7900
Fax: 020 7487 7950

The IPPF is the world's leading voluntary healthcare organisation whose aim is to promote on a worldwide basis sexual and reproductive health, provide family planning services, and to develop public support for sustainable population, development and environment policies.

INTERSTITIAL CYSTITIS SUPPORT GROUP

76 High Street
Stony Stratford
Bucks MK11 1AH
Tel: 01908 569169
Fax: 01908 569169
Email: info@interstitialcystitis.co.uk
Website: www.interstitialcystitis.co.uk

This group provides a support network for sufferers of interstitial cystitis, works to relieve suffering from this illness and promotes the advancement of education of the public and health professionals into the causes and treatments of interstitial cystitis.

IRRITABLE BOWEL SYNDROME NETWORK (IBS NETWORK)

St John's House
Hither Green Hospital
Hither Green Lane
London SE13 6RU
Helpline: 020 8698 4611 ext 8194
Tel: 020 8698 4611 ext 8194
Fax: 020 8698 5655

The IBS Network is run by sufferers of IBS for other sufferers and aims to help alleviate the distress caused by this condition.

ISSUE (NATIONAL FERTILITY ASSOCIATION)

114 Litchfield Street
Walsall
West Midlands WS1 1SZ
Helpline: 01922 722 888
Tel: 01922 722 888
Fax: 01922 640070
Email: webmaster@issue.co.uk
Website: www.issue.co.uk

Issue provides information and support for people with fertility problems and those who work with them.

J

JUSTICE FOR ALL VACCINE DAMAGED CHILDREN

Erin's Cottage
Fussell's Buildings
Whiteway Road
Bristol BS5 7QY
Helpline: 0117 955 7817
Tel: 0117 955 7818

Justice for All Vaccine Damaged Children offers a contact for parents of children damaged by vaccination. It deals with enquiries from health authorities, social services, doctors and solicitors and gives advice on when and how to claim and tribunal procedures etc.

L

LA LECHE LEAGUE
BM 3424
London WC1N 3XX
Helpline: 020 7242 1278
Tel: 020 7242 1278

La Leche League aims to encourage breast feeding of infants.

THE LEONARD CHESHIRE FOUNDATION
30 Millbank
London SW1P 4QD
Tel: 020 7802 8200
Fax: 020 7802 8250

The Leonard Cheshire Foundation is a charitable trust presiding over 75 Cheshire Homes in the UK and overseas, and is affiliated to a further 147. The homes accommodate predominantly the physically handicapped, although several homes cater for mentally handicapped children and adults. The common aim of all homes is to provide shelter and care in an atmosphere as close as possible to that of a family home. Family support services are also offered for handicapped people who prefer to remain in their own homes.

LEUKAEMIA CARE SOCIETY
2 Shrubbery Avenue
Worcester
Worcestershire WR1 1QH
Tel: 01905 330003
Fax: 01905 330090
Website: leukaemia.care.org

A national organisation that aims to provide befriending, hospital visits, limited financial assistance, and caravan holidays to those whose lives are affected by cancer.

LEUKAEMIA RESEARCH FUND
43 Great Ormond Street
London WC1N 3JJ
Helpline: 020 7405 0101
Tel: 020 7405 0101
Fax: 020 7242 1488
Email: info@laekaemia-research.org.uk
Website: www.leukaemia-research.org.uk

The Leukaemia Research Fund is the national charity for the support of research into leukaemia and allied blood disorders. It is advised by a medical and scientific panel. The fund is currently supporting research at more than 60 hospitals and university medical centres in the UK. It promotes international symposia, research meetings and workshops. It also provides patient support through an information service.

LIMBLESS ASSOCIATION
31 The Mall
Ealing
London W5 2PX
Tel: 020 8579 1758

The Limbless Association provides information and advice for people born without upper and lower limbs or who have had amputations. It makes representations on policy matters to government departments, local authorities and health authorities and promotes rehabilitation through its home and hospital visiting service.

LONDON LIGHTHOUSE
111–117 Lancaster Road
London W11 1QT
Tel: 020 7792 1200
Fax: 020 7229 1258

London Lighthouse is a residential and support centre for people affected by HIV and AIDS. It provides a drop-in centre, café, community services, education, training, consultancy, complementary therapies, day care, residential care, convalescent and terminal care.

LUPUS UK
1 Eastern Road
Romford
Essex RM1 3NH
Tel: 01708 731251
Fax: 01708 731252
Email: headoffice@lupus-uk.freeserve.co.uk

Lupus UK aims to educate the public and health professionals about systemic lupus erythematosus (SLE), to support those diagnosed and to raise funds for research.

LYMPHOEDEMA SUPPORT NETWORK
St Luke's Crypt
Sydney Street
London SW3 6NH
Helpline: 020 8748 2403; 020 8647 6456; 020 8650 2154
Tel: 020 7351 4480
Fax: 020 7351 4480

The Lymphoedema Support Network provides advice and support for sufferers of lymphoedema.

M

MACMILLAN CANCER RELIEF
Anchor House
15–19 Britten Street
London SW3 3TZ
Tel: 020 7351 7811
Fax: 020 7376 8098
Website: www.macmillan.org.uk

Macmillan Cancer Relief is a registered charity (as The National Society for Cancer Relief) and was founded by Douglas Macmillan in 1911 to bring care and support to cancer patients. Specially trained nurses are provided to look after cancer patients in their own homes. The Fund also provides help to cancer patients by building continuing care homes which provide in-patient and day care; giving cash grants to patients and families in financial need; and funding an education programme in the new skills of pain relief.

MANIC DEPRESSION FELLOWSHIP
Castle Works
21 St Georges Road
London SE1 6ES
Tel: 020 7793 2600
Fax: 020 7793 2639
Email: mdf@mdf.org.uk

Manic Depression Fellowship helps people with manic depression, their families and carers. It produces a large range of publications and aims to educate the public and caring professions about the condition and to encourage research.

MANIC DEPRESSION SCOTLAND
19 Elmbank Street
Glasgow G2 4PB
Helpline: 0141 331 0440
Tel: 0141 331 0440
Fax: 0141 331 0440

MARFAN ASSOCIATION UK
Rochester House
5 Aldershot Road
Fleet, Hants GU13 9NG
Helpline: 01252 810472
Tel: 01252 810472
Fax: 01252 810473
Website: www.thenet.co.uk/marfan

Marfan Association UK supports people with Marfan syndrome, provides education to the public and health professionals and encourages research.

MARIE CURIE CANCER CARE
28 Belgrave Square
London SW1X 8QG
Tel: 020 7235 3325
Fax: 020 7823 2380
Website: www.mariecurie.org.uk

Marie Curie Cancer Care is a registered charity which provides nursing care for cancer patients through its 11 Marie Curie Homes throughout the UK, and through its nationwide community nursing service. This service is administered on behalf of the Foundation through the local health authority, and is completely free of charge. The Foundation also runs its own cancer research institute in Surrey, and training courses for health professionals involved in cancer care.

MARIE STOPES INTERNATIONAL
153–157 Cleveland Street
London W1P 5PG
Tel: 020 7574 7400
Abortion helpline: 0845 300 8090
Vasectomy and female sterilisation information: 0845 300 0212

Marie Stopes International is run by a registered charity and offers a comprehensive birth control service on a private, fee-paying basis. It advises on all aspects of contraception, gynaecological advice, full health checks for women, menopause and PMS consultations, male and female sterilisation, abortion advice and referral, and an advisory service for slimmers. There are three centres in England, and 12 regional vasectomy centres.

MATERNITY ALLIANCE
45 Beech Street
London EC2P 2LX
Helpline: 020 7588 8582
Tel: 020 7588 8583
Fax: 020 7588 8584
Email: info@maternityalliance.org.uk

Maternity Alliance offers advice and information on maternity rights and benefits.

MEDIC-ALERT FOUNDATION
1 Bridge Wharf
156 Caledonian Road
London N1 9UU
Helpline: 0800 581420
Tel: 020 7833 3034
Fax: 020 7278 0647
Email: info@medicalert.co.uk
Website: www.medicalert.co.uk

The Medic-Alert Foundation is a registered charity whose services are funded by a once-only life-membership fee, and voluntary contributions from friends, members and companies. The Medic-Alert emblem is worn as a bracelet or necklet, and is engraved with the wearer's special medical condition and a 24-hour emergency telephone number, which may be contacted by emergency service personnel.

MEDICAL ADVISORY SERVICE FOR TRAVELLERS ABROAD (MASTA)
London School of Hygiene and Tropical Medicine
Keppel Street
London WC1E 7HT
Helpline: 0891 224100
Tel: 0906 822 4100
Website: www.masta.org

MASTA provides specific information on immunisations, malaria prophylaxis, the latest health news and any Foreign Office advice.

MEDICAL COUNCIL ON ALCOHOLISM
3 St Andrew's Place
London NW1 4LB
Helpline: 020 7487 4445
Tel: 020 7487 4445
Fax: 020 7935 4479

The Medical Council on Alcoholism aims to educate health professionals about the effects of alcohol on health for the benefit of themselves and their patients. In addition, it will also help confidentially with a drink/drug problem.

MENCAP (THE ROYAL SOCIETY FOR MENTALLY HANDICAPPED CHILDREN AND ADULTS)
MENCAP National Centre
123 Golden Lane
London EC1Y 0RT

Helpline: 020 7696 5593
Tel: 020 7454 0454
Fax: 020 7668 3254
Website: www.mencap.org.uk

MENCAP is a registered charity with 55 000 members, most of whom are parents and friends of people with a mental handicap. A constantly expanding service is provided through eight divisional offices, with approximately 550 local affiliated groups. Services include: welfare and legal advice and counselling for families with a mentally handicapped member; holiday services; trustee visitors service; education, training and pathway employment service; Gateway leisure clubs; and residential services and training establishments. MENCAP National Centre can provide local contacts for new parents to meet other families with mentally handicapped children. A wide range of literature outlining MENCAP's services is available from the information department.

MENINGITIS RESEARCH FOUNDATION

Midland Way
Thornbury
Bristol BS35 2BS
Helpline: 0808 800 3344
Tel: 01454 281811
Fax: 01454 281094
Email: info@meningitis.org
Website: www.meningitis.org

Meningitis Research Foundation works to prevent death and disability from meningitis and related infections by promoting awareness of the disease and raising funds for research into its prevention, detection and treatment.

MENTAL HEALTH FOUNDATION

20–21 Cornwall Terrace
London NW1 4QL
Tel: 020 7535 7400
Fax: 020 7535 7474
Website: www.mentalhealth.org.uk

The Mental Health Foundation covers both mental health and learning disabilities and helps to pioneer new approaches to prevention, treatment and care. It allocates grants for research and community projects, contributes to public debate, strives to reduce prejudice and educates and influences health professionals and policy makers.

MIGRAINE ACTION ASSOCIATION

178a High Road
Byfleet
Weybridge
Surrey KT14 7ED
Helpline: 01932 352468
Fax: 01932 351257
Email: info@migraine.org.uk
Website: www.migraine.org.uk

The Migraine Action Association (formerly the British Migraine Association) is a registered charity run for migraine sufferers by migraine sufferers, their families and friends. It encourages and supports research into the causes and treatment of the condition, and provides information on all aspects to sufferers, all branches of the medical profession and the media. It also aims to provide friendly, cheerful reassurance and understanding to sufferers.

THE MIGRAINE TRUST

45 Great Ormond Street
London WC1N 3HZ
Helpline: 020 7831 4818
Tel: 020 7831 4818
Fax: 020 7831 5174
Website: www.migrainetrust.org

The Migraine Trust aims to provide assistance for furthering research into the causes, alleviation and treatment of migraine. It promotes, assists and encourages schemes for research, education, technical training and treatment, and promotes the exchange of information relating to the condition. It makes grants for research into the causes and treatment of migraine as universities and research institutions throughout the world. It is a national organisation, with local groups, and also funds the Princess Margaret Migraine Clinic in London.

MIND (NATIONAL ASSOCIATION FOR MENTAL HEALTH)

15–19 Broadway
Stratford
London E15 4BQ
Helpline: 020 8522 1728; 0845 7660163
Fax: 020 8522 1725

MIND is a registered charity which aims to uphold the rights and represent interests of people with mental health problems. It provides advice and information, a legal casework service, and training courses and conferences. MIND is also a specialist publisher on mental health subjects. There is a national headquarters, seven regional offices and approximately 200 local associations which provide a range of services (e.g. employment schemes, accommodation projects, day centres, advice and information).

MISCARRIAGE ASSOCIATION

c/o Clayton Hospital
Northgate
Wakefield
West Yorkshire WF1 3JS
Helpline: 01924 200799
Tel: 01924 200795
Fax: 01924 298834
Website: www.thema.org.uk

This national charity provides support and information on all aspects of miscarriage and pregnancy loss. It gathers information about causes and management and promotes good management of pregnancy loss by professionals.

MOTOR NEURONE DISEASE ASSOCIATION

PO Box 246
Northampton NN1 2PR
Helpline: 08457 626262
Tel: 01604 250505
Fax: 01604 624726
Email: enquiries@mndassociation.org
Website: www.mndassociation.org

The Motor Neurone Disease Association is a registered charity which aims to promote and encourage research into the disease, and to improve the provision of care of patients in liaison with the statutory services. The organisation covers the UK with 43 local branches around the country.

THE MULTIPLE SCLEROSIS SOCIETY

25 Effie Road
Fulham
London SW6 1EE
Helpline: 0808 800 8000
Tel: 020 7610 7171
Fax: 020 7736 9861
Email: info@mssociety.org.uk
Website: www.mssociety.org.uk

The Multiple Sclerosis Society is a registered charity which exists to promote and encourage research into finding the cause of and cure for multiple sclerosis (MS), and to provide a welfare and support service for families with a sufferer. Headquarters are based in London, supporting 390 local branches which provide practical assistance and support to those with MS. It also supports hospital and university research into the disease, and there are short-stay and holiday centres for those more severely affected.

MULTIPLE SCLEROSIS SOCIETY IN SCOTLAND

The Rural Centre
Hallyards Road
Inglestone EH28 8NZ
Helpline: 0808 800 8000
Tel: 0131 472 4106
Fax: 0131 472 4099
Email: admin@mssociety-scotland.org.uk

MUSCULAR DYSTROPHY GROUP OF GREAT BRITAIN AND NORTHERN IRELAND

7–11 Prescott Place
Clapham
London SW4 6BS
Helpline: 020 7720 8055
Tel: 020 7720 8055
Fax: 020 7498 0670
Email: info@muscular-dystrophy.org
Website: www.muscular-dystrophy.org

The Muscular Dystrophy Group is a registered charity with the prime aim of funding research to find the cause, an effective treatment and a cure for all neuromuscular diseases. It is an entirely voluntary organisation, with nine professional regional organisers and 450 local branches and representatives. It is also concerned with patient welfare and medical services.

MYALGIC ENCEPHALOMYELITIS (ME) ASSOCIATION

Stanhope House
High Street
Stanford-le-Hope
Essex SS17 0HA
Helpline: 01375 351013
Tel: 01375 642466
Fax: 01375 360256
Website: www.meassociation.org.uk

The ME Association provides information and support to ME sufferers, their families, friends and carers.

MYASTHENIA GRAVIS ASSOCIATION

Keynes House
Chester Park
Alfreton Road
Derby DE21 4AS
Tel: 01322 290219
Fax: 01322 293641
Website: www.crabby.demon.co.uk/mga

The Myasthenia Gravis Association provides care and support for sufferers and their families and carers and funds research into the disease.

N

NARCOTICS ANONYMOUS

202 City Road
London EC1V 2PH
Helpline: 020 7730 0009
Tel: 020 7251 4007
Fax: 020 7251 4006

Narcotics Anonymous is a contact group that aims to help members encourage one another in recovery and rehabilitation.

NATIONAL ABORTION CAMPAIGN

The Print House
18 Ashwin Street
London E8 3DL
Tel: 020 7923 4976
Fax: 020 7923 4979

The National Abortion Campaign works to ensure that all women have equal access to safe, free abortion on request. It also aims to raise awareness of the need for free, safe abortion and that a woman's right to such is crucial for her equality and autonomy.

NATIONAL AIDS HELPLINE

Healthwise Helpline
1st Floor Caven Court
8 Mathew Street
Liverpool L2 6RE
Helpline: 0800 567123
Tel: 0151 227 4150
Fax: 0151 227 4019
Email: info@healthwise.org.uk

The National Aids Helpline provides confidential and consistent information on all aspects of HIV and associated illnesses, including AIDS, including the routes of transmission. It also offers a UK-wide referral service.

NATIONAL ANKYLOSING SPONDYLITIS SOCIETY (NASS)

PO Box 179
Mayfield
East Sussex TN20 6ZL

Tel: 01435 873527
Fax: 01435 873027

The National Ankylosing Spondylitis Society is a registered charity concerned with sufferers from the disease, their families, friends and doctors. It is also involved in promotion of research into the disease. The Society aims to provide a forum for sufferers and to educate patients, professions and the public in the problems of the disease. The Society is managed by an elected council which is advised by a Medical Advisory Council, who also provide medical information and articles for the NASS Newsletter.

NATIONAL ASSOCIATION FOR COLITIS AND CROHN'S DISEASE (NACC)

4 Beaumont House
Sutton Road
St Albans
Hertfordshire AL1 5HA
Helpline: 01727 844296
Tel: 01727 862550
Fax: 01727 862550
Email: nacc@nacc.org.uk
Website: www.nacc.org.uk

The National Association for Colitis and Crohn's Disease is a registered charity and gives general support to sufferers from inflammatory bowel diseases, their families, and others concerned. It publishes information and raises funds for research into the causes and the cure of inflammatory bowel disease. The Association consists of a national executive and 40 area groups, which arrange meetings (e.g. medical information lectures and social events). It publishes six booklets and a biannual newsletter is sent free to members.

NATIONAL ASSOCIATION FOR PREMENSTRUAL SYNDROME (NAPS)

PO Box 72
Sevenoaks
Kent TN13 1XQ
Helpline: 01732 760012
Tel: 01732 760011
Fax: 01732 760011
Website: www.pms.org.uk

NAPS aims to ensure that all women suffering from premenstrual syndrome have access to help and treatment where appropriate. NAPS also runs training courses for prospective group leaders and telephone contacts and organises seminars and lectures for health professionals.

NATIONAL ASSOCIATION FOR THE CARE AND RESETTLEMENT OF OFFENDERS (NACRO)

169 Clapham Road
London SW9 0PU
Helpline: 020 7582 6500
Tel: 020 7582 6500
Fax: 020 7735 4666
Email: communications@nacro.og.uk

NACRO works to promote the resettlement of offenders in the community by providing a wide range of practical services to both offenders and those at risk of becoming offenders. It also works to prevent crime and aims to help communities suffering from the effects of crime.

NATIONAL ASSOCIATION FOR THE RELIEF OF PAGET'S DISEASE

323 Manchester Road
Walkden
Worsley
Manchester M28 3HH
Tel: 0161 799 4646
Fax: 0161 799 6511
Email: 106064,1032@compuserve.com
Website: www.paget.org.uk

The National Association for the Relief of Paget's Disease offers advice and support for sufferers of Paget's disease. It also aims to raise awareness of the disease and promote research into its causes and treatment.

NATIONAL ASSOCIATION OF HOSPITAL AND COMMUNITY FRIENDS

2nd Floor, Fairfax House
Couston Road
Colchester CO1 1RJ
Tel: 01206 761227
Fax: 01206 560244
Email: info@hc-friends.org.uk
Website: www.info@hc-friends.org.uk

The National Association of Hospital and Community Friends is the representative body, support and advice centre for friends' groups working for the health, dignity and comfort of patients in hospital and the community. It also provides insurance, grants, training, publications, conferences and local support networks.

NATIONAL ASSOCIATION OF LARYNGECTOMEE CLUBS

Ground Floor
6 Rickett Street
London SW6 1RU
Helpline: 020 7381 9993
Tel: 020 7381 9993
Fax: 020 7381 0025

The National Association of Laryngectomee Clubs promotes the welfare of patients with laryngectomy and offers advice and help to all patients and their friends, families and carers.

NATIONAL ASSOCIATION OF WIDOWS (NAW)

48 Queens Road
Coventry CV1 3EH
Helpine: 024 7663 4848
Tel: 024 7663 4848

The National Association of Widows is a registered charity and offers advice, information and friendly support to all widows. There are branches throughout the country which provide the basis for a social life for widows; a specialist advice and information service is available from the head office.

NATIONAL ASSOCIATION OF WOMEN PHARMACISTS (NAWP)

Please contact:
enquiries@nawp.org.uk
Website: www.nawp.org.uk

The National Association of Women Pharmacists was founded to provide a service designed to keep women pharmacists well-informed. NAWP organises an annual national weekend refresher course which is especially designed for those women who have stopped working to raise a family and wish to re-enter the profession. The Association produces a quarterly newsletter supplemented by factsheets on specific subjects. Local branches of the NAWP hold informal meetings with guest speakers, covering a variety of subjects. Some branches help organise locums in their area. The affairs of the Association are administered by an executive elected from membership.

NATIONAL ASTHMA CAMPAIGN

National Asthma Campaign
Providence House
Providence Place
London N1 0NT
Tel: 020 7226 2260
Fax: 020 7704 0740
Website: www.asthma.org.uk

Aims to promote public awareness of asthma and raises money to fund research projects into diagnosis, treatment and prevention. Provides information and support to sufferers and their families and carers. Publishes an information booklet and a quarterly newsletter.

NATIONAL AUTISTIC SOCIETY

393 City Road
London EC1V 1NE
Helpline: 020 7833 2299
Tel: 020 7833 2299
Fax: 020 7833 9666
Website: www.oneworld.org/autism-uk/

The National Autistic Society is a registered charity and the only organisation working specifically for autistic people. It aims to provide and promote day and residential centres for the care, education and training of autistic children and adults. It encourages research into the problems of the autistic and aims to stimulate greater understanding among doctors, teachers and the general public. It provides an advisory service for parents and interested professionals on the nature of childhood autism, and publishes and distributes literature on the management and education of autistic children.

NATIONAL CANCER ALLIANCE

PO Box 579
Oxford OX4 1LB
Tel: 01865 793566
Fax: 01865 251050
Website: www.nationalcanceralliance.co.uk

The National Cancer Alliance is an alliance of patients and health professionals working to improve the care of all patients with cancer. They also provide a directory of information on cancer services and a list of cancer specialists.

NATIONAL CHILDBIRTH TRUST

Alexandra House
Oldham Terrace
London W3 6NH
Helpline: 020 8992 8637
Tel: 020 8992 8637
Fax: 020 8992 5929
Website: www.nct-online.org

The National Childbirth Trust is a registered charity concerned with education for pregnancy, birth and parenthood. It aims to help parents achieve greater enjoyment and satisfaction before, during and following childbirth through antenatal classes, support with breast feeding, and friendly encouragement after the baby is born. The Trust publishes a wide range of leaflets, and maternity goods are also supplied through its offices. There are seven NCT regions, with over 300 local branches.

NATIONAL CHILDREN'S BUREAU

8 Wakley Street
London EC1V 7QE
Tel: 020 7843 6000
Fax: 020 7278 9512
Website: www.ncb.org.uk

The National Children's Bureau is a registered charity which aims to identify and improve awareness and understanding of issues affecting children and young people.

NATIONAL CONSUMER COUNCIL (NCC)

20 Grosvenor Gardens
London SW1W 0DH
Tel: 020 7730 3469
Fax: 020 7730 0191

The National Consumer Council represents the interests of consumers when they buy or use goods and services (including health services). It particularly watches over the interests of inarticulate and disadvantaged consumers; promotes advice services for consumers nationwide; and encourages consumer representation in nationalised industries. Scottish and Welsh Consumer Councils also exist, and there is a General Consumer Council in Northern Ireland. It does not deal directly with individual consumer enquiries, but does monitor problems taken to other agencies (e.g. Citizens Advice Bureaux).

NATIONAL COUNCIL FOR ONE-PARENT FAMILIES

255 Kentish Town Road
London NW5 2LX
Helpline: 0800 0185026
Fax: 020 7482 4851
Email: helpdesk@oneparentfamilies.org.uk

The National Council for One-Parent Families works to improve the economic, social and legal position of one-parent families. It researches and campaigns to improve the position of lone parents and their children and offers an information service and training for professionals working with such families.

NATIONAL DEAF CHILDREN'S SOCIETY

15 Dufferin Street
London EC1Y 8UR
Helpline: 0800 252380
Tel: 020 7250 0123
Fax: 020 7251 5020

The National Deaf Children's Society is a registered national charity concerned with the needs of parents and families of deaf children. It specialises in advice and information on education, health and social services. The Society gives grants to parents and families for equipment, holidays and education. It also operates a lending library of radio hearing aids and other equipment. There are 140 local groups run by parents and interested professionals.

NATIONAL DEAF-BLIND LEAGUE

100 Bridge Street
Peterborough PE1 1DY
Tel: 01733 358100
Fax: 01733 358356

The National Deaf-Blind League aims to enable people who are both deaf and blind to live full and active lives. It works to raise awareness of deaf-blindness among the public and professionals and to ensure needs are met in community care planning. It visits deaf-blind people for assessment, development of care plans and to enhance social activities and rehabilitation services.

NATIONAL ECZEMA SOCIETY

16 Eversholt Street
London NW1 1BU
Helpline: 020 7388 3444
Tel: 020 7388 4097
Fax: 020 7388 5882
Email: eczema@nes.comu-netcom
Website: www.eczema.org

The National Eczema Society is a registered charity which aims to help people with eczema and their families. It has a research fund and also has established an NES Research Fellowship as the Hospital for Sick Children, Great Ormond Street, London. The NES has branches and local support groups throughout the country, and organises an annual holiday scheme for children and for young people.

NATIONAL ENDOMETRIOSIS SOCIETY

Suite 50
Westminster Palace Gardens
1–7 Artillery Row
London SW1P 1RL
Helpline: 020 7222 2776
Tel: 020 7222 2781
Fax: 020 7222 2786
Email: endoinfo@comuserve.com
Website: www.endo.org.uk

The National Endometriosis Society works to enable sufferers and their families to live with the condition. It offers advice and has self-help groups, workshops and specialist publications.

NATIONAL FEDERATION OF THE BLIND OF THE UK

The Old Surgery
215 Kirkgate
Wakefield WF1 1JG
Tel: 01924 291313
Fax: 01924 200244
Email: nfbuk@globalnet.co.uk
Website: www.users.globalnet.co.uk/~NfBUK

The National Federation of the Blind campaigns for the integration of blind or partially sighted children into ordinary schools, for blindness allowance in people over 16 and for better employment opportunities for blind people.

NATIONAL FEDERATION OF RETIREMENT PENSIONS ASSOCIATIONS

Thwaites House
Railway Road
Blackburn
Lancashire BB1 5AY
Helpline: 01254 52606
Tel: 01254 52606
Fax: 01254 52606

The National Federation of Retirement Pensions Associations works to improve state pensions and other state benefits for pensioners by convening annual conferences and lobbying all party group for pensioners in the House of Commons.

NATIONAL HEART FORUM

Tavistock House South
Tavistock Square
London WC1H 9LG
Tel: 020 7383 7638
Fax: 020 7387 2799
Website: www.heartforum.org.uk

The National Heart Forum is the leading alliance of national agencies who work to try to reduce the UK's high incidence of coronary heart disease.

NATIONAL INSTITUTE OF MEDICAL HERBALISTS

56 Longbrook Street
Exeter EX4 6AH
Tel: 01392 426022
Fax: 01392 498963

The National Institute of Medical Herbalists is the professional body of practising herbalists. It supplies information on herbal medicine, and a list of qualified practitioners may be obtained by sending a SAE. All members of the Institute are graduates of the School of Herbal Medicine as Tunbridge Wells.

NATIONAL KIDNEY FEDERATION

6 Stanley Street
Worksop
Nottinghamshire S81 7HX
Helpline: 0845 6010209
Tel: 01909 487795
Email: mks@kidney.org.uk
Website: www.kidney.org.uk

The National Kidney Federation is the only national organisation in the UK run by kidney patients for the benefit of kidney patients. It has several member organisations and the central office provides advice and information for patients and families, students, the general public and health professionals. It represents patients' interests to the media and government, encourages the public to look on kidney donation as a gift of life and campaigns to improve treatment facilities for patients.

THE NATIONAL KIDNEY RESEARCH FUND AND KIDNEY FOUNDATION

Cirrus Court
Glebe Road
Huntingdon
Cambridgeshire PE29 7EL
Helpline: 01480 398301
Tel: 01480 356086
Fax: 01480 398303
Website: www.nkrf.org.uk

The National Kidney Research Fund raises money for research and for patients' care and welfare.

NATIONAL MENINGITIS TRUST

Fern House
Bath Road
Stroud
Gloucestershire GL5 3TJ
Helpline: 0845 6000 800
Tel: 01453 768000
Fax: 01453 768001
Email: support@meningitis-trust.org.uk
Website: www.meningitis-trust.org.uk

The National Meningitis Trust offers advice and support to sufferers and their families, provides information to health professionals and the public on meningitis and funds research into the disease.

NATIONAL ORGANISATION FOR COUNSELLING ADOPTEES AND PARENTS (NORCAP)

112 Church Road
Wheatley
Oxfordshire OX33 1LU
Helpline: 01865 875000
Tel: 01865 875000
Fax: 01865 875686

NORCAP works to provide advice, support and understanding to adoptees and their birth and adoptive parents. It offers counselling services and acts as an intermediary for adoptees and birth families seeking renewed contact. It provides liaison with local authorities, government and adoption and fostering agencies.

NATIONAL OSTEOPOROSIS SOCIETY

PO Box 10
Radstock
Bath BA3 3YB
Helpline: 01761 472721
Tel: 01761 472721
Fax: 01761 471104
Email: info@nos.org.uk
Website: www.nos.org.uk

The National Osteoporosis Society works to improve the prevention, diagnosis and treatment of osteoporosis. It provides information and advice through its helpline, a network of local groups and specialist publications. It has its own specialist medical advisors.

NATIONAL PHARMACEUTICAL ASSOCIATION (NPA)

Mallinson House
38–42 St Peter's Street
St Albans
Herts AL1 3NP
Tel: 01727 832161
Fax: 01727 840858
Website: www.npa.co.uk
Consumer website: www.askyourpharmacist.co.uk

The National Pharmaceutical Association is the trade association and parent body of a group of organisations serving pharmacy proprietors. Membership, which is voluntary, comprises 96% of all retail pharmacies in the UK (excluding those of Boots and the Co-operative Societies). As the Retail Pharmacists Union and later the National Pharmaceutical Union (NPU), the NPA was formed in 1921 to champion the interests of pharmacy proprietors and to serve as an organisation for the promotion, improvement and protection of its members. Soon after its foundation, it joined forces with the Chemists Defence Association, thus conferring on NPA members automatic insurance against claims for which they are liable as retail pharmacists, entitlement to legal defence against certain prosecutions, legal representation before industrial and other tribunals, and legal defence.

NATIONAL REGISTER OF HYPNOTHERAPISTS AND PSYCHOTHERAPISTS

12 Cross Street
Nelson
Lancashire BB9 7EN
Helpline: 01282 716839
Tel: 01282 699378
Fax: 01282 698633
Email: nrhp@btconnect.com
Website: www.nrhp.co.uk

The National Register of Hypnotherapists and Psychotherapists acts as a referral service for members of the public seeking a qualified hypnotherapist or psychotherapist. People on the register are qualified from the National College of Hypnosis & Psychotherapy and must abide by a code of ethics and have appropriate insurance.

NATIONAL REYE'S SYNDROME FOUNDATION OF THE UK

15 Nicholas Gardens
Pyrford
Woking
Surrey GU22 8SD
Helpline: 01932 346843
Tel: 01932 346843
Fax: 01932 343920

The National Reye's Syndrome Foundation works to support parents of children who have suffered from this disease, to inform both the public and health professionals and to fund research into the cause, prevention and treatment of Reye's syndrome.

NATIONAL SCHIZOPHRENIA FELLOWSHIP (NSF)

Head Office
30 Tabernacle Street
London EC2AA 4DD
Helpline: 020 8974 6814
Tel: 020 7330 9100
Fax: 020 7330 9102
Email: info@nsf.org.uk
Website: www.nsf.org.uk

NSF is the largest national voluntary organisation for people with severe mental illness, their families, friends and carers. It campaigns for better treatment and services and better understanding of the problems caused by severe mental illness, particularly schizophrenia. It has a number of core offices throughout England, Wales and Northern Ireland, many self-help groups and community projects, and it also carries out research and organises training courses and conferences. It provides advice and a range of publications.

NATIONAL SCHIZOPHRENIA FELLOWSHIP (SCOTLAND)

Claremont House
130 East Claremont Street
Edinburgh EH7 4LB
Helpline: 0131 557 8969
Tel: 0131 557 8969
Fax: 0131 557 8968
Email: info@nsfscot.org.uk
Website: www.nsfscot.org.uk

THE NATIONAL SOCIETY FOR EPILEPSY (NSE)

Chalfont Centre for Epilepsy
Chalfont St Peter
Gerrards Cross
Bucks SL9 0RJ
Helpline: 01494 601400; 01494 873991
Tel: 01494 601300; 01494 873991
Fax: 01494 871927

The National Society for Epilepsy is a registered charity which caters for the needs of people suffering from epilepsy, offering assessment, treatment, rehabilitation and long-term care. Research is also carried out into new drugs at the centre. The assessment centre is run in conjunction with the National Hospital for Nervous Diseases. An education department produces a range of leaflets and videos for teaching purposes.

NATIONAL SOCIETY FOR PHENYLKETONURIA AND ALLIED DISORDERS

PO Box 26642
London N14 4ZF
Helpline: 0845 6039136
Website: http://web.ukonline.co.uk/nspku

The National Society for Phenylketonuria and Allied Disorders is an organisation which aims to assist the parents of children born with phenylketonuria (PKU) to manage the problems of the condition. It achieves this by arranging meetings with parents of other children similarly affected, producing and distributing booklets and leaflets, and publishing a comprehensive cookery book to allow the use of a varied and interesting diet in the management of PKU. It also explores holiday opportunities for families with particular dietary needs.

NATIONAL SOCIETY FOR THE PREVENTION OF CRUELTY TO CHILDREN (NSPCC)

National Centre
42 Curtain Road
London EC2A 3NH
Helpline: 0808 800 500
Tel: 020 7825 2775
Fax: 020 7825 2763
Email: infounit@nspcc.org.uk
Website: www.nspcc.org.uk

The NSPCC helps children and their families through its child protection teams, projects and national helpline. It also emphasises the need to identify the causes of child abuse and to work towards its prevention.

NATURAL MEDICINES SOCIETY

PO Box 232
East Moseley
Surrey KT8 1YF
Tel: 020 8974 1166
Fax: 020 8974 1166
Email: NMS@charity-vfree.com

The Natural Medicines Society represents the consumer voice for freedom of choice in medicine. It aims to protect and develop the status of complementary medicine and to ensure that the consumer has genuine freedom of choice in treatment of healthcare.

NEUROFIBROMATOSIS ASSOCIATION (NFA)

82 London Road
Kingston upon Thames
Surrey KT2 6PX
Helpline: 020 8547 1636
Tel: 020 8547 1636
Fax: 020 8974 5601
Email: nfa@zetnet.co.uk
Website: www.nfa.zetnet.co.uk

The NFA provides information for sufferers of neurofibromatosis, the general public and health professionals. It aims to build a network of support workers to provide a supportive/counselling service to sufferers and their families. It supports research into the condition.

NHS DIRECT

Helpline: 08457 4647
Website: www.nhsdirect.nhs.uk

NHS Direct provides free health information to the public and health professionals on maintaining and improving health, managing and treating illness, NHS and related services, self-help groups, waiting times for treatment, local NHS charter standards and how to complain about NHS services.

NORTHERN IRELAND CENTRE FOR POSTGRADUATE PHARMACEUTICAL EDUCATION AND TRAINING (NICPPET)

NICPPET FREEPOST
BeL 3149
Belfast BT9 7BR
Tel: 028 9027 2005
Fax: 028 9027 2368
Website: www.nicppet.org

NICPPET provides education and training for pharmacists in Northern Ireland.

NORTHERN IRELAND CHEST, HEART AND STROKE ASSOCIATION

21 Dublin Road
Belfast BT2 7FJ
Helpline: 0345 697299
Tel: 028 9032 0184
Fax: 028 9033 3487

The Northern Ireland Chest, Heart and Stroke Association works to try to prevent and alleviate chest, heart and stroke illnesses through health promotion, rehabilitation, welfare services and research.

NORTHERN IRELAND COMMUNITY ADDICTION SERVICE

40 Elmwood Avenue
Belfast BT9 6AZ
Helpline: 02890 664434
Tel: 028 9066 4434
Fax: 028 9066 4090
Email: nicas@dial.pipex.com

The Northern Ireland Cummunity Addiction Service is a charity providing a service for people who are abusing alcohol and drugs and people who are concerned about alcohol abuse. Working at a community level, it aims to prevent problems in society and to provide a treatment service.

NURSING HOME FEES AGENCY (NHFA)

Old Bank House
95 London Road
Headington
Oxford OX3 9AE
Helpline: 01865 750665
Tel: 01865 750665
Fax: 01865 742157
Email: admin-nhfa@msn.com
Website: www.nhfa.co.uk

The NHFA provides free specialist/legal advice on entering nursing homes and residential care. This includes advice on investments, local authority support and duties, eligibility for benefits. It aims to help older people to meet care costs for life, while preserving their capital, their independence, dignity and freedom of choice.

O

OBSESSIVE ACTION

Aberdeen Centre
22–24 Highbury Grove
London N5 2EA
Tel: 020 7226 4000
Fax: 020 7288 0828
Email: obsessive-action@demon.co.uk
Website: www.obsessive-action.demon.co.uk

Obsessive Action is a national charity for sufferers of obsessive compulsive disorder, their carers and interested professionals.

OFFICE OF FAIR TRADING

Field House
15–25 Bream's Buildings
London EC4 1PR
Tel: 020 7211 8000
Fax: 020 7211 8000

The Office of Fair Trading is a government department which keeps a watch on trading matters in the UK and protects both consumers and businessmen against unfair practices. This is achieved through the publication of information to help people get to know their rights and obligations; and the encouragement of Codes of Practice drawn up by trade organisations.

OFFICE OF HEALTH ECONOMICS

12 Whitehall
London SW1A 2DY
Tel: 0207 930 9203

The Office of Health Economics was founded by the Association of the British Pharmaceutical Industry in 1962. It exists to undertake research on the economic aspects of medical care, and to investigate health and social problems. It also collects data from other countries, and publishes its findings, data and conclusions.

OVACOME

St Bartholomew's Hospital
West Smithfield
London EC1A 7BE
Tel: 07071 781861
Email: ovacome@ovacome.org.uk
Website: www.ovacome.org.uk

Ovacome is a UK-wide support group for all those concerned with ovarian cancer, including sufferers, friends, families and carers. It aims to share personal experiences, link sufferers, provide information on treatments, screening and research and raise awareness of the condition.

OVEREATERS ANONYMOUS

PO Box 19
Stretford
Manchester M32 9EB
Helpline: 0762 6984674

Overeaters Anonymous works to encourage abstinence from compulsive eating and to help sufferers recover.

P

PAIN INTEREST GROUP

c/o RPSGB
1 Lambeth High Street
London SE1 7JN
Tel: 020 7735 9141

The Pain Interest Group aims to promote pharmaceutical involvement in pain control and to increase the knowledge base of the RPSGB membership. It does this by organising meetings with top level speakers and by disseminating the experience of other pharmacists to the rest of the membership. This is mainly achieved by case history presentations at meetings and via the newsletter, which is circulated as irregular intervals.

PAIN RELIEF FOUNDATION

Clinical Science's Centre
University Hospital
Aintree
Lower Lane
Liverpool L9 7AL
Tel: 0151 523 1486
Fax: 0151 521 6155
Email: pri@liv.ac.uk
Website: www.liv.ac.uk/pri

The Pain Relief Foundation supports clinical research into chronic pain conditions and post-graduate medical education into chronic pain management.

PAIN SOCIETY

9 Bedford Square
London WC1B 9RA
Tel: 020 7636 2750
Fax: 020 7323 2015
Email: painsoc@compuserve.com
Website: www.staff.ncl.ac.uk/r.j.hayes/painsoc.html

The Pain Society was established to help relieve suffering from pain by promotion of education, research and training in raising the standards of pain management.

PARKINSON'S DISEASE SOCIETY OF THE UNITED KINGDOM (PDS)

215 Vauxhall Bridge Road
London SW1V 1EJ
Tel: 020 7931 8080
Fax: 020 7233 9908
Email: mailbox@pdsnk.demon.co.uk
Website: www.parkinsons.org.uk

The Parkinson's Disease Society is a registered charity which helps patients and their relatives with the problems arising from Parkinson's disease. It also collects and disseminates information, and encourages and provides funds for research into the disease. The national headquarters are in London, with approximately 150 local voluntary branches. Medical and welfare advisory panels exist to help patients in the management of their condition.

PARTIALLY SIGHTED SOCIETY

9 Plato Place
72–74 St Dionis Road
London SW6 4TU
Tel: 020 7371 0289
Fax: 020 7371 0289

The Partially Sighted Society provides support, advice and information to visually impaired people and their families.

PATIENTS ASSOCIATION

PO Box 395
Harrow
Middlesex HA1 XJ
Helpline: 0845 6084455
Tel: 020 7423 9111
Fax: 020 7423 9119
Email: mailbox@patients-association.com
Website: www.patients-association.com

The Patients Association is a registered charity and provides an advice service and collective voice for patients, independent of government, the health professions and the drug industry. It is financed by members' subscriptions, donations and a government grant. The Association promotes and protects the interests of patients. It gives information and advice to individuals, and aims to promote understanding and good will between patients and those in medical and paramedical activities. Information leaflets are distributed free to members.

PHARMACEUTICAL SERVICES NEGOTIATING COMMITTEE (PSNC)

59 Buckingham Street
Aylesbury
Bucks HP20 2PJ
Tel: 01296 432823
Fax: 01296 392181
Website: www.psnc.org.uk

The Pharmaceutical Services Negotiating Committee is a statutory body representing the interests of pharmacy contractors who dispense NHS prescriptions. Pharmacists' fees and other payments are negotiated with the Department of Health, and cover, in addition to dispensing, a number of other services (e.g. appliance fitting and the oxygen therapy service). It is independent of the Royal Pharmaceutical Society of Great Britain and the National Pharmaceutical Association.

PHOBICS SOCIETY

4 Cheltenham Road
Chorlton-cum-Hardy
Manchester M21 9QN
Helpline: 0161 881 1937
Tel: 0161 881 1937

The Phobics Society offers help and support to people suffering from panic attacks, phobias and obsessive compulsive disorders.

POSITIVELY WOMEN

347–349 City Road
London EC1V 1LR
Helpline: 020 7713 0222

Tel: 020 7713 0444
Fax: 020 7713 1020
Email: positivelywomen@dircon.org.uk

Positively Women offers peer support, information and advocacy for women with HIV. It also offers crèche facilities and therapeutic services for children affected by HIV. It aims to empower women with HIV to make informed choices and to ensure that the voice of women with HIV is heard.

POST-ADOPTION CENTRE

5 Torriano Mews
Torriano Avenue
London NW5 2RZ
Helpline: 020 7485 2931
Tel: 020 7284 0555
Fax: 020 7482 2367
Email: advice@postadoptioncentre.org.uk
Website: www.postadoptioncentre.org.uk

The Post-Adoption Centre provides advice and counselling with the aim of meeting the needs of both children and adults experiencing problems which arise from adoption. It also provides workshops and professional training.

PRADER-WILLI SYNDROME ASSOCIATION (UK)

2 Wheatsheaf Close
Horsell
Woking
Surrey GU21 4BP
Helpline: 01483 724784
Tel: 01483 724784
Fax: 01483 724784
Website: www.pwsa-uk.demon.co.uk

PWSA(UK) works to provide information and support to people with Prader-Willi syndrome, their parents, friends and carers and to improve knowledge of the syndrome among the public and professionals.

PRE-ECLAMPSIA SOCIETY (PETS)

17 South Avenue
Hullbridge
Hockley
Essex S65 6DQ
Tel: 01702 232533

PETS provides support for sufferers of pre-eclamptic toxaemia. It has a lending library service, and publishes a quarterly newsletter and several booklets. It maintains a national network of women who are affected by pre-eclampsia and willing to talk over the telephone.

PREGNANCY ADVISORY SERVICE

17 Rosslyn Road
Twickenham
Middlesex TW1 2AR
Tel: 020 8891 6833
Fax: 020 8892 2633

The Pregnancy Advisory Service is a registered charity which provides counselling, support and termination of pregnancy. It also offers pregnancy testing, post-coital contraception, sterilisation, cervical smears and artificial insemination by donors.

PROPRIETARY ARTICLES TRADE ASSOCIATION (PATA)

5 Caxton Way
Watford Business Park
Watford WD1 8UA
Tel: 01923 211647
Fax: 01923 211648

The Proprietary Articles Trade Association was formed to ensure that pharmacists received a fair remuneration for their services through the operation of resale price maintenance. It does this through the support of the majority of manufacturers, wholesalers and community pharmacists.

PROPRIETARY ASSOCIATION OF GREAT BRITAIN (PAGB)

Vernon House
Sicilian Avenue
London WC1A 2QH
Tel: 020 7242 8331
Fax: 020 7405 7719
Website: www.pagb.org.uk

The Proprietary Association of Great Britain represents the manufacturers of medicines intended for use without a medical prescription, and is involved in all matters which affect the marketing and use of non-prescription medicines. It represents its members interests in negotiations with all government departments over legislation or other requirements which could influence these products. It administers Codes of Standards which require all labels, leaflets and advertising be accepted by the Association before publishing.

PROSTATE ASSOCIATION

Stanley House
22 Paradise Street
Rugby
Warwickshire CV21 3SZ
Helpline: 01788 643176
Tel: 01788 330054
Fax: 01788 330056
Email: philip@pha.u-net.com
Website: www.pha.u-net.com

The Prostate Association provides advice, help and information on prostate problems for sufferers, their families and carers and the media. It also aims to educate the public and professionals about support and treatment.

PROSTATE CANCER CHARITY

3 Angel Walk
Hammersmith
London W6 9HX
Tel: 0845 300 8383
Fax: 020 8222 7639
Email: info@prostate-cancer.org.uk
Website: www.prostate-cancer.org.uk

The Prostate Cancer Charity works to improve the care and welfare of people whose lives are affected by prostate cancer. It provides support and information to sufferers, their families and carers and funds patient oriented prostate cancer research.

PSORIASIS ASSOCIATION

7 Milton Street
Northampton NN2 7JG
Helpline: 01604 711129
Tel: 01604 711129
Fax: 01604 792894

The Psoriasis Association is a registered charity which provides support and mutual aid for those affected with psoriasis. It provides information on all aspects of the condition, and supports research into its causes, treatment and cure. Through a network of over 60 branches and groups, it supports individuals and provides a point of social contact. The Association also publishes a journal three times a year.

PSORIATIC ARTHROPATHY ALLIANCE (PAA)

PO Box 11
St Albans
Hertfordshire AL2 3JQ
Helpline: 01923 672837
Tel: 01923 672837
Fax: 01923 672837
Website: www.paalliance.org

The Psoriatic Arthropathy Alliance works to raise awareness and help people with psoriatic arthritis and psoriasis.

Q

QUEEN ELIZABETH'S FOUNDATION FOR DISABLED PEOPLE

Woodlands Road
Leatherhead
Surrey KT22 0BN
Helpline: 01306 742282
Tel: 01372 842204
Fax: 01372 844072

Queen Elizabeth's Foundation offers a variety of services to severely physically disabled adults, such as day care, vocational training, holidays, rehabilitation, assessment, accommodation, employment, mobility advice, respite care and further education.

QUIT

Victory House
170 Tottenham Court Road
London W1P 0HA
Helpline: 0800 002200
Tel: 020 7388 5775
Fax: 020 7388 5995
Email: quit-projects:clara.co.uk
Website: www.quit.org.uk

Quit is a national charity helping smokers to quit.

R

THE UK RADIOPHARMACY GROUP

Website: www.ukrg.org.uk

The Radiopharmacy Group brings together practising radiopharmacists and aims to develop close contacts with colleagues in medical physics and nuclear medicine. This has been formally acknowledged by incorporation of the group into the British Nuclear Medicine Society (BNMS) as the Radiopharmacy Group. The President of the group is a member of the Council of the BNMS.

RAYNAUD'S AND SCLERODERMA ASSOCIATION

112 Crewe Road
Alsager
Cheshire ST7 2JA
Helpline: 01270 872776
Tel: 01270 872776
Fax: 01270 883556
Email: webmaster:raynauds.demon.co.uk
Website: www.raynauds.demon.co.uk

Raynaud's and Scleroderma Association provides advice, support and information for people with Raynaud's scleroderma and similar conditions and also funds research to find better treatments.

RELATE

Herbert Gray College
Little Church Street
Rugby
Warwickshire CV21 3AP
Helpline: 01372 464100
Tel: 01788 573241
Fax: 01788 535007
Website: www.relate.org.uk

RELATE offers counselling and psychosexual therapy to adults who seek advice with relationships. Local centres exist throughout England, Wales and Northern Ireland and can be found in the telephone directory.

RELEASE

388 Old Street
London EC1V 9LT
Tel: 020 7729 9904 (10 am–4 pm); 020 7603 8654 (out of hours); 0800 776600

Release is the national drugs helpline.

RE-SOLV

30a High Street
Stone
Staffordshire ST15 8AW
Tel: 01785 817885
Fax: 01785 813205

Re-Solv (the Society for the Prevention of Solvent and Volatile Substance Abuse) provides information and education on all aspects of solvent abuse.

RESTRICTED GROWTH ASSOCIATION

PO Box 8
Countesthorpe
Leicester LE8 5ZS
Tel: 0116 247 8913

The Restricted Growth Association works to remove the prejudice experienced by individuals of restricted growth and to improve their quality of life. It also aims to reduce the fear and distress in a family when a child of restricted growth is born.

ROYAL ASSOCIATION FOR DISABILITY AND REHABILITATION (RADAR)

12 City Forum
250 City Road
London EC1V 8AF
Helpline: 020 7250 3222
Tel: 020 7250 3222
Fax: 020 7250 0212
Email: radar@radar.org.uk
Website: www.radar.org.uk

RADAR is an umbrella organisation with more than 400 local associations in membership. It provides advice and information concerning access, holidays, housing, and mobility. It also gives welfare advice and help, and provides skill and disability training.

ROYAL NATIONAL INSTITUTE FOR THE BLIND (RNIB)

224 Great Portland Street
London W1W 5AA
Helpline: 0845 766 9999
Tel: 020 7388 1266
Fax: 020 7388 2034
Website: www.rnib.org.uk

The Royal National Institute for the Blind is a registered charity and works for all Britain's 135 000 blind people. It provides an education advisory service, schools and colleges; further education for school leavers, commercial college and a school of physiotherapy; a rehabilitation centre; residential care homes for the elderly; hotels and a hostel; a conference centre; shops; careers advice and employment services; advice services on social security benefits and monitors developments in legislation affecting the interests of visually handicapped people; braille and tape libraries for students; and the talking-book library. It gives advice and practical help to blind people and their families, and to teachers, social workers, health-care staff and others. It also supports research into the prevention of blindness, and into the needs of the visually handicapped.

ROYAL NATIONAL INSTITUTE FOR THE DEAF (RNID)

19–23 Featherstone Street
London EC1Y 8SL
Tel: 020 7296 8000
Fax: 020 7296 8199
Email: helpline@rnid.org.uk
Website: www.rnid.org.uk

The Royal National Institute for the Deaf is a voluntary organisation concerned with all aspects of deafness and hearing impairment, in all age groups. It provides a wide range of services to hearing-impaired people, their families and to professional people working with them. Services include education and employment information, a library, medical research, rehabilitative and longer term residential care services, and scientific and technical services.

THE ROYAL SOCIETY OF HEALTH (RSH)

RSH House
38a St George's Drive
London SW1V 4BH
Tel: 020 7630 0121
Fax: 020 7321 0523

The Royal Society of Health is a registered charity and its aims are to promote the protection and preservation of health and to advance health-related sciences. Members are recruited from all health and health-related professions (including pharmacy), and the level of entry is based upon the qualifications held. The Society holds examinations in a wide range of health subjects, and promotes conferences, lectures and visits. A bi-monthly journal containing papers on health matters, nutrition, and environmental and social services is published by the Society.

RURAL PHARMACISTS' ASSOCIATION

c/o South Dene
Gratton Lane
Yelverton
Devon PL20 6AW
Tel: 01822 853515
Fax: 01822 855337

The Rural Pharmacists' Association exists to ensure that all rural patients receive the same professional standards of pharmaceutical supervision and care as patients in urban areas, to protect and improve the position of the rural pharmacist by all legal means, and to advance the profession of pharmacy in rural areas. It also gives counsel and advice to rural pharmacists, and advises the Council of the Royal Pharmaceutical Society on matters affecting rural pharmacy. Membership is open to any pharmacist who is engaged in, or actively considering engaging in, rural pharmacy, or pharmacists who show interest in and work for the benefit of rural pharmacy.

S

SAD (SEASONAL AFFECTIVE DISORDER) ASSOCIATION

PO Box 989
Steyning
West Sussex BN44 3HG
Helpline: 01903 814942
Fax: 01903 879939
Website: www.sada.org.uk

SAD Association informs the public and professionals about SAD in order to provide support for sufferers and their families. It also promotes research into causes and treatment of SAD.

ST JOHN AMBULANCE

1 Grosvenor Crescent
London SW1X 7EF
Helpline: 020 7235 5231
Tel: 020 7235 5231
Fax: 020 7235 0796
Email: postmaster@nhgsa.org.uk
Website: www.sja.org.uk

St John Ambulance is a charitable foundation of the Order of St John. Uniformed members attend public events, providing first-aid cover, and first-aid training is given to industry, in schools and to the general public. The St John Ambulance Air Wing provides emergency transport of donor organs for transplant, and the Aeromedical Service provides fully trained staff to accompany those taken ill while abroad on their journey to Britain. Cadets and Badgers are organisations which give young people the chance to pursue a wide variety of activities, and also learn about first-aid and nursing.

THE SAMARITANS

10 The Grove
Slough
Berkshire SL1 1QP
Helpline: 0345 909090
Tel: 01753 216500
Fax: 01753 819004
Email: admin@samaritans.org.uk
Website: www.samaritans.org.uk

The Samaritans is a registered charity, available 24 hours a day to provide confidential support to anyone passing through crisis and at risk of suicide.

SCHIZOPHRENIA ASSOCIATION OF GREAT BRITAIN (SAGB)

Bryn Hyfryd
The Crescent
Bangor
Gwynedd LL57 2AG
Helpline: 01248 354048
Tel: 01248 354048
Fax: 01248 354048
Email: sagb@btinternet.com
Website: www.btinternet.com/~sagb

The Schizophrenia Association of Great Britain is a registered charity and aims to help patients suffering from mental illness and their families in every possible way; and to promote research into the biochemical and nutritional factors involved in producing psychiatric symptoms in the genetically inherited form. It aims to educate the public about schizophrenia through newsletters, conferences, symposia and lectures. Grants are also made available for research work.

SCOLIOSIS ASSOCIATION (UK)

2 Ivebury Court
325 Latimer Road
London W10 6RA
Helpline: 020 8964 1166
Tel: 020 8964 5453
Email: info@sauk.org.uk
Website: www.sauk.org.uk

This association works to support people with scoliosis and to promote knowledge about the disease among the public and professionals.

SCOPE

(Formerly the Spastics Society)
PO Box 833
Milton Keynes
Buckinghamshire MK12 5NY
Helpline: 0808 800 3333
Fax: 01908 321051
Email: cphelpline@scope.org.uk
Website: www.scope.org.uk

SCOPE is a national organisation which supports services, information and advice for children and adults with cerebral palsy, and their families.

SCOTTISH ASSOCIATION FOR THE DEAF

Moray House
Institute of Education
Heriot-Watt University
Holyrood House
Edinburgh EH8 8AQ
Helpline: 0131 558 3390
Tel: 0131 557 0591
Fax: 0131 557 6922

The Scottish Association for the Deaf works to promote the quality of life for all deaf people in Scotland. It assesses the needs of deaf people to enable them to gain more independence and equal opportunities in the workplace.

SCOTTISH ASSOCIATION FOR MENTAL HEALTH

Cumbria House
15 Carlton Court
Glasgow G5 9JP
Helpline: 0141 568 7000
Tel: 0141 568 7000
Fax: 0141 568 7001
Email: enquire@samh.org.uk

The Scottish Association for Mental Health aims to provide services to people with mental health problems and campaigns for recognition of their rights as human beings and citizens.

SCOTTISH CENTRE FOR POST QUALIFICATION PHARMACEUTICAL EDUCATION (SCPPE)

University of Strathclyde
27 Taylor Street
Glasgow G4 0NR
Tel: 0141 548 4273
Fax: 0141 553 4102
Email: scppe@strath.ac.uk
Website: www.scppe.strath.ac.uk

SCPPE provides education and training for hospital and community pharmacists working within the NHS in Scotland.

SCOTTISH COT DEATH TRUST
Royal Hospital for Sick Children
Yorkhill
Glasgow G3 8SJ
Helpline: 0141 357 3946
Tel: 0141 357 3946
Fax: 0141 334 1376
Email: hblw@clinmed.gla.ac.uk

The Scottish Cot Death Trust aims to raise funds for research into cot death, to improve support for bereaved parents and to educate the public and health professionals about cot death.

SCOTTISH COUNCIL ON ALCOHOL
166 Buchanan Street
Glasgow G1 2NH
Tel: 0141 333 9677
Fax: 0141 333 1606
Email: sca@clara.net

The Scottish Council on Alcohol promotes safe and sensible drinking habits among those people who choose to drink and is working to develop a network of local councils on alcohol. It works with courts, employers, prisons and statutory agencies on a national and international basis.

SCOTTISH DOWN'S SYNDROME ASSOCIATION
158 Balgreen Road
Edinburgh EH11 3AU
Helpline: 0131 313 4225
Tel: 0131 313 4225
Fax: 0131 313 4285

The Scottish Down's Syndrome Association supports people with Down's syndrome and their families and carers throughout Scotland.

SCOTTISH MOTOR NEURONE DISEASE ASSOCIATION
76 Firhill Road
Glasgow G20 7BA
Helpline: 0141 945 1077
Tel: 0141 945 1077
Fax: 0141 945 2578

The Scottish Motor Neurone Disease Association aims to offer advice and support to people with motor neuron disease and their families and carers. It also aims to finance research into the cause and treatment of motor neuron disease.

SCOTTISH SPINA BIFIDA ASSOCIATION
190 Queensferry Road
Edinburgh EH4 2BW
Helpline: 08459 111112
Tel: 0131 332 0743
Fax: 0131 343 3651
Email: ssbahq@compuserve.com
Website: http://ourworld.compuserve.com/homepages/SSBAhq

The Scottish Spina Bifida Association works to enhance public awareness and understanding of people with spina bifida/hydrocephalus and related conditions. It aims to obtain provision for the specialist needs of these people and their families.

SENSE (THE NATIONAL DEAFBLIND AND RUBELLA ASSOCIATION)
11–13 Clifton Terrace
Finsbury Park
London N4 3SR
Tel: 020 7272 7774
Fax: 020 7272 6012
Email: enquiries@sense.org.uk
Website: www.sense.org.uk

Sense provides information and support services for children and young adults who are deaf-blind and their families and carers. It works to improve the quality of life for people who are deaf-blind by campaigning and providing services for their specialist needs.

SHELTER
88 Old Street
London EC1V 9HU
Helpline: 0808 800 4444
Fax: 020 7505 2169
Email: info@shelter.org.uk
Website: www.shelter.org.uk

Shelter provides free independent housing advice through a national network of housing aid centres. It campaigns on behalf of the homeless and poorly housed people for a fairer housing system to make affordable housing available to everybody.

SICKLE CELL SOCIETY
54 Station Road
London NW10 4UA
Helpline: 020 8961 7795
Tel: 020 8961 7795
Fax: 020 8961 8346
Email: sicklecellsoc@btinternet.com
Website: www.sicklecellsociety.org

The Sickle Cell Society provides support to sufferers of sickle cell and their families in the form of welfare and educational grants, holiday and recreational facilities. It promotes awareness of the condition through leaflets, books and videos.

SOCIETY FOR THE PROTECTION OF UNBORN CHILDREN
5–6 St Mathew Street
London SW1P 2JT
Helpline: 0845 603 8501
Tel: 020 7222 5845
Fax: 020 7222 0630
Email: enquiry@spuc.org.uk
Website: www.spuc.org.uk

The Society for the Protection of Unborn Children defends and protects the life of unborn children and the welfare of mothers before and after giving birth. It defends the right to live of disabled people before and after birth and provides post-abortion counselling.

SOCIETY OF APOTHECARIES OF LONDON
Blackfriars Lane
London EC4V 6EJ
Tel: 020 7236 1189
Fax: 020 7329 3177
Website: www.apothecaries.org.uk

The Society of Apothecaries was founded in 1617 by Royal Charter as a Guild for Apothecaries in London. In 1815, under the Apothecaries Act, the Society was empowered to set up the first non-university licensing board to examine candidates who wished to practise medicine in England and Wales. The Act also made the Society responsible for running a register of those who were qualified to practice, and was the earliest legislation requiring a candidate to show that he had clinical experience. In the Act, the Society was also made responsible for examining assistants who worked with doctors in dispensing. The Society still conducts examinations 11 times a year for a registerable licence to practise medicine in the UK, and examines candidates for Diplomas in Medical Jurisprudence, Venereology, the History of Medicine and the Philosophy of Medicine.

SOCIETY OF CHIROPODISTS AND PODIATRISTS
53 Wellbeck Street
London W1M 7HE
Tel: 020 7486 3381
Fax: 020 7935 6359
Email: eng@scpod.org
Website: www.feetforlife.org

The Society of Chiropodists and Podiatrists is the professional organisation for state registered chiropodists.

SOTOS SYNDROME GROUP
2 Mayfield Avenue
Chiswick
London W4 1PW
Tel: 020 8994 7625
Fax: 020 8995 9075

The Sotos Syndrome Group offers support and advice to people with Sotos syndrome and their families and carers.

SPINAL INJURIES ASSOCIATION
76 St James' Lane
London N10 3DF
Helpline: 0800 980 00501
Tel: 020 8444 2121
Fax: 020 8444 3761
Email: sia@spinal.co.uk
Website: www.spinal.co.uk

The Spinal Injuries Association is run by people with spinal injuries for other sufferers. It aims to encourage sufferers to return to normal life and it provides information, welfare, a care attendant agency and advice on holidays.

STILLBIRTH AND NEONATAL DEATH SOCIETY (SANDS)
28 Portland Place
London W1N 4DE
Helpline: 020 7436 5881
Tel: 020 7436 7940
Fax: 020 7436 3715
Email: support@uk-sands.org
Website: www.uk-sands.org

SANDS provides support to people bereaved through pregnancy loss, stillbirth and neonatal death. It aims to improve awareness among the public and professionals of the needs and feelings of bereaved parents.

STROKE ASSOCIATION
CHSA House
123–127 Whitecross Street
London EC1Y 8JJ
Helpline: 0845 3033 100
Tel: 020 7566 0300
Fax: 020 7490 2686
Email: stroke@stroke.org.uk
Website: www.stroke.org.uk

The Stroke Association is a registered charity which works to prevent stroke and helps people who suffer from stroke. It offers advice, funds research, organises conferences and publishes books and leaflets.

STURGE WEBER FOUNDATION UK
348 Pinhoe Road
Whipton
Exeter EX4 8AF
Helpline: 01392 464675
Tel: 01392 464675
Fax: 01392 464675
Email: support@sturgeweber.org.uk
Website: www.sturgeweber.org.uk

The Sturge Weber Foundation supports people with this condition and aims to raise public awareness of it.

T

TELANGIECTASIA SELF-HELP GROUP
39 Sunny Croft
Downley
High Wycombe
Buckinghamshire HP13 5UQ
Helpline: 01494 528047
Tel: 01494 528047
Email: tshg@cwcom.net
Website: www.tolangiectasia.cwccom.net

The Telangiectasia Self-help Group maintains a register of sufferers and puts affected sufferers and their families in touch with each other. It publishes a newsletter informing members of developments in the treatment of the disease.

TERRENCE HIGGINS TRUST/BM AIDS
52–54 Grays Inn Road
London WC1X 8JU
Helpline: 020 7242 1010
Tel: 020 7831 0330
Fax: 020 7242 0121
Email: info@tht.org.uk
Website: www.tht.org.uk

The Terrence Higgins Trust is a registered charity which provides information and support for people with AIDS and AIDS-related complex (ARC), and those who are HIV-positive. This is carried out through various groups within the Trust (e.g. buddies, telephone help line, legal services, health education, drugs education group, families support group, and partners support group). Health education to the community at large is also promoted. The drugs education group provides support to intravenous drug users who are either HIV-positive or who have AIDS/ARC. A mobile health education display attends conferences, seminars, pubs and discos.

THALIDOMIDE SOCIETY

19 Central Avenue
Pinner
Middlesex HA5 5BT
Helpline: 020 8868 5309
Tel: 020 8868 5309
Fax: 020 8868 5309
Email: info@thalsoc.demon.co.uk

The Thalidomide Society provides advice, support and information to people with thalidomide-related and similar disabilities.

TOURETTE SYNDROME (UK) ASSOCIATION

Old Grange House
The Twitten
Southview Road
Crowborough
East Sussex TN6 1HF
Helpline: 01892 669151
Tel: 01892 669151
Fax: 01892 669151

The Tourette Syndrome Association provides support for sufferers of this disease and their families. It also maintains a register of physicians familiar with the treatment of this condition.

TRAUMA AFTERCARE TRUST (TACT)

Buttfields
1 The Farthings
Withington
Gloucestershire GL54 4DF
Helpline: 0800 1696814
Tel: 01242 890306
Fax: 01242 890498
Email: tact@tacthq.demon.co.uk
Website: www.tacthq.demon.co.uk

TACT offers support for people suffering from post-traumatic stress disorder.

TURNING POINT

New Loom House
101 Backchurch Lane
London E1 1LU
Helpine: 020 7702 2300
Tel: 020 7702 2300
Fax: 020 7702 1456
Email: tpmail@turningpoint.co.uk
Website: www.turning-point.co.uk

Turning Point is a national charity which helps people with drug and alcohol problems, mental health problems and learning difficulties.

TWINS AND MULTIPLE BIRTHS ASSOCIATION (TAMBA)

Harnott House
309 Chester Road
Little Sutton
Ellesmere Port CH66 1QQ
Helpline: 01732 868000
Tel: 0870 1214000
Fax: 0870 1214001
Website: www.surrey.org.uk/tamba

The Twins and Multiple Births Association is a registered charity which gives encouragement and support to parents of twins and multiple births, and aims to educate the public and medical profession of the incidence, effects and problems of multiple births. It provides information and literature for parents of multiple births. It also promotes the establishment of twins clubs, and maintains a national register of such clubs (currently nearly 200). A medical and education subgroup exists for professionals involved in health, education, social care or research.

U

UNITED KINGDOM BRAIN TUMOUR SOCIETY

22 Cambridge Road
Aldershot
Hampshire GU11 3JZ
Tel: 01252 653807
Fax: 01252 653807
Email: give.hope@virgin.net
Website:http://freespace.virgin.net/give.hope/guest/ukbts.html

The UK Brain Tumour Society is the national support group for people affected by brain tumours and their families and carers.

UNITED KINGDOM CLINICAL PHARMACY ASSOCIATION

C/o Mrs Pat Kennedy
Alpha House
Countesthorpe Road
South Wigston
Leicester LE18 4PJ
Tel: 0116 277 6999
Fax: 0116 277 6272
Email: pkennedy@ukcpa.u-net.com
Website: www.ukcpa.org.uk

The United Kingdom Clinical Pharmacy Association was established in 1981 to further the interests of all pharmacists whose activities are directed towards the patient. The main objectives of the Association are to improve the quality of patient care by encouraging the rational and effective use of medicines and the promotion of an interdisciplinary approach to drug therapy; to stimulate the development of clinical pharmacy in the UK; and to develop means to evaluate the pharmacist's contribution to overall patient care. Student membership is open to all pharmacy students and pre-registration graduates. Ordinary membership is open to all pharmacists working in the UK.

UNITED KINGDOM THALASSAEMIA SOCIETY

19 The Broadway
Southgate Circus
London N14 6PH
Helpline: 020 8882 0011
Fax: 020 8882 8618
Email: office@ukts.org.uk
Website: www.ukts.org.uk

The UK Thalassaemia Society offers support to sufferers of thalassaemia and their families, to raise awareness of the problems it causes, to promote research into the condition, and to bring together affected families.

UROSTOMY ASSOCIATION

Buckland
Beaumont Park
Danbury
Essex CM3 4DE
Tel: 01245 224294
Fax: 01245 227569

The Urostomy Association is a registered charity which aims to assist patients both before and following the formation of a urinary stoma, through counselling. Is also supports them in returning to lead a full life. There are 22 branches nationwide, and a postal branch covers areas not serviced by a local branch and for those unable to attend meetings.

V

VALUES INTO ACTION

Oxford House
Derbyshire Street
London E2 6HG
Tel: 020 7729 5436
Fax: 020 7729 7797

Values into Action campaigns to achieve laws, services and public attitudes which will allow people with learning difficulties to become valued citizens.

VEGAN SOCIETY

Donald Watson House
7 Battle Road
St Leonards on Sea
East Sussex TN37 7AA
Tel: 01424 427393
Fax: 01424 717064
Website: www.vegansociety.com

The Vegan Society offers information on food and related matters to people who are vegans or thinking about becoming so. It publishes a booklet of foods suitable for those who neither consume nor use any animal products.

VEGETARIAN SOCIETY

Parkdale
Dunham Road
Altrincham
Cheshire WA14 4QG
Tel: 0161 925 2000
Fax: 0161 926 9182
Website: www.vegsoc.org

The Vegetarian Society offers information on food and related matters to people who are vegetarians or thinking about becoming so. It publishes a booklet of foods suitable for vegetarians.

VICTIM SUPPORT

Cranmer House
39 Brixton Road
London SW9 6DZ
Helpline: 0845 3030 900
Tel: 020 7735 9166
Fax: 020 7582 5712

Victim Support is a national charity working for the victims of crime. Staff and trained volunteers in local schemes and crown court witness services provide emotional and practical support and information to victims and witnesses of crime. It works to increase awareness of the effects of crime and to gain better recognition of victims' rights.

VITILIGO SOCIETY

125 Kennington Road
London SE11 6SF
Tel: 020 7840 0855
Fax: 020 7840 0866
Website: www.vitiligosociety.org

The Vitiligo Society provides advice and support for sufferers of this skin condition and their families.

W

WALES COUNCIL FOR THE BLIND

Shand House
20 Newport Road
Cardiff CF24 0DB
Helpline: 029 2047 3954
Tel: 029 2047 3954
Fax: 029 2045 5710
Email: staff@wcbnet.freeserve.co.uk
Website: www.wcbnet.freeserve.co.uk

Wales Council for the Blind aims to empower visually impaired people in Wales by promoting and monitoring services, encouraging improvement of services and coordinating and encouraging statutory and voluntary efforts.

WALES COUNCIL FOR THE DEAF

Glenview House
Court House Street
Pontypridd CF37 1JY
Tel: 01443 485687
Fax: 01443 408555

WEIGHT WATCHERS (UK) LTD

Kidwells Park House
Kidwells Park Drive
Maidenhead
Berkshire SL6 8YT
Tel: 0345 123000

Weight Watchers works to help people lose weight, working through local groups.

WELLBEING

27 Sussex Place
Regents Park
London NW1 4SP
Helpline: 020 7262 5337
Tel: 020 7262 5337
Fax: 020 7724 7725
Email: wb239821@aol.com
Website: www.wellbeing.demon.co.uk

Wellbeing is the research arm of the Royal College of Obstetricians and Gynaecologists and a health research charity for women and babies. It funds research into all women's health matters and provides information to women on such matters.

WELSH CENTRE FOR POSTGRADUATE PHARMACEUTICAL EDUCATION (WCPPE)

8 North Road
Cathays
Cardiff CF10 3DY
Tel: 029 2087 4784
Fax: 029 2087 4540
Website: www.cf.ac.uk/phrmy/WCPPE

WCPPE provides a continuing professional development service to all pharmacists and their support staff in Wales.

WILLIAMS SYNDROME FOUNDATION

161 High Street
Tonbridge
Kent TN9 1BX
Tel: 01732 365152

The Williams Syndrome Foundation provides support and advice to families of children affected by Williams syndrome and infant hypercalcaemia. It funds research, offers an advisory service and pays for group holidays for unaccompanied adults and for families.

WOMEN'S HEALTH

52 Featherstone Street
London EC1Y 8RT
Helpline: 020 7251 6580
Tel: 020 7251 6333
Fax: 020 7608 0928
Website: www.womenshealthlondon.org.uk

Women's Health offers information on a wide range of topics affecting women's health, helping women to make informed choices. It also has a library open to the public.

WOMEN'S NATIONWIDE CANCER CONTROL CAMPAIGN (WNCCC)

Suna House
128–130 Curtain Road
London EC2A 3AQ
Tel: 020 7729 4688; 020 7729 1735
Fax: 020 7613 0771
Email: wncc@admin.co.uk
Website: www.wncc.org.uk

The Women's National Cancer Control Campaign is a registered charity and was formed to help women overcome their fears about cancer, and to take simple precautions which could save their lives, through education and early detection. A wide range of literature is produced to educate and inform women about cervical smears and breast self-examination. The Campaign also has several mobile clinics and organises screening for women at their place of work and in local shopping centres. It can also provide enquirers with details of screening facilities throughout the country.

WOMEN'S NUTRITIONAL ADVISORY SERVICE

PO Box 268
Lewes
East Sussex BN7 2QN
Tel: 01273 487366
Fax: 01273 487576
Email: wnas@wnas.org.uk

The Women's Nutritional Advisory Service offers tailor-made nutritional and lifestyle programmes for premenstrual syndrome, menopause, sugar craving, irritable bowel syndrome, myalgic encephalomyelitis and fatigue.

Part C

Symptom and disease identification

Introduction

Although pharmacists are not expected to diagnose disease, it is important that they are aware of the diverse range of conditions which can cause many of the more common symptoms. It will be readily apparent from the descriptions given in the disease monographs that comprise Chapters 1–13 that individual diseases can cause many different symptoms. Some symptoms may be considered characteristic of a particular disease and provide a valuable clue to the correct diagnosis. Other symptoms, however, are non-specific and may become manifest in a wide variety of conditions; in such cases, the symptom may occur as a consequence of generalised ill-health. Pharmacists who are presented with one or more symptoms by members of the public must be aware of the possible causes and, even in the absence of diagnosis, must be able to differentiate between the symptoms of minor illness and those which forebode a more serious condition. The means by which this can be satisfactorily achieved for a wide range of common symptoms has been discussed in Chapter 18.

Part C of this book has been written to provide pharmacists with a quick reference guide to the possible causes of certain symptoms. The information has been derived by extracting the symptoms recorded in the disease monographs, and tabulating the causative conditions under the disease classifications used in this volume. It must be stressed, however, that by virtue of its method of preparation, the disease list stated under each symptom cannot be comprehensive. Other diseases may cause the symptom, and this listing is intended to provide a perspective of the diversity of causative conditions. Equally, no attempt has been made in this reference guide to quantify or qualify the nature of the symptom; if pharmacists are confronted with a patient reporting a particular symptom, use of this guide will indicate many of the possible causes of the symptom and may suggest a suitable course for further questioning. The guide will also enable pharmacists to consult the appropriate monographs to gain a detailed description of the clinical picture in which the reported symptom can occur. It will also be apparent that the description of one symptom does not diagnose a disease; almost all diseases can only be characterised by recognition of two or more symptoms.

To make the guide concise, many individual symptoms have been grouped under a single heading. The list of symptoms incorporated under this umbrella term immediately follows the symptom heading.

A

Abdominal distension

[abdominal mass; abdominal swelling; ascites; hepatomegaly; hepatosplenomegaly; splenomegaly]

Blood and lymph disorders
- amyloidosis
- haemolytic anaemias
- haemolytic disease of the newborn
- polycythaemia vera
- splenomegaly

Cardiovascular system disorders
- cor pulmonale
- right heart failure
- tricuspid regurgitation
- tricuspid stenosis

Gastrointestinal and related disorders
- acute hepatitis
- acute pancreatitis
- ascites
- chronic cholecystitis
- chronic hepatitis
- cirrhosis of the liver
- coeliac disease
- congenital megacolon
- dyspepsia
- focal ischaemia of the small intestine
- haemolytic jaundice
- ileus
- irritable bowel syndrome
- toxic megacolon
- tropical sprue
- tuberculous peritonitis

Gynaecological disorders
- dysmenorrhoea
- premenstrual syndrome

Infections
- American trypanosomiasis
- brucellosis
- chronic fulminating meningococcaemia
- cytomegalovirus infection
- giardiasis
- infectious mononucleosis
- infective endocarditis
- toxocariasis
- toxoplasmosis (congenital)
- trematode infections
- visceral leishmaniasis
- Weil's disease

Malignant disease
- cancer of the liver
- cancer of the stomach
- Hodgkin's disease
- leukaemias
- ovarian tumours
- pancreatic (exocrine) cancer

Metabolic disorders
- galactosaemia
- glycogen storage diseases
- hepatolenticular degeneration
- hereditary fructose intolerance

Musculoskeletal and connective tissue disorders
- systemic lupus erythematosus

Nervous system disorders
- Reye's syndrome

Nutritional disorders
- lactose intolerance

Abdominal pain and discomfort

[abdominal ache; abdominal colic; abdominal fullness; abdominal tenderness; biliary colic; epigastric pain; griping pain; hepatic tenderness; pelvic pain; renal colic; suprapubic pain]

Non-specific causes
- drugs
- hernia
- insect bites
- intestinal obstruction
- ovarian cyst
- psychosomatic causes
- rupture (e.g. of the liver or spleen)

Blood and lymph disorders
- anaphylactoid purpura
- polycythaemia vera
- sickle-cell anaemia
- splenomegaly

Cardiovascular system disorders
- aortic aneurysm
- myocardial infarction
- right heart failure
- tricuspid regurgitation

Endocrine disorders
- Addison's disease
- adrenocortical insufficiency, acute

Gastrointestinal and related disorders
- appendicitis
- ascites
- cholangitis
- cholecystitis
- choledocholithiasis
- chronic persistent hepatitis
- cirrhosis of the liver
- Crohn's disease
- diverticular disease
- dyspepsia
- gallstones
- gastritis
- gastroenteritis
- ileus
- irritable bowel syndrome
- ischaemic gastrointestinal disorders
- pancreatitis
- peptic ulceration
- peritonitis
- toxic megacolon
- tropical sprue
- ulcerative colitis
- Whipple's disease

Gynaecological disorders
- dysmenorrhoea
- endometriosis

Infections
- ascariasis
- botulism
- cestode infections
- cystitis
- dysentery
- epididymitis
- giardiasis
- hookworm infection
- Legionnaire's disease
- leptospirosis
- mumps
- pelvic actinomycosis
- pneumonia
- prostatitis
- pseudomembranous colitis
- pyelonephritis
- salmonellal infections
- salpingitis
- shigellosis
- strongyloidiasis
- trematode infections
- trichiniasis
- trichuriasis
- urinary-tract infections

Malignant disease
- bladder cancer
- cancer of the gall bladder
- cancer of the liver
- cancer of the stomach
- carcinoid syndrome
- cervical cancer
- chronic leukaemias
- colorectal cancer
- ovarian tumours
- pancreatic (exocrine) cancer
- phaeochromocytoma
- renal cancer
- spinal cord tumours
- Zollinger–Ellison syndrome

Metabolic disorders
hypercalcaemia
porphyrias
Musculoskeletal and connective tissue disorders
polyarteritis nodosa
Nervous system disorders
partial seizures
Nutritional disorders
lactose intolerance
Obstetric disorders
ectopic pregnancy
pre-eclampsia and eclampsia
Renal disorders
acute glomerulonephritis
polycystic kidney disease
renal calculi and colic
Skin disorders
hereditary angioedema

Abscess formation *see also* Eye abscess

Ear disorders
mastoiditis
Infections
osteomyelitis
Skin disorders
pilonidal disease

Accident-prone

Nervous system disorders
amphetamine-type drug dependence
barbiturate-type drug dependence
volatile solvent-type drug dependence

Acne *see* Skin lesions

Altered bowel habit *see also* Constipation, Diarrhoea *and* Constipation and diarrhoea
[increased difficulty in bowel evacuation; increased frequency of bowel evacuation; reduced frequency of bowel evacuation]

Endocrine disorders
hyperthyroidism
Gastrointestinal and related disorders
constipation
diarrhoea
diverticular disease
irritable bowel syndrome
proctitis

Amnesia *see also* Memory impairment

Infections
infective endocarditis
Legionnaire's disease
Malignant disease
intracranial tumours
Nervous system disorders
dialysis encephalopathy
partial seizures

Anaemia

Blood and lymph disorders
thrombotic thrombocytopenic purpura
Gastrointestinal and related disorders
coeliac disease
peptic ulceration
polyps
short-bowel syndrome
ulcerative colitis
Infections
abdominal actinomycosis
African trypanosomiasis
hookworm infection
trichuriasis
visceral leishmaniasis
Malignant disease
cancer of the stomach
leukaemias
non-Hodgkin's lymphoma
oesophageal cancer
ovarian tumours
Musculoskeletal and connective tissue disorders
giant cell arteritis
osteopetrosis
rheumatoid arthritis
systemic lupus erythematosus
Nutritional disorders
pyridoxine deficiency
vitamin A deficiency
Renal disorders
interstitial nephritis
renal failure

Anal and rectal bleeding

Gastrointestinal and related disorders
anal fissure
anorectal fistula
Crohn's disease
haemorrhoids
polyps
proctitis

Anal discomfort *see also* Anogenital lesions

Gastrointestinal and related disorders
anal fissure
anorectal fistula
haemorrhoids
proctitis

Anal skin tag

Gastrointestinal and related disorders
anal fissure
haemorrhoids

Anginal pain *see* Chest pain

Anogenital lesions *see also* Anal discomfort and Vaginal discomfort

Infections
herpesvirus infections (HSV 2)
Skin disorders
lichen planus

Anorexia *see* Loss of appetite

Appetite, loss of *see* Loss of appetite

Arthralgia *see* Joint pain and tenderness

Aura

Nervous system disorders
epilepsy
migraine

B

Back pain and tenderness
[back ache; loin pain; loin tenderness; lumbago]

Cardiovascular system disorders
aortic aneurysm
Gynaecological disorders
dysmenorrhoea
endometriosis
Infections
African trypanosomiasis
brucellosis
chickenpox
herpes zoster
influenza
lymphatic filariasis
Marburg disease and Ebola fever
prostatitis
pyelonephritis
salpingitis
tetanus
viral meningitis
yellow fever
Malignant disease
cervical cancer
renal cell carcinoma
Musculoskeletal and connective tissue disorders
ankylosing spondylitis
fibrositis
osteoporosis
sciatica
Nervous system disorders
anxiety
Renal disorders
acute glomerulonephritis
acute renal failure
polycystic kidney disease
renal calculi and colic

Bad breath *see* Breath, abnormal odour

Behaviour disturbances *see also* Emotional disturbances *and* Perception disturbances
[aggression; agitation; confusion; delirium; delirium tremens; exhibitionism; hyperactivity; intolerance of noise; involuntary noises; irrationality; loss of concentration; loss of self-control; obsession; personality disorders; promiscuity; psychoses; resistance to change; restlessness; self-neglect; temper tantrums; unreliability; violence; wild and illogical speech; withdrawn]

Blood and lymph disorders
thrombotic thrombocytopenic purpura
Cardiovascular system disorders
atherosclerosis in cerebral arteries
Endocrine disorders
hypoglycaemia
hypopituitarism
primary aldosteronism
type I diabetes mellitus
Infections
African trypanosomiasis
cryptococcal meningitis
cysticercosis
encephalitis
infective endocarditis
paratyphoid fever
Pontiac fever
postviral fatigue syndrome
psittacosis
pyogenic meningitis
rabies
typhoid fever
typhus fevers
Malignant disease
insulinoma
intracranial tumours
Metabolic disorders
hepatolenticular degeneration
hypercalcaemia
hypernatraemia
hypocalcaemia
hyponatraemia
porphyrias
Musculoskeletal and connective tissue disorders
polyarteritis nodosa
systemic lupus erythematosus
Nervous system disorders
anxiety
autism
cerebral palsy
chorea
dementia
depressive disorders
dialysis encephalopathy
drug dependence
extradural haemorrhage
Gilles de la Tourette syndrome
hepatic encephalopathy
mania and manic-depressive illness
mental retardation
post-tonic-clonic epileptic seizures
schizophrenia
subarachnoid haemorrhage
subdural haemorrhage
tardive dyskinesia
Nutritional disorders
anorexia nervosa
beri-beri
bulimia nervosa
Renal disorders
renal failure

Blinking *see also* Eyelid fluttering

Eye disorders
corneal ulceration

Nervous system disorders
Gilles de la Tourette syndrome

Blister *see* Skin lesions

Blood from the anus *see* Anal and rectal bleeding

Blood from the nipple *see* Breast abnormalities

Blood in saliva *see* Saliva, blood in

Blood in sputum *see* Sputum

Blood in stools *see* Faeces, changes in

Blood in urine *see* Urine abnormalities

Blood in vomit *see* Nausea and/or vomiting

Body odour

Metabolic disorders
phenylketonuria
Skin disorders
bromhidrosis

Bone pain and tenderness *see also* Joint pain and tenderness

Blood and lymph disorders
sickle-cell anaemia
Endocrine disorders
hyperparathyroidism
Gastrointestinal and related disorders
coeliac disease
Infections
osteomyelitis
Malignant disease
acute leukaemias
Hodgkin's disease
myeloma
prostatic cancer
Musculoskeletal and connective tissue disorders
osteitis deformans
osteoporosis
Nutritional disorders
osteomalacia
Renal disorders
renal osteodystrophy

Bone structure abnormalities *see also* Joint abnormalities and Skeletal deformity
[bone destruction; bone weakness; brittle bones; fracture]

Endocrine disorders
hyperparathyroidism
Gynaecological disorders
Turner's syndrome
Infections
osteomyelitis
Malignant disease
myeloma
Musculoskeletal and connective tissue disorders
osteitis deformans
osteopetrosis
osteoporosis
Renal disorders
renal osteodystrophy

Bony projections on fingers
[Heberden's nodes]

Musculoskeletal and connective tissue disorders
osteoarthritis

Breast abnormalities
[blood from the nipple; breast cancer; breast discomfort; breast distortion; breast size, decreased; breast tenderness; gynaecomastia; lump in the breast; retracted nipple]

Endocrine disorders
adrenal virilisation
hyperthyroidism
hypogonadism
Gastrointestinal and related disorders
cirrhosis of the liver
Gynaecological disorders
premenstrual syndrome
Male genital disorders
Klinefelter's syndrome
Malignant disease
breast cancer

Breath, abnormal odour
[halitosis; ketones on the breath]

Endocrine disorders
type I diabetes mellitus
Infections
herpesvirus infections (HSV 1)
Vincent's infection

Breathing difficulties
[apnoea; breathlessness; dyspnoea; hypercapnia; hyperpnoea; hyperventilation; inspiratory 'whoop'; orthopnoea; reduced exercise tolerance; respiratory distress; respiratory failure; sensation of suffocation; stridor; tachypnoea; wheezing]

Blood and lymph disorders
anaemias
pulmonary embolism and infarction
sickle-cell anaemia
Cardiovascular system disorders
angina pectoris
cardiac arrest
cardiomyopathy
circulatory failure, acute
congestive heart failure
cor pulmonale
hypertension
left heart failure
myocardial infarction
myocarditis
pericarditis
pulmonary hypertension
pulmonary oedema
valvular heart disease
Endocrine disorders
hypothyroidism (neonatal)

Gastrointestinal and related disorders
acute intestinal ischaemia
ascites
cystic fibrosis
Infections
ascariasis
aspergillosis
botulism
epiglottitis
laryngeal diphtheria
Legionnaire's disease
malaria
pertussis
Pneumocystis carinii pneumonia
pneumonia
pulmonary anthrax
psittacosis
septicaemia
tonsillar diphtheria
trematode infections
trichiniasis
tuberculosis
visceral leishmaniasis
Malignant disease
cancer of the hypopharynx
cancer of the larynx
cancer of the pleura and peritoneum
carcinoid syndrome
chronic lymphoid leukaemia
lung cancer
Metabolic disorders
acidosis
alkalosis
hypocalcaemia
hypokalaemia
Musculoskeletal and connective tissue disorders
muscular dystrophy
polymyositis and dermatomyositis
rheumatoid arthritis
sarcoidosis
systemic juvenile chronic arthritis
systemic sclerosis
Nervous system disorders
anxiety
cerebral oedema
myasthenia gravis
tonic-clonic epileptic seizures
Nose disorders
rhinitis
Nutritional disorders
beri-beri
Renal disorders
glomerulonephritis
Respiratory system disorders
acute bronchitis
alveolitis
asthma
bronchiectasis
chronic bronchitis and emphysema
croup
pleurisy and pleural effusion
pneumoconioses
pneumothorax
respiratory distress syndrome
sudden infant death syndrome
Skin disorders
angioedema
hereditary angioedema

Bruising *see* Skin haemorrhage

Buboes *see* Swelling, glandular

Bullae *see* Skin lesions

C

Chest pain
[anginal pain; pain around the ribs; tightness in the chest]

Blood and lymph disorders
anaemias
polycythaemia vera
pulmonary embolism and infarction
Cardiovascular system disorders
angina pectoris
aortic aneurysm
aortic regurgitation
aortic stenosis
atherosclerosis in coronary vessels
atrial fibrillation
cardiomyopathy
mitral stenosis
myocardial infarction
myocarditis
pericarditis
pulmonary hypertension
tricuspid stenosis
Endocrine disorders
hyperthyroidism
Gastrointestinal and related disorders
achalasia
acute gastritis
dyspepsia
hiatus hernia
reflux oesophagitis
Infections
cryptococcosis
Lassa fever
legionellosis
Marburg disease and Ebola fever
plague
pneumonia
post-primary pulmonary tuberculosis
trematode infections
Malignant disease
cancer of the pleura and peritoneum
lung cancer
oesophageal cancer
phaeochromocytoma
Musculoskeletal and connective tissue disorders
ankylosing spondylitis
sarcoidosis

Nervous system disorders
anxiety
Respiratory system disorders
asthma
extrinsic allergic alveolitis
pleurisy and pleural effusion
pneumothorax

Chills and sensation of intense cold *see also* Shivering

Gastrointestinal and related disorders
cholangitis
choledocholithiasis
Infections
chickenpox
cutaneous anthrax
Lassa fever
leptospirosis
malaria
mumps
plague
pseudomembranous colitis
psittacosis
salmonellosis
scarlet fever
septicaemia
Obstetric disorders
septic abortion

Clubbing of the fingers

Gastrointestinal and related disorders
cirrhosis of the liver
Whipple's disease

Cold extremities *see also* Cyanosis

Infections
postviral fatigue syndrome
Nutritional disorders
anorexia nervosa

Cold intolerance

Endocrine disorders
hypopituitarism
hypothyroidism

Cold skin *see* Cyanosis

Colic *see* Abdominal pain and discomfort

Coma *see* Consciousness, loss of

Consciousness, impaired *see also* Consciousness, loss of [stupor]

Infections
cholera
encephalitis
psittacosis
septicaemia
tuberculous meningitis
typhus fevers
Malignant disease
intracranial tumours
Metabolic disorders
hypercalcaemia
respiratory acidosis
Nervous system disorders
cerebral oedema
hepatic encephalopathy
hypertensive encephalopathy
subarachnoid haemorrhage
subdural haemorrhage
tonic-clonic epileptic seizures

Consciousness, loss of *see also* Consciousness, impaired [coma]

Cardiovascular system disorders
cardiac arrest
heart block
Endocrine disorders
hypoglycaemia
hypothyroidism
type I diabetes mellitus
Gastrointestinal and related disorders
cirrhosis of the liver
Infections
acquired immune deficiency syndrome
African trypanosomiasis
cholera
encephalitis
paratyphoid fever
pyogenic meningitis
rabies
tuberculous meningitis
typhoid fever
Malignant disease
insulinoma
Metabolic disorders
hepatolenticular degeneration
hypercalcaemia
hypernatraemia
respiratory acidosis
Nervous system disorders
absence seizures
cerebral oedema
hepatic encephalopathy
hypertensive encephalopathy
Reye's syndrome
stroke
subarachnoid haemorrhage
tonic-clonic epileptic seizures
Nutritional disorders
beri-beri
Obstetric disorders
pre-eclampsia and eclampsia
Renal disorders
renal failure

Constipation *see also* Altered bowel habit, Diarrhoea *and* Constipation and diarrhoea

Non-specific causes
change from breast to bottle feeding
drugs
inadequate dietary fibre
incomplete bowel emptying

insufficient exercise
lack of response to defecation stimulus
painful anal conditions

Blood and lymph disorders
anaemias

Endocrine disorders
hypothyroidism
type I diabetes mellitus

Gastrointestinal and related disorders
anal fissure
appendicitis
diverticular disease
haemorrhoids
ileus
pyloric stenosis

Infections
botulism

Malignant disease
cancer of the bile ducts

Metabolic disorders
hypercalcaemia
porphyrias

Nervous system disorders
parkinsonism

Nutritional disorders
anorexia nervosa

Constipation and diarrhoea *see also* Altered bowel habit, Constipation *and* Diarrhoea

Gastrointestinal and related disorders
congenital megacolon
diverticular disease
irritable bowel syndrome

Infections
paratyphoid fever
typhoid fever

Convulsions *see also* Seizures

Blood and lymph disorders
thrombotic thrombocytopenic purpura

Endocrine disorders
hypoglycaemia

Gastrointestinal and related disorders
kernicterus

Infections
acquired immune deficiency syndrome
African trypanosomiasis
cholera
encephalitis
listeriosis
meningococcal infections
mumps
pertussis
rabies
toxoplasmosis (congenital)
tuberculous meningitis

Malignant disease
insulinoma

Metabolic disorders
hepatolenticular degeneration
hypocalcaemia
hyponatraemia
maple-syrup urine disease
phenylketonuria
porphyrias
respiratory alkalosis

Musculoskeletal and connective tissue disorders
systemic lupus erythematosus

Nervous system disorders
alcohol withdrawal
barbiturate withdrawal
dementia
dialysis encephalopathy
hydrocephalus
hypertensive encephalopathy
mental retardation
Reye's syndrome
subarachnoid haemorrhage

Nutritional disorders
bulimia nervosa
pyridoxine deficiency

Obstetric disorders
pre-eclampsia and eclampsia

Renal disorders
renal failure

Coordination, impaired *see also* Movement difficulties

Endocrine disorders
hypoglycaemia

Infections
encephalitis

Malignant disease
intracranial tumours

Nervous system disorders
alcohol-type drug dependence
cannabis-type drug dependence
chorea
Guillain-Barré syndrome
multiple sclerosis
parkinsonism
volatile solvent-type drug dependence

Corneal changes *see also* Eye pain and discomfort
[corneal thickening; corneal ulceration; dry cornea; keratomalacia]

Eye disorders
dry eye
ectropion and entropion
exophthalmos

Infections
ophthalmia neonatorum
trachoma

Nutritional disorders
vitamin A deficiency

Cough
[dry cough; productive cough]

Non-specific causes
inhalation of irritants (e.g. tobacco smoke)

Cardiovascular system disorders
aortic aneurysm
heart failure
mitral stenosis

Infections
ascariasis
aspergillosis
common cold
cryptococcosis
influenza
laryngeal diphtheria
Lassa fever
legionellosis
leptospirosis
Marburg disease and Ebola fever
measles
paratyphoid fever
pertussis
plague
Pneumocystis carinii pneumonia
pneumonia
psittacosis
pulmonary actinomycosis
pulmonary anthrax
strongyloidiasis
toxocariasis
trematode infections
tuberculosis
typhoid fever
visceral leishmaniasis
Malignant disease
cancer of the pleura and peritoneum
lung cancer
Musculoskeletal and connective tissue disorders
sarcoidosis
Nose disorders
rhinitis
Oropharyngeal disorders
laryngitis
Respiratory system disorders
acute bronchitis
alveolitis
asthma
bronchiectasis
chronic bronchitis and emphysema
croup
pleurisy
pneumoconioses
pulmonary oedema

Cramp *see* Muscle spasm

Cyanosis *see also* Cold extremities

Blood and lymph disorders
pulmonary embolism and infarction
Cardiovascular system disorders
acrocyanosis
left heart failure
pulmonary hypertension
Raynaud's syndrome
right heart failure
shock
Gastrointestinal and related disorders
acute intestinal ischaemia
Infections
cholera
laryngeal diphtheria
Pneumocystis carinii pneumonia
psittacosis
Malignant disease
carcinoid syndrome
phaeochromocytoma
Nervous system disorders
tonic-clonic epileptic seizures
Respiratory system disorders
pneumothorax
pulmonary oedema
respiratory distress syndrome

Cyst

Endocrine disorders
hyperparathyroidism
Gynaecological disorders
benign mammary dysplasia
Skin disorders
acne vulgaris
pilonidal disease

D

Dehydration
[fluid loss]

Endocrine disorders
diabetes insipidus
type I diabetes mellitus
Gastrointestinal and related disorders
ascites
gastroenteritis
ileus
peritonitis
pyloric stenosis
toxic megacolon
ulcerative colitis
Infections
cholera
dysentery
shigellosis
Metabolic disorders
galactosaemia
Nervous system disorders
motion sickness
Renal disorders
renal failure
Skin disorders
exfoliative dermatitis

Dental abnormalities

Endocrine disorders
hypoparathyroidism
Nutritional disorders
scurvy

Developmental abnormalities *see also* Failure to thrive
[growth rate accelerated; growth rate slowed; impaired intellectual development; impaired physical development; impaired sexual development; late onset of walking and crawling; latent development; premature sexual development; retarded development]

Blood and lymph disorders
beta thalassaemia
Endocrine disorders
adrenal virilisation
Cushing's syndrome
growth hormone deficiency
hypogonadism
hypopituitarism
precocious puberty
Gynaecological disorders
Turner's syndrome
Infections
ascariasis
cytomegalovirus infection (congenital)
hookworm infection
Lyme disease
Metabolic disorders
glycogen storage diseases
pseudohypoparathyroidism
Musculoskeletal and connective tissue disorders
muscular dystrophy
osteopetrosis
Nutritional disorders
acrodermatitis enteropathica
rickets
vitamin A deficiency
zinc deficiency
Renal disorders
renal osteodystrophy

Diarrhoea *see also* Altered bowel habit, Constipation *and* Constipation and diarrhoea

Non-specific causes
allergic reaction to food or drugs
drugs (e.g. antibacterials)
excessive dietary sugar
excessive use of laxatives
excessive use of sugar substitutes
Blood and lymph disorders
amyloidosis
anaemias
lymphangiectasia
Endocrine disorders
Addison's disease
adrenocortical insufficiency, acute
hyperthyroidism
Gastrointestinal and related disorders
acute intestinal ischaemia
chronic pancreatitis
coeliac disease
Crohn's disease
cystic fibrosis
diverticular disease
gastroenteritis
short-bowel syndrome
toxic megacolon
tropical sprue
ulcerative colitis
Gynaecological disorders
endometriosis
primary dysmenorrhoea
Infections
acquired immune deficiency syndrome
acute fulminating meningococcaemia
amoebiasis
ascariasis
botulism
cestode infections
cholera
dracontiasis
dysentery
giardiasis
Lassa fever
legionellosis
listeriosis
malaria
Marburg disease and Ebola fever
measles
poliomyelitis
pseudomembranous colitis
septicaemia
shigellosis
strongyloidiasis
toxic shock syndrome
trematode infections
trichiniasis
trichuriasis
upper respiratory-tract infections
urinary-tract infections
visceral leishmaniasis
Malignant disease
cancer of the bile ducts
carcinoid syndrome
colorectal cancer
glucagonoma
Zollinger–Ellison syndrome
Metabolic disorders
galactosaemia
porphyrias
Nervous system disorders
anxiety
diabetic neuropathy
opiate withdrawal
Nutritional disorders
acrodermatitis enteropathica
lactose intolerance
pellagra
Renal disorders
renal failure

Dizziness

Blood and lymph disorders
anaemias
polycythaemia vera
Cardiovascular system disorders
atrial fibrillation
hypertension
orthostatic hypotension
Ear disorders
labyrinthitis
Ménière's disease
otosclerosis
Infections
botulism
cestode infections
influenza
Lassa fever

Malignant disease
intracranial tumours
Nervous system disorders
anxiety
motion sickness
multiple sclerosis
partial seizures
syringobulbia
transient ischaemic attacks
vertigo

Dribbling, persistent

Metabolic disorders
hepatolenticular degeneration
Nervous system disorders
Bell's palsy
cerebral palsy
parkinsonism

Dry cough *see* Cough

E

Ear discharge

Ear disorders
acute otitis media
chronic otitis media
otitis externa
Infections
myiasis

Ear pain

Non-specific causes
hard wax
injury
referred pain (e.g. in herpes zoster)
unerupted lower molars
Ear disorders
acute otitis media
chronic otitis media
mastoiditis
otitis externa
Infections
myiasis
tonsillitis
upper respiratory-tract infections
Malignant disease
cancer of the pharynx
cancer of the tongue

Eczema

Cardiovascular system disorders
varicose veins
Infections
scabies
Metabolic disorders
phenylketonuria
Nutritional disorders
acrodermatitis enteropathica

Emotional disturbances *see also* Behaviour disturbances *and* Perception disturbances
[anxiety; apathy; apprehension; depression; elation; excitement; insomnia; irritability; loss of interest; monotonous and slowed speech; nervousness; neurosis; panic reactions; sensation of fear; sleep disturbance; stress; waking early]

Blood and lymph disorders
anaemias
Cardiovascular system disorders
myocardial infarction
Endocrine disorders
adrenocortical insufficiency, acute
Cushing's syndrome
hyperparathyroidism
hyperthyroidism
hypoglycaemia
hypoparathyroidism
type I diabetes mellitus
Gastrointestinal and related disorders
acute intestinal ischaemia
Gynaecological disorders
menopause
premenstrual syndrome
Infections
cestode infections
enterobiasis
poliomyelitis
pneumonia
post-primary pulmonary tuberculosis
postviral fatigue syndrome
rabies
Malignant disease
intracranial tumours
myeloma
phaeochromocytoma
Metabolic disorders
metabolic alkalosis
porphyrias
Musculoskeletal and connective tissue disorders
systemic lupus erythematosus
Nervous system disorders
anxiety
chorea
dementia
depressive disorders
dialysis encephalopathy
drug dependence
hepatic encephalopathy
mania and manic-depressive illness
parkinsonism
partial seizures
Reye's syndrome
schizophrenia
subarachnoid haemorrhage
Nutritional disorders
anorexia nervosa
bulimia nervosa
Renal disorders
renal failure
Respiratory system disorders
pulmonary oedema

Eructation *see* Flatulence and eructation

Erythema *see* Skin redness

Eye abscess

Eye disorders
dacryocystitis

Eye closure, inability

Nervous system disorders
Bell's palsy

Eye discharge

Eye disorders
conjunctivitis
Infections
ophthalmia neonatorum
trachoma

Eye discoloration

Eye disorders
chalazion
scleritis and episcleritis

Eye inflammation and congestion

Eye disorders
conjunctivitis
entropion
uveitis
Infections
herpesvirus infections
Lassa fever
leptospirosis
measles
myiasis
ophthalmia neonatorum
rubella
toxic shock syndrome
trachoma
yellow fever
Nervous system disorders
cluster headache

Eye movement restricted

Eye disorders
exophthalmos
Infections
tuberculous meningitis

Eye pain and discomfort *see also* Corneal changes
[dry eye; eye irritation; eye movement, painful; retro-orbital pain]

Non-specific causes
eyelid defects
local infection
reduced tear flow caused by:
ageing
inflammation of the lachrymal glands
Eye disorders
closed-angle glaucoma
corneal ulceration
dacryocystitis
dry eye
ectropion and entropion
optic neuropathies
scleritis and episcleritis
uveitis
Infections
common cold
trachoma
viral meningitis
Musculoskeletal and connective tissue disorders
rheumatoid arthritis
systemic lupus erythematosus
Nervous system disorders
Bell's palsy

Eye swelling

Endocrine disorders
hypothyroidism
Infections
infectious mononucleosis
ophthalmia neonatorum

Eye, watery
[epiphora; lachrymation]

Non-specific causes
foreign body
irritants
obstruction of the lachrymal duct
Eye disorders
blepharitis
corneal ulceration
dacryocystitis
ectropion and entropion
scleritis and episcleritis
uveitis
Infections
trachoma
Nervous system disorders
Bell's palsy
opiate withdrawal
Nose disorders
rhinitis

Eyelid discharge

Infections
stye

Eyelid fluttering *see also* Blinking
[blepharospasm]

Eye disorders
dry eye
Nervous system disorders
absence seizures

Eyelid lag and retraction

Endocrine disorders
hyperthyroidism

Eyelid pain

Infections
stye

Eyelid scaling and crusting

Eye disorders
blepharitis

Eyelid swelling

Eye disorders
blepharitis
chalazion
conjunctivitis
Infections
myiasis
stye
trachoma
Nervous system disorders
cluster headache
Skin disorders
seborrhoeic dermatitis

Eyelid ulceration

Eye disorders
blepharitis

F

Facial expression, abnormal changes in

Nervous system disorders
absence seizures

Facial features, changed
[blank expression; bloated face; coarsening of facial features; facial distortion; facial mass; facial mooning; facial palsy; facial paralysis and sagging; hollow cheeks; mask-like expression; swelling around the eye]

Endocrine disorders
acromegaly
Cushing's syndrome
hypothyroidism
Infections
lepromatous leprosy
mucocutaneous leishmaniasis
pyogenic meningitis
tuberculous meningitis
Malignant disease
cancer of the salivary glands
Nervous system disorders
Bell's palsy
parkinsonism

Facial flushing *see also* Hot flushes *and* Skin redness
[facial reddening]

Endocrine disorders
Cushing's syndrome
Infections
scarlet fever
typhus fevers
yellow fever
Malignant disease
carcinoid syndrome

Facial pain and discomfort

Malignant disease
cancer of the pharynx
cancer of the salivary glands
Nervous system disorders
Bell's palsy
cluster headache
trigeminal neuralgia
Nose disorders
sinusitis

Faeces, changes in
[blood in the stools; bloody diarrhoea; faecal mucus; faeces, discoloration; melaena; steatorrhoea; stools, unusual]

Blood and lymph disorders
lymphangiectasia
Cardiovascular system disorders
oesophageal varices
Gastrointestinal and related disorders
acute gastritis
acute hepatitis
acute intestinal ischaemia
cholangitis
cholestatic jaundice
chronic pancreatitis
coeliac disease
cystic fibrosis
haemolytic jaundice
irritable bowel syndrome
ischaemic colitis
peptic ulceration
short-bowel syndrome
tropical sprue
ulcerative colitis
Whipple's disease
Infections
amoebiasis
ascariasis
dysentery
giardiasis
Marburg disease and Ebola fever
salmonellal infections
schistosomiasis
shigellosis
trichuriasis
yellow fever
Malignant disease
cancer of the bile ducts
colorectal cancer
Zollinger–Ellison syndrome

Failure to thrive *see also* Developmental abnormalities *and* Feeding and swallowing difficulties

Blood and lymph disorders
beta thalassaemia
Gastrointestinal and related disorders
congenital megacolon
cystic fibrosis
Infections
giardiasis

Metabolic disorders
galactosaemia
hereditary fructose intolerance
Nervous system disorders
mental retardation
Nutritional disorders
lactose intolerance

Fainting
[syncope]

Blood and lymph disorders
pulmonary embolism and infarction
Cardiovascular system disorders
aortic stenosis
atrial fibrillation
cardiomyopathy
heart block
orthostatic hypotension
pulmonary hypertension
shock
tricuspid stenosis
Infections
salmonellosis
Obstetric disorders
ectopic pregnancy

Fatigue *see also* Prostration
[debilitation; drowsiness; exhaustion; lassitude; lethargy; physical depression; somnolence; tiredness; weakness]

Blood and lymph disorders
anaemias
polycythaemia vera
Cardiovascular system disorders
heart failure
mitral regurgitation
myocarditis
pulmonary hypertension
shock
Endocrine disorders
Addison's disease
adrenocortical insufficiency, acute
hyperthyroidism
hypoglycaemia
hypopituitarism
hypothyroidism
subacute thyroiditis
type I diabetes mellitus
Gastrointestinal and related disorders
chronic hepatitis
coeliac disease
Crohn's disease
gastroenteritis
irritable bowel syndrome
kernicterus
ulcerative colitis
Whipple's disease
Gynaecological disorders
premenstrual syndrome
Infections
acquired immune deficiency syndrome
cestode infections
cholera
cryptococcal meningitis
dysentery
encephalitis
giardiasis
infectious mononucleosis
Legionnaire's disease
Lyme disease
plague
pneumonia
poliomyelitis
pyelonephritis
rabies
septicaemia
syphilis
tonsillar diphtheria
toxic shock syndrome
toxoplasmosis
trypanosomiasis
viral meningitis
visceral leishmaniasis
Malignant disease
acute leukaemias
cancer of the pleura and peritoneum
cancer of the stomach
colorectal cancer
insulinoma
intracranial tumours
lung cancer
pancreatic (exocrine) cancer
renal cell carcinoma
Metabolic disorders
acidosis
hypercalcaemia
hypernatraemia
maple-syrup urine disease
Nervous system disorders
amphetamine withdrawal
anxiety
dialysis encephalopathy
hepatic encephalopathy
Huntington's chorea
mania and manic-depressive illness
mental retardation
opiate-type drug dependence
parkinsonism
Reye's syndrome
subarachnoid haemorrhage
Nutritional disorders
scurvy
Renal disorders
chronic glomerulonephritis
interstitial nephritis
renal failure
Respiratory system disorders
asthma
chronic bronchitis and emphysema

Feeding and swallowing difficulties *see also* Failure to thrive *and* Swallowing difficulties
[difficulty in chewing, eating, and speaking; regurgitation of food]

Endocrine disorders
hypothyroidism (neonatal)

Gastrointestinal and related disorders
achalasia
congenital megacolon
hiatus hernia
reflux oesophagitis
Infections
meningococcal infections
Malignant disease
cancer of the mouth
Metabolic disorders
maple-syrup urine disease
Nervous system disorders
Bell's palsy
myasthenia gravis
Oropharyngeal disorders
glossitis

Feeling of satiety
[abdominal fullness]

Blood and lymph disorders
splenomegaly
Gastrointestinal and related disorders
dyspepsia
Malignant disease
cancer of the stomach

Fever
[pyrexia]

Blood and lymph disorders
agranulocytosis
anaphylactoid purpura
thrombotic thrombocytopenic purpura
Cardiovascular system disorders
myocarditis
Ear disorders
acute otitis media
mastoiditis
Endocrine disorders
subacute thyroiditis
Gastrointestinal and related disorders
acute cholecystitis
acute pancreatitis
appendicitis
cholangitis
choledocholithiasis
cirrhosis of the liver
Crohn's disease
diverticular disease
gastroenteritis
peritonitis
toxic megacolon
tropical sprue
ulcerative colitis
Whipple's disease
Infections
amoebiasis
ascariasis
bacterial infections, many
chronic pulmonary aspergillosis
cryptococcosis
filariasis
malaria
Pneumocystis carinii pneumonia
primary amoebic meningo-encephalitis
schistosomiasis
toxocariasis
toxoplasmosis
trichiniasis
trypanosomiasis
viral infections, many
visceral leishmaniasis
Male genital disorders
torsion of the testis
Malignant disease
cancer of the liver
cancer of the pleura and peritoneum
chronic lymphoid leukaemia
lymphomas
renal cancer
Metabolic disorders
gout
Musculoskeletal and connective tissue disorders
giant cell arteritis
polyarteritis nodosa
polymyalgia rheumatica
rheumatoid arthritis
sarcoidosis
systemic juvenile chronic arthritis
Nervous system disorders
malignant hyperthermia
Nose disorders
sinusitis
Obstetric disorders
septic abortion
Oropharyngeal disorders
aphthous stomatitis
pharyngitis
sialadenitis
Renal disorders
acute glomerulonephritis
interstitial nephritis
Respiratory system disorders
croup
extrinsic allergic alveolitis
Skin disorders
erythema nodosum
exfoliative dermatitis
pityriasis lichenoides
Stevens–Johnson syndrome
toxic epidermal necrolysis

Flatulence and eructation

Gastrointestinal and related disorders
cholecystitis
irritable bowel syndrome
dyspepsia
Infections
giardiasis

Foot discomfort

Blood and lymph disorders
sickle-cell anaemia
Endocrine disorders
acromegaly

Musculoskeletal and connective tissue disorders
ankylosing spondylitis
Skin disorders
callosities and corns

G

Gangrene

Blood and lymph disorders
embolism
Cardiovascular system disorders
atherosclerosis in leg arteries
Gastrointestinal and related disorders
acute intestinal ischaemia

Gum disorders *see* Oropharyngeal lesions

H

Hair loss
[alopecia]

Endocrine disorders
hyperthyroidism
hypoparathyroidism
hypopituitarism
Infections
tinea capitis
Musculoskeletal and connective tissue disorders
systemic lupus erythematosus
Nutritional disorders
acrodermatitis enteropathica
Skin disorders
alopecia
exfoliative dermatitis

Hand discomfort

Blood and lymph disorders
sickle-cell anaemia
Endocrine disorders
acromegaly
Musculoskeletal and connective tissue disorders
systemic sclerosis
Skin disorders
callosities

Headache

Non-specific causes
neck stiffness
prolonged car driving
psychogenic causes
Blood and lymph disorders
anaemias
polycythaemia vera
Cardiovascular system disorders
cerebral aneurysm
hypertension (severe)
Endocrine disorders
acromegaly
Eye disorders
glaucoma
Gastrointestinal and related disorders
irritable bowel syndrome
Gynaecological disorders
menopause
premenstrual syndrome
primary dysmenorrhoea
Infections
acquired immune deficiency syndrome
African trypanosomiasis
brucellosis
cellulitis
chickenpox
cryptococcal meningitis
cutaneous anthrax
encephalitis
erysipelas
infectious mononucleosis
influenza
Lassa fever
legionellosis
leptospirosis
Lyme disease
lymphangitis
malaria
Marburg disease and Ebola fever
meningitis
meningococcal infections
mumps
plague
pneumonia
poliomyelitis
postviral fatigue syndrome
psittacosis
rabies
rubella
salmonellal infections
shigellosis
syphilis
tonsillar diphtheria
tonsillitis
toxic shock syndrome
typhus fevers
yellow fever
Malignant disease
insulinoma
intracranial tumours
myeloma
phaeochromocytoma
Metabolic disorders
respiratory acidosis
Musculoskeletal and connective tissue disorders
arthritis
cervical spondylosis
fibrositis
giant cell arteritis
osteitis deformans
osteomyelitis
Nervous system disorders
anxiety
barbiturate withdrawal
hydrocephalus

hypertensive encephalopathy
migraine
post-tonic-clonic epileptic seizures
stroke
subarachnoid haemorrhage
subdural haemorrhage
trigeminal neuralgia

Nose disorders
sinusitis

Obstetric disorders
pre-eclampsia and eclampsia

Renal disorders
acute glomerulonephritis

Respiratory system disorders
chronic bronchitis and emphysema

Skin disorders
pityriasis lichenoides

Hearing impairment *see also* Sensory derangement

Non-specific causes
drugs (e.g. gentamicin and other aminoglycosides)
foreign body
occlusion of the Eustachian tube
wax

Ear disorders
labyrinthitis
mastoiditis
Ménière's disease
otitis externa
otitis media
otosclerosis

Infections
cytomegalovirus infection (congenital)
Lassa fever
pyogenic meningitis
toxoplasmosis (congenital)
tuberculous meningitis
typhus fevers

Malignant disease
cancer of the nasopharynx

Musculoskeletal and connective tissue disorders
osteitis deformans
osteopetrosis

Nervous system disorders
cerebral palsy
syringobulbia
transient ischaemic attacks

Nose disorders
rhinitis

Heart beat abnormalities
[arrhythmias; atrial fibrillation; bradycardia; ECG changes; heart block; heart conduction defects; heart murmurs; palpitations; tachycardia]

Blood and lymph disorders
amyloidosis
anaemias

Cardiovascular system disorders
arrhythmias
atherosclerosis in coronary vessels
cardiomyopathy
congestive heart failure
cor pulmonale
left heart failure
myocardial infarction
myocarditis
pericarditis
valvular heart disease

Endocrine disorders
hyperthyroidism
hypoglycaemia

Gastrointestinal and related disorders
peritonitis
toxic megacolon

Infections
brucellosis
cholera
gas gangrene
hookworm infection
infective endocarditis
lymphangitis
malaria
psittacosis
scarlet fever
tetanus
trichiniasis

Malignant disease
carcinoid syndrome
insulinoma
phaeochromocytoma

Metabolic disorders
hyperkalaemia
hypokalaemia
porphyrias

Musculoskeletal and connective tissue disorders
polyarteritis nodosa
systemic sclerosis

Nervous system disorders
anxiety
barbiturate withdrawal

Respiratory system disorders
asthma

Heat intolerance

Endocrine disorders
hyperthyroidism

Hiccup

Renal disorders
renal failure

Hirsutism
[excessive facial and body hair]

Endocrine disorders
acromegaly
adrenal virilisation
Cushing's syndrome
hyperprolactinaemia

Gynaecological disorders
polycystic ovary syndrome

Hot flushes *see also* Facial flushing *and* Skin redness

Gynaecological disorders
menopause

Infections
malaria
Malignant disease
carcinoid syndrome

Hunger

Endocrine disorders
hyperthyroidism
hypoglycaemia
Gastrointestinal and related disorders
pyloric stenosis
Malignant disease
insulinoma

I

Incontinence
[faecal incontinence; urinary incontinence]

Gastrointestinal and related disorders
acquired megacolon
Infections
typhus fevers
Malignant disease
spinal cord tumours
Nervous system disorders
dementia
multiple sclerosis
spina bifida
tonic-clonic epileptic seizures

Indigestion
[dyspepsia; heartburn]

Non-specific causes
dental:
ill-fitting dentures
deficient teeth
dental caries
overindulgence in food or alcohol
Cardiovascular system disorders
ischaemic heart disease
Endocrine disorders
hyperparathyroidism
Gastrointestinal and related disorders
cholecystitis
chronic gastritis
hiatus hernia
peptic ulceration
reflux oesophagitis
Malignant disease
cancer of the gall bladder
cancer of the stomach
pancreatic cancer

Infection, increased susceptibility to

Blood and lymph disorders
agranulocytosis
aplastic anaemia
haemolytic anaemias
Gastrointestinal and related disorders
cystic fibrosis
Infections
prostatitis
Malignant disease
most types
Musculoskeletal and connective tissue disorders
muscular dystrophy
osteopetrosis
Nervous system disorders
opiate-type drug dependence
Nutritional disorders
vitamin A deficiency
Renal disorders
nephrotic syndrome
polycystic kidney disease
renal calculi and colic
Respiratory system disorders
bronchiectasis
Skin disorders
exfoliative dermatitis

Infertility *see also* Sexual disturbances

Endocrine disorders
hyperprolactinaemia
hypogonadism
hypopituitarism
Gynaecological disorders
endometriosis
polycystic ovary syndrome
Male genital disorders
Klinefelter's syndrome

Itch
[pruritus; pruritus ani; pruritus vulvae]

Non-specific causes
allergy
drugs (e.g. antibacterials)
dry skin (especially in the elderly)
hyperhidrosis
irritants
poor hygiene
pregnancy
psychosexual disorders
rectal prolapse
Blood and lymph disorders
iron-deficiency anaemia
polycythaemia vera
Cardiovascular system disorders
chilblains
varicose veins
Ear disorders
otitis externa
Endocrine disorders
diabetes mellitus
thyroid disorders
Eye disorders
blepharitis
conjunctivitis
Gastrointestinal and related disorders
anal fissure
anorectal fistula
cholangitis
choledocholithiasis

cholestatic jaundice
cirrhosis of the liver
colitis
Crohn's disease
diarrhoea
haemorrhoids
proctitis

Gynaecological disorders
vaginitis
vulvitis

Infections
African trypanosomiasis
cestode infections
chickenpox
cystitis
enterobiasis
filariasis
herpes labialis
hookworm infection
impetigo
Lyme disease
pediculosis capitis
pediculosis corporis
pityriasis versicolor
salpingitis
scabies
schistosomiasis
skin candidiasis
strongyloidiasis
tinea infections
trichomoniasis
vaginal candidiasis

Malignant disease
cancer of the bile ducts
colorectal cancer
Hodgkin's disease
melanoma
vulval neoplasm

Nose disorders
rhinitis

Renal disorders
chronic glomerulonephritis
renal failure

Skin disorders
eczema
lichen planus
pityriasis rosea
urticaria

Urinary-tract disorders
incontinence

J

Jaw pain

Musculoskeletal and connective tissue disorders
giant cell arteritis

Joint abnormalities *see also* Bone structure abnormalities, Joint pain and tenderness, Movement difficulties *and* Skeletal deformity
[ankylosis; joint destruction; joint disease; joint haemorrhages; joint weakness]

Blood and lymph disorders
haemophilia

Infections
infective arthritis

Musculoskeletal and connective tissue disorders
ankylosing spondylitis

Nervous system disorders
diabetic neuropathy

Renal disorders
renal osteodystrophy

Joint inflammation

Infections
infective arthritis
rheumatic fever

Malignant disease
cancer of the bone

Metabolic disorders
gout

Musculoskeletal and connective tissue disorders
ankylosing spondylitis
frozen shoulder
juvenile chronic arthritis
rheumatoid arthritis

Joint pain and tenderness *see also* Bone pain and tenderness *and* Joint abnormalities
[arthralgia]

Blood and lymph disorders
anaphylactoid purpura

Endocrine disorders
acromegaly

Gastrointestinal and related disorders
acute hepatitis
chronic active hepatitis

Infections
chronic fulminating meningococcaemia
disseminated gonococcal infection
infective arthritis
infective endocarditis
Lyme disease
rheumatic fever
syphilis
tonsillitis

Malignant disease
cancer of the bone

Metabolic disorders
gout

Musculoskeletal and connective tissue disorders
ankylosing spondylitis
bursitis
frozen shoulder
osteoarthritis
polyarteritis nodosa
rheumatoid arthritis
sarcoidosis
systemic lupus erythematosus
systemic sclerosis
tendinitis and tenosynovitis

Renal disorders
interstitial nephritis

Respiratory system disorders
fibrosing alveolitis
Skin disorders
erythema nodosum
Stevens–Johnson syndrome

L

Limb discomfort *see also* Muscle spasm

Blood and lymph disorders
deep vein thrombosis
embolism
Cardiovascular system disorders
Raynaud's syndrome
varicose veins
Gynaecological disorders
primary dysmenorrhoea
Metabolic disorders
porphyrias
Nervous system disorders
restless leg syndrome
Nutritional disorders
scurvy

Limping
[intermittent claudication]

Blood and lymph disorders
embolism
Cardiovascular system disorders
atherosclerosis in leg arteries

Lip lesions *see also* Oropharyngeal lesions
[angular stomatitis; cheilitis; cracked lips; swelling of the lips]

Endocrine disorders
type I diabetes mellitus
Infections
anterior nasal diphtheria
yellow fever
Malignant disease
glucagonoma
Nutritional disorders
pyridoxine deficiency
riboflavine deficiency

Loss of appetite
[anorexia]

Blood and lymph disorders
anaemias
Endocrine disorders
Addison's disease
Gastrointestinal and related disorders
appendicitis
congenital megacolon
dyspepsia
gastric ulceration
gastritis
gastroenteritis
hepatitis ileus
kernicterus
tropical sprue
tuberculous peritonitis
ulcerative colitis
Infections
acquired immune deficiency syndrome
actinomycosis
amoebiasis
anthrax
chickenpox
dysentery
enterobiasis
giardiasis
herpesvirus infections (HSV 2)
influenza
legionellosis
malaria
meningitis
psittacosis
pyelonephritis
rabies
salmonellal infections
schistosomiasis
secondary syphilis
shigellosis
tuberculosis
Malignant disease
cancer of the hypopharynx
cancer of the stomach
chronic leukaemias
metastatic carcinoma of the liver
myeloma
oesophageal cancer
pancreatic (exocrine) cancer
Wilms' tumour
Metabolic disorders
hereditary fructose intolerance
hypercalcaemia
hyponatraemia
Nervous system disorders
depressive disorders
motion sickness
Nutritional disorders
scurvy
zinc deficiency
Renal disorders
interstitial nephritis
renal failure
Skin disorders
toxic epidermal necrolysis

M

Memory impairment *see also* Amnesia

Cardiovascular system disorders
atherosclerosis in cerebral arteries
Nervous system disorders
anxiety
dementia
partial seizures

Menstrual disturbances
[amenorrhoea; dysmenorrhoea; menorrhagia; oligomenorrhoea]

Blood and lymph disorders
anaemias
thrombocytopenia
Endocrine disorders
adrenal virilisation
Cushing's syndrome
hyperprolactinaemia
hyperthyroidism
hypogonadism
hypothyroidism
Gastrointestinal and related disorders
chronic active hepatitis
Gynaecological disorders
endometriosis
polycystic ovary syndrome
Turner's syndrome
Infections
gonorrhoea
pelvic actinomycosis
Metabolic disorders
pseudohypoparathyroidism
Nervous system disorders
depressive disorders
Nutritional disorders
anorexia nervosa

Mouth symptoms *see* Oropharyngeal lesions

Movement difficulties *see also* Coordination, impaired and Joint abnormalities
[akinesia; apraxia; arm jerking; ataxia; body rocking; chorea; hemiparesis; hemiplegia; hyperkinesia; immobility; inability to walk; joint stiffness; lip smacking; neuromuscular disturbances; paralysis; persistent chewing; 'ram-rod' posture; repetitive nodding; rigidity; spastic syndromes]

Blood and lymph disorders
haemophilia
Endocrine disorders
primary aldosteronism
Infections
botulism
herpes zoster
Legionnaire's disease
leprosy
osteomyelitis
poliomyelitis
rabies
subacute sclerosing panencephalitis
tetanus
toxoplasmosis (congenital)
Malignant disease
spinal cord tumours
Metabolic disorders
hepatolenticular degeneration
hyperkalaemia
hypokalaemia
phenylketonuria
porphyrias
Musculoskeletal and connective tissue disorders
many disorders
Nervous system disorders
absence seizures
cerebral palsy
chorea
dementia
epilepsy
extradural haemorrhage
Guillain-Barré syndrome
hepatic encephalopathy
hydrocephalus
motor neuron disease
multiple sclerosis
myasthenia gravis
parkinsonism
spina bifida
stroke
subarachnoid haemorrhage
subdural haemorrhage
syringomyelia
tardive dyskinesia
tics
transient ischaemic attacks
Nutritional disorders
beri-beri

Mucus in stools *see* Faeces, changes in

Muscle pain and tenderness *see also* Muscle spasm
[myalgia]
Blood and lymph disorders
anaphylactoid purpura
Endocrine disorders
adrenocortical insufficiency, acute
hypothyroidism
Infections
acquired immune deficiency syndrome
brucellosis
chickenpox
chronic fulminating meningococcaemia
gas gangrene
influenza
Lassa fever
legionellosis
leptospirosis
Lyme disease
malaria
measles
psittacosis
pulmonary anthrax
rabies
secondary syphilis
tonsillitis
toxic shock syndrome
toxoplasmosis
typhus fevers
viral meningitis
yellow fever
Musculoskeletal and connective tissue disorders
fibrositis
polyarteritis nodosa
polymyalgia rheumatica
systemic lupus erythematosus
systemic sclerosis
Nervous system disorders
diabetic neuropathy
motor neuron disease
post-tonic-clonic epileptic seizures

Muscle spasm *see also* Limb discomfort and Muscle pain and tenderness
[cramp; facial twitching; reflex spasms; tetany; unnatural head posture]

Endocrine disorders
primary aldosteronism
type I diabetes mellitus
Infections
cholera
salmonellosis
tetanus
Metabolic disorders
alkalosis
glycogen storage diseases
hypernatraemia
hypocalcaemia
hypokalaemia
Musculoskeletal and connective tissue disorders
many disorders
Nervous system disorders
motor neuron disease
multiple sclerosis
Nutritional disorders
beri-beri
bulimia nervosa
Renal disorders
renal failure

Muscle stiffness *see also* Muscular rigidity

Infections
tetanus
Musculoskeletal and connective tissue disorders
fibrositis
polymyalgia rheumatica

Muscle wasting
[emaciation; muscle atrophy]

Endocrine disorders
Cushing's syndrome
hypogonadism (male)
Gastrointestinal and related disorders
ascites
cirrhosis of the liver
Infections
actinomycosis
dysentery
visceral leishmaniasis
Malignant disease
spinal cord tumours
Metabolic disorders
hepatolenticular degeneration
Musculoskeletal and connective tissue disorders
cervical spondylosis
polymyositis and dermatomyositis
Nervous system disorders
carpal tunnel syndrome
motor neuron disease
syringomyelia
Nutritional disorders
anorexia nervosa

Muscle weakness

Endocrine disorders
acromegaly
Cushing's syndrome
hyperthyroidism
primary aldosteronism
Infections
botulism
postviral fatigue syndrome
Malignant disease
spinal cord tumours
Metabolic disorders
glycogen storage diseases
hepatolenticular degeneration
hypercalcaemia
hypokalaemia
hyponatraemia
Musculoskeletal and connective tissue disorders
muscular dystrophy
polymyositis and dermatomyositis
Nervous system disorders
carpal tunnel syndrome
motor neuron disease
multiple sclerosis
myasthenia gravis
subdural haemorrhage
Sydenham's chorea
Nutritional disorders
bulimia nervosa
rickets and osteomalacia

Muscular rigidity *see also* Muscle stiffness

Infections
subacute sclerosing panencephalitis
tetanus
Nervous system disorders
malignant hyperthermia
parkinsonism
tonic-clonic epileptic seizures

N

Nail lesions
[crumbling nails; deformed and/or discoloured nail body; nail pitting and ridging; swelling of the nail fold]

Endocrine disorders
hypoparathyroidism
Gastrointestinal and related disorders
cirrhosis of the liver
Infections
paronychia
tinea unguium
Malignant disease
glucagonoma
Musculoskeletal and connective tissue disorders
psoriatic arthritis
Skin disorders
lichen planus

Nail loss

Skin disorders
exfoliative dermatitis

Nasal congestion

Infections
common cold
influenza
lepromatous leprosy
Malignant disease
cancer of the nasopharynx
Nervous system disorders
cluster headache
Nose disorders
rhinitis
sinusitis

Nasal discharge
[rhinorrhoea]

Infections
anterior nasal diphtheria
common cold
lepromatous leprosy
measles
Nervous system disorders
opiate withdrawal
Nose disorders
rhinitis
sinusitis

Nasal irritation *see also* Sneezing

Infections
anterior nasal diphtheria
common cold
Nose disorders
rhinitis

Nausea and/or vomiting

Non-specific causes
diet
drugs
intestinal obstruction
pregnancy
psychological factors
unpleasant smells or sights
Blood and lymph disorders
anaemias
Cardiovascular system disorders
angina pectoris
myocardial infarction
oesophageal varices
syncope
tricuspid regurgitation
Ear disorders
acute otitis media
labyrinthitis
Ménière's disease
Endocrine disorders
Addison's disease
adrenocortical insufficiency, acute
hyperthyroidism
Eye disorders
closed-angle glaucoma
Gastrointestinal and related disorders
acute hepatitis
acute intestinal ischaemia
appendicitis
cholangitis
cholecystitis
choledocholithiasis
cirrhosis of the liver
congenital megacolon
dyspepsia
focal ischaemia of the small intestine
gastritis
gastroenteritis
ileus
ischaemic colitis
kernicterus
pancreatitis
peptic ulceration
peritonitis
pyloric stenosis
Gynaecological disorders
dysmenorrhoea
Infections
acquired immune deficiency syndrome
acute fulminating meningococcaemia
botulism
cestode infections
chickenpox
cholera
cryptococcal meningitis
cutaneous anthrax
dracontiasis
dysentery
erysipelas
giardiasis
influenza
Lassa fever
leptospirosis
liver fluke disease
Lyme disease
malaria
Marburg disease and Ebola fever
meningitis
pelvic actinomycosis
pertussis
poliomyelitis
Pontiac fever
psittacosis
salpingitis
scarlet fever
secondary syphilis
septicaemia
shigellosis
tonsillar diphtheria
toxic shock syndrome
trichiniasis
urinary-tract infections
yellow fever
Male genital disorders
torsion of the testis
Malignant disease
cancer of the bile ducts

cancer of the stomach
carcinoid syndrome
intracranial tumours
myeloma
Wilms' tumour

Metabolic disorders
galactosaemia
hypercalcaemia
metabolic acidosis
porphyrias

Nervous system disorders
barbiturate withdrawal
hypertensive encephalopathy
migraine
motion sickness
Reye's syndrome
subarachnoid haemorrhage
transient ischaemic attacks
vertigo

Nutritional disorders
lactose intolerance

Obstetric disorders
hydatidiform mole
pre-eclampsia and eclampsia

Renal disorders
glomerulonephritis
interstitial nephritis
renal calculi and colic
renal failure

Skin disorders
hereditary angioedema

Neck pain

Infections
postviral fatigue syndrome
tetanus

Musculoskeletal and connective tissue disorders
cervical spondylosis
torticollis

Neck stiffness

Infections
encephalitis
Lyme disease
poliomyelitis
pyogenic meningitis
tetanus
viral meningitis

Musculoskeletal and connective tissue disorders
cervical spondylosis
torticollis

Nervous system disorders
subarachnoid haemorrhage

Neck swelling
[bull neck; goitre; neck oedema]

Endocrine disorders
hyperthyroidism
hypothyroidism
thyroiditis

Infections
epiglottitis
tonsillar diphtheria

Nodules *see also* Skin lesions

Infections
African trypanosomiasis
cutaneous leishmaniasis
rheumatic fever
sporotrichosis
tinea capitis
tinea corporis

Malignant disease
basal cell carcinoma
Kaposi's sarcoma
melanoma

Musculoskeletal and connective tissue disorders
polyarteritis nodosa
rheumatoid arthritis

Skin disorders
erythema nodosum
keloid
pyoderma gangrenosum

Nosebleed
[epistaxis]

Blood and lymph disorders
thrombocytopenia

Infections
Marburg disease and Ebola fever
paratyphoid fever
typhoid fever
yellow fever

Malignant disease
acute leukaemias

Nutritional disorders
scurvy

O

Odour, body *see* Body odour

Oedema *see* Swelling, oedematous

Oral pain

Infections
oral candidiasis

Skin disorders
lichen planus
pemphigus

Oropharyngeal exudate

Infections
cervicofacial actinomycosis
diphtheria
tonsillitis

Oropharyngeal disorders
pharyngitis

Oropharyngeal lesions *see also* Lip lesions, Throat discomfort, Tongue changes and Tongue pain
[aphthous stomatitis; gingival bleeding; gingival infection; gingival inflammation; gingival patches; mouth ulcers; oral bleeding; oral candidiasis; oral hairy leucoplakia; plaques; throat ulcers; tongue patches]

Blood and lymph disorders
agranulocytosis
Gastrointestinal and related disorders
coeliac disease
tropical sprue
Infections
acquired immune deficiency syndrome
cervicofacial actinomycosis
diphtheria
herpesvirus infections (HSV 1)
measles
oral candidiasis
syphilis
Vincent's infection
yellow fever
Malignant disease
cancer of the mouth
Musculoskeletal and connective tissue disorders
systemic lupus erythematosus
Nutritional disorders
scurvy
Oropharyngeal disorders
aphthous stomatitis
gingivitis
oral leucoplakia
pharyngitis
Skin disorders
lichen planus
pemphigus

P

Pain during defecation
[tenesmus]

Gastrointestinal and related disorders
anal fissure
haemorrhoids
ulcerative colitis
Gynaecological disorders
endometriosis
Infections
dysentery
shigellosis

Palpitations *see* Heart beat abnormalities

Perception disturbances *see also* Behaviour disturbances *and* Emotional disturbances
[delusions; disorientation; distorted perception of time; hallucinations; nightmares; psychoses; sense of déja-vu; sense of unreality; sensitivity to light or noise]

Blood and lymph system disorders
thrombotic thrombocytopenic purpura
Infections
African trypanosomiasis
cysticercosis
Legionnaire's disease
rabies
Metabolic disorders
hypocalcaemia
porphyrias
Musculoskeletal and connective tissue disorders
polyarteritis nodosa
systemic lupus erythematosus
Nervous system disorders
depressive disorders
drug dependence
mania and manic-depressive illness
partial seizures
Reye's syndrome
schizophrenia

Productive cough *see* Cough

Prostration *see also* Fatigue

Blood and lymph disorders
agranulocytosis
Eye disorders
closed-angle glaucoma
Gastrointestinal and related disorders
gastroenteritis
Infections
brucellosis
disseminated gonococcal infection
malaria
Marburg disease and Ebola fever
typhus fevers

Pupilary changes

Cardiovascular system disorders
cardiac arrest
Eye disorders
uveitis
Nervous system disorders
cerebral oedema
cluster headache
subdural and extradural haemorrhage

R

Rash *see* Skin lesions

Rectal pain, cyclic

Gynaecological disorders
endometriosis

S

Saliva, blood in

Malignant disease
oropharyngeal cancer

Salivation, excessive

Gastrointestinal and related disorders
gastric ulceration
Infections
epiglottitis
herpesvirus infections (HSV 1)
Vincent's infection
Malignant disease
cancer of the mouth

Nervous system disorders
motion sickness

Scrotal changes
[orchitis; scrotal discoloration; scrotal inflammation; scrotal mass; testicular mass]

Infections
epididymitis
lymphatic filariasis
Marburg disease and Ebola fever
mumps
Male genital disorders
Klinefelter's syndrome
torsion of the testis
varicocele
Malignant disease
choriocarcinoma
testicular cancer

Scrotal pain
[testicular pain and tenderness]

Malignant disease
choriocarcinoma
testicular cancer

Seizures *see also* Convulsions

Nervous system disorders
epilepsy

Sensory derangement *see also* Hearing impairment
[acroparaesthesia; agnosia; burning sensations; dysaesthesia; neuralgia; numbness; 'pins and needles'; prickling sensation; taste impairment]

Cardiovascular system disorders
Raynaud's syndrome
Endocrine disorders
acromegaly
primary aldosteronism
type I diabetes mellitus
Gastrointestinal and related disorders
acute hepatitis
cirrhosis of the liver
Infections
encephalitis
herpes zoster
leprosy
loiasis
postviral fatigue syndrome
Malignant disease
spinal cord tumours
Metabolic disorders
hypocalcaemia
respiratory alkalosis
Musculoskeletal and connective tissue disorders
cervical spondylosis
Nervous system disorders
Bell's palsy
carpal tunnel syndrome
dementia
diabetic neuropathy
Guillain-Barré syndrome
migraine
multiple sclerosis
restless leg syndrome
spina bifida
stroke
syringomyelia
tardive dyskinesia
transient ischaemic attacks
Nutritional disorders
beri-beri

Sexual disturbances *see also* Infertility
[absence of erection or ejaculation; dyspareunia; impotence; loss of libido]

Blood and lymph disorders
anaemias
Endocrine disorders
hyperprolactinaemia
hypogonadism
hypopituitarism
Gynaecological disorders
endometriosis
menopause
vaginitis
vulvitis
Infections
trichomoniasis
Malignant disease
cervical cancer
Nervous system disorders
depressive disorders
diabetic neuropathy
multiple sclerosis
Nutritional disorders
anorexia nervosa

Shivering *see also* Chills and sensation of intense cold
[rigors]

Blood and lymph disorders
agranulocytosis
Infections
brucellosis
infective arthritis
influenza
lymphangitis
malaria
pneumonia
pyelonephritis
pyogenic meningitis
typhus fevers
yellow fever
Metabolic disorders
gout
Respiratory system disorders
extrinsic allergic alveolitis
Skin disorders
exfoliative dermatitis

Skeletal deformity *see also* Bone structure abnormalities *and* Joint abnormalities
[bowing of the long bones; cubitus; vertebral collapse]

Blood and lymph disorders
haemophilia
Endocrine disorders
acromegaly
hyperparathyroidism
hypogonadism
Gynaecological disorders
Turner's syndrome
Male genital disorders
Klinefelter's syndrome
Musculoskeletal and connective tissue disorders
ankylosing spondylitis
cervical spondylosis
juvenile chronic arthritis
muscular dystrophy
psoriatic arthritis
rheumatoid arthritis
osteitis deformans
osteoarthritis
osteopetrosis
osteoporosis
Nutritional disorders
rickets
Renal disorders
renal osteodystrophy

Skin depigmentation

Infections
onchocerciasis
Metabolic disorders
phenylketonuria
Skin disorders
albinism
ischaemic ulcers
pityriasis alba
pityriasis lichenoides
vitiligo

Skin desquamation
[exfoliating lesions]

Infections
Marburg disease and Ebola fever
measles
scarlet fever
toxic shock syndrome
Malignant disease
glucagonoma
Skin disorders
exfoliative dermatitis
toxic epidermal necrolysis

Skin haemorrhage
[bruising; ecchymoses; petechiae]

Blood and lymph disorders
haemophilia
thrombocytopenia
Endocrine disorders
Cushing's syndrome
Infections
infectious mononucleosis
infective endocarditis
Marburg disease and Ebola fever
scabies
scarlet fever
typhus fevers
yellow fever
Malignant disease
leukaemias
superficial spreading melanoma
Skin disorders
pityriasis lichenoides
strawberry naevus

Skin healing, impaired

Nutritional disorders
scurvy
zinc deficiency

Skin inflammation *see also* Skin pain and discomfort *and* Skin redness

Infections
myiasis
tinea infections
Malignant disease
superficial spreading melanoma
Skin disorders
acne vulgaris
eczema
erythema nodosum
folliculitis
lichen planus
sunburn

Skin lesions *see also* Skin, non-specific changes in characteristics, Skin ulcers *and* Nodules
[blackheads; bullae; blisters; comedones; livid striae; macules; naevi; papules; rash; vesicles; wheals; whiteheads]

Cardiovascular system disorders
chilblains
varicose veins
Endocrine disorders
adrenal virilisation
Cushing's syndrome
Gastrointestinal and related disorders
acute hepatitis
chronic active hepatitis
Gynaecological disorders
Turner's syndrome
Infections
acquired immune deficiency syndrome
cellulitis
chancroid
chickenpox
condylomata acuminata
cutaneous anthrax
cutaneous leishmaniasis
erysipelas
filariasis
furunculosis

gas gangrene
herpes zoster
impetigo
infectious mononucleosis
leprosy
listeriosis
Lyme disease
lymphangitis
Marburg disease and Ebola fever
measles
meningococcal infections
myiasis
paratyphoid fever
pediculosis corporis
pediculosis pubis
pityriasis versicolor
rheumatic fever
rubella
scabies
scarlet fever
schistosomiasis
skin candidiasis
sycosis barbae
syphilis
tinea infections
toxic shock syndrome
toxoplasmosis
typhoid fever
typhus fevers

Malignant disease
chronic lymphoid leukaemia
glucagonoma
Kaposi's sarcoma
melanoma

Musculoskeletal and connective tissue disorders
dermatomyositis
juvenile chronic arthritis
polyarteritis nodosa
systemic lupus erythematosus

Nutritional disorders
pellagra

Oropharyngeal disorders
pharyngitis

Skin disorders
acne vulgaris
angioedema
decubitus ulcer
eczema
erythema multiforme
folliculitis
lichen planus
pemphigus
photosensitivity
pityriasis alba
pityriasis lichenoides
pityriasis rosea
psoriasis
pyoderma gangrenosum
sebaceous cyst
Stevens–Johnson syndrome
sunburn
telangiectasia
toxic epidermal necrolysis
ulcers
urticaria

Skin, non-specific changes in characteristics *see also* Skin lesions
[cracked skin; dry skin; greasy skin; lichenification; reduced skin turgor; scaling; shiny skin; skin atrophy; skin coarsening; skin crusting; skin growth; skin maceration; skin necrosis; skin thickening]

Cardiovascular system disorders
chilblains
Raynaud's syndrome

Ear disorders
otitis externa

Endocrine disorders
acromegaly
Cushing's syndrome
hypoparathyroidism
hypothyroidism

Infections
cholera
gas gangrene
impetigo
lepromatous leprosy
pityriasis versicolor
scabies
scarlet fever
skin candidiasis
tinea infections

Metabolic disorders
hypernatraemia
hyponatraemia

Musculoskeletal and connective tissue disorders
dermatomyositis
systemic sclerosis

Nutritional disorders
anorexia nervosa
pellagra

Skin disorders
callosities
eczema
haemangiomas
hyperhidrosis
ichthyosis
mole
photosensitivity
pityriasis
psoriasis
sunburn

Skin pain and discomfort *see also* Skin inflammation *and* Skin redness

Infections
erysipelas
furunculosis
gas gangrene
myiasis
warts

Musculoskeletal and connective tissue disorders
giant cell arteritis

Skin disorders
acne vulgaris
angioedema
callosities and corns
decubitus ulcer
eczema
erythema multiforme

erythema nodosum
folliculitis
hereditary angioedema
lichen planus
pemphigus
photosensitivity
pityriasis alba
pityriasis lichenoides
pityriasis rosea
pruritus
psoriasis
pyoderma gangrenosum
sunburn
toxic epidermal necrolysis
ulcers
urticaria

Skin pigmentation

Cardiovascular system disorders
varicose veins
Endocrine disorders
Addison's disease
Gastrointestinal and related disorders
tropical sprue
Whipple's disease
Infections
gas gangrene
Musculoskeletal and connective tissue disorders
dermatomyositis
systemic sclerosis
Renal disorders
chronic renal failure
Skin disorders
lichen planus
mole
pilonidal disease
sunburn
telangiectasia

Skin redness *see also* Facial flushing, Hot flushes, Skin inflammation *and* Skin pain and discomfort
[erythema]

Blood and lymph disorders
deep vein thrombosis
superficial thrombophlebitis
Cardiovascular system disorders
Raynaud's syndrome
Gastrointestinal and related disorders
cirrhosis of the liver
Infections
cellulitis
erysipelas
impetigo
Lyme disease
paratyphoid fever
rheumatic fever
skin candidiasis
sycosis barbae
typhoid fever
Metabolic disorders
respiratory acidosis
Musculoskeletal and connective tissue disorders
bursitis
dermatomyositis
giant cell arteritis
systemic lupus erythematosus
Nervous system disorders
cluster headache
Nutritional disorders
pellagra
Skin disorders
angioedema
decubitus ulcer
eczema
erythema multiforme
erythema nodosum
photosensitivity
pityriasis alba
pruritus
sunburn
toxic epidermal necrolysis
ulcers
urticaria

Skin ulcers *see also* Skin lesions

Blood and lymph disorders
embolism
Cardiovascular system disorders
chilblains
Raynaud's syndrome
varicose veins
Infections
carbuncles
chancroid
cutaneous anthrax
cutaneous diphtheria
cutaneous leishmaniasis
sporotrichosis
syphilis
Malignant disease
basal cell carcinoma
breast cancer
nodular melanoma
Musculoskeletal and connective tissue disorders
polyarteritis nodosa
Skin disorders
decubitus ulcer
napkin rash
strawberry naevus
ulcers

Skin yellowing

Gastrointestinal and related disorders
jaundice
Metabolic disorders
hyperlipidaemias

Sneezing *see also* Nasal irritation

Non-specific causes
dust
smoking
Infections
common cold
influenza
measles
Nervous system disorders
opiate withdrawal

Nose disorders
rhinitis

Speech disturbances *see also* Voice abnormalities
[aphasia; aphonia; difficulty in eating and speaking; dysarthria; hoarseness; loss of voice; stuttering]

Infections
botulism
epiglottitis
laryngeal diphtheria
Legionnaire's disease
trichiniasis
Malignant disease
cancer of the hypopharynx
cancer of the larynx
cancer of the mouth
oropharyngeal cancer
Metabolic disorders
hepatolenticular degeneration
Nervous system disorders
autism
Bell's palsy
cerebral palsy
dementia
dialysis encephalopathy
Gilles de la Tourette syndrome
hepatic encephalopathy
motor neuron disease
multiple sclerosis
parkinsonism
stroke
Sydenham's chorea
syringobulbia
transient ischaemic attacks
Nutritional disorders
beri-beri
Oropharyngeal disorders
glossitis
laryngitis
pharyngitis

Spots, facial *see* Skin lesions

Sputum

Blood and lymph disorders
pulmonary embolism and infarction
Cardiovascular system disorders
left heart failure
mitral stenosis
pulmonary hypertension
tricuspid stenosis
Infections
aspergillosis
cryptococcosis
leptospirosis
lung fluke disease
plague
pneumonia
post-primary pulmonary tuberculosis
psittacosis
pulmonary actinomycosis
Malignant disease
lung cancer
Respiratory system disorders
bronchiectasis
chronic bronchitis and emphysema
productive cough

Stools, unusual *see* Faeces, changes in

Swallowing difficulties *see also* Feeding and swallowing difficulties *and* Throat discomfort
[dysphagia]

Blood and lymph disorders
agranulocytosis
Cardiovascular system disorders
thoracic aortic aneurysm
Endocrine disorders
subacute thyroiditis
Gastrointestinal and related disorders
achalasia
reflux oesophagitis
Infections
botulism
epiglottitis
infectious mononucleosis
Lassa fever
scarlet fever
tetanus
tonsillar diphtheria
tonsillitis
Malignant disease
cancer of the hypopharynx
cancer of the larynx
oesophageal cancer
oropharyngeal cancer
thyroid cancer
Metabolic disorders
hepatolenticular degeneration
Musculoskeletal and connective tissue disorders
polymyositis and dermatomyositis
systemic sclerosis
Nervous system disorders
cerebral palsy
motor neurone disease
myasthenia gravis
parkinsonism
syringobulbia
transient ischaemic attacks
Oropharyngeal disorders
glossitis
laryngitis
pharyngitis

Sweating abnormalities
[hyperhidrosis; night sweats; sweating, loss of]

Cardiovascular system disorders
acrocyanosis
angina pectoris
circulatory failure, acute
myocardial infarction
Endocrine disorders
acromegaly
hyperthyroidism
hypoglycaemia
subacute thyroiditis

Gastrointestinal and related disorders
acute intestinal ischaemia
Gynaecological disorders
menopause
Infections
acquired immune deficiency
brucellosis
gas gangrene
malaria
post-primary pulmonary tuberculosis
visceral leishmaniasis
Malignant disease
chronic myeloid leukaemia
insulinoma
lymphomas
phaeochromocytoma
Nervous system disorders
cluster headache
diabetic neuropathy
motion sickness
parkinsonism

Swelling, glandular *see also* Swelling, oedematous
[adenopathy; buboes; lymphadenopathy]

Gastrointestinal and related disorders
cirrhosis of the liver
Whipple's disease
Infections
acquired immune deficiency syndrome
American trypanosomiasis
cellulitis
chancroid
cutaneous anthrax
herpesvirus infections
Lyme disease
lymphangitis
lymphatic filariasis
mumps
pediculosis capitis
plague
rubella
syphilis
tonsillar diphtheria
toxoplasmosis
trypanosomiasis
Malignant disease
breast cancer
cancer of the nasopharynx
chronic lymphoid leukaemia
lymphomas
Musculoskeletal and connective tissue disorders
juvenile chronic arthritis
rheumatoid arthritis
sarcoidosis
systemic lupus erythematosus
Oropharyngeal disorders
sialadenitis
sialolithiasis

Swelling, oedematous *see also* Swelling, glandular
[oedema]

Blood and lymph disorders
anaemias
anaphylactoid purpura
lymphangiectasia
superficial thrombophlebitis
Cardiovascular system disorders
cardiomyopathy
cor pulmonale
heart failure
myocarditis
tricuspid stenosis
varicose veins
Endocrine disorders
Cushing's syndrome
hypothyroidism
Gastrointestinal and related disorders
cirrhosis of the liver
coeliac disease
tropical sprue
Gynaecological disorders
premenstrual syndrome
Infections
American trypanosomiasis
cellulitis
cutaneous anthrax
erysipelas
gas gangrene
hookworm infection
trichiniasis
yellow fever
Malignant disease
breast cancer
Hodgkin's disease
Metabolic disorders
hyponatraemia
Musculoskeletal and connective tissue disorders
dermatomyositis
systemic lupus erythematosus
Nutritional disorders
beri-beri
Obstetric disorders
pre-eclampsia and eclampsia
Renal disorders
glomerulonephritis
nephrotic syndrome
oedema
renal failure
Respiratory system disorders
chronic bronchitis and emphysema
Skin disorders
angioedema
decubitus ulcer
eczema
photosensitivity
pityriasis lichenoides
sunburn
urticaria

T

Thirst
[polydipsia]

Endocrine disorders
diabetes insipidus
primary aldosteronism
type I diabetes mellitus

Infections
cholera
Metabolic disorders
hypercalcaemia
Renal disorders
renal failure

Throat discomfort *see also* Oropharyngeal lesions *and* Swallowing difficulties
[dry throat; laryngeal spasm; lump in the throat; oedema of the throat; sore throat; tonsillar enlargement]

Non specific causes
irritants
Gastrointestinal and related disorders
neurotic dysphagia
Infections
common cold
diphtheria
herpes simplex virus infections
infectious mononucleosis
influenza
Lassa fever
legionellosis
Marburg disease and Ebola fever
measles
poliomyelitis
rabies
scarlet fever
tonsillitis
toxic shock syndrome
Malignant disease
oropharyngeal cancer
Metabolic disorders
hypocalcaemia
Oropharyngeal disorders
laryngitis
pharyngitis
Respiratory system disorders
dry cough

Tongue changes *see also* Oropharyngeal lesions *and* Tongue pain
[dry tongue; furred tongue; glossitis; macroglossia; red tongue; tongue atrophy]

Blood and lymph disorders
amyloidosis
megaloblastic anaemias
Endocrine disorders
acromegaly
hypothyroidism
type I diabetes mellitus
Gastrointestinal and related disorders
cirrhosis of the liver
tropical sprue
Infections
paratyphoid fever
scarlet fever
typhoid fever
Malignant disease
glucagonoma
Nervous system disorders
syringobulbia
Nutritional disorders
pyridoxine deficiency
riboflavine deficiency
Oropharyngeal disorders
glossitis

Tongue pain *see also* Oropharyngeal lesions *and* Tongue changes

Oropharyngeal disorders
glossitis

Tremor

Endocrine disorders
hyperthyroidism
hypoglycaemia
Metabolic disorders
hepatolenticular degeneration
Nervous system disorders
anxiety
opiate withdrawal

Urethral discharge

Infections
gonorrhoea
prostatitis
urethritis

Urination abnormalities
[anuria; dysuria; nocturia; oliguria; polyuria; strangury; tenesmus; urinary frequency; urinary hesitancy; urinary obstruction; urinary retention; urinary urgency]

Non-specific causes
irritants
urethral trauma
uterovaginal prolapse
Blood and lymph disorders
haemolytic anaemias
Cardiovascular system disorders
hypertension
shock
Endocrine disorders
adrenocortical insufficiency, acute
diabetes insipidus
hyperparathyroidism
hypopituitarism
primary aldosteronism
type I diabetes mellitus
Gastrointestinal and related disorders
acute intestinal ischaemia
appendicitis
Gynaecological disorders
dysmenorrhoea
endometriosis
vaginitis
vulvitis
Infections
botulism
gonorrhoea

herpesvirus infections (HSV 2)
prostatitis
schistosomiasis
urinary-tract infections
Male genital disorders
benign prostatic hypertrophy
torsion of the testis
Malignant disease
bladder cancer
prostatic cancer
urothelial tumours
Metabolic disorders
hypercalcaemia
Musculoskeletal and connective tissue disorders
cervical spondylosis
Nervous system disorders
anxiety
diabetic neuropathy
multiple sclerosis
Renal disorders
interstitial nephritis
renal calculi and colic
renal failure
Skin disorders
napkin rash

Urine abnormalities
[blood in urine; chyluria; haematuria; pyuria]

Blood and lymph disorders
anaphylactoid purpura
Gastrointestinal and related disorders
acute hepatitis
cholangitis
cholestatic jaundice
Infections
infective endocarditis
lymphatic filariasis
urinary-tract infections
Weil's disease
Malignant disease
bladder cancer
cancer of the bile ducts
prostatic cancer
renal cancer
Metabolic disorders
maple-syrup urine disease
porphyrias
Nutritional disorders
scurvy
Renal disorders
glomerulonephritis
polycystic kidney disease
renal calculi and colic

Uterine abnormalities
[uterine bleeding, abnormal; uterine contractions; uterine enlargement; uterine prolapse]

Gynaecological disorders
menopause
Malignant disease
choriocarcinoma
endometrial cancer
Obstetric disorders
abortion
hydatidiform mole

V

Vaginal bleeding, abnormal

Malignant disease
cervical cancer
Obstetric disorders
abortion
ectopic pregnancy
hydaditiform mole
postpartum haemorrhage

Vaginal discharge

Gynaecological disorders
vaginitis
Infections
gonorrhoea
pelvic actinomycosis
salpingitis
trichomoniasis
urethritis
vaginal candidiasis
Malignant disease
cervical cancer
endometrial cancer

Vaginal discomfort *see also* Anogenital lesions

Gynaecological disorders
menopause
vaginitis

Visual disturbances
[astigmatism; blindness, temporary; blurred vision; diminished acuity; diplopia; flashes of light; 'floaters' in the field of vision; haloes around lights; loss of accommodation; loss of central vision; loss of peripheral vision; night blindness; photophobia; photosensitivity; retinopathy; sensitivity to light]

Blood and lymph disorders
polycythaemia vera
Cardiovascular system disorders
hypertension
orthostatic hypotension
Endocrine disorders
acromegaly
hypoglycaemia
diabetes mellitus
Eye disorders
blepharitis
cataract
corneal ulceration
dry eye
exophthalmos
glaucoma
keratitis
macular degeneration
optic neuropathies

papilloedema
retinal detachment
scleritis and episcleritis
strabismus
uveitis

Infections
acquired immune deficiency syndrome
botulism
cryptococcal meningitis
measles
myiasis
postviral fatigue syndrome
subacute sclerosing panencephalitis
trachoma
viral meningitis

Malignant disease
intracranial tumours
myeloma

Musculoskeletal and connective tissue disorders
giant cell arteritis

Nervous system disorders
cerebral palsy
hydrocephalus
migraine
multiple sclerosis
myasthenia gravis
stroke
transient ischaemic attacks

Nutritional disorders
vitamin A deficiency
zinc deficiency

Obstetric disorders
pre-eclampsia and eclampsia

Skin disorders
albinism

Voice abnormalities *see also* Speech disturbances
[deepening of the voice; failure of the voice to break]

Endocrine disorders
acromegaly
adrenal virilisation (in females)
hypogonadism (in males)

Vomiting *see* Nausea and/or vomiting

Vulval changes
[vulval atrophy; vulval swelling]

Gynaecological disorders
menopause
vulvitis

Infections
trichomoniasis

W

Weight changes
[obesity; weight gain; weight loss]

Endocrine disorders
Addison's disease
Cushing's syndrome
hyperthyroidism
hypogonadism (in adult males)
hypothyroidism
type I diabetes mellitus

Gastrointestinal and related disorders
chronic intestinal ischaemia
cirrhosis of the liver
coeliac disease
Crohn's disease
gastric ulceration
pyloric stenosis
tropical sprue
tuberculous peritonitis
ulcerative colitis
Whipple's disease

Gynaecological disorders
polycystic ovary syndrome
premenstrual syndrome

Infections
acquired immune deficiency syndrome
brucellosis
cestode infections
dysentery
enterobiasis
shigellosis
trichuriasis
tuberculosis
visceral leishmaniasis

Malignant disease
many diseases

Musculoskeletal and connective tissue disorders
giant cell arteritis
muscular dystrophy
polyarteritis nodosa
polymyalgia rheumatica
rheumatoid arthritis
sarcoidosis

Nervous system disorders
depressive disorders
mania and manic-depressive illness

Nutritional disorders
anorexia nervosa

Obstetric disorders
pre-eclampsia and eclampsia

Renal disorders
interstitial nephritis
oedema

Respiratory system disorders
chronic bronchitis and emphysema
fibrosing alveolitis

Wind *see* Flatulence and eructation

Wrist pain

Nervous system disorders
carpal tunnel syndrome

Part D

Glossary of medical terms

Glossary

Introduction

The glossary provides information on terms that have been used without explanation in the text. It is not intended to act as a comprehensive medical dictionary.

Where appropriate, the combining forms, prefixes and suffixes that make up a word have been listed in brackets after the term itself; the hyphens appended to these forms illustrate their position within that particular term. An explanation of the meaning of the combining forms, prefixes and suffixes is appended as a separate list after the main glossary.

The reader's attention has been drawn to terms that are related by the use of cross-references. The relationship may be that the terms are antonyms, or that they represent varying degrees or stages of the same concept. Synonymous terms have been defined under one term only, and all other synonyms are referred to that term.

For those terms that have more than one definition, any cross-reference follows immediately after the definition to which it applies. If the cross-reference applies to all of the stated definitions, it starts on a new line after the last definition.

The reader should consult the index for a term encountered in the text that has not been included in the glossary, as it will usually be explained elsewhere.

A

Aberrance (ab-) An abnormal course.

Abrasion (ab-) An area where skin or mucous membrane has been removed by a mechanical process (e.g. rubbing).

Abscess A pus-filled cavity formed by tissue disintegration. *See also* COLD ABSCESS *and* MICRO-ABSCESS.

Accommodation Adaptation (e.g. the changing focus of the lens of the eye).

Acetaldehyde Acetaldehyde (ethanal) is an intermediate in the metabolic oxidation of ethanol. It is converted to acetyl-coenzyme A.

Acetylcholine A neurotransmitter released at nerve terminals of the parasympathetic nervous system, at neuromuscular junctions and in autonomic ganglia.

Acetyl-coenzyme A The principal precursor in the formation of lipids, and an intermediate in the Krebs cycle.

Achilles tendon A tendon connecting the calf muscles to the heel.

Achlorhydria (a-) Absence of hydrochloric acid in gastric juice.

Acholuria (a-, -chol-, -uria) Absence of bile pigment in the urine.

Acid A substance that can combine with a base to form a salt; a proton donor; a liberator of hydrogen ions (H^+) in water. *See also* BASE(2).

Acid–base balance The ratio of acids to bases in body fluids, maintained homeostatically with the aid of buffering systems. It ensures that the concentration of hydrogen ions (H^+) in body fluids remains within defined limits.

Acquired Refers to conditions that develop under the influence of external factors, and which are not of genetic or congenital origin.

Acroparaesthesia (acro-, -aesthesi-) Numbness, tingling or other abnormal sensations (e.g. 'pins and needles') in the extremities, usually affecting the fingers, hands and forearms. *See also* ANAESTHESIA, DYSAESTHESIA *and* PARAESTHESIA.

Active immunisation The process of antibody formation, which may occur naturally following recovery from an infection, or may be induced by inoculation with a vaccine or toxoid. *See also* PASSIVE IMMUNISATION *and* VACCINATION(1).

Acuity Clarity, acuteness, sharpness; used especially to refer to vision.

Acute Refers to a disorder with a relatively severe course and of short duration. *See also* CHRONIC *and* SUBACUTE.

Adenitis (aden-, -itis) Inflammation of a gland.

Adenocarcinoma (aden-, -carcin-, -oma) A malignant neoplasm composed of glandular tissue. *See also* ADENOMA.

Adenoid (aden-, -oid) 1. Similar to a gland. 2. The term adenoids refers to lymphoid tissue in the nasopharynx; the pharyngeal tonsil.

Adenoma (aden-, -oma) A benign neoplasm composed of glandular tissue. *See also* ADENOCARCINOMA.

Adenomatous (aden-, -oma-) Refers to an adenoma or glandular hyperplasia.

Adenopathy (adeno-, -pathy) Enlargement of glands, particularly lymph nodes.

Adenosine triphosphate (tri-) Adenosine triphosphate (ATP) is found in all cells where it acts as an energy store. The energy is released by hydrolysis of the high-energy phosphate bonds.

Adenosis (aden-, -osis) 1. Any disorder of a gland. 2. The abnormal development of glandular tissue.

Adhesion (ad-) The joining of neighbouring surfaces of organs and tissues that are normally separate.

Adjunct (ad-, -junct) A substance that is administered to assist or aid another in its actions or to provide a supportive measure.

Adrenalectomy (adren-, -ectomy) The removal of an adrenal gland by surgery.

Adrenergic Refers to sympathetic nerves or to the characteristics of adrenaline and substances producing similar effects (e.g. catecholamines). *See also* CHOLINERGIC *and* SYMPATHOMIMETIC.

Adrenoceptor (-ceptor) A receptor on an effector organ innervated by postganglionic fibres of the sympathetic nervous system. There are two types of adrenoceptor, classified according to their reaction to noradrenaline and adrenaline, and to other excitatory or inhibitory drugs that interact with these receptors. Alpha-adrenoceptors generally produce excitatory responses while beta-adrenoceptors generally produce inhibitory responses.

Adrenocortical (adreno-, -cortic-) Refers to the adrenal cortex.

Adventitia The external layer of connective tissue surrounding an organ, often applied to the tunica externa of an artery.

Adynamic (a-, -dynami-) Refers to loss of, or reduction in, normal function.

Aerobic (aer-) Occurring in, or requiring the presence of, oxygen. *See also* ANAEROBIC.

Aerophagia (aer-, -phagia) The excessive swallowing of air.

Aetiology (-logy) The study of the cause(s) of a disease.

Affect Feelings, mood, or emotions.

Affective disorder (dis-) A disorder characterised by disturbances of affect.

Afferent (af-, -ferent) Carrying inwards to a centre. *See also* EFFERENT.

Agenesis (a-, -gen-, -sis) Absence of an organ or part as a result of complete failure of embryonic development. *See also* APLASIA, DYSPLASIA *and* HYPOPLASIA.

Agnosia (a-, -gno-, -ia) The inability to recognise or interpret sensory stimuli (e.g. auditory, visual and olfactory).

Agonist 1. An agent that stimulates activity at cell receptors. 2. A muscle that causes movement on contraction while its opposing muscle remains relaxed. *See also* ANTAGONIST.

Airway 1. The passage from the nose or mouth to the alveoli, through which air passes during respiration. 2. A device placed in the nose or mouth to ensure the clear passage of air into, and out of, the lungs.

Akinesia (a-, -kine-, -ia) Difficulty in initiating movement or an inability to move. *See also* BRADYKINESIA, DYSKINESIA *and* HYPOKINESIA.

Albumin (alb-) A water-soluble protein synthesised in the liver, and the major protein of blood plasma. Its principal functions are to maintain the intravascular colloid osmotic pressure and to transport water-insoluble substances.

Albuminuria (alb-, -uria) The presence of albumin in the urine.

Alcohol dehydrogenase (-ol, de-, -hydro-, -ase) An enzyme responsible for the dehydrogenation (oxidation) of alcohols to form an aldehyde or aketone.

Alkaline phosphatase (-ase) An hydrolytic enzyme that liberates inorganic phosphate. It is found in many body tissues, and is active at a high pH.

Allele (all-) One of two or more different forms of a gene located at a given site on homologous chromosomes, and responsible for specific characteristics of an organism.

Allergy (all-) A state of hypersensitivity to certain substances (allergens) that is mediated by the immune system. *See also* ATOPY.

Allograft (allo-) Tissue transplant between two genetically different individuals of the same species.

Alpha-1-antitrypsin (anti-) A plasma protein synthesised in the liver, which inhibits the action of proteolytic enzymes (e.g. trypsin and chymotrypsin).

Ambulant Able to walk and not confined to bed.

Amino acid An organic acid containing an amino group ($-NH_2$) and a carboxyl group (-COOH). Amino acids comprise the basic unit in the structure of proteins.

Amniocentesis (-centesis) Aspiration of amniotic fluid, via the transabdominal route, for analysis.

Amputation The complete or partial removal of an appendage or outgrowth of a body (e.g. limb or breast) by surgery.

Anabolism (ana-) A form of metabolism in which living cells synthesise complex compounds from simpler substances. *See also* CATABOLISM.

Anaerobic (an-, -aer-) Occurring in, or requiring the absence of, oxygen. *See also* AEROBIC.

Anaesthesia (an-, -aesthesi-) Complete or partial loss of sensation. It may be caused by a lesion of the nervous system, or it may be artificially induced to perform painful procedures. *See also* ACROPARAESTHESIA, DYSAESTHESIA *and* PARAESTHESIA.

Anaphylatoxin A substance liberated during activation of the complement system. It induces degranulation of mast cells and the release of histamine.

Anaplasia (ana-, -plasia) Retrogression of cells to a less differentiated, more primitive form, characteristic of neoplasms.

Anastomosis (-stomo-, -sis) 1. A connection between normally separate ducts, vessels or cavities which may be formed by surgery, disease, or as a result of trauma. 2. A natural confluence of similar, usually tubular, structures.

Androgen (andro-, -gen) Any substance capable of producing masculine characteristics in either sex.
Angioblast (angio-, -blast) Embryonic tissue from which blood cells and vessels differentiate.
Angioplasty (angio-, -plasty) Reconstruction of a blood vessel by surgery or by other methods (e.g. balloon dilatation).
Angular stomatitis (stomat-, -itis) Superficial inflammation and erosion at one or more corners of the mouth.
Ankylosis (ankylo-, -sis) Joint immobility caused by pathological changes of the joint or associated structures as a result of trauma, disease, or surgery.
Anogenital (-genit-) Refers to the anus and genitalia.
Anorectal (-rect-) Refers to the anus and rectum.
Anorexia (an-, -ia) Loss of appetite.
Antagonist (ant-) 1. An agent that binds to cell receptors without eliciting a pharmacological response, and which can cancel or reverse the action of another. 2. A muscle that cancels or reverses the action of another. *See also* AGONIST.
Antenatal (ante-) Refers to the period between conception and delivery. *See also* POSTNATAL.
Anterior horn (ante-) The ventral portion of grey matter within the spinal cord containing motor cells. *See also* POSTERIOR HORN.
Antibiotic (anti-, -bio-) An organic compound, produced by microorganisms, that kills or inhibits the growth of other microorganisms, and is used to treat infections. The term may also be applied to synthetic derivatives. *See also* ANTIMICROBIAL.
Antibody (anti-) A specific immunoglobulin produced by the immune system in response to stimulation by an antigen, and which reacts only with that antigen or one that is closely related. *See also* ANTINUCLEAR ANTIBODY *and* AUTO-ANTIBODY.
Anticholinergic (anti-) 1. A substance that antagonises the action of acetylcholine at muscarinic and nicotinic receptors of the parasympathetic nervous system. 2. Inhibition of the passage of impulses through parasympathetic nerves. *See also* ANTIMUSCARINIC.
Antifibrinolytic (anti-, -ly-) A substance that inhibits the enzymatic dissolution of fibrin.
Antigen (anti-, -gen) An agent that, under suitable conditions, induces a specific immune response. It also interacts with antibodies or sensitised T-cells specific to it, or both.
Antigen determinant (anti-, -gen) The chemical structure on the surface of an antigen responsible for the specific interaction with an antibody.
Antimicrobial (anti-, -micro-) An agent that kills or inhibits the growth of microorganisms. *See also* ANTIBIOTIC.
Antimicrobial resistance (anti-, -micro-) A microorganism may be naturally insensitive to an antimicrobial agent. Alternatively, a microorganism may acquire resistance during use of an antimicrobial by natural selection of a resistant strain or by random mutation. Resistance may also be transferred from one microorganism to another.
Antimuscarinic (anti-) An agent that antagonises the action of acetylcholine at muscarinic receptors of the parasympathetic nervous system.
Antinuclear antibody (anti-, -nucle-) An auto-antibody that interacts with specific components of cell nuclei (e.g. DNA).
Antiseptic (anti-, -sep-) A chemical agent used to kill or inhibit the growth of microorganisms on living tissue, in order to prevent or reduce the harmful effects of infection. *See also* DISINFECTANT.
Antiserum (anti-, -ser-) A human or animal serum preparation containing antibodies, whose production is induced by the administration of an antigen or by natural infection. Antisera are used for passive immunisation. *See also* VACCINE.
Antitoxin (anti-, -toxi-) An antibody that acts against a toxin, especially a bacterial exotoxin.
Anuria (an-, -uria) Complete cessation of urine formation by the kidneys, and hence excretion.
Apathy Indifference or lack of concern, interest or emotion.
Aphasia (a-, -pha-, -ia) A reduction in, or loss of, comprehension of spoken or written language, or the ability to speak or write. It is usually caused by a lesion of the speech centre of the brain.
Aphonia (a-, -phon-, -ia) Loss of voice.
Aphtha Small, shallow, and painful ulcer, usually of the oral mucosa.
Aplasia (a-, -plasia) 1. Incomplete development of an organ, tissue, or part, although the basic structure may be present. 2. Incomplete or absent formation of cellular products from an organ or tissue. *See also* AGENESIS, DYSGENESIS, DYSPLASIA *and* HYPOPLASIA.
Apnoea (a-, -pnoea) Cessation of breathing. *See also* DYSPNOEA, HYPERPNOEA, ORTHOPNOEA *and* TACHYPNOEA.
Appendage (ap-, -pend-) An outgrowth from a body or organ.
Appendectomy (-ectomy) The removal of the appendix by surgery.
Apposed (ap-) Two surfaces in contact with each other. *See also* CONTIGUOUS.
Apraxia (a-, -prax-, -ia) Impairment of voluntary muscular movement in the absence of paralysis or other impairment of motor or sensory pathways. *See also* ATAXIA.
Arachidonic acid An essential unsaturated fatty acid found in animal fats, and a precursor of prostaglandins.
Arterial tension (arteri-, tens-) The pressure provoked by blood within an artery.
Arterionecrosis (arterio-, -necro-, -sis) Necrosis of arteries.
Arteritis (arter-, -itis) Inflammation of an artery. *See also* VASCULITIS.
Arthralgia (arthr-, -algia) Joint pain.
Arthropathy (arthro-, -pathy) Any disease of the joints.
Articular (articul-) Refers to a joint.
Artificial respiration (-spirat-) A technique employed to produce respiratory movements when natural movements have ceased. *See also* ASSISTED VENTILATION.
Aschoff nodule A granulomatous lesion with a central necrotic core.
Aseptic (a-, -sep-) Refers to the complete absence of microorganisms.
Asexual reproduction Production of offspring without gametes and fusion. Asexual methods include budding and fission. *See also* SEXUAL REPRODUCTION.

Asphyxia (a-, -ia) Impaired or absent ventilation caused by airway obstruction or lack of oxygen in inspired air. *See also* SUFFOCATION.
Aspiration (-spirat-) 1. To remove fluid from body cavities by applying suction. 2. Inhalation.
Assisted ventilation Respiratory support by mechanical means. *See also* ARTIFICIAL RESPIRATION.
Astigmatism (a-, -stig-, -ism) A focusing abnormality of the eye caused by irregular surfaces of the cornea or lens, resulting in blurred or distorted vision.
Astringent (-stringent) An agent that causes constriction of tissues to lessen secretion or discharge.
Astrocyte (astro-, -cyte) A cell found in the grey and white matter of the central nervous system, and forming part of the supporting network for neurons.
Astrocytoma (astro-, -cyt-, -oma) A malignant neoplasm composed of astrocytes.
Asymptomatic (a-) Symptom-free.
Ataxia (a-, -tax-, -ia) Impaired co-ordination of muscular movements. *See also* APRAXIA.
Atheroma (-oma) Plaques on arterial walls, initially of cholesterol deposits, which may become fibrous or calcified.
Athetosis (-osis) Repetitive, involuntary, slow, writhing movements of the limbs, usually most severe in the hands and feet.
Atony (a-, -ton-) Decreased tone of a tissue, resulting in weakness or loss of normal strength.
Atopic (a-, -top-) 1. Refers to atopy. 2. ECTOPIC(2).
Atopy (a-, -top-) A hypersensitivity to common allergens, involving immunoglobulin E (IgE). It is thought to be familial. *See also* ALLERGY.
ATP ADENOSINE TRIPHOSPHATE.
Atresia (a-, -ia) Abnormal closure of a channel in the body (e.g. bile duct) or an external orifice (e.g. anus).
Atrophy (a-, -trophy) The decrease in size of a cell, organ, tissue, or part of an organism. *See also* HYPERTROPHY *and* INVOLUTION.
Aura The sensations preceding the onset of any paroxysmal attack. The aura may be affective, sensory, or motor. *See also* PRODROMAL.
Auto-antibody (auto-, -anti-) An antibody produced in autoimmune diseases as a result of immunological intolerance of the body's own tissues. Auto-antibodies may be organ-specific or antinuclear.
Auto-immunity (auto-) The immune response directed towards the body's own tissues, which results in the production of auto-antibodies.
Auto-infection (auto-) Infection caused by microorganisms already present in the body, and commonly, but not exclusively, transferred from one site to another.
Autolysis (auto-, -lysis) Destruction of cells or tissues by the action of the organism's own intracellar enzymes. It occurs after death, or it may be pathological.
Autonomous (auto-) Functionally independent.
Autosome (auto-, -some) Any of the chromosomes in a cell, excluding the sex chromosomes. In a human somatic cell there are 44 autosomes (22 pairs) and 2 sex chromosomes (1 pair).
Autotrophic (auto-, -trophic) A type of nutrition in which carbon dioxide is the sole source of carbon for synthesis of organic compounds. *See also* HETEROTROPHIC.
Avascular (a-, -vas-) Lack of blood supply to a tissue. *See also* VASCULAR.
Avirulent (a-) Not pathogenic.
Axon The long specialised process of a neuron along which impulses travel away from the cell to other neurons and tissues.
Azoospermia (a-, -zoo-, -sperm-, -ia) Absence of spermatozoa in the semen.

B

Bacteraemia (bacter-, -aemia) The presence of bacteria in the blood.
Bacteriophage (bacterio-, -phag-) A virus that causes lysis of bacteria, usually specific for a particular strain or species.
Bacteriuria (bacteri-, -uria) The presence of bacteria in the urine.
Balanitis (balan-, -itis) Inflammation of the glans penis and the prepuce in the male, or the clitoris in the female.
Barrier nursing The nursing techniques applied to prevent the spread of infection from the affected patient to others. Reverse barrier nursing comprises the nursing techniques applied to infection-prone patients who are kept in isolation to prevent the acquisition of infection.
Basal (bas-) Refers to, or situated near, the base.
Base (bas-) 1. The lowest part of a structure or organ. 2. A non-acid that can combine with an acid to form a salt; a proton acceptor; a liberator of hydroxyl ions (OH^-) in water. *See also* ACID.
Behaviour disorder (dis-) A disorder of behaviour often associated with psychoses and related disorders, characterised by abnormal actions (e.g. disinhibition, hyperactivity or mannerisms).
Behaviour therapy (therap-) Psychological treatment to alleviate the symptoms of abnormal behaviour produced by certain stimuli.
Benign A condition that is mild, favouring recovery and not recurrent or malignant.
Betacarotene A provitamin found in some vegetables (e.g. carrots) and converted to vitamin A by the liver.
Betz cells Large pyramidal neurons of the Betz cell area in the motor cortex. They form part of the pyramidal tract and control voluntary movement.
Bicarbonate A salt of carbonic acid in which the anionic portion is HCO_3^-. Administered as sodium bicarbonate infusion to correct acid–base imbalance.
Biliary (bili-) Refers to the gall bladder, bile ducts, or bile.
Biopsy (bio-) The removal of living tissue, diseased or normal, for examination, used as an aid in diagnosis.
Biosynthesis (bio-, -syn-, -sis) The formation of substances within a living organism by the process of synthesis, often under the control of enzymes.
Bipolar (bi-) 1. Possessing two poles, or processes at both ends. 2. At both ends of a cell. 3. Used to describe affective disorders characterised by both manic and depressive periods. *See also* UNIPOLAR.
Birth asphyxia (neo-, a-, -ia) Birth asphyxia (neonatal asphyxia) occurs at, or during, birth, usually due to disorders *in utero*.

Birth canal Comprises the cervix, vagina, and vulva, and through which the fetus passes during birth.

Blepharospasm (blepharo-, -spas-) Tonic muscular spasm of the eyelid, resulting in complete or partial closure of the eye.

Blind antimicrobial treatment (anti-, -micro-) Antimicrobial therapy administered to a patient with pyrexia of unknown origin (PUO), before microbiological confirmation of infection and antimicrobial sensitivity. *See also* BROAD-SPECTRUM ANTIMICROBIAL DRUG.

Bone marrow Specialised tissue found in the cavity of long bones and the spongy tissue of all bones. It consists of a network of reticular fibres and cells, including blood cells at different stages of development, fat cells, and macrophages. Its functions include the production of erythrocytes, leucocytes, and platelets.

Bone reabsorption (re-) Loss of bone tissue mediated by osteoclasts, which may be physiological or pathological.

Boss A round protruding part of a structure or tissue.

Bradykinesia (brady-, -kine-, -ia) Abnormally slow movement, and physical and mental response. *See also* AKINESIA, DYSKINESIA, and HYPOKINESIA.

Bradykinin A polypeptide, and one of a group of kinins.

Broad-spectrum antimicrobial drug (anti-, -micro-) Describes the activity of an antimicrobial drug to which a wide range of microorganisms are sensitive. *See also* BLIND ANTIMICROBIAL TREATMENT.

Bronchopulmonary (broncho-, -pulmon-) Refers to the lungs and the airways into them (i.e. the bronchi and bronchioles).

Bronchoscopy (broncho-, -scopy) Examination of the bronchi using a fibreoptic bronchoscope, which is also a tool for biopsy.

Bronchospasm (broncho-, -spas-) Spasmodic smooth muscle contraction of the bronchi.

Bunion A swelling of the first metatarsophalangeal joint caused by a bursa. It results in displacement of the great toe.

C

Cachexia (cac-, -ia) Severe generalised ill-health caused by chronic disorders or malnutrition, and marked by emaciation and general weakness.

Cadaver A corpse. The term usually refers to a human body used for medical study or other procedures (e.g. transplantation).

Caesarean section (sect-) Surgical delivery of a fetus by incision through the abdominal and uterine walls.

Calcification (calci-) The physiological or pathological deposition of calcium salts in tissues, resulting in hardening.

Calculus (calc-) A hard stone-like deposit of mineral salts or other material, found in certain body cavities and tissues (e.g. kidney, bladder, and gall bladder).

Cancer A malignant neoplasm.

Cannabis Part of any plant of the genus *Cannabis*. Its various forms are known by many names, including bhang, ganja, hashish and marijuana.

Capsule (caps-) 1. Outer covering of an organ or structure. 2. A shell, usually made from a gelatin basis, containing glycerol in proportions that may be varied to regulate the degree of hardness. Capsules are used to enclose one or more drugs and excipients.

Capsulitis (caps-, -itis) Inflammation of a capsule.

Carbohydrate (carbo-, -hydrat-) A member of a large and diverse group of organic compounds containing carbon, hydrogen and oxygen. Carbohydrates include sugars, starches, celluloses and gums, and are classified as monosaccharides (e.g. glucose), disaccharides (e.g. sucrose), and polysaccharides (e.g. glycogen). They act as the principal source of metabolic energy in living cells.

Carbonic anhydrase (carbo-, -an-, -hydr-, -ase) An enzyme that catalyses the conversion of carbon dioxide and water to carbonic acid, which further dissociates into hydrogen ions (H^+) and bicarbonate ions (HCO_3^-).

Carcinogen (carcino-, -gen) An agent capable of inducing a malignant neoplasm.

Carcinoid (carcin-, -oid) Histologically similar to a malignant neoplasm but clinically benign.

Cardiac (cardi-) 1. Refers to the heart. 2. Refers to the opening between the oesophagus and the stomach.

Cardiac massage, external (cardi-) Rhythmic manual compression of the heart to maintain the circulation by applying pressure over the sternum.

Cardiac output (cardi-) The amount of blood expelled per minute into the aorta from the left ventricle. It is equal to the stroke volume multiplied by the number of beats per minute.

Cardiac reserve (cardi-) The capacity of the heart for increased function in response to greater demands, expressed as the maximum percentage that the cardiac output can increase above normal.

Cardiac tamponade (cardi-) Compression of the heart as a result of the accumulation of fluid or blood within the pericardium.

Cardiogenic (cardio-, -genic) 1. Arising from the heart or as a result of its abnormal function. 2. Refers to the embryonic development of the heart.

Cardiomyocyte (cardio-, -myo-, -cyte) A cell of the myocardium.

Cardiomyotomy (cardio-, -myo-, -tomy) Incision through the muscle layer at the junction of the oesophagus and the stomach, but excluding the mucous membrane.

Cardioversion (cardio-, -vers-) Synchronised transthoracic electric shock applied under general anaesthesia to restore sinus rhythm of the heart.

Carditis (card-, -itis) Inflammation of the heart.

Carotid artery (arter-) An artery supplying the head and neck. There are two common carotid arteries, designated left and right. Each passes upwards through the neck, where they divide to form the internal and external carotid arteries.

Carotid sinus (sinu-) The small dilated region in the internal carotid artery. It contains baroreceptors that are sensitive to blood pressure fluctuations, and which are involved in the reflex control of blood pressure and heart-rate.

Carpal tunnel (carp-) The passage in the wrist between the carpal bones and ligaments, through which the median nerve passes.

Carrier 1. An individual who harbours (and is thus capable of transmitting) the microorganisms capable of causing an infection, without showing any signs or symptoms of illness. *See also* RESERVOIR OF INFECTION. 2. An individual capable of transmitting a hereditary disease to offspring. 3. A substance used to transport a drug as an aid to efficacy.

Caseation 1. The precipitation of casein during the coagulation of milk. 2. A degeneration or necrosis in which morbid tissues are changed into a dry cheese-like mass.

Catabolism (cata-) A form of metabolism in which complex compounds are broken down by living cells to form simpler substances. *See also* ANABOLISM *and* FERMENTATION.

Catalase (cata-, -ase) An enzyme present in most cells, except some anaerobic bacteria, and responsible for the breakdown of hydrogen peroxide to water and oxygen.

Catarrh Inflammation of a mucous membrane (particularly one in the upper respiratory tract) causing an increased flow of mucus.

Catecholamine A sympathomimetic compound containing a catechol and an amine group. Physiological examples include adrenaline, noradrenaline and dopamine.

Catheter A flexible tube inserted into a body cavity to withdraw or introduce fluids. *See also* INDWELLING CATHETER.

Caudaequina (caud-) The nerve roots arising from the lower part of the spinal cord and forming a tail-like structure.

Cauterisation The therapeutic destruction of tissue using heat, an electric current or caustic agents. *See also* CRYOSURGERY.

Cavernous (cav-, -ous) Refers to a structure or tissue containing hollow spaces.

Cavitation (cav-) 1. The formation of hollow spaces within tissues. 2. A cavity.

Central vision Vision produced through stimulation of the macula lutea by light. *See also* PERIPHERAL VISION.

Cercaria The final free-swimming larval stage of flukes.

Cerebellum A motor area of the brain involved in the involuntary control of co-ordination, posture and balance.

Cerebral (cerebr-) Refers to the cerebrum.

Cerebrovascular (cerebro-, -vas-) Refers to the blood vessels that supply the brain, and especially the cerebral hemispheres.

Cervical smear (cervic-) A cervical smear (Pap test) is the microscopic examination of cells obtained from the cervix of the uterus, and used to detect cervical cell abnormalities.

Cervicitis (cervic-, -itis) Inflammation of the cervix of the uterus.

Cervicofacial (cervic-, -faci-) Refers to the face and neck.

Cervix The neck of an organ or body, but generally refers to the neck of the uterus.

Chalone 1. A hormone that exerts an inhibitory effect. 2. A tissue-specific reversible inhibitor of mitosis produced by the tissue itself.

Chancre A primary ulcer-like lesion at the point of entry of an infection, usually applied to the primary lesion seen in syphilis.

Cheilitis (cheil-, -itis) Inflammation of the lips.

Chelate To form a complex with a metal ion, incorporating it into a ring and rendering it inactive.

Chemoprophylaxis (chemo-) The use of a chemotherapeutic agent as a preventive measure against disease.

Chemosurgery (chemo-) 1. The combined use of surgery and chemical agents to remove diseased tissue. 2. The therapeutic destruction of tissue using chemical agents.

Chemotaxis (chemo-, -tax-) The directional movement of a cell or organism in response to a chemical stimulus.

Chemotherapy (chemo-, -therap-) The treatment of disease using drugs.

Cheyne-Stokes respiration (-spirat-) An abnormal respiratory rhythm characterised by alternating periods of hyperpnoea and apnoea.

Chiasma The crossing of two elements or structures in an X-formation.

Cholecystectomy (chole-, -cyst-, -ectomy) The removal of the gall bladder by surgery.

Choledochotomy (choledocho-, -tomy) Surgical incision of the bile duct for investigation or the removal of gallstones.

Cholestasis (chole-, -stasis) The complete or partial inhibition of the flow of bile.

Cholesterol (chole-, -ster-, -ol) A steroid alcohol synthesised in the liver and used in the formation of bile acids and steroid hormones (e.g. oestrogens). Cholesterol may also be ingested in the diet (e.g. in animal fats, milk, egg-yolk, liver and kidneys).

Cholinergic Refers to parasympathetic nerves or to the characteristics of acetylcholine and substances producing similar effects. *See also* ADRENERGIC.

Chondritis (chondr-, -itis) Inflammation of cartilage.

Chordae tendineae (chord-, ten-) The tendinous cords connecting each cusp of the tricuspid and mitral valves to the papillary muscles in the heart.

Chorionic gonadotrophin (gon-, -trophin) A hormone produced by placental tissue, and which stimulates the gonads. It is also found in the urine of pregnant females.

Chromaffin cell (chrom-) A specialised cell that readily stains with chromium salts, and is found in the adrenal medulla and other parts of the sympathetic nervous system. It is responsible for the storage and secretion of catecholamines.

Chromatolysis (chromato-, -lysis) The disintegration of the Nissl granules within a nerve cell body, caused by injury or cell fatigue.

Chromophobe cell (chromo-, -phobe) A cell that does not stain easily, if at all. In particular, it refers to some agranular cells in the anterior lobe of the pituitary gland.

Chromosome (chromo-, -some) A structure present in all cell nuclei, formed of chromatin and containing DNA. Animals have a characteristic number of chromosomes present in all somatic cells. In humans, this number is 46 (23 pairs). *See also* AUTOSOME.

Chronic (chron-) Refers to a disorder which persists. *See also* ACUTE *and* SUBACUTE.

Chyluria (-uria) The presence of chyle in the urine.

Cicatrix The new tissue formed on healing of a wound; a scar.

Cilia (cili-) 1. Hair-like projections from a cell that facilitate movement. 2. Eyelashes. 3. Eyelids.

Circadian rhythm (circa) The cycle of about 24 hours that marks repetitive biological activities and functions in living organisms. *See also* DIURNAL *and* NOCTURNAL.

Claudication Limping.

Clitoris A part of the female external genitalia situated at the anterior end of the vulva and corresponding to the male penis in structure, position, and origin. The clitoris is normally less than 2 cm long.

Clonus Muscular contraction and relaxation occurring in rapid succession. *See also* MYOCLONUS.

Clubbing Enlargement of the soft tissue of the fingers and toes, resulting in a characteristic deformity. The nails are curved and have a shiny appearance.

Coarctation Narrowing or stricture. *See also* STENOSIS.

Coccidioidomycosis (-myco-, -sis) A fungal infection caused by *Coccidioides immitis*, and affecting the skin, bone, viscera or respiratory tract.

Codon A set of three nucleotides in one strand of DNA or RNA, and which carries the code for one amino acid.

Coenocytic (coeno-, -cyt-) Refers to a cell or mass of cytoplasm in which there is more than one nucleus.

Coenzyme (co-, -zym-) A non-protein organic substance that activates an enzyme.

Coitus Sexual intercourse between a male and a female.

Cold abscess An abscess that is not inflamed and warm, and develops slowly.

Colectomy (col-, -ectomy) The complete or partial removal of the colon by surgery.

Colitis (col-, -itis) Inflammation of the colon.

Collagen The constituent protein of the white fibres of connective tissue.

Collagenase (-ase) An enzyme that catalyses collagen degradation.

Collateral (col-) Secondary, subordinate, or alternative.

Colloid cyst A cyst containing material that resembles jelly, and which is sometimes found in the brain.

Colonoscopy (col-, -scopy) Examination of the colon using a fibreoptic colonoscope, which is also a tool for biopsy.

Colorectal (col-, -rect-) Refers to the colon and the rectum.

Colostomy (col-, -stomy) A surgical procedure to establish an opening (stoma) from the colon to the surface of the abdomen, and through which faeces may be eliminated. It may be temporary or permanent. The term may also be applied to the opening itself. *See also* ILEOSTOMY and UROSTOMY.

Coma A state of deep unconsciousness with no voluntary response to external stimuli. Some reflex actions may also be impaired. *See also* STUPOR.

Common bile duct The duct that transports bile to the duodenum. It is formed by the merging of the cystic duct from the gall bladder and the common hepatic duct from the liver.

Complement A series of nine components (C1 to C9) activated in a specific sequence (cascade) by certain antigen–antibody complexes. Activated complement binds to the complex and destroys the antigen by several possible mechanisms (e.g. chemotaxis and inflammation, cell lysis, and phagocytosis). The system is regulated by inhibitory factors (e.g. C1-esterase inhibitor).

Compliance 1. A measure of the ability of an organ (e.g. heart, bladder, or lungs) to alter shape and size in response to varying demands. 2. Agreement, consent, or yielding to the wishes of another.

Computerised tomography Computerised tomography (CT) is a technique which uses X-rays and detectors to scan the body in cross-section. Visual images are produced by computer processing of the data.

Conception The start of pregnancy, marked by the fertilisation of an ovum.

Concretion 1. The formation of a solid mass. 2. CALCULUS.

Congenital (-gen-) Refers to any condition existing before or at birth. *See also* HEREDITARY.

Conidium An asexual spore formed at the tip of a conidiophore (a specialised branch of a mycelium). The conidium is non-motile and is produced by some species of fungi and filamentous bacteria.

Conjugated hyperbilirubinaemia *See* HYPERBILIRUBINAEMIA.

Consolidation The process of becoming firm or solid. *See also* CONCRETION.

Contagious May be transmitted from one individual to another.

Contiguous (con-) Two parts that are adjacent or in contact. *See also* APPOSED.

Contraction (-tract-) A shortening or reduction in overall size that is usually temporary, or an increase in tension (e.g. muscle contraction to facilitate movement).

Contracture (-tract-) A sustained shortening or contraction of muscle(s), caused by pathological changes in muscle tissue.

Contraindication (contra-) A condition or disease that renders an otherwise acceptable treatment completely unsuitable.

Contusion A bruise; an injury that does not break the skin.

Convulsion An involuntary, violent, and spasmodic or prolonged contraction of skeletal muscles. *See also* SEIZURE.

Coralline Similar to or branching like coral.

Coronary Refers to vessels, nerves or ligaments that encircle a structure, although usually applied to the arteries that lie over the outer surface of cardiac muscle.

Coronary bypass A surgical procedure to bypass an obstruction in a coronary artery. A vein (usually taken from the leg) or other suitable conduit is grafted between the aorta and coronary arteries and distal to the obstruction.

Cowpox A skin infection affecting the udders and teats of cows, caused by cowpox virus (vaccinia). It may be transmitted to humans. *See also* VACCINATION(2).

Cramp An involuntary and painful spasmodic muscle contraction.

Craniotomy (cranio-, -tomy) A surgical procedure on the cranium.

Creatinine The end-product of metabolism in muscle tissue, excreted by the kidneys.

Creatinine clearance The volume of plasma cleared of creatinine, expressed as millilitres per minute.

Cribriform plate The bony plate at the top of the nasal cavity, which is perforated to allow the passage of the olfactory nerves. *See also* ETHMOID BONE.

Cross tolerance Tolerance acquired to one drug which is exhibited towards other, usually similar, agents.

Cryosurgery (cryo-) The therapeutic destruction of tissue using extremely low temperatures.

Cryotherapy (cryo-, -therap-) The use of low temperatures for therapeutic purposes. *See also* CAUTERISATION.

Crypt A small pocket or recess found on the surface of some tissues.

Cryptogenic (crypto-, -genic) Of unknown origin. *See also* IDIOPATHIC.

Crystalluria (-uria) The presence of crystals in the urine.

Cubitus valgus Deformity of the elbow, marked by a deviation away from the body when the arm is placed by the side.

Curettage The removal of material from a surface or cavity wall using a spoon-shaped instrument (curette).

Cutaneous (cut-) Refers to the skin.

Cuticle (cut-) 1. The epidermis. 2. The epidermis that surrounds the base of the nail. 3. A layer covering the free surface of epithelial cells.

Cyst 1. An enclosed cavity or sac with an epithelial lining, and often containing fluid. 2. A stage in the life-cycle of some parasites, marked by enclosure within a protective covering.

Cystadenoma (cyst-, -aden-, -oma) An adenoma in which fluid-filled cysts form.

Cystectomy (cyst-, -ectomy) 1. The removal of a cyst. 2. The complete or partial removal of the urinary bladder by surgery.

Cystic (cysti-) 1. Refers to a cyst. 2. Refers to the urinary bladder or to the gall bladder.

Cystic duct (cysti-) The duct passing from the gall bladder to the common bile duct, and through which bile passes.

Cystinuria (-uria) A hereditary disorder that results in excessive urinary excretion of cystine, arginine, lysine and ornithine and results in the formation of urinary cystine calculi.

Cytoplasm (cyto-, -plas-) The protoplasm of a cell located outside the nucleus. *See also* NUCLEOPLASM.

Cytoplasmic membrane (cyto-, -plas-) The membrane enclosing the cytoplasm of a cell, composed of phospholipids and proteins.

Cytostatic (cyto-, -stat-) 1. Refers to the suppression of cell growth and multiplication. 2. Refers to the blockage of capillaries by leucocytes in the early stages of inflammation.

Cytotoxic (cyto-, -toxi-) Refers to agents that have an adverse effect on cells.

D

Dacryocystorhinostomy (dacryo-, -cysto-, -rhino-, -stomy) Surgical procedure to create a passage from the lachrymal sac to the nasal cavity.

Danders Scales from animal hair or bird feathers.

Dark adaptation Adjustment by the eye for night vision.

Dead space 1. The regions within the respiratory tract through which air passes, but exchange of oxygen and carbon dioxide does not take place. 2. A cavity that remains after incomplete closure of a wound.

Debility (de-) 1. Generalised weakness and loss of strength. 2. Loss of muscle tone due to illness.

Debridement (de-) The removal of dead, injured, or infected tissue, or foreign material from a wound.

Decerebrate (de-, -cerebr-) Loss of cerebral function as result of brain damage.

Decerebrate posture A position characteristic of damage to the upper part of the brain stem. The patient's legs are rigidly extended with flexed ankles and toes, the arms are internally rotated, and the elbows are extended.

Decompression (de-) A procedure to relieve pressure exerted on or within tissues.

Defecation (de-) The elimination of faeces from the rectum.

Definitive host The host within which a parasite reaches sexual maturity or its adult stage. *See also* INTERMEDIATE HOST.

Dehydration (de-, -hydrat-) The removal or loss of water from a substance or from body tissues.

Delirium A mental disorder of varying severity characterised by hallucinations, delusions, impaired perception, excitement, restlessness and disorientation.

Delirium tremens Delirium caused by alcohol withdrawal in alcohol-dependent subjects.

Delusion A false belief that is firmly held, even in the presence of irrefutable evidence to the contrary. *See also* HALLUCINATION.

Demyelination (de-, -myel-) Loss of the myelin sheath surrounding nerves.

Denature (de-) To alter the nature of a substance; often applied to proteins that are physically changed by the action of heat or chemical agents. Also applied to the adulteration of alcohol to render it unfit for consumption.

Dendritic (dendr-) 1. Branching, like a tree. 2. Refers to the cytoplasmic thread-like extensions (dendrites) of neurons.

Dentition (denti-) The teeth; usually refers to natural teeth and their position.

Deoxyribonucleic acid (-nucle-) Deoxyribonucleic acid (DNA) is found in the nucleus of all living cells and is the store of genetic information. The molecular structure is a double helix, in which each of the two strands is composed of a deoxyribose-phosphate backbone with attached nitrogenous bases (adenine, cytosine, guanine and thymine). The two strands are held together by hydrogen bonds between the bases, which pair in a specific sequence to determine the genetic information. *See also* RIBONUCLEIC ACID.

Dermabrasion (derma-) Skin abrasion using wire brushes or sandpaper, under local anaesthesia, to remove superficial lesions.

Dermatitis herpetiformis (derma-, -itis, herpet-, -form-) A chronic skin disorder with remissions and relapses, which is frequently associated with coeliac disease. It is characterised by intense pruritus and the presence of symmetrical groups of erythematous lesions (e.g. bullae, papules and vesicles) on the buttocks, elbows, knees, scalp and shoulders. Hyperpigmentation is a common feature, although hypopigmentation and scarring may also occur.

Dermatographism (dermato-, -graph-, -ism) Urticaria caused by firm stroking of the skin.

Desquamation (de-, -squam-) The shedding of an outer layer (e.g. epithelial cells of the skin) in the form of scales.

Dialysis (dia-, -lysis) The separation of small non-colloidal molecules from larger colloidal molecules in solution, across a semipermeable membrane. *See also* HAEMODIALYSIS *and* PERITONEAL DIALYSIS.

Diaphragm (dia-, -phrag-) A structure separating one area from another. It usually refers to the muscular structure that separates the thoracic cavity from the abdominal cavity.

Diaphysis The shaft of a long bone. *See also* EPIPHYSIS.

Diarthroidal joint (-arthr-) A joint that is freely movable (e.g. hip, elbow or wrist).

Diastole The period during which the chambers of the heart dilate and fill with blood. *See also* SYSTOLE.

Diastolic pressure The minimum arterial blood pressure, which occurs during ventricular diastole. *See also* SYSTOLIC PRESSURE.

Diathermy (-therm-) The heat treatment of tissues using an electric current, ultrasonic waves or electromagnetic radiation. It may be used to warm tissues or destroy them. *See also* CRYOSURGERY.

Differentiation Applied to cells and tissues as they mature into specialised forms and acquire specificity.

Diffusion (di-, -fus-) The spontaneous movement of molecules, ions or particles in order to reach a uniform concentration throughout the solvent.

Dilatation The increase in volume or enlargement of orifices and hollow organs and structures (e.g. colon, arteries and heart). *See also* DISTENSION.

Diphtheroid (-oid) Similar to diphtheria or the causative microorganism *Corynebacterium diphtheriae*.

Diplegia (di-, -plegia) Paralysis affecting corresponding parts on both sides of the body. *See also* HEMIPLEGIA, PARAPLEGIA *and* QUADRIPLEGIA.

Diploid (di-, -ploid) Having two sets of chromosomes.

Diplopia (dipl-, -opia) Double vision, in which two images of a single object are seen.

Disinfectant (dis-) A chemical agent used to destroy microorganisms, but not necessarily bacterial spores; it may reduce the number to a level below that which is harmful rather than kill all the microorganisms present. The term may be applied to treatment of inanimate objects, as well as body surfaces and cavities. *See also* ANTISEPTIC.

Disseminated (dis-) Dispersed or spread throughout.

Disseminated intravascular coagulation (dis-, intra-, -vas-) A condition in which there is widespread activation of tissue factor, which leads to blood clotting within vessels. A generalised depletion of clotting factors eventually causes haemorrhage. A variety of disorders may allow elements that activate tissue factor to enter the blood. These include obstetric complications, Gram-negative endotoxins, adenocarcinomas, snakebites and major trauma.

Distension Enlargement due to internal pressure. *See also* DILATATION.

Diuresis (-ur-, -sis) An increase in urine production. *See also* ENURESIS *and* INCONTINENCE.

Diurnal Refers to activities that occur during the hours of daylight. *See also* CIRCADIAN RHYTHM *and* NOCTURNAL.

DNA DEOXYRIBONUCLEIC ACID.

Duodenal bulb The first part of the duodenum, adjacent to the pylorus.

Dynamic (dynami-) Refers to force and motion; active.

Dysaesthesia (dys-, -aesthesi-) Impairment of sensory function, particularly touch. *See also* ACROPARAESTHESIA, ANAESTHESIA *and* PARAESTHESIA.

Dyscrasia (dys-) A general term for any abnormal condition, particularly developmental or metabolic disorders.

Dysfunction (dys-, -funct-) Functional abnormality of an organ.

Dysgenesis (dys-, -gen-, -sis) Defective development, often applied to embryonic development. *See also* AGENESIS, APLASIA, DYSPLASIA *and* HYPOPLASIA.

Dyskinesia (dys-, -kine-, -ia) Difficulty in voluntary movement such that movements are partial, incomplete or fragmentary. *See also* AKINESIA, BRADYKINESIA *and* HYPOKINESIA.

Dyslexia (dys-, -ia) A reading abnormality in the presence of normal intellect, which may be caused by a brain lesion. There may also be spelling and handwriting impairment.

Dyspareunia (dys-, -ia) Difficult or painful sexual intercourse.

Dysplasia (dys-, -plasia) Abnormal development of an organ or part. *See also* AGENESIS, APLASIA, DYSGENESIS *and* HYPOPLASIA.

Dyspnoea (dys-, -pnoea) Difficulty in breathing. *See also* APNOEA, HYPERPNOEA, ORTHOPNOEA *and* TACHYPNOEA.

Dysuria (dys-, -uria) Difficult or painful urination. *See also* STRANGURY.

E

ECT ELECTROCONVULSIVE THERAPY

Ectopia (ecto-, -ia) Malposition or displacement of an organ or part. It is usually congenital.

Ectopic (ecto-) 1. Refers to ectopia. 2. Not in its normal location, or originating from an abnormal site.

Eczematous Refers to, or has the characteristics of, eczema.

EEG ELECTROENCEPHALOGRAM.

Efferent (e-, -ferent) Carrying outwards from a centre. *See also* AFFERENT.

Efficacy The capacity to produce a desired effect.

Effusion (e-, -fus-) The discharge or spread of fluid (e.g. blood), usually into parts of the body.

Elastase (-ase) An enzyme that catalyses the hydrolysis of peptide bonds (e.g. of elastin in connective tissue).

Electroconvulsive therapy (electro-, therap-) Electroconvulsive therapy (ECT) involves the passage of an electric current between two electrodes, usually at the anterior temporal regions of the scalp. It is performed under general anaesthesia and muscle relaxation, and a convulsion is induced. Adverse effects include amnesia and learning difficulties, but these are usually temporary. Serious adverse effects are rare.

Electrodesiccation (electro-) Destruction of tissue using an electric current applied with a small electrode. It results in dehydration and charring of tissue. *See also* ELECTROLYSIS.

Electroencephalogram (electro-, -encephalo-, -gram) An electroencephalogram (EEG) is a record of the brain's electrical activity. Characteristic distortion of normal wave patterns is associated with disorders of brain function.

Electrolysis (electro-, -lysis) Destruction of tissue using an electric current. It results in a focal inflammatory reaction. *See also* ELECTRODESICCATION.

Electrolyte balance (electro-) The concentration of plasma electrolytes within normal limits, and maintained by homeostasis.

Emaciation Extreme leanness or wasting of the body with loss of subcutaneous fat, and caused by illness or starvation.

Embolectomy (-ectomy) The removal of an embolus by surgery.

Embolisation 1. Pathological occlusion of a blood vessel by a blood clot, bubble of air, foreign body or fat (i.e. an embolus). 2. Formation of an embolus. 3. Therapeutic occlusion of a blood vessel.

Embryo The stage following fertilisation, usually characterised by the period of most rapid development. In humans, this stage is the first eight weeks of gestation. *See also* FETUS *and* NEONATE.

Embryogenesis (-gen-, -sis) The process of embryo formation and development.

Empyema (em-, -py-) The collection of pus within a body cavity.

Encysted (en-, -cyst-) Enclosed in a resistant capsule. *See also* CYST.

Endarterectomy (end-, -arter-, -ectomy) The removal of the tunica intima of an artery by surgery.

Endemic (end-) Refers to a disease caused by factors constantly present in an affected region or community, but producing clinical symptoms in very few. *See also* EPIDEMIC.

Endocervix (endo-) The inner lining of the neck of the uterus or the opening of the cervix into the uterus.

Endocrine (endo-) Refers to the functions of endocrine glands, which secrete hormones directly into the blood or lymph and not into a duct. *See also* EXOCRINE.

Endocytosis (endo-, -cyto-, -sis) The process by which cells engulf material, which may be liquid (pinocytosis) or solid (phagocytosis). The cytoplasmic membrane folds inwards, carrying the enclosed material into the cell.

Endogenous (endo-, -genous) Arising or developing from within. *See also* EXOGENOUS(1).

Endometritis (endo-, -metr-, -itis) Inflammation of the endometrium.

Endomyocardium (endo-, -myo-, -cardi-) Comprises both the myocardium and endocardium.

Endoneurium (endo-, -neur-) The connective tissue within peripheral nerves that separates individual fibres.

Endoplasmic reticulum (endo-, ret-) A network of membrane-bound channels in the cytoplasm of eukaryotic cells. It is responsible for intracellular transport, and the storage and synthesis of materials.

Endoscopy (endo-, -scopy) Visual examination of hollow organs or cavities of the body (e.g. stomach) using a fibreoptic endoscope, which is also a tool for biopsy.

Endospore (endo-, -spor-) A spore formed within a cell or hypha, by asexual or sexual reproduction. *See also* EXOSPORE(2).

Endothelium (endo-) The inner cellular layer of all body cavities and of the cardiovascular system. *See also* EPITHELIUM.

Endotoxin (endo-, -toxi-) A heat-stable lipopolysaccharide found in bacterial cell walls, especially in those classified as Gram-negative, and which is released after the death of the cell. Endotoxins possess pyrogenic properties. *See also* EXOTOXIN.

Endotracheal (endo-, -trache-) Within or through the lumen of the trachea.

Enophthalmos (en-, -ophthalmo-) Abnormal recession of the eyeball into the orbital cavity.

Enteral feeding (enter-) A method of supplying nutritional support by tube to a patient unable to ingest sufficient quantities of food in the normal way. It may be accomplished via the mouth or nose (nasogastric), or through a fistula (gastric, duodenal, or jejunal). *See also* PARENTERAL FEEDING.

Enteric (enter-) Refers to the small intestine.

Enteritis (enter-, -itis) Inflammation of the mucous membranes of the intestine and, in particular, the small intestine.

Enteropathogenic (entero-, -patho-, -genic) Capable of producing disease of the intestine.

Enteropathy (entero-, -pathy) Any disease or disorder of the intestine.

Enterotoxin (entero-, -toxi-) A bacterial exotoxin affecting the intestine.

Enuresis (-ur-, -sis) Involuntary urination. *See also* DIURESIS *and* INCONTINENCE.

Enuretic alarm An electrical device that responds to a few drops of urine, employed to evoke a conditioned response in those, especially children, affected by nocturnal enuresis.

Enzootic (en-, -zoo-) Refers to a disease endemic in an animal community.

Enzyme (-zym-) A protein involved in biochemical reactions as a catalyst.

Eosinophilia (-phil-, -ia) An excess of eosinophils in the blood.

Epidemic (epi-) Refers to a disease caused by factors not generally present in an affected region or community, often spreading rapidly, and of high morbidity. *See also* ENDEMIC *and* PANDEMIC.

Epidermoid (epi-, -derm-, -oid) Similar to, or part of, the epidermis.

Epididymectomy (epi-, didym-, -ectomy) The removal of the epididymis by surgery.

Epididymo-orchitis (epi-, -didymo-, -orch-, -itis) Inflammation involving the epididymis and the testis.

Epigastrium (epi-, -gastr-) The upper middle region of the abdomen.

Epileptiform (-lep-, -form) A condition resembling epilepsy.

Epiphora (epi-) Abnormal overflow of tears.

Epiphysis (epi-) The end of a long bone containing a secondary ossification centre, which lays down spongy bone. It is separated from the diaphysis by a cartilaginous epiphyseal plate, which is replaced by bone in early adulthood, thus preventing further growth.

Epistaxis (epi-) Bleeding from the nose.

Epithelioid (epitheli-, -oid) Similar to epithelium.

Epithelium (epitheli-) The thin cellular layer covering all internal and external surfaces of the body. *See also* ENDOTHELIUM.

Eructation (e-) Belching; the removal of accumulated gases from the stomach through the mouth. *See also* FLATUS.

Erythema marginatum (eryth-) A red patch in which the centre is faded and the margins raised.

Erythrocyte sedimentation rate (erythro-, -cyte) The erythrocyte sedimentation rate (ESR) is the rate of settling of erythrocytes when a known volume of blood is treated with an anticoagulant and allowed to stand under controlled conditions. The ESR varies in many conditions.

Erythrogenic (erythro-, -genic) 1. The production of erythrocytes. 2. The production of erythema.

Erythropoietin (erythro-, -poie-) A hormone secreted by the kidneys (or liver in the fetus), which stimulates erythropoiesis.

ESR ERYTHROCYTE SEDIMENTATION RATE.

Ethmoid bone Forms the supporting structure for the nasal cavities. It is located on the floor of the cranium and between the orbits. *See also* CRIBRIFORM PLATE.

Euthyroid (eu-) Refers to the normal function of the thyroid gland.

Evanescent Passing quickly, vanishing or unstable.

Exchange transfusion (ex-, trans-, -fus-) Transfusion involving the gradual replacement of blood with that of a donor. Blood is removed from the recipient in small quantities and is replaced by an equal volume transfused simultaneously.

Excision (ex-, -cis-) The removal of tissue or structures by surgery. *See also* RESECTION.

Excrescence (ex-) A growth, usually abnormal, from a surface.

Excretion (ex-) The removal of waste or unwanted material from the body.

Exfoliation (ex-) Peeling in scales or layers.

Exocrine (exo-) Refers to the function of exocrine glands (e.g. sweat glands and the pancreas), which secrete substances via a duct. *See also* ENDOCRINE.

Exogenous (exo-, -genous) 1. Arising or developing from external causes. *See also* ENDOGENOUS. 2. Additions to an outer surface that produce growth.

Exospore (exo-, -spor-) 1. The outer layer of a spore wall. 2. CONIDIUM. *See also* ENDOSPORE.

Exotoxin (exo-, -toxi-) A heat-labile protein secreted by multiplying bacteria, and having effects away from the focus of the infection. Exotoxins are extremely toxic to man. *See also* ENDOTOXIN.

Expectorate (ex-) To remove matter (e.g. mucus and sputum) from the lungs by coughing.

Extensor (ex-, -tens-) A muscle responsible for extending a limb, thereby increasing the angle of the joint. *See also* FLEXOR.

Extracellular fluid (extra-) Fluid found outside cells (e.g. plasma, cerebrospinal fluid, lymph and interstitial fluid).

Extravasation (extra-, -vas-) The escape of fluid, which may often be blood or blood components, from ducts or vessels, and its accumulation in the surrounding tissues. *See also* EXUDATION *and* TRANSUDATION.

Exudation (ex-) The escape of fluid, which may contain cells or cellular debris, from tissues or capillaries into surrounding tissues. It often occurs in inflammatory reactions. *See also* EXTRAVASATION *and* TRANSUDATION.

F

Facultative Refers to the ability to adapt to particular circumstances or perform a function, but which is not obligatory. *See also* OBLIGATE.

Familial Refers to the family, and to disorders that tend to occur more frequently among members of a family.

Fascia Fibrous tissue enclosing and separating groups of muscles and organs.

Fat 1. Adipose tissue. 2. A lipid formed by esterification of glycerol and fatty acids. *See also* TRIGLYCERIDE.

Fatigue Weariness and reduced efficiency resulting from exertion. It may range from lassitude to exhaustion. The threshold of fatigue may be lowered in illness. *See also* LASSITUDE, LETHARGY *and* PROSTRATION.

Fatty acid An acid containing a hydrocarbon chain and a terminal carboxyl group (-COOH). It may be saturated (e.g. stearic acid) or unsaturated (e.g. arachidonic acid). Fatty acids are utilised for fat synthesis (by esterification with glycerol); free fatty acids (FFA) in plasma are metabolised to meet energy requirements.

Fauces The passage from the mouth to the pharynx; the throat.

Febrile Refers to fever; feverish.

Femur The long bone of the thigh.

Fermentation The conversion of complex organic compounds (e.g. carbohydrates) into simpler compounds (e.g. alcohols). Fermentation takes place in anaerobic conditions and in the presence of an enzyme. *See also* CATABOLISM *and* GLYCOLYSIS.

Fertility The capacity for conception.

Fetus An unborn offspring. In humans, the term is used during the period from eight weeks after conception up to birth. *See also* EMBRYO *and* NEONATE.

Fever Raised body temperature above the normal (37°C; 98.6°F). *See also* HYPERPYREXIA, HYPERTHERMIA *and* HYPOTHERMIA.

FFA Free fatty acid. *See* FATTY ACID.

Fibrinoid (-oid) Similar to fibrin.

Fibrinolytic (-ly-) Refers to the enzymatic dissolution of fibrin.

Fibroid (fibr-, -oid) 1. Formed of, or similar to, fibrous tissue. 2. A leiomyoma. Fibroids is a term used colloquially to denote a leiomyoma occurring in the uterus.

Fibrosis (fibro-, -sis) The abnormal formation of fibrous tissue; the degeneration of a tissue into a fibrous mass.

Fibrous (fibr-, -ous) Composed of fibre.

Fibula The outer, smaller bone in the lower leg. *See also* TIBIA.

Filamentous Thread-like.

Filtration angle The angle at the periphery of the anterior chamber of the eye. It is the principal drainage site for aqueous humour.

Fimbria 1. A border; fringe-like. 2. A fine filamentous appendage of some bacteria, which is shorter than a flagellum.

Fission (fiss-) Splitting into two or more components.

Fistula An abnormal or surgically created channel or communication between two internal organs, or leading from an internal organ to the exterior of the body.

Flaccid In a relaxed and weak state.

Flaccid paralysis (para-) Paralysis with loss of tendon reflexes and reduction of muscle tone. *See also* SPASTIC PARALYSIS.

Flagella, flagellum (flagell-) Fine filamentous structures attached to some cells (e.g. spermatozoa), and used for motility.

Flatulence The accumulation of excessive amounts of air or gas in the gastrointestinal tract.
Flatus Gas or air in the gastrointestinal tract, which is expelled from the anus. *See also* ERUCTATION.
Flexor (flex-) A muscle responsible for bending a limb, thereby reducing the angle of a joint. *See also* EXTENSOR.
Floaters Small spots in the field of vision which appear to move, caused by deposits in the vitreous humour of the eye.
Focus The point of concentration or the principal centre of a process.
Follicle A small sac, pouch or cavity.
Follicular carcinoma (carcin-, -oma) A neoplasm of the thyroid gland that is composed of epithelial follicles without formation of papillae.
Fomites Inanimate objects (e.g. clothing) that can harbour microorganisms and act as agents of transmission. *See also* RESERVOIR OF INFECTION.
Free fatty acid *See* FATTY ACID.
Fructosaemia (-aemia) The presence of fructose in the blood.
Fructose (-ose) A ketohexose sugar found in honey and sweet fruits.
Fructosuria (-uria) The presence of fructose in the urine.
Fulminant Refers to a disease that occurs suddenly and with great intensity. *See also* INSIDIOUS.
Functional (funct-) Refers to the function of an organ, as opposed to its structure.
Fungating Indicates a fungus-like appearance with marked proliferation.
Furuncular Resembling a furuncle (boil).
Fusiform (-form) Resembling a spindle.

G

Gag reflex (re-, -flex) The reflex contraction of muscles in the pharynx resulting in the closure of the glottis, cessation of breathing, and retching or vomiting. It may be caused by touching the back of the pharynx.
Galactokinase (galacto-, -ase) An enzyme produced in the liver, which catalyses the formation of galactose 1-phosphate from galactose and ATP.
Galactorrhoea (galacto-, -rrhoea) 1. Spontaneous secretion of milk after the period of breast feeding is completed. 2. Excessive flow of milk.
Galactose (galact-, -ose) An aldohexose sugar, isomeric with glucose, obtained from lactose, milk sugar or sugar beet.
Gall bladder The organ used for storing and concentrating bile produced in the liver. When required, bile leaves the gall bladder via the cystic duct.
Gamete (gam-) A reproductive cell (e.g. ovum and spermatozoon).
Gametocyte (gameto-, -cyte) A cell (e.g. oocyte and spermatocyte) that produces gametes.
Gammaradiation (radi-) Radiation of short wavelength emitted from the nucleus of a radioactive substance.
Gammopathy (-pathy) The abnormal proliferation of lymphoid cells that produce immunoglobulins. *See also* MONOCLONAL GAMMOPATHY *and* POLYCLONAL GAMMOPATHY.
Ganglion (ganglio-) 1. A group of neurons outside the central nervous system. 2. The term ganglia refers to specific centres in the brain (e.g. basal ganglia). 3. A fluid-filled enlargement of the sheath of a tendon.
Gangrene Necrosis and putrefaction of tissues as a result of occlusion of their blood supply.
Gastrectomy (gastr-, -ectomy) The complete or partial removal of the stomach by surgery.
Gastric (gastr-) Refers to the stomach.
Gastric acid (gastr-) The generic term for hydrochloric acid in gastric juice.
Gastric glands (gastr-) The glands found in the mucosal membrane lining the stomach, and which secrete gastric juice.
Gastric juice (gastr-) The fluid secreted by the gastric glands containing hydrochloric acid, enzymes and mucus.
Gastric lavage (gastr-) Lavage performed to remove stomach contents.
General adaptation syndrome The sum of all non-specific responses of the body to prolonged systemic stress.
Genetic (gen-) 1. Refers to birth, reproduction, or origin. 2. Inherited or congenital, as of a disease.
Genetic counselling (gen-) Advice, based on genetic information, given to couples as to the likelihood of passing potentially hereditary anomalies to their children.
Genus A taxonomic category that comprises species of broadly similar characteristics, but which differ in detail. Similar genera belong to the same family.
Germinal cell (germ-) 1. A cell capable of division and differentiation. 2. A cell derived from the epithelial layer lining the seminiferous tubules and involved in spermatogenesis.
Germination (germ-) 1. The developmental process within a fertilised ovum. 2. The developmental beginning of a spore or seed.
Gestation Pregnancy; the period from fertilisation of an ovum to birth.
Gingivae (gingiv-) The gums, consisting of mucous membranes and connective tissue.
Gingival papillae (gingiv-) The portion of the gums between the teeth.
Gingivectomy (gingiv-, -ectomy) The removal of gingival tissue by surgery.
Gland A secretory or excretory cell, or a collection of such cells.
Globus hystericus A subjective sensation of suffocation, often described as a lump in the throat.
Glottis (glott-) The passage between the vocal cords in the pharynx.
Glucose (gluc-, -ose) A monosaccharide hexose utilised as the main source of energy. Excess glucose is converted to glycogen and fat. Glucose is an end-product of carbohydrate metabolism.
Glucose loading (gluc-, -ose) Administration of glucose in sufficient quantities to enable its rate of metabolism to be assessed.
Glucose tolerance (gluc-, -ose) The ability of the body to maintain the plasma glucose concentration within normal limits after glucose loading.
Glucuronide A metabolite formed by the conjugation of glucuronic acid with a compound (e.g. morphine) to facilitate its elimination.

Glutathione A peptide composed of glutamate, cysteine, and glycine, and which takes part in several redox reactions. It also functions in the transport of amino acids across membranes.

Glycogen (glyco-, -gen) Along-chain polysaccharide polymer of glucose. It is formed from excess glucose and stored as an energy reserve. It is stored mainly in the liver, but is also found in the muscles.

Glycolipid (glyco-, -lip-) A lipid containing a carbohydrate component.

Glycolysis (glyco-, -lysis) The enzymatic conversion of glucose into simpler compounds (lactate and pyruvate) carried out in anaerobic conditions. It results in the storage of energy in the form of adenosine triphosphate (ATP). *See also* CATABOLISM *and* METABOLISM.

Glycoprotein (glyco-) A conjugated compound consisting of a protein and a carbohydrate component.

Glycosaminoglycan (glyco-) A polysaccharide compound which is a component of many mucins. It may be combined with a protein.

Glycosuria (glyco-, -uria) The presence of glucose in the urine.

Goitre An enlargement of the thyroid gland, which is usually visible as a swelling at the front of the neck.

Goitrogenic (-genic) Capable of producing a goitre.

Golgi apparatus A specialised structure within a cell. It is situated near the nucleus and provides the site for synthesis of carbohydrate side-chains of substances (e.g. glycoproteins and mucopolysaccharides). Its functions include the transportation of these synthesised products.

Graft 1. To implant or transplant organs or tissues. 2. The organs or tissues used in the procedure. *See also* ALLOGRAFT.

Granulation tissue (gran-) Newly formed tissue associated with healing of wounds or ulcers. It consists of blood vessels and other cells, and has a red appearance.

Granulocyte (gran-, -cyte) A granule-containing cell, especially a leucocyte, which contains basophil, eosinophil and neutrophil granules.

Granuloma (gran-, -oma) A benign neoplasm composed of granulation tissue.

Gravid (grav-) Pregnant; containing a developing fetus.

Grommet A small plastic tube that is inserted through the eardrum to allow air to enter and dry out excessive secretions in the middle ear.

Gustatory Refers to the sense of taste.

Guthrie test An investigative test to detect the presence of elevated concentrations of phenylalanine in the blood of neonates.

Gynaecology (gynaeco-, -logy) The study of disease(s) of the female reproductive system.

Gynaecomastia (gynaeco-, -mast-, -ia) Excessive development of the mammary glands in the male. They may be functional.

H

Haemangioblastoma (haem-, -angio-, -blast-, -oma) A benign neoplasm in the brain consisting of blood-vessel cells or angioblasts.

Haematemesis (haemat-, -sis) The vomiting of blood.

Haematoma (haemat-, -oma) A swelling composed of blood, usually clotted, and resulting from a haemorrhage.

Haematuria (haemat-, -uria) The presence of blood in the urine.

Haemochromatosis (haemo-, -chromato-, -sis) A chronic inherited disorder of iron metabolism in which excessive amounts of iron are deposited in tissues.

Haemodialysis (haemo-, -dia-, -lysis) The removal of water, electrolytes, and waste products (e.g. urea and creatinine) from the blood using a special apparatus. Solutes diffuse across a semipermeable membrane (usually made from cellulose) into a dialysate solution. Diffusion of certain substances (e.g. calcium and acetate) also takes place from the dialysate into the blood. *See also* PERITONEAL DIALYSIS.

Haemoglobinuria (-uria) The presence of haemoglobin in the urine.

Haemolysis (haemo-, -lysis) The destruction or dissolution of erythrocytes, with the resultant liberation of haemoglobin.

Haemopoiesis (haemo-, -poiesis) The process of formation and development of blood cells.

Haemoptysis (haemo-) The coughing up of blood or mucus stained with blood.

Haemorrhage (haemo-, -rrhage) Bleeding; the escape of blood from blood vessels.

Haemorrhoidectomy (-ectomy) The removal of haemorrhoids by surgery.

Haemosiderin (haemo-) An iron–protein complex present in tissues as a storage form of iron and used to form haemoglobin.

Haemostasis (haemo-, -stasis) 1. A process that stops bleeding. It may be physiological or induced. 2. The arrest of blood flow through a vessel or to a particular part of the body.

Half-life The time required for the concentration of a substance to decline by 50%. The half-life of a drug is the time required for plasma concentrations to decline by 50%, provided that elimination occurs by first-order kinetics. It provides a measure of the rate of drug elimination.

Hallucination An apparent sensory perception (e.g. auditory, visual or olfactory) which is not present or is non-existent. *See also* DELUSION.

Hallucinogen (-gen) A substance that produces hallucinations.

Hamartoma (hamart-, -oma) A growth of cells and tissue that resembles a neoplasm, and in which normal cells of the organ show an abnormal degree of proliferation and mixture.

Hamstring Any one of the tendons at the back of the knee.

Heartburn A burning sensation usually felt behind the sternum, but which may rise to the neck. It is caused by reflux of gastric contents into the oesophagus.

Hemiparesis (hemi-) Partial paralysis or muscular weakness affecting one side of the body.

Hemiplegia (hemi-, -plegia) Complete paralysis affecting one side of the body. *See also* DIPLEGIA, PARAPLEGIA *and* QUADRIPLEGIA.

Hepatic (hepat-) Refers to the liver.

Hepatic-portal system (hepat-) The flow of venous blood from the digestive organs to the liver via the hepatic portal vein. After passing through the liver, the blood leaves via the hepatic vein to rejoin the systemic circulation.

Hepatocellular (hepato-) Refers to, or affecting, liver cells.

Hepatocyte (hepato-, -cyte) A liver cell.

Hepatolenticular (hepato-) Refers to the liver in association with the lentiform nucleus (a part of the basal ganglia in the extrapyramidal system).

Hepatoma (hepat-, -oma) A malignant neoplasm of the liver parenchymal cells.

Hepatomegaly (hepato-, -megaly) Enlargement of the liver.

Hepatosplenomegaly (hepato-, -spleno-, -megaly) Enlargement of the liver and the spleen.

Hereditary (hered-) Genetically transmitted from parents to offspring. *See also* CONGENITAL.

Hereditary spherocytosis (hered-, sphero-, -cyto-, -sis) A form of haemolytic anaemia, inherited as an autosomal dominant trait, in which the defective cytoplasmic membranes of erythrocytes are lost as the cells pass through the spleen.

Hermaphrodite Having both male and female sex organs.

Hernia The protrusion of part of an organ through an opening in the surrounding structures. *See also* UMBILICAL HERNIA.

Herpetic Refers to, or having the characteristics of, viruses or herpesvirus infections.

Heterotrophic (hetero-, -trophic) A type of nutrition in which complex organic molecules are required as the source of carbon for synthesis of organic compounds. *See also* AUTOTROPHIC.

Heterozygous (hetero-, -zyg-) Possessing different alleles at a given position on a chromosome pair. *See also* HOMOZYGOUS.

Hiatus A break or gap; an opening.

Hindbrain The posterior part of the embryonic brain that develops into the cerebellum, pons and medulla oblongata. The term may also be applied to these areas in the fully developed brain.

Hippocampus An area of grey matter involved in emotional behaviour and memory.

Hirsute Possessing abundant hair.

Histamine A substance present in most body tissues, especially mast cells, connective tissue, basophils and platelets. Its actions are mediated through two types of receptors, H_1 and H_2. Stimulation of H_1-receptors produces smooth muscle contraction (e.g. in the intestines and bronchioles), vasodilatation of small blood vessels resulting in hypotension, and an increase in capillary permeability causing oedema. Stimulation of H_2-receptors produces an increase in gastric acid secretion.

Histology (histo-, -logy) The study of tissue anatomy and physiology with respect to cellular structure and microscopical evaluation.

Histoplasmosis (-osis) A fungal infection primarily involving the reticulo-endothelial system, and caused by *Histoplasma capsulatum*.

Homeostasis (homeo-, -stasis) The tendency towards stability and equilibrium in the internal environment. This is achieved by dynamic processes and a system of control mechanisms (e.g. negative feedback).

Homogeneous (homo-) Possessing similar or uniform composition.

Homozygous (homo-, -zyg-) Possessing a pair of identical alleles at a given position on a chromosome pair. *See also* HETEROZYGOUS.

Hormone A chemical substance released from one part of the body (usually an endocrine gland) and transported in the bloodstream to another organ where it exerts its action.

Host 1. An animal or plant that harbours a parasitic microorganism. *See also* DEFINITIVE HOST *and* INTERMEDIATE HOST. 2. The recipient of transplanted tissue obtained from a donor.

Hyaline Possessing a glassy translucent appearance.

Hyaline membrane disease A respiratory disease of neonates, characterised by the development of a lining of eosinophilic hyaline material in the terminal respiratory passages.

Hydronephrosis (hydro-, -nephro-, -sis) Distension of the ureter and renal pelvis due to obstruction of the outflow of urine. Atrophy of the kidney may occur.

Hydrops (hydro-) The accumulation of serous fluid in any tissue or body cavity.

Hydrosalpinx (hydro-, -salp-) The accumulation of watery fluid in a Fallopian tube.

Hydrostatic (hydro-, -stat-) Refers to the pressure of a fluid when in a state of equilibrium.

Hydrotherapy (hydro-, -therap-) The treatment of a disorder by immersion in, external application of, or administration of, water.

Hyperactivity (hyper-) An excessive increase in physical activity.

Hyperbaric (hyper-, -bar-) Greater than normal pressure or weight; gases under greater than atmospheric pressure.

Hyperbilirubinaemia (hyper-, -aemia) An excess of bilirubin in the blood. Conjugated hyperbilirubinaemia is an excess in the blood of bilirubin that is combined with glucuronic acid, sulfate or other substances (i.e. conjugated bilirubin). Unconjugated hyperbilirubinaemia is an excess in the blood of free bilirubin.

Hypercalciuria (hyper-, -calci-, -uria) An excess of calcium in the urine.

Hypercapnia (hyper-) An excess of carbon dioxide in the blood.

Hypercholesterolaemia (hyper-, -aemia) An excess of cholesterol in the blood.

Hyperglycaemia (hyper-, -glyc-, -aemia) An excess of sugar in the blood.

Hyperirritability (hyper-) An excessive responsiveness to slight stimuli.

Hyperkeratosis (hyper-, -kerato-, -sis) Hypertrophy of the epidermal layer of the skin.

Hyperkinesia (hyper-, -kine-, -ia) Excessive activity or motor function. *See also* HYPOKINESIA.

Hyperopia (hyper-, -opia) Long-sightedness, in which the focal point of parallel rays of light is behind the retina, so that the near point is further away than normal.

Hyperoxia (hyper-, -ox-, -ia) An increase in the oxygen concentration in tissues caused by breathing hyberbaric oxygen or air.

Hyperphagia (hyper-, -phagia) Excessive eating.

Hyperphosphataemia (hyper-, -aemia) An excess of phosphates in the blood. *See also* HYPOPHOSPHATAEMIA.

Hyperplasia (hyper-, -plasia) The increase in size of, or part of, an organ, as a result of an increase in the number of cells. *See also* HYPERTROPHY *and* HYPOPLASIA.

Hyperpnoea (hyper-, -pnoea) An abnormal increase in the depth and rate of breathing. *See also* APNOEA, DYSPNOEA, ORTHOPNOEA and TACHYPNOEA.

Hyperpyrexia (hyper-, -pyr-, -ia) A very high body temperature of at least 40.5°C (105°F). *See also* FEVER, HYPERTHERMIA *and* HYPOTHERMIA.

Hypersensitivity (hyper-, -sens-) An enhanced and exaggerated response to a foreign substance (allergen). It is usually mediated by the immune system. *See also* ALLERGY *and* ATOPY.

Hyperthermia (hyper-, -therm-, -ia) An abnormally high body temperature, particularly one induced therapeutically. *See also* FEVER, HYPERPYREXIA *and* HYPOTHERMIA.

Hypertonia (hyper-, -ton-, -ia) Enhanced tone of muscles or arteries.

Hypertrophy (hyper-, -trophy) The increase in size of an organ, or part of an organ as a result of an increase in cell size. *See also* ATROPHY *and* HYPERPLASIA.

Hyperuricaemia (hyper-, -uric-, -aemia) An excess of uric acid in the blood.

Hyperventilation (hyper-) 1. Deep breathing which is abnormally prolonged and with increased frequency. 2. An increase in gaseous exchange in the lungs. It causes a fall in the plasma carbon dioxide concentration. *See also* HYPOVENTILATION.

Hyperviscosity (hyper-) Abnormally excessive viscosity.

Hypnotic (hypno-) 1. Produces sleep. 2. Refers to hypnotism.

Hypoalbuminaemia (hypo-, -aemia) An abnormal deficiency of albumin in the blood.

Hypochlorhydria (hypo-, -ia) An abnormal reduction in the secretion of hydrochloric acid in gastric juice.

Hypochondrial Refers to the hypochondrium.

Hypofibrinogenaemia (hypo-, -aemia) An abnormal deficiency of fibrinogen in the blood.

Hypogeusia (hypo-, -ia) Impaired sense of taste.

Hypokinesia (hypo-, -kine-, -ia) An abnormal decrease in activity or motor function. *See also* AKINESIA, BRADYKINESIA, DYSKINESIA *and* HYPERKINESIA.

Hypophosphataemia (hypo-, -aemia) An abnormal deficiency of phosphates in the blood. *See also* HYPERPHOSPHATAEMIA.

Hypophysectomy (-ectomy) The removal of the pituitary gland by surgery.

Hypoplasia (hypo-, -plasia) Underdevelopment of an organ or part, usually implying fewer than the normal number of cells. It is less severe than aplasia. *See also* AGENESIS, APLASIA, DYSPLASIA *and* HYPERPLASIA.

Hypoproteinaemia (hypo-, -aemia) An abnormal deficiency of protein in the blood.

Hypotension (hypo-, -tens-) An abnormally low blood pressure.

Hypothermia (hypo-, -therm-, -ia) A body temperature below normal, which is only usually of clinical significance when it falls below 33°C (91–92°F). It may be therapeutically induced to reduce tissue metabolism and oxygen requirement. *See also* FEVER, HYPERPYREXIA *and* HYPERTHERMIA.

Hypoventilation (hypo-) A reduction in gaseous exchange in the lungs which causes hypercapnia. *See also* HYPERVENTILATION.

Hypovolaemia (hypo-, -aemia) An abnormal decrease in the volume of circulating blood in the body.

Hypoxaemia (hyp-, -ox-, -aemia) A deficiency of oxygen in the blood.

Hypoxidosis (hyp-, -ox-, -sis) An impairment in function of cells caused by a reduction in the supply of oxygen.

Hysterectomy (hyster-, -ectomy) The removal of the uterus by surgery.

Hysterotomy (hystero-, -tomy) 1. Incision of the uterus. 2. CAESARIAN SECTION.

I

Iatrogenic (iatro-, -genic) Produced by doctors; usually applied to adverse conditions produced as a result of treatment by a doctor. Causes may include inappropriate manner, examination, or discussion, and medical or surgical procedures. *See also* NOSOCOMIAL.

Idiopathic (idio-, -path-) 1. Refers to a condition of unknown aetiology. 2. Refers to a primary disease (i.e. one not resulting from another disease).

Idiosyncrasy (idio-) An individual characteristic not shared by others. It includes behaviour, habit and a response to agents that is peculiar to an individual.

Ileac (ile-) 1. Refers to the ileum. 2. Refers to ileus.

Ileostomy (ileo-, -stomy) A surgical procedure to establish an opening (stoma) from the ileum to the surface of the abdomen. The term may also be applied to the opening itself. *See also* COLOSTOMY *and* UROSTOMY.

Iliac (ile-) Refers to the ilium.

Immunisation A process of increasing a subject's resistance to infection. *See also* ACTIVE IMMUNISATION *and* PASSIVE IMMUNISATION.

Immunocompromise A diminished immune response caused by external factors (e.g. immunosuppressants, radiotherapy or malignant disease). *See also* IMMUNODEFICIENCY *and* IMMUNOSUPPRESSION.

Immunodeficiency A disorder characterised by the inability to produce an immune response. It may affect any part of the immune system. *See also* IMMUNOCOMPROMISE.

Immunosuppression Inhibition of the immune system by the administration of immunosuppressants (e.g. azathioprine or corticosteroids) to prevent rejection of transplant tissue. It may be selective, and complete or partial. *See also* IMMUNOCOMPROMISE.

Immunosurveillance The concept of a detection and monitoring function of the immune system. It is responsible for recognising neoplastic cells and their destruction by an immune response.

Immunotherapy (-therap-) Therapeutic measures involving active and passive immunisation, stimulation or suppression of the immune system, or establishing the ability to produce an immune response.

Impaction Firmly packed or wedged.

Impotence (im-) The inability to perform sexual intercourse due to the failure to achieve or maintain an erection.
In utero Within the uterus.
In vitro Occurring outside the living body. *See also* IN VIVO.
In vivo Occurring within the living body. *See also* IN VITRO.
Incision (in-, -cis-) The cut produced by a sharp implement during surgery.
Incontinence (in-) Loss of voluntary control of defecation (faecal or rectal incontinence) or urination (urinary incontinence). *See also* DIURESIS *and* ENURESIS.
Incubate To provide the ideal conditions (e.g. temperature and humidity) for growth and development.
Incubation period The interval of time between exposure to a pathogenic microorganism and the first appearance of clinical features of the infection.
Indolent (in-) 1. Slow-growing. 2. With little or no pain.
Induration (-dur-) The hardening of a tissue or organ.
Indwelling catheter A catheter that remains in position.
Infant Refers to a child from the neonatal period up to 12 months of age. *See also* NEONATE *and* PREMATURE INFANT.
Infection 1. The invasion of a host by pathogenic, or potentially pathogenic, microorganisms, and their subsequent multiplication. *See also* INFESTATION. 2. An infectious disease.
Infestation The invasion or habitation of a host by surface-dwelling parasites. *See also* INFECTION(1).
Infiltration (in-) The accumulation within a tissue of a substance not normally present, or in concentrations in excess of the normal.
Infusion (in-, -fus-) 1. The intravenous administration of a fluid, other than blood, for therapeutic purposes. The fluid flows in by gravity. *See also* INJECTION(1) *and* TRANSFUSION. 2. A dilute solution of a vegetable drug prepared by macerating the drug in hot or cold water, and straining.
Inhalation (in-) The inspiration of air or other substances into the lungs.
Injection (in-, -ject-) 1. The parenteral administration of a fluid for therapeutic purposes. The fluid is forced in using a syringe. *See also* INFUSION(1). 2. Congestion of a part.
Innervation (in-) The nerve supply or distribution to an organ or tissue.
Inoculation (in-) The introduction of microorganisms (or any other antigenic substance) into living tissue or culture media. The process may result in disease, or be used to stimulate an immune response or to study the cultured material.
Inoculum (in-) An agent or substance introduced into tissues by inoculation.
Inotropic Influencing the contractility of muscles, especially the myocardium. There may be a negative influence resulting in reduced contractility, or a positive influence resulting in enhanced contractility.
Insertion (in-) 1. The process of implanting or setting. 2. The site of attachment.
Insidious Refers to a disease that develops or spreads with few signs or symptoms relative to its severity. *See also* FULMINANT.
Interferon A protein produced by most cells in response to viral infection, and which induces the production of antiviral substances by non-infected cells. Interferons also have complex effects on immunity and cell function; they suppress lymphocyte function, lower the threshold for mast-cell histamine release, and may have antineoplastic effects.
Interleukin A specific lymphokine that affects antibody production and influences T-cell differentiation and production.
Intermediate host The host in which a parasite undergoes asexual reproduction or is in the larval stage. *See also* DEFINITIVE HOST.
Interstitial (inter-) Refers to the spaces within or between tissues.
Intestinal flora The bacteria that are normal residents of the intestine.
Intolerance (in-) 1. The inability to endure or withstand. *See also* TOLERANCE. 2. An unfavourable response.
Intracranial pressure (intra-, -crane-) The pressure of the cerebrospinal fluid in the subarachnoid space.
Intractable Uncontrollable and unresponsive to remedial measures.
Intraluminal (intra-) Within the lumen of a tubular tissue or organ.
Intrathecal (intra-, -thec-) 1. Within a sheath. 2. Within the subarachnoid space.
Intrinsic factor A glycoprotein secreted by the mucosal cells of the stomach, and which is necessary for the absorption of vitamin B_{12}.
Intubation (in-) Insertion of a tube into a body cavity, especially into the trachea to maintain the airway.
Involution (in-) 1. A reduction in the size of an organ. It may be degenerative, physiological, or follow enlargement. *See also* ATROPHY. 2. Turning towards the inside.
Ion-exchange resin A polymer of high molecular weight, whose component ions are exchanged for other ions of the same charge in the surrounding medium.
Ionising radiation (rade-) High-energy electromagnetic radiation that is capable of producing ionisation (e.g. X-rays and gamma radiation).
Iridectomy (irid-, -ectomy) The removal of part of the iris by surgery.
Irradiation Exposure (which may be therapeutic) to electromagnetic waves. *See also* RADIATION(1).
Isotonic (iso-, -ton-) 1. Applied to different solutions that exert equal osmotic pressure with respect to a particular membrane. 2. Applied to a solution that exerts the same osmotic pressure as serum (e.g. sodium chloride 0.9%).
Isotope (iso-) A chemical element possessing the same atomic number as another, but having a different atomic mass.

J

Jacksonian epilepsy Jacksonian epilepsy is characterised by seizures that occur on one side of the body and move systematically from one group of muscles to the next. The cause is a discharging focus in the motor cortex of the brain.

K

Kallidin A polypeptide and a member of the group of kinins.

Kallikrein-kinin system The enzymatic cascade system resulting in the formation of the inflammatory mediators, kinins.

Kartagener's syndrome An inherited pulmonary disorder characterised by immotile cilia, which results in defective mucociliary clearance.

Karyolysis (karyo-, -lysis) The destuction of a cell nucleus, in which it swells, lyses, and loses its chromatin. *See also* KARYORRHEXIS *and* PYKNOSIS.

Karyorrhexis (karyo-, -rhex-) Disintegration of the cell nucleus. It results in dispersal of chromatin throughout the cytoplasm in the form of granules which are finally removed from the cell. *See also* KARYOLYSIS *and* PYKNOSIS.

Keratitis (kerat-, -itis) Inflammation of the cornea.

Keratoconjunctivitis (kerato-, -itis) Inflammation of the cornea and the conjunctiva.

Keratolysis (kerato-, -lysis) Separation or loosening of the outermost layer of skin, the stratum corneum.

Keratomalacia (kerato-, -malacia) Dryness and softening of the cornea caused by severe vitamin-A deficiency. Corneal ulceration, night blindness and complete visual loss may occur.

Kerion A raised granulomatous lesion associated with tinea infections, and thought to be caused by an immune response. It is inflamed, pustular and wet and spongy in appearance, and heals in a short time.

Keto acid An organic acid with a ketone group (>C=O) and a carboxyl group (-COOH).

Ketoacidosis (keto-, -osis) Acidosis resulting from the accumulation of ketones in body tissues and fluids.

Ketogenic (keto-, -genic) Refers to the ability to form ketones.

Ketonuria (keto-, -uria) The presence of ketones in the urine.

Kinin A polypeptide (e.g. bradykinin and kallidin) formed in plasma as a result of the action of the enzyme, kallikrein. Kinins have powerful vasodilator properties, increase capillary permeability, cause smooth muscle contraction and stimulate pain receptors.

Krebs' cycle The cyclic process of metabolism resulting in the complete oxidation of acetyl-coenzyme A. Carbon chains of carbohydrate, fat and protein are metabolised to form carbon dioxide, water, and adenosine triphosphate.

Kyphosis (-osis) Excessive curvature of the spine in the thoracic region; hunchback.

L

Labial (labe-) Refers to a lip, or, more commonly, the labia that constitute part of the female external genitalia.

Labyrinthectomy (-ectomy) The removal of the labyrinth of the inner ear by surgery.

Labyrinthine Refers to the labyrinth of the inner ear.

Lachrymation (lachry-) Tear production and flow.

Lactation (lact-) 1. Milk secretion. 2. The period of milk secretion after childbirth.

Lactoferrin (lacto-, -ferr-) An iron-binding protein that possesses antimicrobial activity, and which is found in tissue fluids (e.g. breast milk, saliva and tears) and neutrophils.

Lactose (lact-, -ose) A disaccharide found in milk.

Laminectomy (-ectomy) The removal of the arch of a vertebra by surgery, resulting in exposure of the spinal cord.

Laparotomy (laparo-, -tomy) An incision through the abdominal wall, but also applied to that in the loin.

Large cell carcinoma (carcin-, -oma) A malignant neoplasm composed of large anaplastic cells, and originating especially in a bronchus.

Larva An independent stage in the life-cycle of some organisms, characterised by motility, and in some cases, feeding.

Laryngeal (laryng-) Refers to the larynx.

Laryngectomy (laryng-, -ectomy) The removal of the larynx by surgery.

Laryngospasm (laryngo-, -spas-) Muscle spasm of the larynx, resulting in its closure.

Lassitude Weakness; tiredness. *See also* FATIGUE, LETHARGY *and* PROSTRATION.

Latent Present but not active; dormant.

Lavage Washing-out or irrigation of an organ.

Laxative Having the action of softening and promoting the discharge of faeces.

Lentigo (lent-) A yellowish-brown spot on the skin caused by melanin deposition.

Lesion A pathological condition (e.g. infection, injury or malignant disease).

Lethargy A condition characterised by extreme drowsiness, weakness and complacency. *See also* FATIGUE, LASSITUDE *and* PROSTRATION.

Leucocytosis (leuco-, -cyto-, -sis) An abnormal increase in the number of leucocytes in the blood. *See also* LEUCOPENIA.

Leucopenia (leuco-, -penia) An abnormal deficiency in the number of leucocytes in the blood. *See also* LEUCOCYTOSIS.

Ligation (lig-) The application of a thread-like material (e.g. catgut, wire, cotton or silk) around a vessel or part, used to constrict it.

Lipid (lip-) A member of a large and diverse group of fat and fat-like organic compounds containing carbon, hydrogen and oxygen, and characterised as water-insoluble. They are classified as simple lipids (e.g. oils), compound lipids (e.g. phospholipids), or derived lipids (e.g. fatty acids). They act as a source of energy, constituents of cell structure, and serve other metabolic functions.

Lipoprotein (lipo-) A combination of lipid and protein that renders the lipid water-soluble. The group includes low-density lipoproteins that deposit cholesterol in cells and high-density lipoproteins that remove cholesterol from cells and transport it to the liver for elimination.

Lithotripsy (litho-, -tripsy) A procedure to crush a bladder calculus, with subsequent irrigation and removal of fragments.

Lobectomy (-ectomy) The removal of one or more lobes of an organ (e.g. thyroid gland) by surgery.
Local Confined to a small area; not systemic.
Locomotor (-mot-) Refers to motion, or parts of the body responsible for motion.
Lucid Clear and understandable.
Lung-hilum A depression in the mediastinal surface of each lung at which the bronchus, blood and lymph vessels, and nerve supply enter.
Lymphadenectomy (lymph-, -aden-, -ectomy) The removal of a lymph node by surgery.
Lymphadenopathy (lymph-, -adeno-, -pathy) Any disorder of the lymph nodes.
Lymphoblast (lympho-, -blast) The immature precursor cell of a lymphocyte.
Lymphoreticular (lympho-, -ret-) Refers to the reticulo-endothelial system of the lymph nodes.
Lysis (ly-, -sis) Dissolution or disintegration; decomposition.
Lysosome (lyso-, -some) An organelle enclosed by a double membrane and found in many types of cell. It contains hydrolytic enzymes that have intracellular digestive functions.
Lysozyme (lyso-, -zym-) An enzyme found in various tissue fluids (e.g. saliva and tears) that is capable of breaking down bacterial cell walls.

M

Maceration The softening of tissues caused by soaking.
Macroglossia (macro-, -gloss-, -ia) Enlargement of the tongue.
Maculopapular Characterised by the presence of macules and papules.
Malabsorption (mal-) Defective gastrointestinal absorption of nutrients.
Malaise A non-specific feeling of illness, uneasiness or discomfort, often signifying a disturbance of body function.
Malignant 1. A condition that is life-threatening, virulent or recurrent. 2. Possessing properties of anaplasia, invasive growth and metastasis. *See also* BENIGN.
Malnutrition (mal-, -nutre-) A disorder of nutrition, which may be caused by an insufficient intake of nutrients, unbalanced diet or defective utilisation of nutrients.
Mammography (mammo-, -graphy) Examination of the breasts using X-rays.
Manipulation (man-) 1. Treatment using the hands. 2. In physiotherapy, it refers to the movement of a joint beyond its active limit.
Mantoux test A diagnostic test to determine the sensitivity to tuberculin. A positive hypersensitivity reaction indicates the presence of the tubercle bacillus, although the infection may be inactive. It is carried out prior to BCG (Bacillus Calmette-Guérin) vaccination.
Marfan's syndrome An inherited disorder characterised by partial dislocation of the lenses of the eye, abnormally long and thin hands and feet (especially fingers and toes), and cardiovascular abnormalities.
Mastectomy (mast-, -ectomy) The removal of a breast by surgery.
Mastoidectomy (mast-, -ectomy) The removal of the mastoid process or mastoid air cells by surgery.
Mastopathy (masto-, -pathy) A disorder of a breast.
Maxilla The bone that forms the upper jaw.
Meconium The dark green viscous liquid discharged from the bowels of a neonate. It consists of bile, amniotic fluid, and debris.
Mediastinum (mede-) The mass of tissues in the thoracic cavity, excluding the lungs. It extends from the sternum to the vertebral column, and includes the heart, oesophagus, thymus gland and other structures.
Medulla Refers to the innermost part of a structure. Sometimes called the marrow.
Medulloblastoma (medullo-, -blast-, -oma) A malignant neoplasm of the cerebellum composed of undifferentiated cells resembling the neural tube.
Megaloblast (megalo-, -blast) A large immature nucleated cell, the precursor of an abnormal erythrocyte.
Melaena The passage of dark tarry faeces, which contain occult blood as a result of haemorrhage within the gastrointestinal tract.
Membrane A thin lining or covering tissue of a surface or cavity, or the dividing tissue of a space or organ.
Membrane depolarisation (de-) 1. Neutralisation of polarity across a membrane. 2. In neurons, the reversal of the resting membrane potential when stimulated; the positive potential of a membrane with respect to the potential outside the cell.
Menarche (men-, -arche) The time when the first menstrual period begins.
Mendelian laws The law of segregation which states that allelic pairs of genes segregate from one another and pass to different gametes; the law of independent assortment which states that genes that are not alleles are distributed to the gametes independently of one another.
Meningo-encephalitis (meningo-, -encephal-, -itis) Inflammation of the brain and the meninges.
Menorrhagia (meno-, -rrhagia) Excessive blood loss during regular but possibly prolonged menstruation. *See also* OLIGOMENORRHOEA.
Mesenteric vein (mes-, -enter-) The vein that receives blood from the mesentery.
Mesentery (mes-, -enter-) The portion of the peritoneum that attaches the intestine to the abdominal wall.
Mesothelioma (meso-, -oma) A malignant neoplasm of the mesothelium.
Mesothelium (meso-) The epithelial membrane of the pleura, pericardium and peritoneum.
Metabolism (meta-) The sum of the chemical processes occurring in an organism, including anabolism and catabolism, and the biodegradation of foreign substances and drugs.
Metacarpal (meta-, -carp-) Refers to the bones of the hand, between the wrist and the fingers.
Metatarsal (meta-, -tars-) Refers to the distal part of the foot between the instep and the toes.
Metatarsophalangeal (meta-, -tarso-, -phalang-) Refers to the metatarsal bones and the phalanges.
Micro-abscess (micro-) A very small localised abscess.
Microcephaly (micro-, -cephal-) An abnormally small head.
Microflora (micro-) Microorganisms characteristic of a particular part.

Microsomal enzyme (micro-, -zym-) An enzyme associated with microsomes, especially in liver cells.

Miliary Refers to characteristic lesions that are small and resemble millet seeds.

Milk-alkali syndrome A syndrome caused by an excessive intake of milk or absorbable alkali over a prolonged period.

Mineral An inorganic solid of uniform composition found in the crust of the earth.

Miosis (mio-, -sis) Contraction of the pupil of the eye.

Mitochondria (mito-, -chondre-) Double-membraned intracellular organelles located in the cytoplasm, and which are the principal sites of energy production.

Mitosis (mito-, -sis) Cell divison that results in two daughter cells of identical genetic composition to the parent cell.

Monoclonal gammopathy (mono-, -pathy) Gammopathy in which there is an increase in a single immunoglobulin clone. *See also* POLYCLONAL GAMMOPATHY.

Mononeuropathy (mono-, -neuro-, -pathy) A disorder affecting one nerve only. *See also* POLYNEUROPATHY.

Morbid 1. Diseased; refers to, or affected by, disease. 2. Refers to mental thoughts that are unhealthy or tend towards abnormality.

Morbidity 1. A morbid condition. 2. The ratio of the number of people within a population suffering from a disease to the number unaffected. *See also* MORTALITY(2).

Morphology (morpho-, -logy) The study of the structure and form of living organisms.

Mortality 1. The mortal quality; destined to die. 2. The death rate; the ratio of the total number of deaths to the total population of a specified group. *See also* MORBIDITY(2).

Motor (mot-) Refers to motion or movement, and its nervous and muscle control.

Mucin (muc-) A glycoprotein or mucopolysaccharide compound, constituting the main component of mucus.

Mucinous (muc-, -ous) Resembling or marked by the production of mucin.

Mucocutaneous (muco-, -cut-) Refers to the mucous membranes and the skin.

Muco-epidermoid (muco-, -epe-, -derm-, -oid) Characterised by epithelial cells and cells that produce mucus.

Mucoid (muc-, -oid) Resembling mucus or mucin.

Mucolytic (muco-, -ly-) Refers to the thinning, digestion, or dissolution of mucus.

Mucopeptide (muco-) Any glycosylated peptide derived from a glycoprotein.

Mucopurulent (muco-, -pur-) Characterised by the presence of mucus and pus.

Mucosa (muc-) A mucous membrane.

Mucous (muc-, -ous) Refers to mucus; secreting mucus.

Mucous membrane (muco-) A mucus-secreting membrane lining body cavities that open to the external environment (e.g. gastrointestinal and respiratory tracts).

Mucus (muc-) A viscous secretion of mucous glands and membranes that prevents body cavities from drying out. The main constituent of mucus is mucin.

Muscle tone (ton-) The state of resting tension and contraction of muscle, which maintains form and provides passive resistance to stretch or elongation.

Muscularis mucosa (muc-) The muscle layer of a mucous membrane.

Musculoskeletal Refers to the muscles and the bones.

Mutagenic (-genic) Causing mutation.

Myalgia (my-, -algia) Pain in a muscle or muscles.

Mycosis (myco-, -sis) Any fungal infection.

Myelocyte (myelo-, -cyte) An immature leucocyte formed from a myeloblast, which further develops into a type of granular leucocyte.

Myelogenous (myelo-, -genous) Originating in the bone marrow.

Myeloid (myel-, -oid) 1. Refers to derived from, or similar to, bone marrow. 2. Refers to the spinal cord. 3. Resembles myelocytes.

Myeloproliferative (myelo-) Refers to or characterised by the proliferation of bone marrow or any of the blood cells derived from bone marrow.

Myelosuppression (myelo-) Inhibition of bone-marrow function.

Myoclonus (myo-) Clonus occurring in a particular muscle or group of muscles.

Myopathy (myo-, -pathy) Any muscle disorder.

Myositis (myo-, -itis) Inflammation of voluntary muscles.

Myotomy (myo-, -tomy) Incision or dissection of muscle.

N

Naevocytic (naevo-, -cyt-) Refers to, or composed of, naevus cells.

Naevus (naev-) 1. Any birthmark. 2. A circumscribed, usually hereditary, malformation of the skin and occasionally the oral mucosa. It is caused by hyperplasia of tissue (e.g. blood vessels, epidermis or connective tissue).

Nail fold The fold of skin around the base and sides of a nail.

Navel UMBILICUS.

Nebuliser A device that converts a drug solution into a fine mist, which can be inhaled into the lungs.

Necrolysis (necro-, -lysis) Exfoliation and separation of tissue caused by necrosis.

Neonatal asphyxia BIRTH ASPHYXIA.

Neonate (neo-) A newborn child; usually refers to the first 30 days of life. *See also* EMBRYO, FETUS and INFANT.

Nephrectomy (nephr-, -ectomy) The removal of a kidney by surgery.

Nephritis (nephr-, -itis) Inflammation of the kidneys, affecting the glomeruli, tubules or interstitial tissue.

Nephrogenic (nephro-, -genic) Refers to originating in, or caused by, the kidneys.

Nerve A cord-like structure consisting of a collection of nerve fibres, which emerge from the spinal cord (nerve root) and innervate body structures (nerve terminal).

Neural tube (neur-) The embryonic central nervous system.

Neuralgia (neur-, -algia) Any disorder of a nerve or nerves causing intermittent, but frequently intense, pain.

Neurilemma (neur-) The outer membrane covering the Schwann cell of a nerve fibre.

Neuritis (neur-, -itis) Inflammation of a nerve or nerves. It may result in pain, numbness, paraesthesia, muscle wasting, and loss of reflexes.
Neurofibromatosis (neuro-, -fibr-, -oma-, -osis) An inherited autosomal dominant disorder characterised by multiple skin neurofibromas and pigmentation.
Neurogenic (neuro-, -genic) Refers to, originating in, or caused by, the nervous system.
Neurology (neuro-, -logy) The study of the nervous system and its diseases.
Neuromuscular (neuro-) Refers to nerves and muscles.
Neuromuscular junction (neuro-, junct-) The site of contact between the axon terminal of a motor neuron and the membrane of a skeletal muscle cell.
Neuromuscular transmission (neuro-, trans-) The transfer of a nerve impulse across a neuromuscular junction to a muscle cell, which is mediated by acetylcholine.
Neuron (neuro-) A nerve cell. It consists of the axon, cell body, and dendritic processes.
Neuronitis (neuro-, -itis) Inflammation and degeneration of neurons.
Neuropathy (neuro-, -pathy) Any disease or disorder of the nervous system.
Neurosecretory (neuro-) Refers to the secretory functions of nerve cells.
Neurosis (neuro-, -sis) A mild personality disorder characterised by emotional disturbances and anxiety, but without distortion of reality. *See also* PSYCHOSIS.
Neurotransmitter (neuro-, -trans-) An endogenous substance that is released from the axon terminal of a presynaptic neuron, and diffuses across the synaptic cleft to bind to a receptor site on the target cell. It may have an excitatory or inhibitory effect. *See also* SYNAPSE.
Neurotropic (neuro-, -tropic) Possessing an affinity for nervous tissue.
Neutropenia (-penia) A deficiency in the number of neutrophils in the blood.
Night blindness Poor vision in dim light, especially at night, although vision in brighter light may be good.
Nissl granules (gran-) Granules found in the cell body of neurons, and composed of endoplasmic reticulum and ribosomes.
Nitrogen balance The state of equilibrium between nitrogen intake and excretion.
NMR *See* NUCLEAR MAGNETIC RESONANCE SCANNING.
Nocturia (-uria) Excessive urination at night.
Nocturnal Refers to activities that occur during the night. *See also* CIRCADIAN RHYTHM *and* DIURNAL.
Node (nod-) A normal or pathological swelling, tissue mass, or a collection of cells.
Normal pressure hydrocephalus (hydro-, -cephal-) A syndrome characterised by the clinical manifestations of hydrocephalus, but without an increase in intracranial pressure. It occurs in adults and may be associated with previous episodes of hydrocephalus. Presenting symptoms include dementia, apraxia and urinary incontinence.
Normocalcaemia (normo-, -calc-, -aemia) A normal plasma-calcium concentration.
Nosocomial (noso-) Refers to, or originating in, a hospital. *See also* IDIOPATHIC.
Nuclear magnetic resonance scanning Nuclear magnetic resonance (NMR) scanning is a technique in which images are generated by radio-waves directed at right-angles to protons in a magnetic field.
Nucleic acid (nucle-) A polymeric compound found in a cell nucleus. The two principal nucleic acids are deoxyribonucleic acid (DNA) and ribonucleic acid (RNA).
Nucleoplasm (nucleo-, -plas-) The protoplasm of a cell located within the nucleus. *See also* CYTOPLASM.
Nucleus (nucle-) 1. The distinct part of a cell that contains genetic information. 2. A collection of neurons in the central nervous system.
Nulliparous (-par-) Refers to a woman who has never given birth. *See also* PARITY.
Numb A condition of complete or partial loss of sensation.
Nystagmus Involuntary oscillation of the eyeball in one or more planes.

O

Oat cell A cell that resembles the shape of oat grains.
Obligate Refers to the necessity for particular environmental conditions. *See also* FACULTATIVE.
Obstetrics The medical and surgical management of pregnancy, childbirth and the puerperium.
Occipital Refers to the back of the skull or head.
Occipital artery The artery branching from the carotid artery and located in the occipital region. It supplies the muscles of the neck and scalp, the mastoid process, and the meninges.
Occult Obscured or concealed.
Occupational therapy (therap-) Measures designed to promote recovery from illness or surgery, or to stimulate mental processes. It includes work or hobbies, instruction on the efficient use of recovery aids (e.g. walking sticks), and instruction on the performance of daily functions (e.g. bathing).
Ocular (ocul-) Refers to the eye; ophthalmic.
Oculogyric crisis (oculo-) A crisis in which there is prolonged fixation of the eyeballs in one position.
Oligodendroglioma (oligo-, -dendro-, -gle-, -oma) A malignant neoplasm composed of oligodendrocytes.
Oligomenorrhoea (oligo-, -meno-, -rrhoea) Diminished menstrual flow. *See also* MENORRHAGIA.
Oligospermia (oligo-, -sperm-, -ia) A deficiency of spermatozoa in the semen.
Oliguria (olig-, -uria) Diminished urine production in relation to fluid intake. *See also* POLYURIA.
Omentectomy (-ectomy) The complete or partial removal of the omentum by surgery.
Omentum The folded double-layer of peritoneum connecting the stomach to another organ.
Oncogenic (onco-, -genic) Capable of producing a malignant neoplasm.
Oocyst (oo-, -cyst) The encysted and fertilised stage in the development of protozoa.
Oophoritis (oophor-, -itis) Inflammation of an ovary.
Opacity 1. Being opaque. 2. An opaque spot.
Ophthalmic (ophthalm-) OCULAR.

Ophthalmic tonometer (ophthalm-, ton-) An instrument to measure intra-ocular pressure.
Ophthalmitis (ophthalm-, -itis) Inflammation of an eye.
Opportunistic infection Refers to an infection caused by microorganisms that are not usually pathogenic, but become so under certain conditions (e.g. immunodeficiency).
Optic chiasma The cross-over point of the optic nerves.
Optic nerve The sensory nerve from each eye, which transmits impulses to the visual centre in the occipital lobe of the cerebral cortex.
Orchidectomy (orchid-, -ectomy) The removal of one or both testes by surgery.
Orchitis (orch-, -itis) Inflammation of one or both of the testes.
Orf A viral infection that affects sheep, and produces vesiculopustular dermatitis or stomatitis. It may be transmitted to humans.
Organelle Any permanent membrane-bound structure within a cell that is capable of a specific function involving cellular metabolism.
Organic 1. Refers to an organ. 2. Refers to, or arising from, an organism. 3. Chemical compounds that contain carbon.
Organism An entire living form.
Orifice (or-) An opening to a hollow organ.
Orthopaedics (ortho-) The surgical management of bone and joint disorders.
Orthopnoea (ortho-, -pnoea) Breathlessness that is relieved by assuming a sitting or upright posture. *See also* APNOEA, DYSPNOEA, HYPERPNOEA *and* TACHYPNOEA.
Osmolality (osmo-) Refers to osmotic concentration, expressed as moles of solute particles per kilogram of solvent.
Osmosis (osmo-) The movement of a solvent from a solution of lower concentration to a solution of higher concentration through a semipermeable membrane separating the two solutions.
Osmotic pressure The force that causes osmosis.
Ossification (oss-) The process of bone formation through the action of osteoblasts.
Osteitis (oste-, -itis) Inflammation of bone.
Osteitis fibrosa (oste-, -itis, fibro-) A bone disorder characterised by the deposition of fibrous tissue in marrow spaces and increased bone turnover. It results in disorganised structure of the bone and causes impaired strength.
Osteochondritis (osteo-, -chondr-, -itis) Inflammation of bone and cartilage.
Osteoclast-activating factor (osteo-, -clas-) A lymphokine produced by lymphocytes that activates and facilitates the action of osteoclasts.
Osteodystrophy (osteo-, -dys-, -trophy) Defective formation of bone.
Osteogenic (osteo-, -genic) Refers to tissue involved in the growth and repair of bone.
Osteopathy (osteo-, -pathy) 1. Any bone disease. 2. A form of therapy for bone disease involving manipulative techniques.
Osteotomy (osteo-, -tomy) Incision of a bone.
Otitis (ot-, -itis) Inflammation of the ear.
Oxidising agent (ox-) An oxygen-releasing agent that may be used for its disinfectant and deodorising properties.
Oxygen debt The extra oxygen used in oxidative metabolism to reconvert lactic acid to glucose, and to restore energy stores depleted during exercise or hypoxia.

P

Pacemaker 1. A device or structure that initiates and establishes action and the rate of a process or function. 2. The sino-atrial node. 3. An artificial pacemaker used to replace the action of an impaired sino-atrial node by the application of electronic impulses.
Palliative Refers to the reduction in intensity or severity of a disorder or its symptoms, but not resulting in a cure.
Pallor Paleness.
Palpable Perceived by touching.
Palpitation A rapid and forceful heart beat that may be perceived by the patient. The rhythm can be impaired.
Palsy PARALYSIS.
Pancreatectomy (-ectomy) The complete or partial removal of the pancreas by surgery.
Pancreatin An enzyme mixture obtained from the pancreas of animal source, and containing exocrine pancreatic secretions.
Pandemic (pan-) Refers to an epidemic disease that extends over a very large area.
Pannus Vascularisation and granulation tissue over a membrane or structure.
Papilla A general term for any small nipple-shaped elevated structure.
Papillary carcinoma (carcin-, -oma) A malignant neoplasm with outgrowths of papillae.
Paracentesis (-centesis) The surgical insertion of a cannula into a cavity to aspirate accumulated fluid.
Paraesthesia (par-, -aesthese-) An abnormal sensation (e.g. burning, tingling and 'pins and needles'). *See also* ACROPARAESTHESIA, ANAESTHESIA *and* DYSAESTHESIA.
Paralysis (para-) Loss or impairment of motor or sensory function of a part due to a lesion of the nervous system. *See also* FLACCID PARALYSIS, PARESIS *and* SPASTIC PARALYSIS.
Paranasal (para-, -nas-) Situated on the side of the nose.
Paraplegia (para-, -plegia) Paralysis of the legs and lower part of the body. *See also* DIPLEGIA, HEMIPLEGIA *and* QUADRIPLEGIA.
Parasitology (-logy) The study of parasites.
Parathyroidectomy (-ectomy) The removal of one or more of the parathyroid glands by surgery.
Parenchyma The functional part of an organ, excluding the supporting tissue.
Parenteral (par-, -enter-) Refers to administration by a route other than by the gastrointestinal tract. It usually refers to the administration of injectable preparations for a systemic effect.
Parenteral feeding (par-, -enter-) A method of supplying nutritional support via a peripheral vein, central vein or an arteriovenous shunt. It is used when the enteral route cannot be utilised. It may be given either as a supplement or as the sole source of dietary provision, in which case it is referred to as total parenteral nutrition (TPN). *See also* ENTERAL FEEDNG.

Paresis Partial or incomplete paralysis.
Parietal 1. Refers to the wall of a cavity or organ. 2. Refers to the region near the parietal bone of the skull, which constitutes the greater part of the sides and roof.
Parity (par-) Refers to a woman with respect to her having borne children. *See also* NULLIPAROUS.
Parotid Situated near the ear.
Parotitis (-itis) Inflammation of the parotid gland.
Paroxysm 1. Exacerbation or recurrence of a disease or symptoms of a disease. 2. A spasm.
Partial pressure The pressure exerted by each of the component gases in a mixture. *See also* TENSION(2).
Parturition (part-) The process of giving birth; childbirth, labour or delivery.
Passive immunisation The injection of immune serum containing the required antibodies to provide immediate, although short-lived, protection from infection. *See also* ACTIVE IMMUNISATION.
Pediculate Possessing a peduncle.
Peduncle 1. A stalk-like structure. 2. The stalk of a neoplasm attached to normal tissue.
Pelvic cavity The pelvic cavity contains the urinary bladder, sigmoid colon, rectum and the reproductive organs.
Pelvic floor PERINEUM.
Pelvic inflammatory disease Acute or chronic inflammation of the structures within the pelvic cavity. It especially refers to bacterial infection of the female genital tract.
Pelvis The lower part of the trunk formed by the two hip bones, the sacrum and the coccyx.
Pepsin The proteolytic enzyme found in gastric juice, which catalyses protein hydrolysis. It is formed from its inactive precursor, pepsinogen, by the action of hydrochloric acid.
Peptic A general term referring to the stomach, digestion, or the action of pepsin and gastric juice.
Perception The interpretation and conscious awareness of sensory stimuli.
Perfusion (per-, -fus-) The normal or artificial passage of a liquid through or over an organ or tissue.
Perianal (pere-) Refers to the area around the anus.
Pericellular (pere-) Refers to the area around a cell.
Perihepatitis (pere-, -hepat-, -itis) Inflammation of the peritoneum around the liver and its surrounding tissues.
Perineum (pere-) The muscular area between the anus and the scrotum in the male, or anus and vulva in the female; the pelvic floor.
Periodontium (pere-, -odont-) The connective tissue and bone surrounding a tooth.
Periorbital (pere-, -orb-) Refers to the area around the orbit of the eye.
Periosteum (pere-, -oste-) The connective tissue covering bones.
Periostitis (-itis) Inflammation of the periosteum.
Peripheral (pere-) Refers to a site away from a centre or located on an outer surface or part.
Peripheral vision (pere-) Vision produced through stimulation of areas away from the macula lutea by light. *See also* CENTRAL VISION.
Periportal (pere-) Refers to the area around the portal vein.
Peristalsis (pere-, -stal-, -sis) A wave of contraction that propels the contents of a hollow organ along its length, brought about by the action of longitudinal and circular muscles.
Peritoneal cavity (peritone-, -cav-) The space between the peritoneum lining the abdominal cavity and covering the abdominal organs.
Peritoneal dialysis (peritone-, -dia-, -lysis) The removal of water, electrolytes and waste products (e.g. urea and creatinine) from the blood using the peritoneal membrane as the dialysing membrane. Dialysate solution is introduced into the peritoneal cavity through an indwelling catheter, and subsequently removed after allowing time for substances to be exchanged across the peritoneal membrane. *See also* HAEMODIALYSIS.
Peritoneum (peritone-) The serous membrane in the abdomen that covers the abdominal organs and lines the abdominal cavity. *See also* MESENTERY *and* PERITONEAL CAVITY.
Peritonsillar (pere-) Refers to the region around a tonsil.
Pere-ungual (pere-) Refers to the region around a nail.
Permeable (per-) Allowing the passage of fluids and substances. *See also* SEMIPERMEABLE.
Pernicious A severe and life-threatening disorder.
Personality disorder (dis-) A behaviour disorder characterised by abnormal behaviour, lifestyle and social interaction, which is usually firmly fixed and permanent.
pH An abbreviation that refers to the hydrogen ion (H^+) concentration of a solution. A pH value of 7 represents a neutral solution, a value of less than 7 represents an acidic solution, and a value of greater than 7 represents an alkaline solution.
Phacoanaphylaxis (phaco-) A hypersensitivity reaction to the protein of the lens of the eye.
Phacolytic (phaco-, -ly-) Refers to dissolution of the lens of the eye.
Phagocytosis Endocytosis of solid material.
Phalanges, phalanx (phalang-) The bones of the fingers and toes.
Pharmacodynamics (pharmaco-, -dyname-) The study of drug action with respect to molecular structure, mechanisms of action, and the biochemical and physiological action.
Phenon (pheno-) A term used in some classification systems to denote a group of strains which share similar phenotypic characteristics.
Phenotype (pheno-) 1. The observable characteristics of an organism as determined by both genetic and environmental influences. 2. The expression of a single gene or gene pair.
Phenylalanine An essential aromatic amino acid.
Phimosis (-sis) The inability to retract the prepuce over the glans penis due to the constriction of the orifice of the prepuce. It may be acquired or congenital.
Phlyctenule A small ulcerated nodule, or a vesicle of the cornea or conjunctiva.
Phospholipase (-ase) Any of the several enzymes that catalyse phospholipid hydrolysis.
Photocoagulation (photo-) The controlled coagulation of protein using a high intensity beam of light. It is used primarily to destroy neoplastic cells and in eye surgery.
Photophobia (photo-, -phobia) 1. Visual intolerance of normal light levels. 2. A phobic state caused by well-lit places.

Photosynthesis (photo-, -syn-, -sis) The synthesis of chemicals employing light as a source of energy.

Physiology (physio-, -logy) The study of the chemical and physical factors involved in the functioning of living organisms and their component parts.

Physiotherapy (physio-, -therap-) Physical therapy involving the use of exercise, massage, manipulation and other methods to aid recovery from illness, to improve and alleviate symptoms, and to prevent physical disability.

Phytate A form of inositol found in plants, particularly the seeds; a salt of phytic acid.

Pigmentation Coloration.

Pilo-erection (pilo-) The upright posture of hair.

Pinocytosis Endocytosis of liquid materials.

Placenta The organ that connects the fetus with the inner surface of the maternal uterus. It allows the selective exchange of soluble substances between fetal and maternal blood. *See also* TROPHOBLAST.

Plasmapheresis The separation of blood cells from plasma. The separated cells are mixed with a plasma substitute and transfused back into the bloodstream. The procedure may be used for collecting plasma components or for therapeutic purposes.

Plasmolysis (-lysis) The dissolution of protoplasm due to water loss by osmotic action.

Pleomorphism (pleo-, -morph-) The ability to exhibit more than one distinct form.

Pneumonitis (pneumon-, -itis) Inflammation of the lungs.

Poison A substance that can cause structural or functional damage to body tissues when administered or applied by any route.

Polyarthritis (poly-, -arthr-, -itis) Arthritis affecting several joints simultaneously.

Polyarticular (poly-, -articul-) Involving many joints.

Polyclonal gammopathy (poly-, -pathy) Gammopathy in which there is an increase in two or more immunoglobulins. *See also* MONOCLONAL GAMMOPATHY.

Polydipsia (poly-, -ia) Excessive thirst.

Polymenorrhoea (poly-, -meno-, -rrhoea) Abnormally frequent menstruation.

Polymyalgia (poly-, -my-, -algia) Myalgia affecting several muscles.

Polyneuropathy (poly-, -neuro-, -pathy) Neuropathy involving several nerves. *See also* MONONEUROPATHY.

Polypharmacy (poly-, -pharmac-) The concurrent administration of several drugs.

Polyposis (-osis) A disorder characterised by the presence of multiple polyps.

Polyuria (poly-, -uria) Excessive urine production. *See also* OLIGURIA.

Porphyrin A molecular structure consisting of four 5-membered heterocyclic rings. It is found naturally as a chelate with metal ions (e.g. haemoglobin or chlorophyll).

Portal 1. Entrance. 2. Refers to the region of the liver where the portal vein and hepatic artery enter, and the hepatic ducts leave.

Portal hypertension (hyper-, -tens-) An abnormally high blood pressure in the hepatic portal vein. The normal pressure is 5–10 mmHg.

Posterior horn (post-) The dorsal portion of grey matter within the spinal cord containing sensory cells. *See also* ANTERIOR HORN.

Postnatal (post-) Refers to the period after birth. *See also* ANTENATAL, POSTPARTUM *and* PUERPERIUM.

Postpartum (post-, -part-) Refers to the mother in the period immediately after parturition. *See also* POSTNATAL *and* PUERPERIUM.

Postprandial (post-) Refers to the period immediately following a meal.

Postural Refers to posture or position.

Precursor (pre-) That which precedes a specific form, usually in a less developed inactive form.

Premature infant A premature infant is an infant that is born between the 27th week of gestation and full term, with a low birth weight.

Prepatellar (pre-) In front of the patella.

Preservative A substance added to a product to prevent decomposition, by killing or inhibiting the growth of microorganisms or preventing specific chemical reactions (e.g. oxidation).

Pressor Refers to the tendency to increase blood pressure.

Presynaptic (pre-) Situated or occurring before a synapse.

Priapism A persistent and painful erection of the penis attained without sexual stimulation.

Primary First or of most importance.

Procreation The process of producing offspring.

Proctocolectomy (procto-, -col-, -ectomy) The removal of the rectum and colon by surgery.

Prodromal (pro-, -drom-) Refers to the early, often premonitory, symptoms of a disease. *See also* AURA.

Proglottides The segments comprising the body of a cestode.

Prognosis (pro-, -gno-, -sis) A prediction of the course and outcome of a disease.

Progressive (pro-) Advancing, or increasing in severity.

Projectile vomiting The forceful ejection of vomit.

Prolactinoma (-oma) A benign pituitary neoplasm that secretes prolactin.

Prolapse (pro-) Forward or downward displacement; protrusion.

Proliferate Cellular multiplication resulting in growth.

Prolymphocyte (pro-, -lympho-, -cyte) An immature cell in the intermediate stage between a lymphoblast and lymphocyte.

Prone Lying down, facing downwards. *See also* SUPINE.

Prophylaxis The prevention of disease. *See also* CHEMOPROPHYLAXIS.

Prostacyclin A substance synthesised by vascular endothelial cells that prevents platelet aggregation on normal vascular tissue. It is also a potent vasodilator.

Prostaglandin A lipid derived from unsaturated 20-carbon fatty acids present in most body tissues. The actions of prostaglandins include increasing or reducing blood pressure, bronchoconstriction or bronchodilatation, reducing gastric secretion, altering platelet adhesiveness, altering intestinal and uterine muscle tone, and mediating inflammation.

Prostatectomy (-ectomy) The complete or partial removal of the prostate gland by surgery.

Prosthesis An articial replacement for a limb or body part, which may be functional or for cosmetic purposes.

Prostration Extreme exhaustion. *See also* FATIGUE, LASSITUDE *and* LETHARGY.

Protease (-ase) PROTEOLYTIC ENZYME.

Protein A member of a large and diverse group of organic compounds containing carbon, hydrogen, oxygen and nitrogen, and occasionally sulfur and phosphorus. Proteins are composed of amino acids linked by peptide bonds in a specific genetically determined sequence.

Proteinase (-ase) PROTEOLYTIC ENZYME.

Proteinuria (-uria) The presence of plasma proteins in the urine.

Proteolytic enzyme (-ly-, -zym-) An enzyme that catalyses the splitting of peptide bonds of proteins by hydrolysis to form smaller polypeptides.

Protoplasm (-plas-) The main constituent of all animal and plant cells. It is a viscous, translucent, water-based liquid composed mainly of nucleic acids, proteins, fats, carbohydrates and inorganic salts. *See also* CYTOPLASM *and* NUCLEOPLASM.

Pseudocyst (pseudo-, -cyst) Resembling a cyst, but without a distinct wall of epithelial cells.

Pseudomembrane (pseudo-) A false membrane; resembling a membrane but consisting of a thick fibrinous exudate.

Pseudopodium (pseudo-, -pod-) A temporary protrusion of cytoplasm in amoebic protozoa, formed to facilitate movement and phagocytosis.

Pseudopolyp (pseudo-) Resembling a polyp, but caused by hypertrophy of the mucous membrane as a result of ulceration.

Pseudopolyposis (pseudo-, -osis) A disorder characterised by the presence of multiple pseudopolyps.

Psychiatry (psych-) The study, treatment and prevention of mental illness.

Psychic (psych-) Refers to the mind, mental thoughts and emotions, including conscious and unconscious manifestations.

Psychogenic (psycho-, -genic) Having a psychic origin.

Psychomotor (psycho-, -mot-) 1. Refers to combined psychic and motor events (e.g. sensory auras and seizures). 2. Refers to the cerebral origin of voluntary movement.

Psychosis (psycho-, -sis) A general term for a profound psychiatric disorder of organic or psychic aetiology, and characterised by personality disorders, loss of reality, and often delusions or hallucinations. *See also* NEUROSIS.

Psychosomatic (psycho-, -somat-) Refers to the appearance or exacerbation of physical symptoms as a result of psychic causes.

Psychotherapy (psycho-, -therap-) The treatment of certain psychiatric disorders by psychological methods. It includes the use of recollection techniques, group therapy, listening and talking to the patient, offering reassurance and encouragement, developing and increasing self-confidence, and other more complex forms of treatment (e.g. hypnosis).

Puberty The period during which the secondary sexual characteristics develop, the sex organs become active, and the capability for sexual reproduction is attained.

Puerperium A period of about six weeks after parturition, during which time the reproductive organs of the mother return to their pre-pregnancy state. *See also* POSTNATAL *and* POSTPARTUM.

Pulmonary (pulmon-) Refers to the lungs.

Pulse 1. The rhythmic arterial dilatation produced by ventricular systole. The pulse-rate is the number of pulsations per minute, the normal being between 50 and 100. 2. Rhythmic and recurrent.

Purine A widely distributed compound occurring as a derivative form in the body. The purines or purine bases (e.g. adenine, guanine and xanthine) are constituents of caffeine, theophylline, and the nucleic acids.

Purulent (pur-) Forming, containing, or discharging pus.

Putrefaction The enzymatic decomposition of animal and plant tissues by microorganisms. Protein decomposition is characterised by a foul smell resulting from the formation of putrefaction products (e.g. ammonia and hydrogen sulfide).

Pyaemia (py-, -aemia) The presence of pyogenic microorganisms in the blood, resulting in the formation of multiple abscesses.

Pyknosis (pykno-, -sis) A thickening. It refers especially to cellular degeneration in which the cell nucleus condenses to form a homogenous mass. *See also* KARYOLYSIS *and* KARYORRHEXIS.

Pyoderma (pyo-, -derma) Any skin disorder characterised by purulent lesions.

Pyosalpinx (pyo-, -salp-) Accumulation of pus in a Fallopian tube.

Pyramidal cell A large pyramid-shaped neuron located in the grey matter of the cerebral cortex.

Pyrexia (pyr-) FEVER.

Pyrimidine A widely distributed compound occurring as a derivative form in the body. The pyrimidines or pyrimidine bases (e.g. uracil, thymine and cytosine) are constituents of the nucleic acids.

Pyrogen (pyro-, -gen) A substance that causes a rise in body temperature.

Pyuria (py-, -uria) The presence of pus in the urine.

Q

Quadriplegia (quadre-, -plegia) Paralysis of both arms and both legs. *See also* DIPLEGIA, HEMIPLEGIA *and* PARAPLEGIA.

Quarantine The detention and isolation of sources of contagious or communicable disease as a routine procedure, or in suspected or definite cases.

R

Radiation (rade-) 1. Electromagnetic waves. *See also* IRRADIATION. 2. Spreading from a central point.

Radioactivity (radio-) The property of emitting radiation.

Radiobiology (radio-, -bio-, -logy) The study of the effect of radiation on living cells and tissues.

Radiography (radio-, -graphy) Examination of internal structures using radiation, which is passed through the body onto sensitised photographic film.

Radioisotope (radio-, -iso-, -top-) A radioactive isotope.

Radiolabel (radio-) A radioactive isotope that is used to replace a stable chemical element in a compound. It is introduced into the body to study the distribution of a compound with the aid of a radiation detecting device.

Radiotherapy (radio-, -therap-) The therapeutic use of ionising radiation.
Rarefaction Reduction in density and mass but not volume.
Rash A skin eruption.
Receptor (-ceptor) 1. A molecular structure on or within a cell that allows the binding of a specific agent to elicit a specific response. 2. A specialised nerve terminal that responds to sensory stimuli. *See also* SYNAPSE.
Recrudescence (re-) The recurrence of symptoms within days or weeks of their subsidence. *See also* RELAPSE.
Rectosigmoid (recto-) Refers to the region at the end of the sigmoid colon and the beginning of the rectum.
Rectovaginal (recto-, -vagin-) Refers to the rectum and the vagina.
Reflex (re-, -flex) The involuntary and rapid response to a stimulus.
Reflux (re-, -flux) Backward flow or regurgitation.
Refractory Resistant to treatment.
Regurgitation (re-) The return or backward flow of contents.
Rehydration (re-, -hydrat-) The administration of fluids to correct dehydration.
Relapse (re-) The recurrence of a disease after apparent cure, usually within weeks or months. *See also* RECRUDESCENCE.
Remission (re-) The subsidence and cessation of disease symptoms; the period of subsidence.
Replacement therapy (therap-) The treatment of deficiency disorders by the administration of natural or synthetic derivatives of the deficient substance.
Resection (-sect-) The complete or partial removal of an organ or structure by surgery. *See also* EXCISION.
Reservoir of infection A host that carries pathogenic microorganisms, usually without any harmful effects, and serves as a source of infection. Non-living material may also act as a reservoir. *See also* CARRIER(1) *and* FOMITES.
Residual volume The volume of air in the lungs following maximum expiration. *See also* VITAL CAPACITY.
Resistance 1. An opposite force; counteraction. 2. The ability of an organism to remain unaffected by microorganisms or their toxins. *See also* ANTIMICROBIAL RESISTANCE. 3. In psychotherapy, the conscious and active opposition to prevent unconscious thoughts from emerging.
Respiration (-spirat-) The complete process of gaseous interchange between the tissues and the external environment. It includes ventilation, and gaseous exchange between the lungs and the blood, and between the blood and the cells.
Respirator (-spirat-) 1. An apparatus to prevent the inhalation of harmful environmental substances. 2. An apparatus to provide artificial respiration or assisted ventilation.
Resuscitation (re-) The emergency treatment to restore life in an apparently deceased patient (e.g. using cardiac massage and artificial respiration).
Retch To make an involuntary and ineffectual attempt to vomit.
Reticulin (ret-) The protein from reticular connective tissue.
Reticulo-endothelial system (ret-) A functional system of potent phagocytic cells found throughout the body, and serving as a defence mechanism. The cells include macrophages and are concentrated in the spleen, liver, bone marrow and lymph nodes.
Retinopathy (-pathy) Any non-inflammatory disease of the retina.
Retrobulbar (retro-) Situated behind the eyeball.
Retrograde (retro-, -grad-) Backwards; in an opposite direction.
Retroperitoneum (retro-, -peritone-) The area behind the peritoneum.
Retrosternal (retro-, -stern-) Situated behind the sternum.
Rheumatism A general term applied to any disorder characterised by inflammation or degeneration of connective tissue, particularly of joints and muscles.
Rhinorrhoea (rhino-, -rrhoea) A profuse discharge of mucus from the nose.
Ribonucleic acid (-nucle-) Ribonucleic acid (RNA) is found in the nucleus and cytoplasm of all living cells, and processes information from DNA for cellular protein synthesis. The molecular structure is similar to DNA except that ribose replaces deoxyribose, and uracil replaces thymine. Three types exist: messenger RNA (mRNA), transfer RNA (tRNA), and ribosomal RNA (rRNA). *See also* DEOXYRIBONUCLEIC ACID.
Ribosome (-some) A granule composed of ribosomal RNA (rRNA) bound to specific proteins. Ribosomes are found in the cytoplasm of all living cells.
Rigor 1. Rigidity. 2. A chill or shivering fit, with fever and cold skin.
RNA RIBONUCLEIC ACID.
Rosacea An inflammatory skin disorder characterised by extensive facial erythema, often with papules, pustules and telangiectasia.
Rubefacient (rub-, -facient) Producing erythema.
Rupture 1. A break or tear. 2. HERNIA.

S

Sac A pouch or bag-like structure.
Saccular Resembling a sac.
Sacral Refers to, or situated near, the sacrum.
Sacrococcygeal (sacro-) Refers to the region of the sacrum and coccyx.
Saturated fat A fat composed of a fatty acid that contains only single bonds in the carbon chain. It is found in animal products (e.g. meat and milk).
Scan A visual display of body tissues produced by moving a sensing device over the body, or body part, or by a series of observations to produce a complete image.
Schizogony A type of asexual reproduction in which the nucleus undergoes multiple fission, followed by separation of the cytoplasm into discrete masses around each daughter nucleus.
Sclerosis (sclero-, -sis) Hardening, especially of the nervous system due to connective tissue hyperplasia, and also applied to blood vessels. It is usually of chronic inflammatory origin.
Sclerotherapy (sclero-, -therap-) The injection of a sclerosant.
Scotoma An area of diminished vision surrounded by an area of less diminished or normal vision.

Sebaceous (-aceous) Refers to sebum.

Seborrhoea (sebo-, -rrhoea) Excessive sebum secretion from the sebaceous glands.

Secondary 1. Occurring in second place, or as a result of a primary disorder. 2. Often used to denote metastasis.

Secretin A hormone secreted by the intestinal mucosa, whose actions include inhibition of gastric juice secretion, stimulation of pancreatic juice and bile secretion, and stimulation of intestinal juice.

Secretion The production and release of a specific functional substance by a cell or a gland.

Seizure 1. An epileptic attack. *See also* CONVULSION. 2. A sudden occurrence of a disease and its symptoms.

Self-limiting Refers to a disease that follows a definite course, and is restricted in duration as a result of its own characteristics and not by external factors.

Seminal duct Any of the ducts of the male reproductive organs.

Seminoma (-oma) A malignant neoplasm of the testis, arising from germ cells.

Semipermeable (semi-, -per-) Refers to the selective passage of certain molecules. *See also* PERMEABLE.

Semipermeable membrane (semi-, -per-) A membrane that allows the passage of solvent (e.g. water), but not solutes.

Senility A generalised physical and mental dysfunction associated with ageing.

Sensorineural (sens-, -neur-) Refers to a sensory nerve or the sensory mechanism.

Sensory (sens-) Refers to sensations or to sensory nerves.

Sepsis (sep-, -sis) A condition caused by the presence of pathogenic microorganisms, or their toxins, in the blood or tissues.

Septic (sep-) Refers to sepsis or putrefaction.

Septum (sept-) A dividing structure or partition.

Sero-mucinous (ser-, -muc-) Refers to serum and mucin.

Serotonin Serotonin (5HT, 5-hydroxytryptamine) is a widely distributed compound found in most body tissues and in high concentration in platelets. Its actions include inhibition of gastric juice secretion, stimulation of smooth muscle and acting as a neurotransmitter in the central nervous system.

Serous (ser-) 1. Refers to or resembling serum. 2. Containing or producing serum.

Serous membrane (ser-) A membrane that covers structures not exposed to the external environment, and which secretes serum.

Serum (ser-) 1. The clear watery portion of body fluids. 2. The clear liquid part of blood, excluding blood cells and clotting factors.

Serum sickness (ser-) A hypersensitivity reaction occurring 7–12 days after administration of a foreign serum or some drugs (e.g. penicillin). It is characterised by arthralgia, fever, lymphadenopathy, skin rashes, oedema and urticaria.

Sexual reproduction Production of offspring by fusion of male and female gametes. *See also* ASEXUAL REPRODUCTION.

Shear Refers to the distortion of an object caused by two oppositely directed parallel forces.

Shunt 1. To divert or bypass. 2. An anastomosis between two vessels, especially blood vessels.

Shy-Drager syndrome A progressive disorder characterised by orthostatic hypotension and symptoms of autonomic nervous system insufficiency. Generalised neurological dysfunctions follow and include parkinsonism, cerebellar ataxia and paralysis of the extrinsic ocular muscles.

Sialorrhoea (sialo-, -rrhoea) Excessive salivation.

Sibling Brother or sister; having one or both parents in common.

Sigmoidoscopy (-scopy) Examination of the rectum and sigmoid colon using a fibreoptic sigmoidoscope, which is also a tool for biopsy.

Sinus (sinu-) 1. A cavity or channel. 2. A natural cavity within a bone or other tissue, especially the air cavities within the skull communicating with the nostrils. 3. A venous cavity, channel or receptacle of blood. 4. A fistula or tract permitting the escape of pus from a suppurating cavity.

Sinus rhythm Normal heart rhythm.

Sinusoidal (sinu-, -oid-) Resembling a sinus.

Slough 1. To separate, shed or cast off. 2. Necrotic tissue separating from living tissue.

Somatic (somat-) 1. Refers to the body. 2. Refers to body structure excluding the viscera.

Somnolence (somn-) Abnormal drowsiness or inclination to sleep.

Sorbitol A hexahydric alcohol and a sweetening agent. It is metabolised to fructose.

Spasm (spas-) A sudden involuntary painful muscle contraction.

Spastic paralysis (spas-, para-) Paralysis with increased tendon reflexes and spasticity of the muscles. It is commonly caused by motor neuron lesions. *See also* FLACCID PARALYSIS.

Spasticity (spas-) A non-specific condition of increased muscular tone with exaggeration of the reflexes.

Species A taxonomic category that comprises strains possessing common features. Similar species belong to the same genus.

Sphincter A circular muscle that constricts and closes an orifice or passage.

Splenectomy (splen-, -ectomy) The removal of the spleen by surgery.

Sputum The substance expelled from the respiratory passages by coughing.

Squamous (squam-) Scaly, or covered in scales.

Stasis The stoppage or slowing of the flow of a fluid.

Stasis eczema A chronic inflammatory skin disorder of the lower legs caused by venous insufficiency. It is characterised by brown pigmentation, oedema and ulceration.

Steatorrhoea (steato-, -rrhoea) An excessive amount of fat in the faeces.

Stenosis (steno-, -sis) The narrowing or constriction of a vessel, passage, or duct. *See also* COARCTATION and STRICTURE.

Stomatitis (stomat-, -itis) Inflammation of the oral mucosa. *See also* ANGULAR STOMATITIS.

Stopple GROMMET.

Strangulated Tightly constricted and with diminished blood supply.

Strangury Painful and slow urination caused by spasm of the bladder and urethra. *See also* DYSURIA.

Stress 1. Exerted pressure; force. 2. The total response to adverse stimuli, which elicits homeostatic mechanisms. The stimule may be of any origin, and if the compensatory mechanisms are inadequate, they could cause or precipitate disorders. *See also* GENERAL ADAPTATION SYNDROME.

Stricture (strict-) The closure or abnormal narrowing of a vessel, passage, or duct. *See also* COARCTATION *and* STENOSIS.

Stridor A harsh and loud breathing sound caused by a constricted airway. *See also* WHEEZE.

Strip 1. To apply pressure along a vessel, using the finger, to move the contents. 2. To remove a large vein by surgery.

Stroke volume The amount of blood pumped out of a ventricle in each heart beat. *See also* CARDIAC OUTPUT.

Stupor Almost complete unconsciousness, in which the subject responds only to forceful and vigorous stimuli. *See also* COMA.

Subacromial (sub-, -acro-) Beneath the acromion, which is the lateral projection of the scapula over the shoulder joint.

Subacute (sub-) Refers to a disorder with characteristics intermediate between acute and chronic.

Subconjunctival (sub-) Beneath the conjunctiva.

Subcutaneous (sub-, -cut-) Beneath the skin.

Sublingual (sub-, -lingu-) Beneath the tongue.

Submandibular (sub-) Beneath the bone of the lower jaw.

Submucosa (sub-, -muc-) The areolar tissue layer beneath a mucous membrane.

Subperiosteal (sub-, -pere-, -oste-) Beneath the periosteum.

Subphrenic (sub-, -phren-) Beneath the diaphragm.

Sucrose (-ose) A disaccharide found in sugar cane, sugar beet and other plants. It is used as a food and sweetening agent.

Suffocation Cessation of breathing caused by airway obstruction. *See also* ASPHYXIA.

Superficial (super-) Refers to, or occurring near, the surface.

Supine Lying down, facing upwards. *See also* PRONE.

Supportive therapy (therap-) Measures directed towards maintaining the patient's strength.

Suprapubic (supra-) Situated above the pubic bone, which is the anterior inferior part of the hip bone.

Supraventricular (supra-, -ventricul-) Above the ventricles, referring especially to the atria and atrioventricular node.

Surfactant A substance that reduces the surface tension of fluids.

Suture A surgical stitch.

Sympathectomy (-ectomy) The excision or interruption of sympathetic nerves by surgery.

Sympathomimetic Having an action which mimics that produced by stimulation of sympathetic nerves. *See also* ADRENERGIC.

Symptomatic 1. Refers to a symptom or symptoms. 2. Indicative of a specific disorder. 3. Refers to treatment directed towards alleviating symptoms.

Synapse The site of functional proximity between neurons, at which transmission of an impulse occurs. *See also* NEUROTRANSMITTER *and* RECEPTOR(2).

Syndrome A set of distinct and characteristic symptoms that occur together; a symptom complex.

Syrinx A tube or fistula.

Systemic Refers to the whole body. *See also* LOCAL.

Systole The period during which the heart, and especially the ventricles, contract. *See also* DIASTOLE.

Systolic pressure The maximum arterial blood pressure which occurs during ventricular systole. *See also* DIASTOLIC PRESSURE.

T

Tachypnoea (tachy-, -pnoea) Abnormally rapid breathing, *See also* APNOEA, DYSPNOEA, HYPERPNOEA *and* ORTHOPNOEA.

Tactile (tact-) Refers to the sense of touch.

Taxonomy (tax-, -nom-) The structured classification and naming of organisms.

Temporal (tempor-) 1. Refers to the lateral portion on both sides of the head, in the region of the temple. 2. Refers to time; temporary.

Tenesmus Straining, particularly on defecation or urination, which may be accompanied by pain.

Tension (tens-) 1. The state and degree of stretch or strain. *See also* ARTERIAL TENSION. 2. The partial pressure of a gas in a fluid (e.g. the pressure of oxygen (PaO_2) or carbon dioxide ($PaCO_2$) in arterial blood).

Teratogenesis (terato-, -gen-, -sis) The production of developmental abnormalities in the fetus.

Teratoma (terat-, -oma) A malignant neoplasm composed of several tissue types, which are usually foreign to the site in which it occurs. Teratomas form most commonly in the ovaries or testes.

Terminal 1. Refers to an end or extremity. 2. Refers to the last stages of a fatal disease.

Tertiary In third place

Testicular feminisation syndrome A syndrome affecting males and characterised by the development of external secondary female characteristics, but with the testes present. It is thought to be caused by target-organ resistance to testosterone.

Tetany 1. Excessive neuromuscular excitability caused by abnormal calcium metabolism. It is characterised by flexion of the wrists and ankles, muscle twitching, cramp, laryngospasm and convulsions. 2. Sustained tonic muscle contraction.

Therapeutics (therap-) The branch of medicine that is concerned with the treatment of disease.

Thoracotomy (thoraco-, -tomy) Incision of the chest wall.

Thrombectomy (thromb-, -ectomy) The removal of a thrombus by surgery.

Thromboplastin (thrombo-) A substance that promotes coagulation of blood.

Thymectomy (thym-, -ectomy) The removal of the thymus gland by surgery.

Thymoma (thym-, -oma) A malignant neoplasm consisting of thymic tissue.

Thyroid storm A rare and life-threatening disorder caused by the sudden exacerbation of hyperthyroidism.

Thyroidectomy (-ectomy) The complete or partial removal of the thyroid gland.

Tibia The inner, larger bone in the lower leg. *See also* FIBULA.
Tinnitus A sensation of noises in the ear (e.g. ringing, buzzing, or clicking).
Tolerance Refers to the ability to endure, or become less responsive to, a drug or toxin, especially during a period of continued exposure. *See also* CROSS TOLERANCE *and* INTOLERANCE(1).
Tone (ton-) The state of organs and tissues in which function and firmness is normal. *See also* MUSCLE TONE.
Tonsil A small aggregation of large lymph nodes within a mucous membrane. The pharyngeal tonsil (adenoid) is found in the nasopharynx, the two palatine tonsils are found on the sides of the oropharynx, and the two lingual tonsils are found at the base of the tongue. The term tonsils usually refers to the palatine tonsils.
Tonsillectomy (-ectomy) The removal of one or more tonsils by surgery, usually referring to the palatine tonsils and sometimes also the lingual tonsils.
Topical (top-) Refers to a specific area of a surface.
Total parenteral nutrition *See* PARENTERAL FEEDING.
Toxaemia (tox-, -aemia) 1. The presence of bacterial toxins in the blood. *See also* ENDOTOXIN *and* EXOTOXIN. 2. Metabolic disturbances.
Toxic (toxe-) Refers to a poison or toxin.
Toxicology (toxico-, -logy) The study of the preparation, identification and action of poisons and toxins, and their antidotes.
Toxigenic (toxe-, -genic) Producing a toxin.
TPN Total parenteral nutrition. *See* PARENTERAL FEEDING.
Trabecula A term for connective tissue that anchors or supports.
Tracheitis (trache-, -itis) Inflammation of the trachea.
Tracheobronchial (tracheo-, -bronch-) Refers to the trachea and bronchi.
Tracheostomy (tracheo-, -stomy) A surgical procedure to establish an opening into the trachea through the neck. The term may also be applied to the opening itself.
Traction (tract-) The application of a longitudinal pulling force to a structure.
Transcription The transfer of genetic information, with reference to the process by which a single strand of DNA serves as a template for the formation of the messenger RNA (mRNA) base sequence. *See also* TRANSLATION.
Transferase (trans-, -ase) An enzyme capable of transferring a chemical entity from one molecule to another, such that the chemical entity does not exist in a free state during the transfer.
Transfusion (trans-, -fus-) The administration of donor blood or blood products (e.g. plasma, serum, or blood substitutes) into the circulatory system. Prior to transfusion of whole blood, selection and cross-matching is carried out. The same blood group is selected and tested by cross-matching with the recipient's serum. Both the recipient and donor blood is tested for atypical antibodies. *See also* EXCHANGE TRANSFUSION *and* INFUSION(1).
Transitional cell A cell of the transitional epithelium, which lines some hollow organs (e.g. bladder). The cells are large and round and are capable of distension. This property prevents rupture and allows the organ to expand.
Transitional epithelium *See* TRANSITIONAL CELL.
Translation The production of a specific protein on the ribosome of a cell, as determined by the base sequence on the messenger RNA (mRNA) molecule. *See also* TRANSCRIPTION.
Transplantation (trans-) A procedure to graft tissues or organs from one part of the body to another, or from one person to another. *See also* ALLOGRAFT.
Transudation (trans-) The outflow of serum or other body fluids through a tissue membrane or surface as a result of inflammation or other causes. The transudate has a low content of protein, cells and cellular debris. *See also* EXTRAVASATION *and* EXUDATION.
Transurethral (trans-, -urethr-) Refers to a procedure performed through the urethra.
Trauma 1. A physical wound or injury. 2. An emotional shock, especially one having a lasting psychic effect.
Tremor Involuntary shaking or trembling.
Trichotillomania (tricho-, -mania) A compulsive impulse to pull out the hair.
Trigeminal nerve The fifth cranial nerve, the sensory portion of which innervates the face, nasal cavity, mouth, and teeth, while the motor portion innervates the muscles involved in chewing.
Triglyceride (tre-, -glyc-) A fat composed of three molecules of fatty acid esterified with glycerol. It is stored in adipose tissue.
Trimester (tre-) A three-month period of time.
Trophoblast (tropho-, -blast) The cell layer through which a developing fetus receives nourishment from the mother, and which forms part of the placenta.
Trophozoite (tropho-, -zo-) The active and feeding stage in the life-cycle of a protozoal microorganism.
Tunica A covering.
Turgor Refers to a state of fullness or swelling; normal appearance and fullness.

U

Ulcer An open lesion on an external or internal surface of the body, produced by sloughing of necrotic tissue usually as a result of inflammation.
Ulceration 1. The formation of an ulcer. 2. ULCER.
Ultrasound (ultra-) Sound with a frequency above 20 000 Hz and inaudible to the human ear. Its properties are dependent on the power level used. It may be used for diagnostic purposes using echo reflection techniques, physiotherapy, or to selectively destroy tissues.
Ultraviolet radiation (ultra-, rade-) Radiation emitted from beyond the violet end of the visible spectrum.
Umbilical hernia The protrusion of part of the intestine through the abdominal wall at the umbilicus, but under the skin and subcutaneous tissue.
Umbilicus The navel, marking the attachment site of the umbilical cord, which connected the developing fetus to the placenta.
Unconjugated hyperbilirubinaemia *See* HYPERBILIRUBINAEMIA.
Underwater seal drainage A closed drainage system in which a tube leading from the pleural cavity is

immersed in a container of water. This allows air, blood and fluid to be drained from the pleural cavity, and lung expansion to be maintained.

Ungual Refers to a nail or nails.

Unipolar (une-) 1. Possessing only one pole or process. 2. At one end of a cell. 3. Used to describe affective disorders characterised by depressive periods only. *See also* BIPOLAR.

Urate A salt of uric acid (e.g. sodium urate).

Ureteric (ureter-) Refers to the ureter.

Urethral (urethr-) Refers to the urethra.

Uricosuric (urico-, -ur-) Refers to the promotion of uric acid excretion.

Urostomy (uro-, -stomy) A surgical procedure to divert the flow of urine from the bladder to an opening (stoma) created on the surface of the abdomen. A length of intestine is isolated, usually from the ileum, and inserted between the ureters and the stoma, thus acting as a drainage channel for urine. The term may also be applied to the opening itself. *See also* COLOSTOMY *and* ILEOSTOMY.

Urothelial (uro-) Refers to the epithelium of the urinary bladder.

Uterine (uter-) Refers to the uterus.

Uterorectal (utero-, -rect-) Refers to the uterus and the rectum, or to a communication between them.

Uvula A pendent fleshy structure, referring especially to the cone-shaped structure within the oropharynx descending from the soft palate.

V

Vaccination 1. The injection or oral administration of a vaccine to induce active immunity. *See also* ACTIVE IMMUNISATION. 2. Historically, the term was applied to inoculation with cowpox virus (vaccinia) to induce immunity to smallpox.

Vaccine A preparation of antigenic material used for active immunisation against specific bacteria or viruses. *See also* ANTISERUM.

Vacuole A cavity formed in the protoplasm of a cell.

Vagotomy (-tomy) The complete or selective interruption of the vagus nerve by surgery.

Vagus nerve The tenth cranial nerve, which consists of motor and sensory fibres. It innervates the muscles of the pharynx, larynx, respiratory system, oesophagus, stomach, small intestine, gall bladder, part of the large intestine and the heart.

Valvotomy (-tomy) Incision of a valve, especially a heart valve.

Varicose (varic-, -ose) Refers to, or characterised by, a distended and tortuous vein, artery or lymph vessel.

Vascular (vas-) 1. Refers to blood vessels. 2. Implies a profuse blood supply. *See also* AVASCULAR.

Vasculitis (vas-, -itis) Inflammation of a vessel, especially of a blood or lymph vessel. *See also* ARTERITIS.

Vasoactive (vaso-) Refers to an effect on the tension and internal diameter of blood vessels. *See also* VASOCONSTRICTION, VASODILATATION *and* VASOMOTOR.

Vasoconstriction (vaso-) A reduction in the diameter of blood vessels, especially the arterioles. *See also* VASODILATATION.

Vasodilatation (vaso-) An increase in the diameter of blood vessels, especially the arterioles. *See also* VASOCONSTRICTION.

Vasodilation VASODILATATION.

Vasomotor (vaso-, -mot-) Refers to the contractility of the muscular walls of the blood vessels. *See also* VASOACTIVE, VASOCONSTRICTION *and* VASODILATATION.

Vasospasm (vaso-, -spas-) Spasm of blood vessels, resulting in vasoconstriction.

Vector A carrier of an infective agent, which promotes the transfer of infection.

Vegetation 1. Any plant-like or fungus-like growth. 2. A clot attached to a diseased heart valve, and composed of blood platelets, fibrin and infecting microorganisms.

Vegetative 1. Refers to nutrition and growth. 2. Refers to involuntary or unconscious function. 3. Refers to the cellular resting phase, in which the cell is not involved in replication. 4. Refers to asexual reproduction.

Venesection (ven-, -sect-) Incision of a vein.

Ventilation The breathing process resulting in the gaseous exchange between the lungs and the external environment. *See also* HYPERVENTILATION, HYPOVENTILATION *and* RESPIRATION.

Ventricle A cavity, especially of the brain and heart.

Ventriculo-atrial shunt (ventriculo-, -atre-) An anastomosis created between a cerebral ventricle and a cardiac atrium using a plastic tube, to allow drainage of cerebrospinal fluid.

Ventriculo-peritoneal shunt (ventriculo-, peritone-) An anastomosis created between a cerebral ventricle and the peritoneum using a plastic tube, to allow drainage of cerebrospinal fluid.

Vermiform (verme-, -form) Resembling the shape of a worm.

Vernal Refers to the spring.

Vesiculation (vesic-) The formation of vesicles.

Vesiculopustular (vesic-) Refers to vesicles and pustules.

Vestigial Refers to the degenerated remnants of a structure which was functional during embryonic or fetal development, or in primeval species.

Villus A small projection or protrusion, especially from a mucous membrane of the small intestine.

Viraemia (-aemia) The presence of viruses in the blood.

Virilisation The development of male secondary sexual characteristics, especially applied to such changes in females.

Viscera (viscer-) The organs within the body cavities, especially those of the abdomen. *See also* SOMATIC(2).

Viscosity The resistance to flow caused by molecular cohesion, commonly applied to liquids as the resistance to shear forces.

Vital capacity (vit-) The total volume of gas expired from the lungs after maximum inspiration and expiration. *See also* RESIDUAL VOLUME.

Vitamin (vit-) An organic compound required by the body in small amounts for metabolism. Vitamins are generally obtained from the diet and are classified as water-soluble (e.g. vitamin C) or fat-soluble (e.g. vitamin D).

Volvulus A knot or twist in the gastrointestinal tract, resulting in obstruction.

Vomitus 1. The forcible ejection of the contents of the stomach through the mouth. 2. The matter ejected by vomiting.

W

Wheeze A whistling sound made during breathing, especially that associated with asthma or the mechanical obstruction of the trachea or bronchi. *See also* STRIDOR.

X

X-rays Radiation of short wavelength produced by electrons emitted at high speed from a heated cathode and bombarding a heavy metal anode.

Z

Zoonosis (zoo-, -sis) An animal disease capable of being transmitted to humans under natural conditions.

Zygote (zygo-) A term applied to a fertilised ovum (formed by the union of a male and female gamete) before it divides.

Combining forms, prefixes and suffixes

Introduction

Many words, including medical terms, are composed from one or more word roots derived from classical Greek and Latin. A knowledge of these word roots may facilitate the comprehension of a wide range of terms, without the need to consult a dictionary.

The following list comprises combining forms, prefixes and suffixes of some of the most commonly used word roots that make up many of the medical terms used throughout this publication. It is not, however, intended to be a comprehensive etymological list.

A hyphen following a term indicates that the term is used in the prefix position, while a hyphen preceding a term indicates the suffix position. Combining forms may appear in any position within a word, and are identified in this list by hyphens at both ends.

A definition is given under the form that bears the closest resemblance to the actual word root. Some forms which are merely deviations in spelling have been listed, with a cross-reference to the main entry. There may be several combining forms of the same word root, and those most commonly used have been grouped together as one entry, although it should be noted that this list is not exhaustive. If a particular form differs significantly and would appear in the alphabetical listing at a distance from the main entry, it has been listed separately with a cross-reference to the main entry. The reader's attention has been drawn to terms that have the same meaning but are derived from different word roots, by the use of cross-references. In these cases, the definitions have been given under all the terms.

For those terms that have more than one definition, any cross-reference follows on immediately after the definition to which it applies. If the cross-reference applies to all of the stated definitions, it starts on a new line after the last definition.

The reader should consult the glossary for examples of the breakdown of words into combining forms, prefixes, and suffixes, which have, where appropriate, been listed in brackets after the word itself.

A

a- Without, not. The prefix becomes an- before a vowel or h.

ab- From, off, away from.

-able Capable of.

ac- *See* ad-.

-aceous Of the nature of, resembling, forming.

-acou- Hear. Alternative spelling, -acu-.

-acro- At an extremity, topmost.

-acu- 1. Needle. 2. *See* -acou-.

ad- To, toward. The prefix becomes ac-, af-, ag-, ap-, as-, or at- before words beginning with c, f, g, p, s, or t respectively.

-aden-, -adeno- Gland.

-adip-, -adipo- Fat. *See also* -lip- and -stear-.

-adren-, -adreno- Adrenal gland.

-aemia Of or in the blood. Alternative spelling, -emia.

-aer- Air, gas.

-aesthesi-, -aesthesio- Perception, feeling, sensation. Alternative spellings, -esthesi-, -esthesio-.

af- *See* ad-.

ag- *See* ad-

-agra Painful seizure.

-alb- White. *See also* -leuc-(1).
-alg-, -algesi-, -algio-, -algo- Pain. *See also* -odyn-.
-algia Painful condition. *See also* -odynia.
-algio- *See* -alg-.
-algo- *See* -alg-.
-all-, -allo- Other, different, abnormal.
-alve- Channel, cavity.
amb-, ambi- On both sides.
-ambly- Dullness, dimness.
-amyl-, -amylo- Starch.
an- 1. *See* a-. 2. *See* ana-.
ana- 1. Up, upward, positive. 2. Back, backward. 3. Excessive, again. The prefix becomes an- before a vowel.
-ancyl-, -ancylo- *See* -ankyl-.
-andr-, -andro- Male, man.
-angi-, -angio- A vessel, usually a blood vessel. *See also* -vas-.
-anis-, -aniso- Unequal, dissimilar, asymmetric.
-ankyl-, -ankylo- Bent, crooked, looped. Alternative spellings, -ancyl-, -ancylo.
ant-, anti- Against, opposed to.
ante- Before, in front of.
-anthrop-, -anthropo- Human.
anti- *See* ant-.
ap- 1. *See* ad-. 2. *See* apo-.
apo- 1. Detached, separated. 2. Formed from. The prefix becomes ap- before a vowel.
-appendic-, -appendico- Appendix.
-arachn-, -arachno- 1. Arachnoid membrane. 2. Spider.
-arch-, -archae-, -arche-, -archi- 1. Original, first, primitive. 2. Leader.
-arter-, -arteri-, -arterio- Artery.
-arthr-, -arthro- Joint. *See also* -articul-.
-articul- Joint. *See also* -arthr-.
as- *See* ad-.
-ase Enzyme. *See also* -zym-.
-asis Condition, state of, process. *See also* -ia, -iasis, -ism, -osis, and -sis.
-astro- Star.
at- *See* ad-.
-atel-, -atelo- Incomplete, not perfect.
-atri-, -atrio- Atrium of the heart.
-aur-, -auri- Ear. *See also* -ot-.
aut-, auto- Self, self-induced.
-axi-, -axio- Axis.
azo- Signifies the presence of -N=N- in a molecule.

B

-bact-, -bacter-, -bacteri-, -bacterio- Bacteria.
-balan-, -balano- Glans penis or glans clitoridis.
-bar- Weight.
-bas-, -basi-, -basio-, -baso- 1. Base, foundation. 2. Chemical base.
bi- Two. *See also* -dipl- and dis-(2).
-bili- Bile. *See also* -chol-.
-bio- Life. *See also* -vit- and -zo-.
-blast-, -blasto- Germ, bud, embryonic cell.
-blenn-, -blenno- Mucus. *See also* -muc- and -myx-.
-blephar-, -blepharo- Eyelid. *See also* -cili-(2).
-brachi-, -brachio- Arm.
-brachy- Short.
-brady- Slow.
-brom-, -bromo- 1. The presence of bromine. 2. Smell.
-bronch-, -broncho- Bronchus.
-bucc-, -bucco- Cheek.

C

-cac-, -caco- Bad, abnormal. *See also* -dys- and mal-.
-caec-, -caeco- 1. Blind. 2. Caecum. Alternative spellings, -cec-, -ceco-. *See also* -typhl-.
-calc- 1. Stone. *See also* -lith-. 2. Heel. 3. Calcium. *See also* -calci-.
-calci-, -calco- Calcium or its salts. *See also* -calc (3).
-canth-, -cantho- The angle of the eye.
-caps- Container.
-carb-, -carba-, -carbo- Charcoal, coal, carbon.
-carcin-, -carcino- Cancer, malignancy.
-card-, -cardi-, -cardio- 1. Heart. 2. The cardiac orifice of the stomach.
-carp- Wrist.
cata- Down, lower, under, against, negative.
-caud- Tail.
-cav- Hollow. *See also* -cel-(2), -cen-
-cec-, -ceco- *See* -caec-.
-cel-, -celo- 1. Hernia, swelling, tumour. 2. Cavity, hollow. *See also* -cav-. 3. Abdomen. *See also* -celi- and -ventr-(1).
-cele 1. Tumour, swelling, hernia. 2. Cavity.
-celi-, -celio- Abdomen. *See also* -cel-(3) and -ventr-(1).
-celo- *See* -cel-.
-cen-, -ceno- Hollow, empty. *See also* -coen-.
-centesis Piercing, puncturing, perforating.
-cephal-, -cephalo- Head.
-ceptor Receiver, taker.
-cerebr-, -cerebro- Brain.
-cervic- Neck. *See also* -trachel-.
-cheil-, -cheilo- Lip. *See also* -labi-
-chem-, -chemi-, -chemo- Chemical.
-chol-, -chole-, -cholo- Bile. *See also* -bili-.
-choledoch-, -choledocho- Common bile duct.
-cholo- *See* -chol-.
-chondr-, -chondro- Cartilage.
-chondri-, -chondrio- Granule.
-chondro- *See* -chondr-.
-chord-, -chordo- Cord.
-chrom-, -chromo- 1. Chromium. 2. Colour. *See also* -chromat-(2).
-chromat-, -chromato- 1. Chromatin. 2. Colour. *See also* -chrom-(2).
-chromo- *See* -chrom-.
-chron-, -chrono- Time.
-cide Killing, destroying. *See also* -cis-(2).
-cili-, -cilio- 1. Cilia, hair-like. 2. Eyelid. *See also* -blephar-. 3. Some internal structures of the eye.
circa-, circum- Around.
-cis- 1. Cut. *See also* -sect- and -tomy. 2. Kill. *See also* -cide.
-clas- Break.
co- *See* con-.
-coen-, -coeno- Common feature, shared. Alternative spellings, -cen-, -ceno-.

-col- 1. Colon. 2. *See* con-.
-colp-, colpo- Vagina. *See also* -vagin-.
com- *See* con-.
con- With, together. The prefix becomes co- before h or a vowel; col- before l; com- before b, m, or p; and cor- before r. *See also* syn-.
contra- Against, opposite.
-copr-, -copro- Faeces.
cor- *See* con-.
-corp-, -corpor- Body. *See also* -somat-.
-cortic-, -cortico- Cortex, rind.
-cost-, -costa- Rib. *See also* -pleur-(3).
-crani-, -cranio- Skull.
-crescent Grow, increase. *See also* -cret-(2).
-cret- 1. Separate, distinguish. 2. Grow, increase. *See also* -crescent.
-cry-, -cryo- Cold.
-crypt-, -crypto- Hidden, concealed.
-cut- Skin. *See also* -derm and -derma-.
-cyan-, -cyano- Blue.
-cycl-, -cyclo- 1. Round, circle, cycle. 2. Recurring.
-cyst-, -cysti-, -cysto- Bladder, cyst, sac. *See also* -vesic-.
-cyt-, -cyto- Cell.
-cyte Cell.
-cyto- *See* -cyt-.

D

-dacry-, -dacryo- Tears. *See also* -lachry-.
-dactyl-, -dactylo- Finger, toe. *See also* -phalang-.
de- Down, away, removal from.
-deca- Ten.
-dendr-, -dendro- Tree, tree-like structure.
-dent-, -denti-, -dento- Tooth. *See also* -odont-.
-derm Germ layer, skin. *See also* -cut- and -derma-.
-derma-, -dermat-, -dermato-, -dermo- Skin. *See also* -cut- and -derm.
-desis Binding, fusion.
-dextr-, -dextro- To the right.
di- 1. *See* dia-. 2. *See* dis-.
dia- Across, apart, between, completely, through. The prefix becomes di- before words beginning with a vowel.
-didym-, -didymo- Testis. *See also* -orch-.
-dipl-, -diplo- Twice. *See also* bi- and dis-(2).
dis- 1. Reversal, separation, apart. 2. Duplication. *See also* bi- and -dipl-. The prefix becomes di- before words beginning with a consonant.
-dors-, -dorsi-, -dorso- 1. Back. 2. Back of the body.
-drom-, -dromo- Course, running, conduction.
-dur- Hard. *See also* -scirrh- and -scler-(1).
-dynam-, -dynami- Power.
-dys- Bad, difficult, disordered, painful. *See also* -cac- and mal-.

E

e- Out from, away from, expel. *See also* ex-.
ect-, ecto- Outside, outer, outermost.
-ectasia, -ectasis Dilatation, distension, expansion.
ecto- *See* ect-.
-ectomise, -ectomy Removal of.
-ede- *See* -oede-.
em- *See* en-.
-emia *See* -aemia.
en- Into, on, inside. The prefix becomes em- before b, p or ph.
-encephal-, -encephalo- Brain.
end-, endo- Within, inner.
-enter-, -entero- Intestine.
ep- *See* epi-.
epi- Upon, over, above, in addition, outer. The prefix becomes ep- before a vowel.
-epitheli-, -epithelio- Epithelium.
-eryth-, -erythr-, -erythro- Red, redness. *See also* -rub-.
-eso- Within, inside. *See also* intra-
-esthesi-, -esthesio- *See* -aesthesi-.
-eu- Good, well, easily.
ex- Out of. *See also* e-.
exo- External, outward.
extra- Outside, beyond, in addition to.

F

-faci- Face.
-facient Make, causing to become.
-febr- Fever. *See also* -pyr- and -pyret-.
-ferent Carry.
-ferr-, -ferro- Iron.
-fibr-, -fibro- Fibre.
-fiss- Split.
-flagell- Whip.
-flect- Bend, divert. *See also* -flex-
-flex- Bend, divert. *See also* -flect-
-flu- Flow. *See also* -flux-.
-flux- Flow. *See also* -flu-.
-form Shape, resembling. *See also* -oid.
-funct- Perform, serve.
-fund- Pour. *See also* -fus-.
-fus- Pour. *See also* -fund-.

G

-galact-, -galacto- Milk. *See also* -lact-(1).
-gam-, -gamo- Marriage, sexual union. *See also* -gamet- and -zyg-.
-gamet-, -gameto- Refers to a gamete. *See also* -gam-.
-gamo- *See* -gam-.
-gangli-, -ganglio- Swelling.
-gastr-, -gastro- Stomach.
-ge-, -geo- Soil, earth.
-gen-, -geno- 1. Reproduction, producing. *See also* -genic, -genous(2) and -gon-(3). 2. Gene. 3. Race.
-genic Producing. *See also* -gen-(1), -genous(2) and -gon-(3).
-genit-, -genito- Reproductive organs. *See also* -gon-(2).
-geno- *See* -gen-.

-genous 1. Produced by, arising from. 2. Producing. *See also* -gen-(1), -genic, and -gon-(3).
-geo- *See* -ge-.
-ger-, -gero- Old age. *See also* -presby-.
-germ- Bud.
-gero- *See* -ger-.
-gingiv-, -gingivo- Gingivae, gums.
-gli-, -glio- 1. Glue-like. *See also* -glutin-. 2. Neuroglia.
-glomerul-, -glomerulo- Glomeruli of the kidneys.
-gloss-, -glosso- Tongue. *See also* -glott- and -lingu-.
-glott- Tongue. *See also* -gloss- and -lingu-.
-gluc-, -gluco- Sweet, glucose. *See also* -glyc-(1).
-glutin- Glue. *See also* -gli-(1).
-glyc-, -glyco- 1. Sweet, sugar. *See also* -gluc-. 2. Glycerin. 3. Glycogen.
-gnath-, -gnatho- Jaw.
-gno- Know.
-gon-, -gono- 1. Seed. *See also* -sperm-. 2. Reproductive organs. *See also* -genit-. 3. Reproduction. *See also* -gen-(1), -genic, and -genous(2).
-grad- Step, walk.
-gram Recorded, written. *See also* -graph- and -graphy.
-gran- Grain.
-graph-, -grapho- Write, record. *See also* -gram and -graphy.
-graphy Write, record. *See also* -gram and -graph-.
-grav- Heavy.
-gyn-, -gynaeco-, -gyne-, -gyno- Female, woman.

H

-haem-, -haemat-, -haemato-, -haemo- Blood. Alternative spellings, -hem-, -hemat-, -hemato-, -hemo-. *See also* -sangui-.
-hamart-, -hamarto- Fault.
-hapl-, -haplo- Single, simple. *See also* -mon- and uni-.
-hem-, -hemat-, -hemato- *See* -haem-.
-hemi- Half. *See also* -semi-.
-hepat-, -hepato- Liver.
-hept-, -hepta- Seven. *See also* -sept-(1).
-hered- Heir.
-herpet-, -herpeto- 1. Herpes. 2. Reptile.
-heter-, -hetero- Other, different.
-hex-, -hexa- Six.
-hidr-, -hidro- Sweat.
-hist-, -histio-, -histo- Tissue.
-homeo- *See* -homo-.
-homo-, -homoeo- Unchanging, same, steady. Alternative spelling, -homeo-.
-hydr-, -hydro- Water, hydrogen.
hyp-, hypo- Under, beneath, below, deficient, less than normal. *See also* infra- and sub-.
hyper- Above, beyond, excessive, over, above normal. *See also* super- and ultra-.
-hypn-, -hypno- Sleep. *See also* -somn-.
hypo- *See* hyp-.
-hyster-, -hystero- 1. Uterus. *See also* -metr-(2). 2. Hysteria.

I

-ia Condition, state. *See also* -asis, -iasis, -ism, -osis and -sis.
-iasis Condition, process, particularly a morbid one. *See also* -asis, -ia, -ism, -osis and -sis.
-iatr-, -iatric-, -iatro- Physician, medicine, medical treatment.
-ichthy-, -ichthyo- Fish.
-idio- Self, one's own.
il- *See* in-.
-ile-, -ileo- Ileum.
-ili-, -ilio- Ilium.
im- *See* in-.
in- 1. In, on. 2. Implies a negative. The prefix becomes il- or ir- before words beginning with l or r respectively, and im- before words beginning with b, m or p.
infra- Below, beneath. *See also* hyp- and sub-.
inter- Between, among.
intra- Within, on the inside. *See also* -eso-.
ir- *See* in-.
-irid-, -irido- Iris of the eye, iridescent.
-isch-, -ischo- Deficiency, suppression.
-ism Condition, state, action. *See also* -asis, -ia, -iasis, -osis and -sis.
iso- Equal, alike.
-itis Inflammation.

J

-ject- Throw.
-jejun-, -jejuno- 1. Jejunum. 2. Hunger.
-junct- Join.

K

-kary-, -karyo- Nucleus.
-kerat-, -kerato- 1. Horn. 2. Cornea.
keto- Signifies the presence of the carbonyl group (>C=O) in a molecule.
-kine-, -kinesi-, -kinesio- Motion.

L

-labi-, -labio- Lip. *See also* -cheil-.
-lachry- Tears. *See also* -dacry-.
-lact-, -lacto- 1. Milk. *See also* -galact-. 2. Lactic acid.
-laev-, -laevo- To the left. Alternative spellings, -lev-, -levo-.
-lal-, -lalo- Speech, talk, babble. *See also* -lexis and -pha-.
-lapar-, -laparo- Flank, loins, abdomen.
-laryng-, -laryngo- Larynx.
-later-, -latero- Side.
-legia Reading. *See also* -lexis.

-leio- Smooth.
-lent- Lentil.
-lep- Seize.
-lepsis, -lepsy Seizure.
-leuc-, -leuco- 1. White. *See also* -alb-. 2. Leucocyte. Alternative spellings, -leuk-, -leuko-.
-leuk-, -leuko- *See* -leuc-.
-lev-, -levo- *See* -laev-.
-lexis, -lexy Speech. Often used instead of -legia to denote reading. *See also* -lal- and -pha-.
-lig- Bind, tie.
-lingu- Tongue. *See also* -gloss- and -glott-.
-lip-, -lipo- Fat. *See also* -adip- and -stear-.
-lith-, -litho- Stone, calculus. *See also* -calc-(1).
-logy Study of, science of.
-ly-, -lys-, -lyso- Loose, dissolve.
-lymph-, -lympho- 1. Lymph, lymphatic system, lymphocytes, or lymphoid tissue. 2. Water.
-lys- *See* -ly-.
-lysis Loosening, dissolving.
-lyso- *See* -ly-.

M

-macr-, -macro- Large. *See also* -mega-(1) and -megal-.
mal- Bad, abnormal. *See also* -cac- and -dys-.
-malacia Softening.
-mamm-, -mammo- Breast. *See also* -mast-(1).
-man- Hand.
-mania An abnormal preoccupation.
-mast-, -masto- 1. Breast. *See also* -mamm-. 2. Mastoid process.
-medi-, -medio- Middle. *See also* -mes-.
-medullo- Medulla.
-mega- 1. Great, large. *See also* -macro- and -megal-. 2. One million or a million times.
-megal-, -megalo- Large. *See also* -macro- and -mega-(1).
-megaly Enlarged.
-meio- Less, smaller. Alternative spelling, -mio-.
-melan-, -melano- Black, dark.
-men-, -meno- 1. Month. 2. Menses.
-mening-, -meningo- Membrane, meninges.
-meno- *See* men-.
-mer-, -mero- 1. Part. 2. Thigh.
-mere Part, segment.
-mero- *See* -mer-.
-mes-, -meso- Middle. *See also* -medi-.
meta- 1. After, beyond. 2. Change.
-metr- 1. Measure. 2. Uterus. *See also* -hyster-(1).
-metra-, -metro- *See* -metr-(2).
-micro- 1. Small. 2. One-millionth.
-mio- *See* -meio-.
-mit-, -mito- Thread-like.
-mne-, -mnem-, -mnes- Memory, remember.
-mon-, -mono- Single. *See also* -hapl- and uni-.
-morph-, -morpho- Form, shape.
-mot- Move.
-muc-, -muco- Mucus. *See also* -blenn- and -myx-.
multi- Many. *See also* poly-.
-my-, -myo- Muscle.
-myc-, -mycet-, -myceto-, -myco- Fungus.
-myel-, -myelo- 1. Bone marrow. 2. Spinal cord. 3. Myelin.
-myo- *See* -my-.
-myring-, -myringo- Tympanic membrane.
-myx-, -myxo- Mucus, slime. *See also* -blenn- and -muc-.

N

-naev-, -naevo- Mole, naevus. Alternative spellings, -nev-, -nevo-.
-narc-, -narco- Stupor, numbness.
-nas-, -naso- Nose.
-ne-, -neo- New.
-necr-, -necro- Dead.
-neo- *See* -ne-.
-nephr-, -nephro- Kidney. *See also* -ren-.
-neur-, -neuro- Nerve.
-nev-, -nevo- *See* -naev-.
-nod- Knot.
-nom-, -nomo- Law, usage, custom.
non- Implies a negative.
-non-, -nona- Nine.
-norm-, -normo- Usual, normal.
-nos-, -noso- Disease. *See also* -path- and -pathy.
-nucl-, -nucle-, -nucleo- Kernel, nucleus.
-nutri- Nourish. *See also* -troph- and -trophic.

O

-octa- Eight.
-ocul-, -oculo- Eye. *See also* -ophthalm-.
-odont-, -odonto- Tooth. *See also* -dent-.
-odyn-, -odyno- Pain, distress. *See also* -alg-.
-odynia Painful condition. *See also* -algia.
-odyno- *See* -odyn-.
-oede- Swell. Alternative spelling, -ede-.
-oid Having the form of, resembling. *See also* -form.
-ol Denotes an alcoholic or phenolic compound.
-ole-, -oleo- Oil.
-olig-, -oligo- Little, few, scanty. *See also* -pauci-.
-oma Abnormal growth, neoplasm, tumour.
-omphal-, -omphalo- Umbilicus, navel.
-onc-, -onco- Swelling, mass, tumour.
-onych-, -onycho- Nails of fingers or toes.
-oo- Egg, ovum. *See also* -ov-.
-oophor-, -oophoro- Ovary.
-ophthalm-, -ophthalmo- Eye. *See also* -ocul-.
-opia Vision.
-or-, -oro- Mouth. *See also* -stom-.
-orb- 1. Circle, sphere. *See also* -spher-. 2. Eyeball.
-orch-, -orchi-, -orchid-, -orchido-, -orchio- Testis. *See also* -didym-.
-oro- *See* -or-.
-orth-, -ortho- Straight, upright, normal, correct.
-ose 1. Full of. *See also* -ous. 2. Carbohydrate.

-osis Action, condition, process, especially a morbid one. Often used to denote an abnormal increase. *See also* -asis, -ia, -iasis, -ism, and -sis.
-osm-, -osmo- 1. Osmosis. 2. Odour.
-oss- Bone. *See also* -ost-.
-ost-, -oste-, -osteo- Bone. *See also* -oss-.
-ot-, -oto- Ear. *See also* -aur-.
-ous Possessing, full of. *See also* -ose(1).
-ov-, -ovi-, -ovo- Egg, ovum. *See also* -oo-.
-ox-, -oxy- 1. Oxygen. 2. Pointed. 3. Acid.

P

-paed-, -paedo- Child. Alternative spellings, -ped-, -pedo-.
pan- All, completely, entire.
par- *See* para-.
-par- To give birth to; bear. *See also* -part-.
para- Near, beyond, apart from, beside, abnormal. The prefix becomes par- before a vowel.
-part- To give birth to; bear. *See also* -par-.
-path-, -patho- Disease. *See also* -nos- and -pathy.
-pathy Disease. *See also* -nos- and -path-.
-pauci- Few. *See also* -olig-.
-ped-, -pedo- 1. Foot. *See also* -pod- 2. *See* -paed-.
-pend- Hang down.
-penia Deficiency of.
-pent-, -penta- Five.
-pep-, -peps-, -pept- Digest.
per- Through. *See also* trans-.
peri- Around, about, surrounding.
-peritone-, -peritoneo- Peritoneum.
-pexy Fixing, fixation.
-pha- Speak. *See also* -lal- and -lexis.
-phac-, -phaco- 1. The lens of the eye. 2. Freckle, mole. Alternative spellings, -phak-, -phako-.
-phag-, -phago- Eat, ingest, engulf.
-phagia, -phagy Eating, swallowing.
-phago- *See* -phag-.
-phagy *See* -phagia.
-phak-, -phako- *See* -phac-.
-phalang-, -phalango- The bones of the fingers or toes. *See also* -dactyl-.
-pharmac-, -pharmaco- Drug, medicine.
-pharyng-, -pharyngo- Pharynx.
-phen-, -pheno- 1. Show, display. 2. Refers to benzene.
-phil, -phile, -philia, -philic Like, have an affinity for, attraction. *See also* -tropin.
philo- Affinity for, attraction.
-phleb-, -phlebo- Vein. *See also* -ven-.
-phobe, -phobia Abnormal fear of, aversion to.
-phon-, -phono- Sound.
-phore Denotes a carrier.
-phot-, -photo- Light.
-phrag- Fence in, block.
-phren-, -phreno- 1. Mind. *See also* -psych- and -thym-(1). 2. Diaphragm.
-physio- 1. Nature. 2. Physiology. 3. Physical.
-phyt-, -phyto- Plant.
-phyte 1. Plant. 2. Pathological growth.
-phyto- *See* -phyt-.
-pil-, -pilo- Hair. *See also* -trich-.
-plas- Mould, shape.
-plasia Development, formation.
-plasty Moulding, shaping; plastic surgery.
-plegia Paralysis, stroke.
-pleo- More.
-pleur-, -pleuro- 1. Pleura. 2. Side. 3. Rib. *See also* -cost-.
-ploid Refers to the degree of multiplication of chromosome sets.
-pnea *See* -pnoea.
-pneo- Breath, blowing, respiration. *See also* -pneuma-(2), -pneumo-(2), -pnoea, -spir-(2), and -spirat-.
-pneuma-, -pneumat-, -pneumato- 1. Air, gas. *See also* -pneumo-(1). 2. Breath, respiration. *See also* -pneo-, -pneumo-(2), -pnoea, -spir-(2), and -spirat-.
-pneumo-, -pneumon-, -pneumono- 1. Air, gas. *See also* -pneuma-(1). 2. Respiration. *See also* -pneo-, -pneuma-(2), -pnoea, -spir-(2), and -spirat-. 3. Lungs. *See also* -pulmo-.
-pnoea Breathing, respiration. Alternative spelling, -pnea. *See also* -pneo-, -pneuma-(2), -pneumo-(2), -spir-(2), and -spirat-.
-pod-, -podo- Foot. *See also* -ped-.
-poie- Make.
-poiesis Formation, production.
poly- Much, many. *See also* multi-.
post- After, beyond, behind.
prae-, pre- Before, in front of. *See also* pro-.
-prax- Conduct, action.
pre- *See* prae-.
-presby-, -presbyo- Old age. *See also* -ger-.
pro- Before, in front of. *See also* prae-.
-proct-, -procto- Anus, rectum. *See also* -rect-.
-pseud-, -pseudo- False, spurious, apparent.
-psych-, -psycho- Mind. *See also* -phren-(1) and -thym-(1).
-ptosis Falling, sinking down, drooping.
-pulmo-, -pulmon-, -pulmono- Lungs. *See also* -pneumo-(3).
-pur- Pus. *See also* -py-.
-pyel-, -pyo- Pus. *See also* -pur-.
-pyel-, -pyelo- Pelvis of the kidney.
-pykn-, -pykno- Thick, frequent, compact.
-pylor-, -pyloro- Pylorus.
-pyo- *See* -py-.
-pyr-, -pyro- Fire, heat. *See also* -febr- and -pyret-.
-pyret-, -pyreto- Fever. *See also* -febr- and -pyr-.
-pyro- *See* -pyr-.

Q

quadr-, quadri- Four.

R

-rachi-, -rachio- Spine.
-radi-, -radio- Ray, radiation.
re- Back, again.
-rect-, -recto- Rectum. *See also* -proct-.
-ren-, -reno- Kidney. *See also* -nephr-.
-ret- Net.
retro- Backwards, back, lying, situated behind.
-rhea, -rrhea *See* -rhoea.

-rhex- Burst, break.
-rhin-, -rhino- Nose.
-rhoea, -rrhoea Flowing, running. Alternative spellings, -rhea, -rrhea.
-rrhage, -rrhagia Excessive or unusual flow or discharge.
-rrhea *See* -rhoea.
-rrhoea *See* -rhoea.
-rub-, -rubr- Red. *See also* -eryth-.

S

-sacr-, -sacro- Sacrum.
-salp-, -salping-, -salpingo- Tube. *See also* -syring-.
-sangui-, -sanguin- Blood. *See also* -haem-.
-sapr-, -sapro- Decaying, putrid, rotten.
-sarc-, -sarco- Flesh, substance of muscles.
-scirrh-, -scirrho- Hard. *See also* -dur- and -scler-(1).
-scler-, -sclero- 1. Hard. *See also* -dur- and -scirrh-. 2. Sclera.
-scope Instrument for examining.
-scopy Examining.
-seb-, -sebi-, -sebo- Sebum, sebaceous.
-sect- Cut. *See also* -cis-(1) and -tomy.
-semi- Half. *See also* -hemi-.
-sens- Feel, perceive.
-sep- Decay, rot.
-sept- 1. Seven. *See also* -hept-. 2. Septum, partition.
-ser- Whey, watery.
-sial-, -sialo- Saliva, salivary glands.
-sin-, -sinu- Hollow, fold.
-sis Condition, state. *See also* -asis, -ia, -iasis, -ism, and -osis.
-somat-, -somato- Body. *See also* -corp-.
-some Body.
-somn-, -somni- Sleep. *See also* -hypn-.
-spas- pull, draw. *See also* -tract-.
-sperm-, -spermat-, -spermato-, -spermo- Seed. *See also* -gon-(1).
-spher-, -sphero- Ball, sphere. *See also* -orb-(1).
-sphygmo- Pulse.
-spir-, -spiro- 1. Spiral, coil. 2. Breath, breathing. *See also* -pneo-, -pneuma-(2), -pneumo-(2), -pnoea, and -spirat-.
-spirat- Breathe. *See also* -pneo-, -pneuma-(2), -pneumo-(2), -pnoea, and -spir-(2).
-spiro- *See* -spir-.
-splen-, -spleno- Spleen.
-spondyl-, -spondylo- Vertebra.
-spor-, -sporo- Spore.
-squam-, -squamo- Scale.
-stal-, -stol- Send.
-stasis 1. Stand still. 2. Slowing, stopping.
-stat Stationary, fixed.
-stear-, -stearo-, -steat-, -steato- Fat. *See also* -adip- and -lip-.
-steat-, -steato- *See* -stear-.
-sten-, -steno- Narrow, contracted.
-ster- Solid.
-sterco- Faeces.
-stern-, -sterno- Sternum.
-stig- Spot, mark.
-stol- *See* stal-.
-stom-, -stomat-, -stomato-, -stomo- Mouth, orifice. *See also* -or-.
-stomy Making an opening; an artificial opening created surgically.
-strict- Compress, tighten, cause pain. *See also* -stringent.
-stringent Compress, tighten, cause pain. *See also* -strict-.
sub- Under, near, almost, support. The prefix becomes suf- or sup- before words beginning with f or p respectively. *See also* hyp- and infra-.
suf- *See* sub-.
sup- *See* sub-.
super- Above, beyond, excess. *See also* hyper-, supra-, and ultra-.
supra- Above, over. *See also* super-.
sym- *See* syn-.
syn- With, together, merging, together, joined, alike. The prefix becomes sym- before b, m, or p. *See also* con-.
-syndesm-, -syndesmo- Ligament.
-synovi-, -synovio- Synovial membrane.
-syring-, -syringo- Pipe, tube, cavity, fistula. *See also* -salp-.

T

-tachy- Rapid, swift.
-tact- Touch.
-tars-, -tarso- 1. Margin of the eyelid. 2. Instep of the foot.
-tax- Arrange, order.
-tempor- 1. Time. 2. Refers to the temple.
-ten-, -teno-, -tenont- Tendon.
-tens- Stretch. *See also* -ton-(1).
-terat-, -terato- Monster.
-thec- Sheath, case.
-therap- Treatment.
-therm-, -thermo- Heat.
-thorac-, -thoraco- Chest.
-thromb-, -thrombo- Clot, thrombus.
-thym-, -thymo- 1. Mind, soul, emotions. *See also* -phren-(1) and -psych-. 2. Thymus gland.
-thyr-, -thyro- Thyroid gland, shield-shaped.
-tomy Cutting; surgical cutting or incision. *See also* -cis-(1) and -sect-.
-ton- 1. Stretch, under tension. *See also* -tens-. 2. Tone.
-top-, -topo- Place.
-tors- Twist.
-tox-, -toxi-, -toxico-, -toxo- Poison.
-trache-, -tracheo- Trachea, windpipe.
-trachel-, -trachelo- Neck, constriction. *See also* -cervic-.
-tracheo- *See* trache-.
-tract- Draw, drag. *See also* -spas-.
trans- Across, through, beyond. *See also* per-.
-traumat-, -traumato- Wound.
-tri- Three.
-trich-, -tricho- Hair. *See also* -pil-.
-tripsy Crushed.
-troph-, -tropho- Nutrition. *See also* -nutri-.
-trophic, -trophin, -trophy Nutrition, growth. *See also* -nutri-.
-trophin *See* -trophic.
-tropho- *See* -troph-.
-trophy *See* -trophic.
-tropic Turning towards, influencing.
-tropin Having an affinity for. *See also* -phil.

-typhl-, -typhlo- 1. Blind. 2. Caecum (blind gut). *See also* -caec-.
-tyr-, -tyro- Cheese.

U

ultra- Excess, beyond. *See also* hyper- and super-.
uni- One. *See also* -hapl- and -mon-.
-ur-, -uro-, -uron-, -urono- 1. Urine. *See also* -uria and -uric-(1). 2. Urinary tract.
-ureter-, -uretero- Ureter.
-urethr-, -urethro- Urethra.
-uria Of or in the urine. *See also* -ur-(1) and -uric-(1).
-uric-, -urico- 1. Urine. *See also* -ur-(1) and -uria. 2. Uric acid.
-uro-, -uron-, -urono- *See* -ur-.
-uter-, -utero- Uterus.

-vagin-, -vagino- Sheath, vagina. *See also* -colp-.
-varic-, -varico- 1. Twisted, swollen. 2. Varicose vein.
-vas-, -vaso- Vessel, duct. *See also* -angi-.
-ven-, -veno- Vein. *See also* -phleb-.
-ventr-, -ventri-, -ventro- 1. Abdomen. *See also* -cel-(3) and -celi-. 2. Front of the body.
-ventricul-, -ventriculo- Ventricle of the heart or brain.
-ventro- *See* ventr-.
-vermi- Worm.
-vers- Turn. *See also* -vert-.
-vert- Turn. *See also* -vers-.
-vertebr-, -vertebro- Vertebra, vertebral column.
-vesic, -vesico- Bladder, blister. *See also* -cyst-.
-viscer-, -viscero- Organ.
-vit- Life. *See also* -bio- and -zo-.

-xanth-, -xantho- Yellow.
-xen-, -xeno- Strange, foreign.
-xer-, -xero- Dry.
-xyl-, -xylo- Wood.

Z

-zo-, -zoo- Animal, life. *See also* -bio- and -vit-.
-zyg-, -zygo- Union, joining. *See also* -gam-.
-zym-, -zymo- 1. Enzyme. *See also* -ase. 2. Fermentation.

Selected bibliography and reference sources

This section provides a list of books to enable pharmacists to study the background details relevant to the topics covered in this book. It also serves as a guide to further reading and provides reference sources. Details are included under the following classification:

- Anatomy and physiology
- Diagnostic techniques
- Medical dictionaries
- Medicine
- Paediatrics
- Pharmacy
- Pregnancy
- Professional and self-help organisations

Price bands

Price bands provide an indication of the relative cost of books. They serve as a basis of comparison, and have been checked prior to going to press.

A	Up to £9.99
B	£10 to £19.99
C	£20 to £29.99
D	£30 to £39.99
E	£40 to £49.99
F	Over £50

Anatomy and physiology

Gray's Anatomy, 38th edition
P L Williams *et al.*
Edinburgh: Churchill Livingstone, 1995
Price band: F

Principles of Anatomy and Physiology, 9th edition
G J Tortora
New York: John Wiley & Son Inc, 1999
Price band: D

Diagnostic techniques

A Guide to Laboratory Investigations, 3rd edition
Michael McGee
Abingdon: Radcliffe Medical Press, 2000
Price band: C

Diagnostic Procedures, 2nd edition
Franklin A Michota Jr
Hudson, Cleveland: Lexi-Comp, 2001
Price band: C

Understanding Laboratory Investigations
Christopher Higgins
Oxford: Blackwell Science, 2000
Price band: C

Medical dictionaries

Black's Medical Dictionary, 39th edition
Gordon MacPherson
London: Adam & Charles Black, 1999
Price band: C

Concise Medical Dictionary, 5th edition
E A Martin (ed.)
Oxford: Oxford Paperbacks, 1998
Price band: A

Dorland's Illustrated Medical Dictionary, 29th edition
Philadelphia: W B Saunders, 2000
Price band: D

Stedman's Medical Dictionary, 27th edition
Philadelphia: Lippincott, Williams & Wilkins, 1998
Price band: D

Textbook of Dermatology, 6th edition (3 vols)
R Champion *et al.* (eds)
Oxford: Blackwell Scientific Publications, 1998
Price band: F

Medicine

Cecil Textbook of Medicine, 21st edition
Russell Cecil, Lee Goldman, Claude Bennett (eds)
Philadelphia: W B Saunders, 1999
Price band: F

Clinical Medicine, 4th Edition
P J Kumar and M L Clark (eds)
Edinburgh: W B Saunders, 1998
Price band: B

Davidson's Principles and Practice of Medicine, 18th edition
Christopher Haslett (ed.)
Edinburgh: Churchill Livingstone, 1999
Price band: D

The Merck Manual of Diagnosis and Therapy, 17th edition
M H Beers and R Berkow (eds)
Pennsylvania: Merck & Co., 1999
Price band: B

Oxford Handbook of Clinical Medicine, 5th edition
J Longmore, M Longmore, I Wilkinson, E Torok
Oxford: Oxford University Press, 2001
Price band: A

Oxford Handbook of Clinical Specialities, 2nd edition
J A B Collier, M Longmore, T Hodgetts
Oxford: Oxford University Press, 1999
Price band: B

Oxford Textbook of Medicine, 3rd edition (3 vols)
D J Wetherall, J G G Ledingham, D A Warrell (eds)
Oxford: Oxford University Press, 1996
Price band: F

Shorter Oxford Textbook of Psychiatry, 4th edition
M Gelder, R Mayou, P Cowen
Oxford: Oxford University Press, 2001
Price band: D

Roxburgh's Common Skin Diseases, 16th edition
R Marks (Reviser)
London: Arnold, 1993
Price band: C

Paediatrics

Essential Paediatrics, 4th edition
D Hull and D I Johnson
Edinburgh: Churchill Livingstone, 1999
Price band: C

Nelson's Textbook of Paediatrics
Richard E Behrman *et al.*
Philadelphia: W B Saunders, 1999
Price band: F

Pharmacy

British National Formulary, Number 43
Royal Pharmaceutical Society of Great Britain and the British Medical Association
London: Pharmaceutical Press, 2001 (twice yearly)
Price band: B

Clinical Pharmacy and Therapeutics, 2nd edition
Roger Walker and Clive Edwards
Edinburgh: Churchill Livingstone
Price band: D

Drug Interactions, 5th edition
Ivan H Stockley
London: Pharmaceutical Press, 1999
Price band: F

Drugs of Abuse
Simon Wills
London: Pharmaceutical Press, 1997
Price band: B

Handbook of Non-Prescription Drugs, 13th edition
American Pharmaceutical Association
Washington: American Pharmaceutical Association, 2002
Price band: F

Martindale: The Extra Pharmacopoeia, 33rd edition
Sean C Sweetman (ed.)
London: Pharmaceutical Press, 1999
Price band: F

Medicines in the Elderly
David Armour and Chris Cairns
London: Pharmaceutical Press, 2001
Price band: C

Minor Illness or Major Disease?, 2nd edition
C Edwards and P Stillman
London: Pharmaceutical Press, 2000
Price band: C

Non-Prescription Medicines
Alan Nathan
London: Pharmaceutical Press, 1998
Price band: C

Pathology and Therapeutics for Phamacists, 2nd edition
Russell Greene and Norman Harris
London: Pharmaceutical Press, 2000
Price band: E

Patient Care in Community Practice, 2nd edition
R J Harman (ed.)
London: Pharmaceutical Press, 2002
Price band: C

USP DI: Vol I: *Drug Information for the Health Care Professional*; Vol II: *Advice for the Patient*, 22nd edition
Rockville, MD: USP Corporation, 2002
Price band: F

Pregnancy

Prescribing in Pregnancy, 3rd edition
Peter Rubin (ed.)
London: BMJ Books, 2000
Price band: B

Therapeutics in Pregnancy and Lactation
Anne Lee, Sally Inch, David Finnigan (eds)
Abingdon: Radcliffe Medical Press, 2000
Price band: B

Professional and self-help organisations

The Health Address Book: A Directory of Health Support Groups, 3rd edition
The RSM Press in collaboration with the Patients Association
London: The Royal Society of Medicine Press, 2001
Price band: B

The Patient's Internet Handbook
Robert Kiley and Elizabeth Graham
London: The Royal Society of Medicine Press, 2002
Price band: A

Index

Page numbers in **bold** refer to main entries; page numbers in *italics* refer to figures and tables.